AF669451

Anesthesia *for* Transplant Surgery

Anesthesia *for* Transplant Surgery

Jayashree Sood MD FFARCS PGDHHM FICA
Senior Consultant and Chairperson
Department of Anesthesiology, Pain and Perioperative Medicine
Sir Ganga Ram Hospital, New Delhi, India

Vijay Vohra MD FRCA FICA
Senior Consultant, Chairman
Department of Liver Transplant, GI Anesthesia and Intensive Care
Institute of Liver Transplantation
Medanta The Medicity, Gurgaon, Haryana, India

Foreword
DS Rana

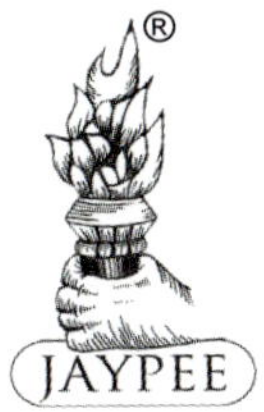

JAYPEE BROTHERS MEDICAL PUBLISHERS (P) LTD.

New Delhi • London • Philadelphia • Panama

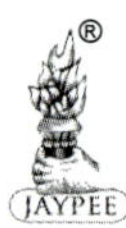

Jaypee Brothers Medical Publishers (P) Ltd

Headquarters
Jaypee Brothers Medical Publishers (P) Ltd
4838/24, Ansari Road, Daryaganj
New Delhi 110 002, India
Phone: +91-11-43574357
Fax: +91-11-43574314
Email: jaypee@jaypeebrothers.com

Overseas Offices

J.P. Medical Ltd
83 Victoria Street, London
SW1H 0HW (UK)
Phone: +44-2031708910
Fax: +02-03-0086180
Email: info@jpmedpub.com

Jaypee-Highlights Medical Publishers Inc.
City of Knowledge, Bld. 237, Clayton
Panama City, Panama
Phone: +1 507-301-0496
Fax: +1 507-301-0499
Email: cservice@jphmedical.com

Jaypee Medical Inc.
The Bourse
111 South Independence Mall East
Suite 835, Philadelphia, PA 19106, USA
Phone: +1 267-519-9789
Email: jpmed.us@gmail.com

Jaypee Brothers Medical Publishers (P) Ltd
17/1-B Babar Road, Block-B, Shaymali
Mohammadpur, Dhaka-1207
Bangladesh
Mobile: +08801912003485
Email: jaypeedhaka@gmail.com

Jaypee Brothers Medical Publishers (P) Ltd
Bhotahity, Kathmandu, Nepal
Phone: +977-9741283608
Email: kathmandu@jaypeebrothers.com

Website: www.jaypeebrothers.com
Website: www.jaypeedigital.com

Inquiries for bulk sales may be solicited at: jaypee@jaypeebrothers.com

Anesthesia for Transplant Surgery

First Edition: **2014**

ISBN: 978-93-5152-139-6

Printed at : Ajanta Offset & Packagings Ltd., New Delhi

Contributors

Amitabh Dutta MD PGDHR (Human Rights)
Consultant
Department of Anesthesiology,
Pain and Perioperative Medicine
Sir Ganga Ram Hospital
New Delhi, India

Anil Jain MD
Senior Consultant and Vice Chairperson
Department of Anesthesiology,
Pain and Perioperative Medicine
Sir Ganga Ram Hospital
New Delhi, India

Anjali Gera MD
Consultant
Department of Anesthesiology,
Pain and Perioperative Medicine
Sir Ganga Ram Hospital
New Delhi, India

Anjeleena Kumar Gupta DA FRCA
Consultant
Department of Anesthesiology
Pain and Perioperative Medicine
Sir Ganga Ram Hospital
New Delhi, India

Archna Koul MD
Consultant
Department of Anesthesiology,
Pain and Perioperative Medicine
Sir Ganga Ram Hospital
New Delhi, India

Arun Maheshwari MD
Senior Consultant and Chairperson
Department of Cardiac Anesthesia
Sir Ganga Ram Hospital
New Delhi, India

Bhuwan Chand Panday MD
Associate Consultant
Department of Anesthesiology,
Pain and Perioperative Medicine
Sir Ganga Ram Hospital
New Delhi, India

Bimla Sharma MD DGO MBAHCS FICA
Senior Consultant
Department of Anesthesiology,
Pain and Perioperative Medicine
Sir Ganga Ram Hospital
New Delhi, India

Chand Sahai DA MD
Senior Consultant
Department of Anesthesiology,
Pain and Perioperative Medicine
Sir Ganga Ram Hospital
New Delhi, India

Deepanjali Pant MD
Senior Consultant
Department of Anesthesiology,
Pain and Perioperative Medicine
Sir Ganga Ram Hospital
New Delhi, India

Dinesh Gautam DA DNB
Consultant
Department of Anesthesiology,
Pain and Perioperative Medicine
Sir Ganga Ram Hospital
New Delhi, India

Harsha Jauhari MS FRCS FICS FAIS
Senior Consultant and Chairperson
Department of Renal Transplant
Sir Ganga Ram Hospital
New Delhi, India

Jayashree Sood MD FFARCS PGDHHM FICA
Senior Consultant and Chairperson
Department of Anesthesiology,
Pain and Perioperative Medicine
Sir Ganga Ram Hospital
New Delhi, India

Manish Gupta MD
Consultant
Department of Anesthesiology,
Pain and Perioperative Medicine
Sir Ganga Ram Hospital
New Delhi, India

Manish Kohli DA DNB
Associate Consultant
Department of Anesthesiology,
Pain and Perioperative Medicine
Sir Ganga Ram Hospital
New Delhi, India

Monish S Raut MD FNB (Cardiac Anesth)
Clinical Assistant
Department of Cardiac Anesthesia
Sir Ganga Ram Hospital
New Delhi, India

Naimish Mehta MS FACRSI FEBS
Consultant
Department of Anesthesiology,
Pain and Perioperative Medicine
Sir Ganga Ram Hospital
New Delhi, India

Naresh Dua MD
Consultant
Department of Anesthesiology,
Pain and Perioperative Medicine
Sir Ganga Ram Hospital
New Delhi, India

Neetu Jain MD DNB
Consultant
Department of Anesthesiology,
Pain and Perioperative Medicine
Sir Ganga Ram Hospital
New Delhi, India

Nitin Sethi DNB
Associate Consultant
Department of Anesthesiology,
Pain and Perioperative Medicine
Sir Ganga Ram Hospital
New Delhi, India

Prabhat Kumar Choudhary MD
Associate Consultant
Department of Anesthesiology,
Pain and Perioperative Medicine
Sir Ganga Ram Hospital
New Delhi, India

Pradeep Jain MD FICA
Senior Consultant
Department of Anesthesiology,
Pain and Perioperative Medicine
Sir Ganga Ram Hospital
New Delhi, India

Pramoj Jindal DNB MNAMS
Consultant
Department of General Surgery
Sir Ganga Ram Hospital
New Delhi, India

Rachna Bhutani DA DNB
Consultant
Department of Anesthesiology,
Pain and Perioperative Medicine
Sir Ganga Ram Hospital
New Delhi, India

Rahul Bhayana DNB
Consultant
Department of Anesthesiology and Critical Care
Kailash Hospital
Noida, Uttar Pradesh, India

Raminder Sehgal MD FICA
Senior Consultant
Department of Anesthesiology,
Pain and Perioperative Medicine
Sir Ganga Ram Hospital
New Delhi, India

Ranju Gandhi MD
Assistant Professor
Department of Anesthesiology and Critical Care
Safdarjung Hospital and Vardhman Mahavir Medical College
New Delhi, India

Rashmi Jain DNB
Senior Consultant
Department of Anesthesiology,
Pain and Perioperative Medicine
Sir Ganga Ram Hospital
New Delhi, India

Savitar Malhotra MD
Associate Consultant
Department of Anesthesiology,
Pain and Perioperative Medicine
Sir Ganga Ram Hospital
New Delhi, India

Shashank Pandey MD DIP (Cardiac Anesth)
Senior Consultant
Department of Anesthesiology,
Pain and Perioperative Medicine
Sir Ganga Ram Hospital
New Delhi, India

Shikha Sharma MD
Senior Consultant
Department of Anesthesiology,
Pain and Perioperative Medicine
Sir Ganga Ram Hospital
New Delhi, India

Subhash Gupta MD
Senior Consultant
Department of Anesthesiology,
Pain and Perioperative Medicine
Sir Ganga Ram Hospital
New Delhi, India

Sudhir Chadha MS MCh
Senior Consultant
Department of Renal Transplant and Urology
Sir Ganga Ram Hospital
New Delhi, India

Sumir Dubey MS MCh
Consultant
Department of Cardiac Surgery
Sir Ganga Ram Hospital
New Delhi, India

Vibha Varma MS DNB
Consultant
Department of Surgical
Gastroenterology and Liver Transplant
Sir Ganga Ram Hospital
New Delhi, India

Vijay Vohra MD FRCA FICA
Senior Consultant and Chairman
Department of Liver Transplant
GI Anesthesia and Intensive Care
Institute of Liver Transplantation
Medanta The Medicity
Gurgaon, Haryana, India

Vinay Kumaran MS MCh FEBS
Consultant
Department of Surgical Gastroenterology and Liver Transplant
Sir Ganga Ram Hospital
New Delhi, India

Vipin Tyagi MS DNB
Associate Consultant
Department of Renal Transplant and Urology
Sir Ganga Ram Hospital
New Delhi, India

Foreword

Since the first successful kidney transplantation between identical twins in the US almost six decades ago, the field of solid organ transplantation has made progress by leaps and bounds and despite setbacks along the way, the spirit of the transplant surgeons, the immunologists and others in transplantation has never flagged. However, these transplantations would not have seen the light of day without parallel development in anesthesiology and critical care; since the process of physically transplanting an organ in the recipient is one cog in the wheel.

The anesthesiologist posted with transplantation units in any hospital in any part of the world plays a key role in the good outcome of these patients who are in end stage organ failure. In our hospital we have a dedicated team of anesthesiologists who are involved in the perioperative care of this special group of patients.

Our hospital has been involved in transplantation surgery since 1985, first for kidney transplantation and then from 2001 for liver. We have in fact trained many anesthesiologists who are in practice elsewhere, thus widening the specialized services which have become available in India.

With the experience of many years and several cases (more than 2700 renal and 800 liver transplants, at the time of writing this book) the Department of Anesthesiology, Pain and Perioperative Medicine felt the time had come to put it all in a book so that others may share in the journey that they have undertaken so far, and influence a new generation of anesthesiologists with a special interest in anesthesia for organ transplantation.

I hope the reading of this book will increase your knowledge and spark your interest in this field of medicine.

DS Rana
Chairman-Board of Management
Sir Ganga Ram Hospital
New Delhi, India

Preface

Transplantation has been 'referred to' since ages in mythology. The results of transplant surgery in the initial years were not encouraging due to 'rejection' and 'infection'. However with improved knowledge of immunosuppression and availability of newer and better immunosuppressive drugs, transplant of almost all organs is possible, with improved results.

In this book we have tried to cover all aspects related to 'transplantation'. Beginning from history to physiology, immunosuppression, to surgical and anesthetic technique and finally postoperative pain relief. We have included transplantation pertaining to all organs. We have tried to give a very simple and practical approach to the management of this group of patients.

All the contributing authors are experts in their respective fields.

We do hope the readers will enjoy and benefit reading this book.

Jayashree Sood
Vijay Vohra

Acknowledgments

I am greatly indebted to Dr VP Kumra, Emeritus Consultant, Department of Anesthesiology, Pain and Perioperative Medicine, Sir Ganga Ram Hospital, New Delhi, India who has always been a guiding force behind my academic achievements. I am grateful to Dr DS Rana, Chairman, Board of Management, Sir Ganga Ram Hospital, for writing a foreword and for his continuous support to our academic endeavors.

I would like to take this opportunity to acknowledge my colleagues who have contributed to this book. Their expertise has surely added to the scientific quality of the book.

My heartfelt thanks to Dr Vijay Vohra, my colleague and friend who has co-edited this book with me.

A special thanks to Ms Silvi Philips and Mr Prakash Bisht for their secretarial help. Their untiring efforts have made it possible to complete this book.

This book would not have been possible without the constant inspiration and support of my husband, Dr Subhash Sood and my blue eyed children Rahul, Ruchi and Dheeraj, and my grand daughters 'Ayra' and 'Samaira'

Jayashree Sood

Acknowledgments

This is probably the first effort in India to publish a book on Anesthesia for organ transplantation. Internationally also there are not many who had ventured into this subject and therefore, there is no book with consolidated material on organ transplantation and anesthesia. Finally, this is a book which covers all aspects of organs transplantation and Dr Jayashree Sood must be complimented in the polarizing forces to get this book together. She has unending energy and huge respect in the anesthetic community.

All the authors should be complimented for their hard work. Ms Silvi Philips and Mr Prakash Bisht need a special mention for their secretarial help and for following up on all the contributors. It has been a pleasure to have been associated with all the contributors and hope the book will be well accepted by the readers.

Vijay Vohra

Contents

1 CHAPTER

History of Transplantation

Chand Sahai

Scientific reasoning is a kind of dialogue between the possible and the actual, between what might be and what is in fact the case. The human mind treats a new idea the way the same body treats a strange protein; it rejects it

Sir Peter B Medawar

INTRODUCTION

Since ancient times there have been references to man's interest in transplantation as seen in religion, literature and the arts. An example of xenotransplantation (where the recipient and donor are from different species) is from India: Lord Ganesha, the elephant-headed god (Fig. 1.1).

The Phoenicians paid obeisance to Gods who had animal heads, while Greek mythology is rife with creatures concocted from various combinations of human and animal parts. In fact the Chimera (serpent's tail, lion's head and feet, and goat's head arising from the middle of the body) is the modern symbol of clinical transplantation (Fig. 1.2).

A legendary example of an allograph where both donor and recipient are from the same species may be found in Jacopo da Varazze's *Legenda Aurae* (the Golden Legend): in 348 AD the martyred saints Cosmas and Damian returned to perform miracles, they are shown in the painting replacing the gangrenous leg of Justinian, a Roman deacon, with a leg taken from a recently deceased Ethiopian. The transplanted

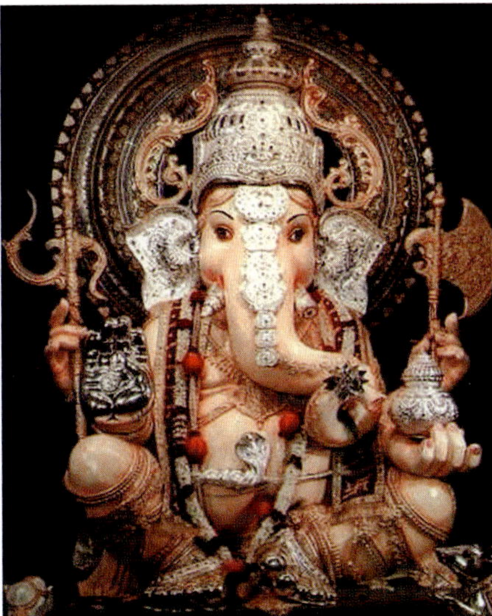

Fig. 1.1: Ganesha was guarding the entrance to the room where the goddess Parvati was bathing. On being denied access Lord Shiva, Parvati's consort was infuriated and decapitated Ganesha. Parvati wanted Ganesha back, so Shiva replaced his head with the first sleeping being found, in this case an elephant

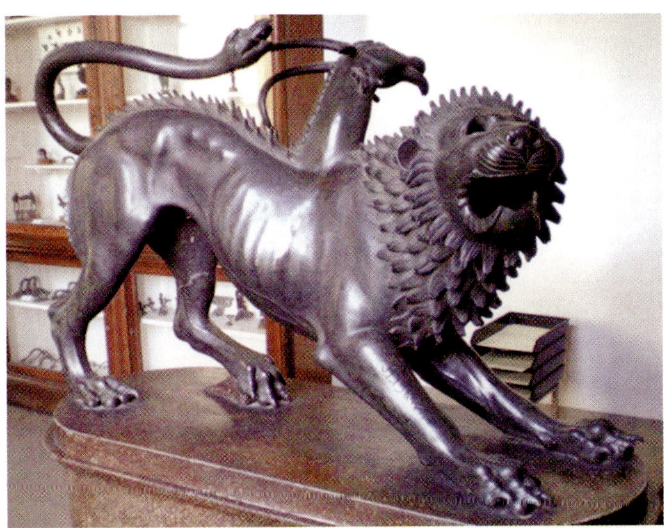

Fig. 1.2: Bronze statue of Chimera, 4th century BC in the Museo-Archeologico, Florence, Italy

limb is conspicuous by the color contrast with the recipient (Fig. 1.3).

In the *Susruta Samhita,* susruta famed surgeon of ancient India (Fig. 1.4), described a technique for reconstruction of a new nose in those punished by cutting off the olfactory organ. This involved rotating a skin flap from the forehead to cover the defect and to refashion a new nose. Susruta's technique was further developed by Gasparo Tagliacozzi in 16th century Bologna a time of syphilis and swordplay. John Hunter, a Scotsman, carried out several experimental studies including some relating to transplantation, an example of which is shown in Figure 1.5.

During the polio epidemics of the 1940s and 1950s, improved pulmonary support led to several patients being successfully resuscitated. Some of these survivors however, were in a vegetative brain-dead state, alive only because of physiologic life support. A historic outcome of this, at least as far as transplantation was concerned, was that the old criterion of cessation of heartbeat and respiration to define death was in time changed to mean intractable brain damage, leading to the harvest of organs from brain-dead donors with intact circulatory systems.[1]

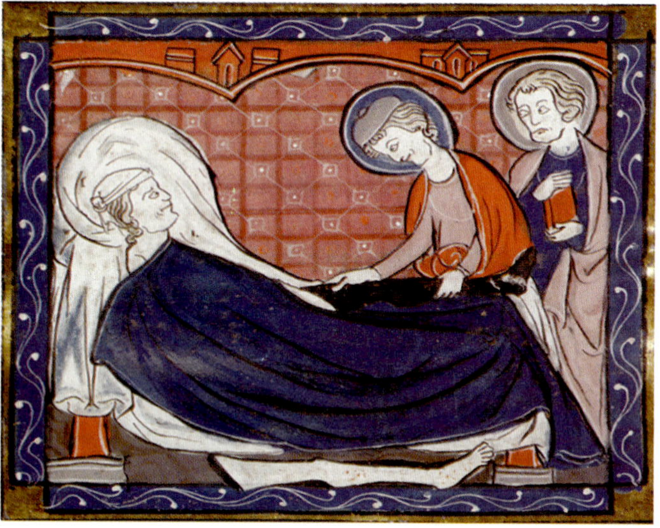

Fig. 1.3: The saints Cosmas and Damian performing the miracle of transplantation. This item is reproduced by permission of The Huntington Library, San Marino, California

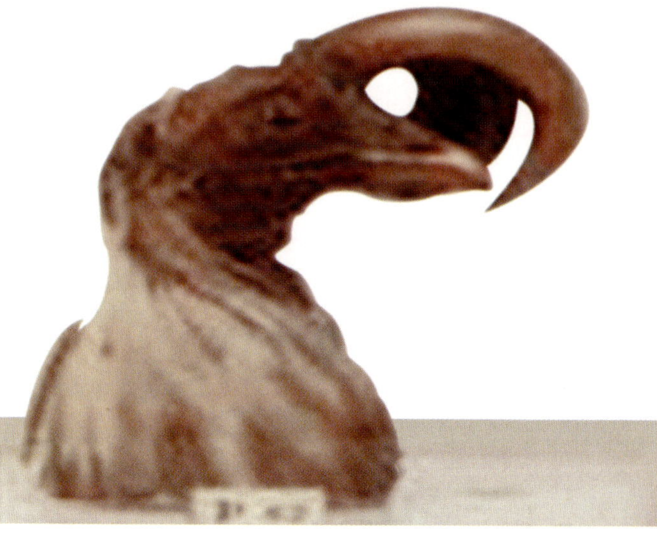

Fig. 1.5: Photograph of a specimen where a spur has been transplanted into a cock's comb, housed in London's Hunterian Museum. © The Hunterian Museum at the Royal College of Surgeons

The swift progression in the field of transplantation in the 20th century was feasible because of concurrent developments in the fields of anesthesia, medicine, surgery, dialysis, immunology, antibiotics, intensive care medicine, open heart surgery and the cardiopulmonary bypass machines. But it is Alexis Carrel (1873-1944) (Fig. 1.6), Nobel Prize winner for

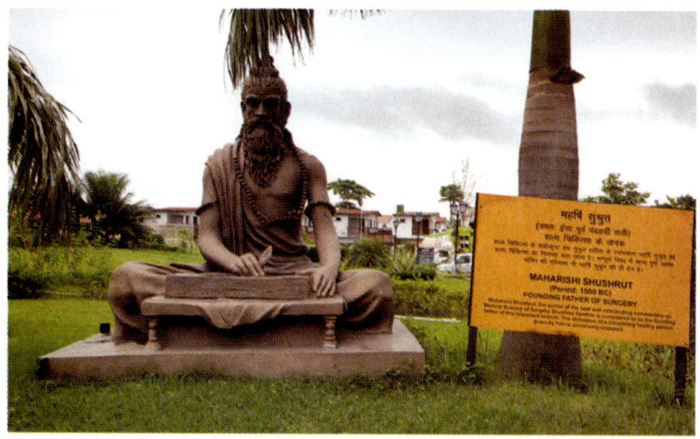

Fig. 1.4: Susruta surgeon of ancient India. © Gagan Mehta

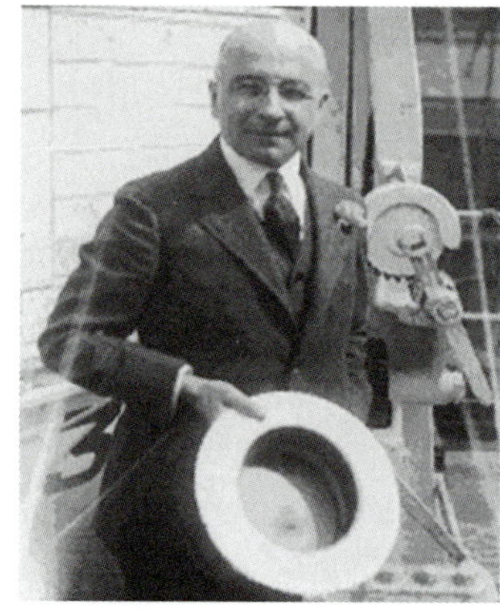

Fig. 1.6: Alexis Carrel (1873-1944) Nobel Prize winner for Medicine in 1912

Medicine in 1912, who recognized that vascular anastomoses would play a pivotal role in organ transplantation.[2] His methods of vascular anastomosis using fine thread and needles, learnt from professional seamstresses is still in use today with hardly any modifications.[3] His promising results with the new technique of vascular anastomosis led to animal experimentations like transplanting kidneys into the necks of dogs.[4] In "*The Transplantation of Veins and Organs*"[5] Carrel described several experiments including the first heterotopic heart transplant. He is known as the father of transplant vascular surgery.

One of the great stumbling blocks to successful transplantation was the fact that donor tissues were not recognized by the immune system of the recipient and soon rejected, with disastrous results. Another Nobel Prize winner, Peter Medawar (Fig. 1.7), hypothesised that graft rejection was an immunological event encompassing both memory and specificity and carried out numerous experiments on acute rejection and immunologic tolerance.[6,7]

In the early days of immunosuppression in patients, who had undergone organ transplantation, donor organ rejection was kept at bay using corticosteroids or total body irradiation. In the late 1950s and early 1960s, 6-mercaptopurine and azathioprine stepped into the immunosuppression field.[7] A watershed in the field of immunosuppression was the introduction of the drug cyclosporine in 1974 by Borel and associates.[9] Cyclosporine, a polypeptide binds to a specific cell protein, 'cyclophilin', which is present in high concentrations in organs like the kidney and liver.

KIDNEY TRANSPLANT

The kidney was the first organ to be successfully transplanted in humans. This singular achievement was possible because of several factors, like the development of dialysis for the treatment of acute renal failure and later on of chronic renal failure, which kept end stage renal failure patients alive while they waited for a kidney donor or for a donor kidney graft to start functioning. Other constructive factors: the kidney being a paired organ meant that one could be donated; technical simplicity of the actual surgery, reliable monitoring of the graft via urine production and rapid improvement of physiological parameters in the recipient. History was made in December 1954 (Fig. 1.8), at the Brigham and Women's Hospital in Boston, USA. One of identical twin brothers was in renal failure and his healthy brother wanted to donate one of his kidneys to save the life of his ailing sibling. The Brigham group led by Dr Joseph Murray (another Nobel Prize winner) took a normally functioning kidney from the healthy twin and placed it retroperitoneally in the twin brother who was, dying of renal failure. The results were sensational to say the least, the uremic twin recovered dramatically. He passed away nine years later, not from renal failure, but from a myocardial infarction.[10]

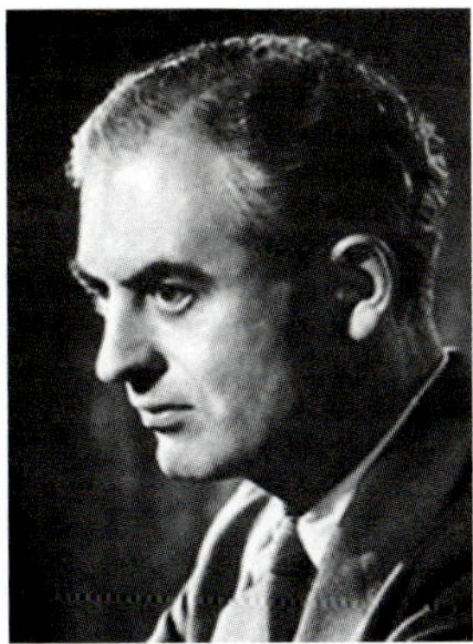

Fig. 1.7: Peter Medawar (1915-1987) pioneer in immunology who hypothesized that graft rejection was an immunological event. With permission of Magdalen College website

LIVER TRANSPLANT

The first attempts at liver transplant were made without cover of immunosuppression, obviously no transplant could survive for long. The first liver transplantation using a cadaveric organ was done by Thomas Starzl (Fig. 1.9) in March 1963 in Denver, which was a failure, with the patient dying intra-operatively due to massive hemorrhage.[11] Four years later, however, a

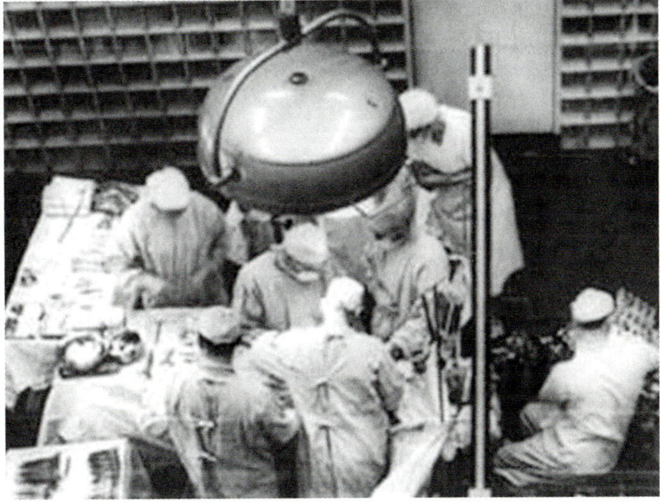

Fig. 1.8: The historic operation, at the Brigham and Women's Hospital where a brother donated one of his kidneys to save the life of his twin who was dying of renal failure. Performed by Dr Joseph Murray (image courtesy of Brigham and Women's Hospital)

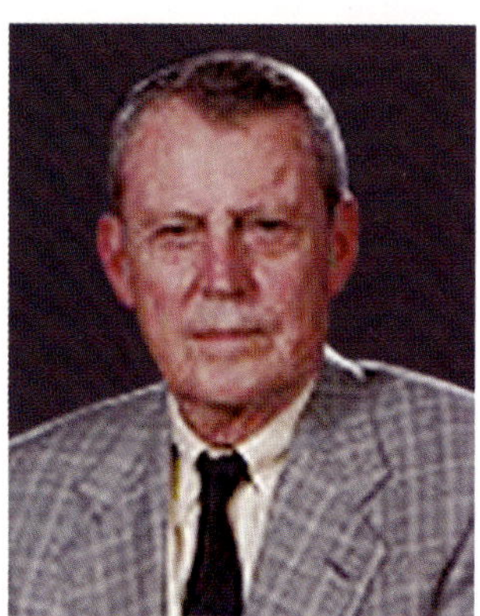

Fig. 1.9: Thomas Starzl, liver transplant pioneer

successful liver transplantation was performed, again by Starzl.[12] Oddly enough, even though liver transplant mortality in the first year after surgery was extremely high in the early days of this treatment for end stage liver disease, many recipients from this time survived 20 to 29 years, having been immunosuppressed using azathioprine, prednisolone and antilymphocyte globulin.[13] Poor long-term survival almost brought liver transplantation to a standstill in the 1970s, apart from teams led by Starzl in Colorado (USA) and Sir Roy Calne in Cambridge (UK) who tested cyclosporine in the clinical scenario in 1978.[14] The use of cyclosporine, improved surgical techniques and perioperative care, as well as better donor and recipient selection and venous bypass, all generated a renewed interest in liver transplantation. Cyclosporine use increased the survival rates at one year in the Starzl group from 33% to more than 70%.[15] Cyclosporine has powerful immunologic effects on both cell-mediated T-helper lymphocyte and lymphocyte-derived antibody synthesis without the bone marrow suppression of azathioprine and the side effects seen with steroids.[16]

HEART TRANSPLANT

Heart transplant surgery was the fruition of decades of work by early pioneers including Alexis Carrel and Norman Shumway among others. But it was Dr Christian Barnard, who performed the first human to human cardiac transplant in South Africa in December 1967.[17] The patient survived only 18 days on his new heart. A few days later Norman Shumway (Fig. 1.10) carried out the first successful heart transplant in the US in January 1968.[18] Over the years the methods of donor and recipient selection have improved, there is better management of the donor organ and advances in immunosuppression and cardiopulmonary bypass, which have all combined to improve the survival of heart transplant patients.

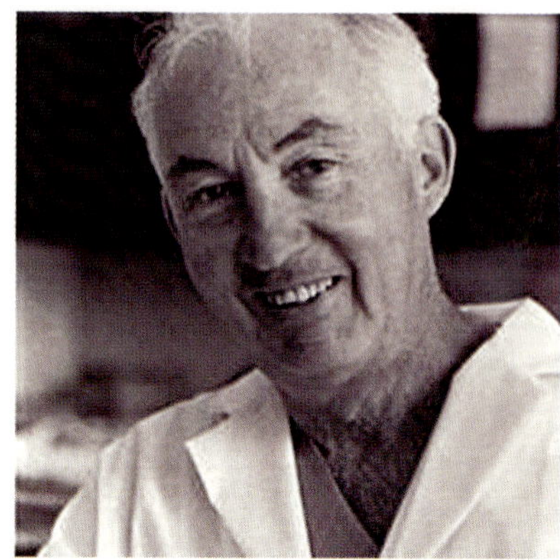

Fig. 1.10: Norman Shumway, MD, PhD, was the father of heart transplantation and one of the pre-eminent heart surgeons of his time. (Image courtesy of Stanford University School of Medicine's Office of Communication & Public Affairs)

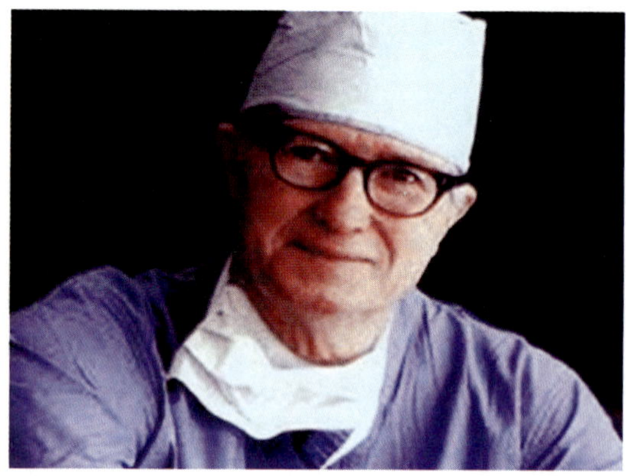

Fig. 1.11: James D Hardy, MD May 14, 1918–February 19, 2003. Used with permission of the University of Mississippi Medical Center

LUNG TRANSPLANT

James D Hardy (Fig. 1.11) at the University of Mississippi performed the very first lung transplant (June 11, 1963) in a patient with carcinoma of the lung. The patient however died of kidney failure 18 days later.[19] In the seventeen years between 1963 and 1980 forty lung transplantations were attempted worldwide, unfortunately only two of the patients survived for more than a month. The introduction of cyclosporine on the transplant scene changed this depressing state of affairs, and in 1981, Dr Bruce Reitz of Stanford University carried out the first successful heart lung transplant in a patient with pulmonary vascular disease.[20,21]

Dr Joel Cooper (Fig. 1.12) of the Toronto General Hospital performed the first successful single lung transplant on a patient with pulmonary fibrosis.[22] Six years post transplant the patient passed away as a result of renal failure. In 1986

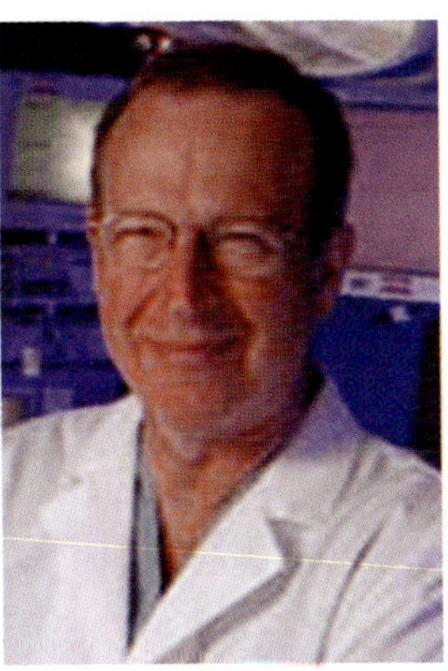

Fig. 1.12: With permission of Dr Joel Cooper. Image from Academy Fellows , at http://www.uphs.upenn.edu/surgery/faculty/jdc.html

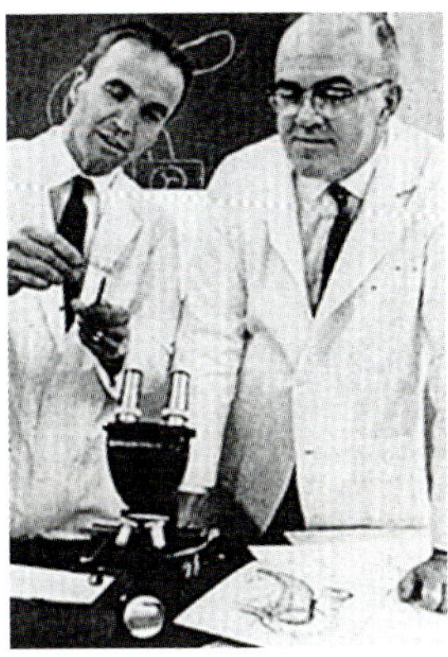

Fig. 1.13: Drs Kelly and Lillehei

Dr Cooper performed a double lung transplant.[23] It must be mentioned here that cyclosporine is not free from significant side effects like nephrotoxicity, neurotoxicity, opportunistic infection, de novo diabetes, and B-cell lymphoma. Another star in the immunosuppressive drugs armamentarium was compound FK-506, later known as tacrolimus which was used in liver recipients who had cyclosporine refractory rejection.[24] Of course other immunosuppressant drugs are being manufactured now.

PANCREAS TRANSPLANT

Pancreas transplantation is used to provide patients with Type 1 diabetes mellitus another source of insulin, offering normal glucose metabolism and independence from the frequent injections of exogenous insulin. Though experimental pancreas transplantation preceded the discovery of insulin, it was not until December 17, 1966 that Drs Kelly and Lillehei (Fig. 1.13) of the University of Minnesota carried out the first human pancreatic transplant in conjunction with a kidney transplant.[25] The patient received a pancreatic allograft and a cadaveric kidney and azathioprine and prednisone were used for immunosuppression. Unfortunately the patient developed a pancreatic fistula and died of a pulmonary embolism about two and a half months post-transplant. The major problem in these patients was the management of the exocrine secretion.[26] Other postoperative difficulties are complications from infection, a high incidence of thrombosis, acute rejection and pancreatitis.

INTESTINAL TRANSPLANT

Lillehei and coworkers at the University of Minnesota were the first to show that intestinal transplantation was possible, by successful experimental transplantation in a canine model in 1959.[27] In the 1960s intestinal transplantation was attempted in humans for the first time, by Deterling in Boston in 1964, unpublished. The first published human intestinal transplantation was by, again, Lillehei and coworkers who transplanted the whole of the small intestine and right colon. The superior mesenteric vessels were anastomosed to the left common iliac vessels.[28] This and many other of the early intestinal transplant patients did not survive long.[29] Death was from technical complications such as: rejection or infection. The advent of cyclosporine renewed interest in the procedure even though the first intestinal transplant where cyclosporine was used was a failure.[30] Successful intestinal transplants were not performed until the mid-1980s when improved immunosuppressive drugs like tacrolimus became available along with better methods to prevent infection.[31,32]

As a result of these improvements, today intestinal transplantation has become the treatment of choice for patients with life-threatening complications of intestinal failure. As part of a multivisceral graft (including the liver) or as small bowel alone, transplantation of the intestine alone has progressed from a completely experimental procedure to one that appears destined to replace chronic total parenteral nutritional support as the preferred method of treatment. According to the Intestine Transplant Registry Report Washington, DC September 15–18, 2011 with 79 contributing centers, a total of 2611 transplants were performed which included small bowel, small bowel with liver and multivisceral transplantations. Of these 1341 were survivors at the time of the publishing of the registry.[33]

Corneal transplant procedures were developed during the 19th century. In 1837, the Irishman Samuel Bigger performed a successful transplant of a full-thickness cornea into the blind eye of a pet gazelle. Continuing improvement in the grafting procedure and increasing success rates in experimental animals led to the first successful human corneal transplant in 1906. Corneal transplantation became a standard procedure in ophthalmology practice; its success was in marked contrast to the high failure rate of skin grafts.

The success story of tissue and organ transplantation is not something that emerged overnight. It has been built up bit by bit over a long period of time, made up of interlocking ideas, fantasy and unsuccessful experiments, culminating in a medical specialty which appears to have no limitations. As superior techniques in surgery, anesthesia and tissue preservation develop, as do better immunosuppression regimens and advanced postoperative care, more parts of the human body will become amenable to transplantation. As for the indications for organ replacement, they have already evolved from that of saving patients with end stage organ disease to cosmetic indications and improving motor functions, as the recent hand transplants and face transplants show.

Transplant technology fulfills the human desire to live longer... the flame of human desire grows gradually, and it is hard to put it out.

T Awaya[34]

CLINICAL PEARLS

- Interest in organ transplant goes back many centuries.
- Hit and trial experiments on humans and animals, and between species, all unsuccessful.
- Donor organ rejection by host and also the means of safe vascular anastomoses main problems.
- Alexis Carrel developed a method for vascular anastomoses still in use today.
- Peter Medawar and others unravel the mysteries of the immune system, which is the cause of donor organ rejection.
- The first successful human kidney transplantation was between identical twin brothers, where immunosuppression was not required. Other solid organ transplants followed.
- Steroids, azathioprine, whole body irradiation and antilymphocyte globulin used in the early days to suppress the immune response in organ transplantation. Later cyclosporine spearheaded the newer immunosuppressant drugs, which greatly improved the life of the donor organ.
- Present day level of success in organ transplantation has been due to the simultaneous development in anesthesia management, intensive care units, vastly improved equipment (e.g. cardiopulmonary bypass, dialysis machines) superior immunosuppressant regimens and improved selection and preoperative preparedness of donors and recipients.
- Indications for transplants have changed from end stage organ disease to improving motor functions and for cosmetic appearance.

REFERENCES

1. Machado C, Korein J, Ferrer Y, et al. The Declaration of Sydney on human death. J Med Ethics. 2007;33:699-703.
2. Carrel A. The transplantation of organs: a preliminary communication. JAMA 1905;45:1645.
3. Carrel A. La technique operatoire des anastomoses vasculaires et la transplantation des visceres. Lyons Med 1902;98:859-64.
4. Patterson C, Patterson KB. The history of heart transplantation. Am J Med Sci 1997;314:190-7.
5. Carrel A, Guthrie CC. The transplantation of veins and organs. Am Med 1905;10(1):101-2.
6. Medawar PB. Second study of behavior of skin homografts in rabbits. J Anat 1945;79:157.
7. Medawar PB. The behavior and fate of skin autografts and skin homografts in rabbits. J Anat 1944;78:176.
8. Starzle TE. History of liver and other splanchnic organ transplantation. In Busuttil RW, Klintmalm GB (eds). Transplantation of the liver. Philadelphia, W B Saunders, 1996;pg 3.
9. Borel JF, Feurer C, Magnee C, et al. Effects of the new antilymphocytic peptide cyclosporine in animals. Immunology 1977;32:1017.
10. Merrill JP, Murray JE, Harrison JH, et al. Successful homotransplantations of the human kidney between identical twins. JAMA 1956; 160:277-82.
11. Starzl TE, et al. Homotransplantation of the liver in human. Surg Gynecol Obstet 1963;117:659-76.
12. Starzl TE, et al. Orthoptic homotransplantations of the human liver Ann Surg 1968;168:392-415.
13. Groth CG, Brent LB, Calne RY, Dausset JB, Good RA, Murray JE, et al. Historic landmarks in clinical transplantation: conclusions from the consensus conference at the University of California, Los Angeles. World J Surg 2000;24:834-43.
14. Calne RY, et al. Cyclosporin A initially as the only immunosuppressant in 34 patients of cadaveric organs; 32 kidneys, 2 pancreases, and 2 livers. Lancet 1979;2:1033-36.
15. Starzl TE, et al. Liver transplantation with the use of cyclosporine A and prednisone. N Engl J Med 1981;305:266-69.
16. Borel JF, Feurer C, Gubler HU. Biological effects of cyclosporin A: a new antilymphocytic agent. Agents Actions 1976;6:468-75.
17. Barnard CN. The operation. A human cardiac transplant:an interim report of a successful operation performed at Groote Schuur Hospital, Cape Town. S Afr Med J 1967;41:1271-4.
18. Stinson EB, Dong E Jr, Schroeder JS, Harrison DC, Shumway NE. Initial clinical experience with heart transplantation. Am J Cardiol 1968;22:791-803.
19. Blumenstock DA, Lewis C. The first transplantation of the lung in a human revisited. Ann Thorac Surg 1993;56:1423-25.
20. Reitz BA, Wallwork JL, Hunt SA, et al. Heart- lung transplantation: successful therapy for patients with pulmonary vascular disease. N Engl J Med 1982;306:557-64.
21. Toronto Lung Transplant Group. Unilateral lung transplantation for pulmonary fibrosis. N Engl J Med 1986;314:1140-45.

22. Cooper JD, Pearson FG, Patterson GA, et al. Technique of successful lung transplantation in human. J Thorac Cardiovasc Surg 1987;93(2):173-81.
23. Cooper JD, Patterson GA, Grossman, et al. Double-lung transplant for advanced chronic obstructive lung disease. Am Rev Respir Dis 1989;139(2):303-7.
24. Fung JJ, Todo S, Jain A, et al. Conversion of liver allograft recipients with cyclosporine related complications from cyclosporine to FK 506. Transplant Proc 1990;22(1):6-12.
25. Kelly WD, Lillehei RC, Merkel FK, et al. All transplantation of the pancreas and duodenum along with the kidney in diabetic nephropathy. Surgery 1967;61(6):827-37.
26. Mai ML, Ahsan N, Gonwa T. The long-term management of pancreas transplantation. Transplantation 2006;82(8):991-1003.
27. Lillehei R, Goott B, Miller F. The physiological response of the small bowel of the dog to ischemia including prolonged in vitro preservation of the bowel with successful replacement and survival. Ann Surg 1959;150:543.
28. Lillehei RC, Idezuki Y, Feemster JA, et al. Transplantation of stomach, intestine, and pancreas: experimental and clinical observation. Surgery 1967;62:721.
29. Margreiter R. The history of intestinal transplantation. Transplant Rev 1997;11(1):9.
30. Cohen Z, Silverman R,Wassef R, et al. Small intestine transplantation using cyclosporine: report of a case. Transplantation 1986;42:613.
31. Deltz E, Schroeder P, Gebhardt H, et al. Successful clinical small bowel transplantation: report of a case. Clin Transplant 1989;3:89s.
32. Goulet O, Revillon Y, Jan D, et al. Two and one-half-year follow-up after isolated cadaveric small bowel transplantation in an infant. Transplant Proc 1992;24:1224.
33. Intestine Transplant Registry Report Washington, DC September 2011;15-18.
34. Awaya T. Organ transplantation and the human revolution. Trans Proc. 1999;31:1317-19.

2 CHAPTER Ethics in Human Organ Transplantation

Amitabh Dutta

Organ transplantation in human subjects became a reality in around the mid-twentieth century. The proven ability of an organ transplant to positively impact longevity has fuelled unprecedented growth of transplantation science. Currently, organ transplantation has evoluted into a truly globalized entity owing to growing awareness, newer safe techniques (anesthesia, surgery, post-transplantation care, rehabilitation), development of infrastructural healthcare resources, presence of proactive formative regulatory guidelines (local, state) and most importantly, the availability of willing donors. With the result, organ transplantation, over the past three decades, has been a notable aspect of medical advancement that has saved innumerable lives and improved quality of life of many. However, there have been issue-based impediments to the relative growth and uniform dissemination of organ transplantation as an accepted independent system. The specific hurdles in regard to above stated include, scarce donor resource (live, cadaveric), the controversy surrounding absolute diagnosis of brain death, conflict of interest (financial, legal, social, psychological), associated specific organ transplant-related implications for the recipient, priorities (social, community, national) and intricacies of human rights issues (right to safe transplantation, right to donate an organ, right to receive an organ). These issues, which otherwise were seemingly abstract outliers hitherto, are threateningly complex whenever an overlap, conflict, or decision-making encroaches the domain of actual process of transplantation.

The current organ transplantation science is elaborate, contentious and has contradictions that mandate debate. Interestingly, the debate matter is not specifically related to the technicality involving the organ transplantation itself, but the more generic and contextual influences that relate organ transplantation science to the general public at large. Ethics, a complex conglomerate of value-based factors (veracity, fidelity, duty, religious/cultural teachings, etc.) seems to be the most significant element that critically impacts, controls and streamlines the contemporary transplantation metrics.

HISTORICAL OVERVIEW

Human organ transplantation began with a series of pioneering experimental studies by a French surgeon, Alexis Carrel (Nobel Laureate, 1912) at the beginning of this century.[1] Surgical transplantation of human organs from donors (living person/deceased) to the sick recipients started around the Second World War. In the late 20th century, with the establishment of safe and effective organ transplantation techniques, introduction of the anti-rejection agent cyclosporine (FDA, 1983), and arousal of public interest vis-à-vis longevity potential the transplantation process offered, the frequency of organ transplantation witnessed an accelerative development. The explosive arrival of structured ethics (Nuremberg Code, 1946) following the Nuremberg War trials (1946) changed the way the patients got treated. Interestingly, the specialty of 'Ethics' kept an exclusive parallel pace with the transplantation science throughout the latter half of the last century (Table 2.1). It veered incisively into the science of human organ transplantation primarily because of the progressive scarcity[2] of the donor organ secondary to enormous growth of sick individuals who were willing-and-waiting for the prospective organ transplantation.

ETHICS AND TRANSPLANTATION

The three facets of the ethics tripod that umbrellas the modern-day transplantation science stems from the need of an individual (the organ recipient), the inter-individual understanding (organ donor ↔ recipient) and the societal/social expectations (public control, community benefit, state regulations/guidelines). The first facet emanates from a super-conscious human process namely, *Altruism*; the second originates from the age-old family/society-driven morality, i.e. '*duty-towards-others*' (*Deontology*, 'Duty Ethics'); the last one involves a community-specific ethical philosophy, known as *Utilitarianism ('greatest good for greatest number of individuals')*. Although in the strictest ethical sense, the

Table 2.1: Organ transplantation and ethics milestones

Organ Transplantation	*Ethics Milestones*
	1946-The Nuremberg Code
	1948-UDHR
1954-First organ transplant (kidney)	
1962-First cadaveric kidney transplant	
1963-First lung transplant	
	1964-DoH-WMA
1967-First liver transplant	
1968-First heart transplant	
	1978-Belmonte report
	1980-ICMR guidelines
1981-First heart-lung transplant	
1983-FDA approves cyclosporin	
	1991- CIOMS

UDHR, Universal declaration of human rights; DoH-WMA, Declaration of Helsinki–World Medical Association; FDA, Food and Drug Administration; CIOMS, Council for International Organizations of Medical Sciences; ICMR, Indian Council of Medical Research.

three facets of the tripods remain separated to maintain a fine balance, there are variable overlaps depending on the abstract situation(s). The broad-fronted principles of modern-day medical ethics (given below) has lent a structured and operational facelift to the above stated basis of conceptual western ethics. An explorative ethical discussion is therefore warranted whenever an organ transplant procedure is activated in order to specifically balance the aspects related to socio-cultural sensitivity, human ergonomics, legal/regulatory oversight, and above all, financial considerations. Introduced in the year 1979, the famous four principles of Beauchamp and Childress have been in the forefront in catalyzing the understanding between high-level moral concepts and the low-level common morality.[3]

1. Principle of autonomy *(informed consent)*
2. Principle of beneficence *(the patient must get the benefit, risk: benefit ratio)*
3. Principle of Non-maleficence ***(Do no harm,** risk: benefit ratio)*
4. Principle of justice *(comparative/distributive)*

The recently introduced principle of *totality of responsibility* (ICMR, 2006, *collective responsibility*) has a holistic stance, which entails professional and moral responsibility for due observance of all the principles.[4]

The ethical governance of human organ transplantation, therefore, is a key to problem solving, decision-making, regulation formulation, and overall success of the organ transplantation procedure. However, the ethical optimization of organ transplantation system may give rise to new case-to-case subtle intra-ethics conflicts (e.g. 'deontology' versus 'utilitarianism'), which demands precision approach that is both inclusive and objective.

The 'Donation-Allocation-Transplantation' (DAT) Protocol

Almost every organ transplantation procedure involves an elaborate expanse that encompasses far greater and more significant zones than the transplantation surgery itself. It probably begins with the 'pre-transplant period' followed by the actual 'operative transplantation phase'. The 'post-transplantation phase' including the 'follow-ups' and 'outcome analyses', completes the range.

ETHICS OF ORGAN DONATION

Altruism and Living Organ Donation

Altruism, an unselfish concern for the welfare of others, or 'selflessness', plays a crucial role in related and the unrelated living organ donations. It forms the basis of motivation that propels the donor to go ahead with organ donation despite knowing the adverse implications of a major surgical intervention and the life after that. Only after the altruistic instincts get makeover of what is called '*Altruistic realization*', the donation can take place. There are subtle ethical conflicts that arise within and between the prospective donor-recipient pair. The catalyst for the altruistic realization to decision for organ donation is influenced by literacy, socio-economic status, need-dependence, cultural/religious aspects, and most importantly, the money-related intricacies. In a recent cross-cultural study, a group of French and Canadian transplant physicians deduced that altruism plays a central yet enigmatic role in promotion of organ donation.[5] In addition, they reiterated that although there is always a cost associated with altruism, it should not be that great enough that it involves sacrificing ones' life. As the evolutionary changes impact human population and individuals, there is a definitive surge in the knowledge among the literates and operational wisdom among semi/illiterates. Richard Dawkins, an eminent evolutionary biologist and author *('The Selfish Gene', 'The God Delusion')*, speculates that with the availability of common knowledge and overriding distractions the humans are confronted with, the belief in god and religion will recede and would continue to be on the decline. With the result, the altruistic instincts as well as related realization will have vanishing erosion. The living organ donations, which although are more altruistic than ever, seems be interspersed with disturbing financial undertones.

The recent decline in the number of altruistic living related organ donors might have to do with the above. However, a new type of altruistic living donors is available, i.e. living altruistic donors (LAD) or the non-directed donors (NDD). They come forward on their own to the organ procurement agencies and offer their organ. They typically remain anonymous as well as are not seemingly interested to know as to who got the organ they donated.

In light of the above we may have to confront different shades of altruism (Flow chart 2.1)[6-10] that dictates and lends pre-regulatory approval to the most significant event in organ transplantation system, i.e. an organ donation.

Cadaveric Organ Donation

Since the first 'cadaveric' organ transplant (kidney) happened in the year 1962, it remained the major contributor of organs for transplantation until the beginning of the 21st century when the living organ donation outnumbered the cadaveric organ donation.[11] The primary source of cadaveric organ donors is brain-dead individuals or the recently deceased persons. The significant aspect of the cadaveric donation is that one cadaveric donor can provide different organs (liver, kidneys, cornea, heart, lungs) for different recipients on the wait list. Upon availability of a cadaveric donor, it is a mammoth coordinative exercise to call up and allocate the respective organs to the needy waiting recipients. The process of collective allocation involves certain ethical conflicts that require critical attention.

The three ethical issues pertinent to the cadaveric (*Latin*: *Cadaver*, 'a dead body') organ donation/transplantation are:

1. The definition of 'death'
2. Advance directives
3. Transplantation-related factors that may adversely affect the risk: benefit ratio

   (Organ (type, size, blood type), distance/time gap from transplant center, waiting list).

The definition and legal quantification of '*death*' is a

Table 2.2: Definition of death

Socio cultural	Kind of dead
Medical death	Brain/cortical death, irreversible loss of function of entire brain (Harvard Medical School Consensus, 1968)
Legal death	Irreversible loss of function of the entire brain as well as the brainstem (US Presidents' Commission, 1981)

Flow chart 2.1: Shades of altruism

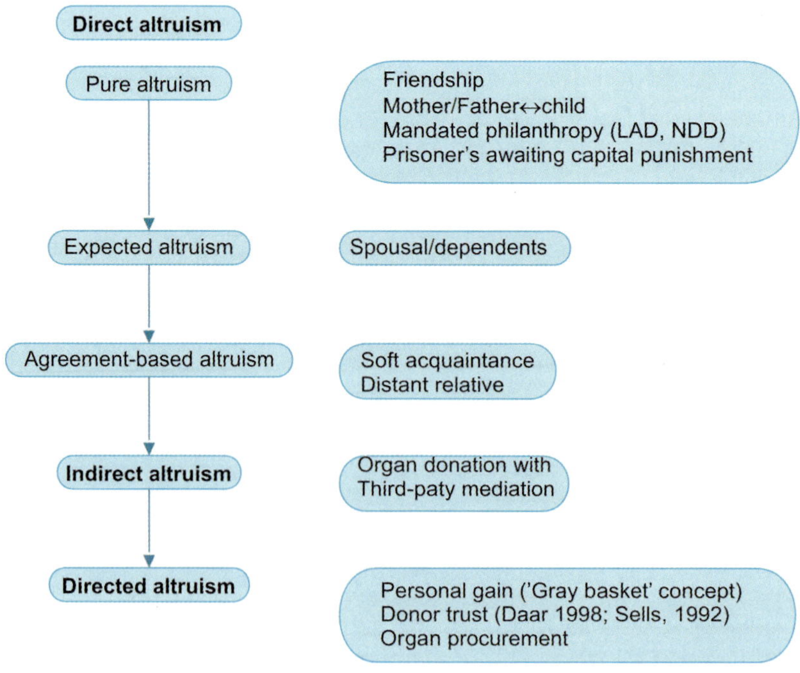

must before one can proceed with organ procurement and transplantation (Table 2.2). In the same regard, it is very important that the family member, close relatives, or legal guardian takes the responsibility of the informed consent admissible under such circumstances vis-à-vis institutional/state regulatory requirements. In case the patient had secured '*advanced directives*', i.e. the 'medical will' for the future course of medical treatment when he/she no longer can be part of the decision-making process for self, legal experts control the procurement of organ.[12] If advanced directives support organ donation, one can go ahead following supplementary family consent. In the absence of advanced directives, the family solely controls the decision to donate.

The institutional/state policy takes its own recourse (*Automatic enforcement*) in the absence of advanced directives and/or when the family/relatives cannot be traced.[13]

As per the WHO draft guidelines for human organ transplantation, there are two consent systems that regulates cadaveric organ retrievals, including. (i) The 'opting in'(explicit consent) consent wherein the deceased persons have had expressed (before death) their desire to donate their organs after their death, or a family member approves the organ removal, particularly in the absence of advanced directives of the deceased person, and (ii) The 'opting out' (presumed consent) consent, which presumes that organs may be removed for transplantation from the bodies of deceased persons until unless their advanced directive suggests objections and/or in absence of such directives, when the close family members actively informed the transplantation team of expressed verbal objections of the deceased person when living.

The persons who wish to be cadaveric organ donors after life can register themselves with local transplant centers. They get a donor card that expresses their organ donation preferences. In Minnesota (USA), it is legally binding to have ones' donation preferences in the driving licenses.[14] With ethical deliberations, new organ donation advocacy systems are in place that takes the responsibility of ethical explanation of cadaveric donation to the family members and facilitate organ donation in a timely manner.

ETHICS IN ORGAN ALLOCATION

After donor availability is secured, the difficult question arises, as to how and whom to allocate the organ for transplantation. Although there are number of ways to allocate organ(s) to the prospective recipients, the allocation decisions are more often than not, conflicting and can be contested.[15] Ethics-based allocations seem to be a unifying process within the standard approach wait-list, the socio-cultural structure of the contemporary local society and, the state regulations (Fig. 2.1). The allocation can be '*duty*'-centric or a '*justice*' (distributive)-oriented process (Flow chart 2.2).[16-18] While the former is more individualistic (related living organ donor) the latter caters to the need specifics/dynamics of a larger society/state and covers living anonymous donation (LAD) by a non-directed donor (NDD) and cadaveric organ donations.[19]

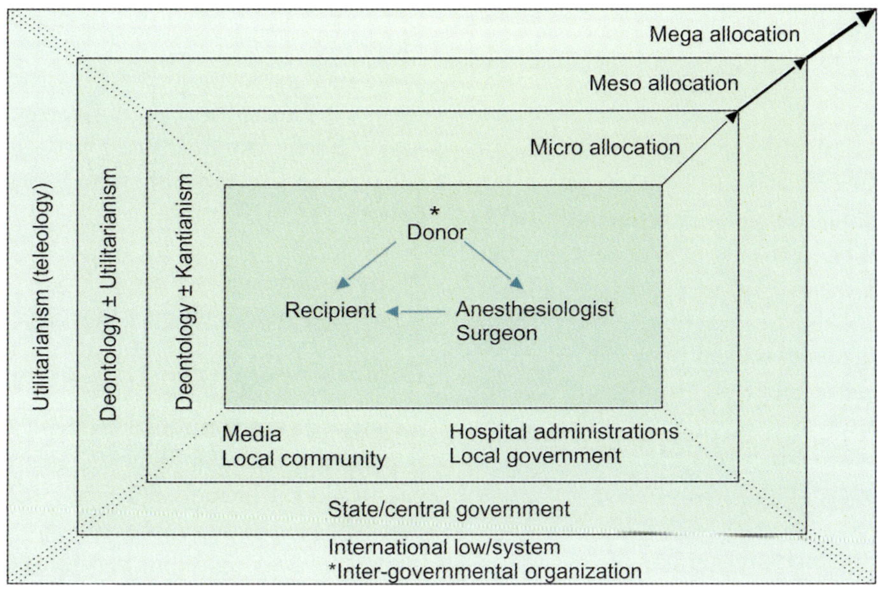

Fig. 2.1: Allocation principles for organ transplantation

Flow chart 2.2: Distributive Justice in organ allocation

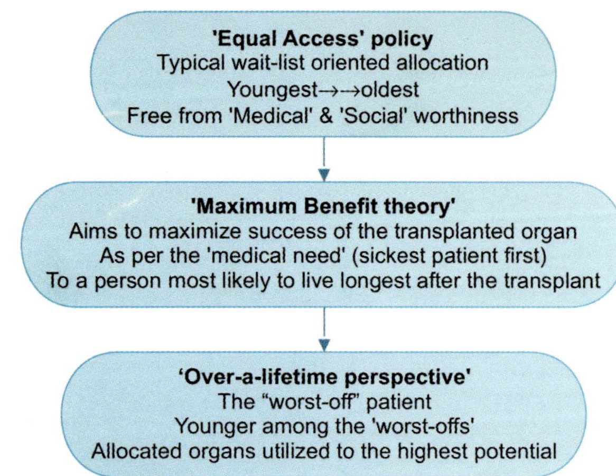

After the ethics-driven allocation of organs to be transplanted is considered, it enters a final rigorous selection trail (Fig. 2.1). The final selection fine-tunes the organ allocation and acts as a socio-scientific bridge between the ethics-directed organ allocation and the social expectations. In the United States, United Network for Organ Sharing (UNOS)[20] has proposed criteria to be considered by organ donation/procurement centers for deliberation on organ allocation and reaching a decision. The criteria include:

1. Medical need for the transplantation
2. Transplant success in terms of number of life-years gained
3. Length of time on the wait list.

In short, ethically, policies need to be aimed at both increasing organ donations and empowering a system that allocates them in the fairest way possible.[21]

ETHICAL ISSUES RELATED TO ORGAN TRANSPLANT PROCEDURE

Domino Transplantation

The 'domino' or the 'double' transplant is a possibility when two 'donor-recipient' sets who are non-matching (ABO incompatibility) within the pair agrees to a cross-matching within them to overcome the incompatibility and facilitate transplantation. The general ethical concern is that it requires participatory agreement and 'informed consent' of all the four (2 donors + 2 recipients) individuals. In addition, there are specific ethical conflicts/dilemma that can mar the above stated double donor-recipient cross-match, including:

1. *Conflict-of-Interest:* (financial, relational)
2. *Donor organ function gradient:* between the two donors (donor specifics (age, co-morbid illness))
3. *Disclosure compliance*: after the first transplantation has started, the donor waiting to donate may refuse donation once he/she gets the current knowledge that the transplant has got affected. This may be secondary to maleficent intention, acute inability to hold altruistic realization to donate the organ, or under duress of financial compulsion. In view of the above, the domino transplant should start together or the current details be kept under the wraps till the second donor gets anesthetized.

Split Transplants

Split transplants are 'splitting of one organ to (e.g. liver) into portions such that it suffices for more than one prospective recipient'. The ethical issue that haunts the split transplants is the risk of a donor portion proving inadequate thereby enhancing risk of transplant failure for the recipients.

Retransplantation

Re-transplantation has evoked intriguing ethical issues because of the obvious imperatives it threatens to draw every single time a retransplantation is considered. In terms of distributive justice, since retransplant recipients at similar level of urgency do significantly worse than primary transplant recipients,[22] a difference that increases with each successive transplant, we need to tread with extreme caution and objective considerations to ensure that the retransplantation will maximize the utility of the retransplanted organ. Irrespective of every requisite procedure in place, the society views every retransplant with reservations and construes the recipient to be a wealthy and powerful personality. Typically society is at its reactive best when a liver retransplant is effected upon a recipient who is considered for transplantation for organ system failure caused by negative lifestyle choices/ behavior (e.g. an alcoholic who re-initiated alcohol after the first transplant).[23, 24]

SPECIFIC ETHICAL ISSUES IN THE CONTEMPORARY ORGAN TRANSPLANTATION SCIENCE

Commerce of Organ Transplantation

Financial incentivization of the living organ donation process is currently the most difficult issue the medical bioethicist has to face, deliberate and give a solution.[25] Primarily, the ethicists around the globe have a consensus opinion that commerce (buying/selling) of human organs is an immoral and disrespectful practice.[26] The most likely affected will be the economically weaker sections of the society. In one way, they may be lured into selling their organs, and in the other, they will never be in a position to buy one for themselves if and when needed. The economic disparity and the money getting utilized as an organ-buying tool have grave implications on donor safety and the ultimate success of the transplantation process. As per John Dossetor, in the contemporary social systems, buying-n-selling human organs will continue to be reflected in negative light.[27]

Whilst the financial implications of organ transplantation proceed seems all but natural, it becomes troublesome when the economic prospects displace the intricacies involving organ transplantation from the center-fold only to render it a 'driven' rather a 'need' based medical intervention. It possibly stems from state policy that actually allows for regulated/controlled 'medical tourism' wherein organ transplantation is considered an attractive entity both for the healthcare provider (financial gain, fame) and the patients (availability of transplant option, cheaper than their own country). The corrupt practice that undermines the ethical homeostasis of the organ transplantation system is more complicated than one can comprehend. Typically, transition from 'tourism' to 'trading' and from 'trading' to 'trafficking' remains non-descript and opaque. A new ethical problem has emanated from overactive, ambitious and motivated organ transplant coordinators who continually 'track' the donor-recipient pair during the pre-transplant preparation phase. When the transplant scheduling is imminent, the pair gets 'jacked' off by them with some or the other lure (financial [cheaper alternative, incentives], promise of greater expertize, long-term care, etc.). Intriguingly, although this phenomenon seems to be in the common knowledge, it is deliberately under-investigated owing to stakeholders' conflict-of-interest. It is very possible that the '*tracking-jacking*' may cut across city/state boundaries unless an effective identification and block mechanism gets in place.

Alternative Organ Sources for Transplantation

Xenotransplantation

Following the positive impact of the immunosuppressant drug cyclosporine on the uptake of the transplanted organ, the demand for donor organ increased dramatically. In the last two decades of the 20th century, with an anticipated actuarial increase for the demand of donor organs in foresight, the possibility of using animal organs for human transplantation became an intensive study matter. In the year 1986, first xenotransplantation was carried out successfully. However, it drew reactions from bioethicists as well as animal ethicists from around the world. The major ethical issues[28] related to xenotransplantation may include, (i) Exploitation of a healthy living animal, and (ii) The possibility that one or the other species of animal may be targeted and pushed toward extinction, and (iii) Risk to the recipient as well as the whole human species form possible transfer of animal bacteria/viruses to the humans.[29]

Animals are vertebrates, who, like the humans, have a body system that gives rise to adverse consequences when subjected to intervention. The Bentham's advocacy of humane treatment of animals (1780), arrogating rights to animals (Singer, 1975),[30] and the speciesism concept (Regan, 1983)[31] are all in direct conflict with the Kantian deontologists who do not consider animals as moral agents. The Council for Interntional Organizations of Medical Sciences (CIOMS) has formed international guiding principles that propagate the efforts aimed to be critical about every xenotransplantation and that the medical community should look forward to transplantation science that is based on the alternatives to animal use.

Artificial Organs

The first artificial heart transplant (1980) was closely followed by the world. Ethically, the stilted risk: benefit ratio for the transplant recipient, conflict-of-interest related to the procedure itself (surgeons' inclination, related research) and the financial implications (manufacture of artificial organ), has long been a matter of debate. In addition, for the risk involved, and possibility of repeat transplant due to transplanted artificial organ dysfunction, artificial organ transplant may prove to be cost-ineffective.

Stem Cells

Stem cells are next big thing in organ transplantation and the way to overcome organ donor shortage in the future. Stem cells are the ones who have natural ability to form different specialized cells in the human body. Currently, stem cells can be found in human adults. But the most consistent and effective stem cells can be retrieved from a growing human embryo. The ethical conflict is that the practice of using embryo for stem-cells lines may promote termination of pregnancy.

Savior Sibling

A savior sibling is a child who is born to provide an organ or cell transplant to a sibling that is affected with a fatal disease, such as cancer or Fanconi anemia that can best be treated by hematopoietic stem cell transplantation.

Ethical considerations related to a savior sibling selection involve the following:

1. Commodification of the donor child
2. Possible exploitation of the donor child.

REGULATORY/LEGAL ASPECTS OF ORGAN TRANSPLANTATION

"As Biomedicine and Biotechnology catch the investments of Governments all over the world the need for ethical scrutiny, policy advice and possibly, new regulatory and governance structures is widely recognized."

Alastair Y Campbell, Professor in Medical Ethics

International Efforts

Early Regulations/Laws

The United States made early inroads into legalities of human organ transplantation that facilitated the formation of regulations worldwide in time to come. They came out with following enactments:

The *Anatomical Gift Act (1972)* established 'Uniform organ donor card', which empowered anyone over the age of eighteen years to make decisions regarding their organ donation preferences.[32]

National Organ Transplant Act (NOTA) (1984)-brought the formation of United Network for Organ Sharing (UNOS). It was established to maintain a list of people awaiting organ transplant. UNOS suggested:

1. Financial compensation for organ procurement organizations
2. Prohibition of sale of organs for transplantation.

The WHO Guiding Principles: Based on the 40th World Health Assembly (1987) resolution proposal: "*to study, in collaboration with other organizations concerned, the possibility of developing appropriate guiding principles for human organ transplants*", and its adoption in the 42nd World Health Assembly (1989), the World Health Organization (WHO) came out with 'guiding principles on human organ transplantation'. These guiding principles (Table 2.3) are intended to provide an orderly, ethical, and acceptable framework for regulating the acquisition and transplantation of human organs for therapeutic purposes.[33] The term "human organ" includes organs and tissues but does not relate to human reproduction, and accordingly does not extend to reproductive tissues, namely ova, sperm, ovaries, testicles or embryos. In addition, it does not deal with blood/blood constituents for transfusion purposes.

National Endeavors

The Human Organ Transplantation Act (HOTA), India, 1994 (revised in 2007)

The 'Transplantation of Human Organ Act' (1994), in essence, proposed three important legislative elements:

1. To accept brain death as also a definition of death
2. To stop commercial dealing in organs
3. To define the 'near relative' (father, mother, brother, sister, son, daughter and wife) who could donate organs without permission from the government.

Table 2.3: WHO guiding principles on human organ transplantation

WHO Guiding Principles (WGP)	*Ethics/Transplant Element in Question*	*Sub-details*
WGP-1	Autonomy	▪ Lawful Informed Consent must be secured
WGP-2	Conflict-of-Interest	▪ Transplant physicians determining 'death' for cadaveric donations must not be involved in actual transplantation procedure
WGP-3	Organ donation	▪ Guidelines to promote living organ donations and improve cadaveric organ procurement.
WGP-4	Living organ donation	▪ To establish 'free informed consent' ▪ Minors should be exempted from living organ donations
WGP-5	Commerce related to organ donation	▪ Prohibition of Human organ trafficking ▪ Allows admissible expenditure incurred in transplantation
WGP-6	Advertisement and organ donation	▪ Allows for advertisements for living altruistic donation ▪ Prohibition of advertisement as a profit-sharing tool
WGP-7	Duty of organ transplant physicians	▪ Advises the transplantation physicians to refrain from transplantation if there is knowledge that financial irregularities have taken place
WGP-8	Entrepreneurial practices in organ transplantation	▪ Aims to restrict/abolish entrepreneurial practices for organ 'recovery' as well as 'implantation'
WGP-9	Distributive justice	▪ Supports 'Justice' and the medical need as a basis for transplantation over financial/other considerations

WHO, World Health Organization

THOA was adopted by all the states and Union Territories except for Jammu and Kashmir and Andhra Pradesh, which have their own organ-regulation legislations.

The revised 'Transplantation of Human Organ Act' (THOA) (2007) has amendment in place for that has expanded the definition of 'near relative' to include grandparents, grandchildren, uncles and aunts. Also, not-so-close relatives who have stayed with the patient can donate organs, provided there are no commercial dealings.

Organ Procurement and Distribution Centers

Under a new plan, Union Ministry of Health, India has proposed organ procurement and distribution centers at the national (National Organ Procurement and Distribution Organization (NOPDO)) and the state (State Organ Procurement and Distribution Organization (SOPDO)) level. Their primary aim is to:

- Increase availability of organs from cadaver donors
- Build capacity for retrieval of organs and transplantation and
- Roll out post-transplant services to both recipients and living donors.

In addition to the above efforts, Ministry of Health plans to initiate an *Organ Donor Register.*

A *National Organ Transplantation Program* is also under consideration.

RECENT ENDEAVORS

An Organ Retrieval Banking Organization (ORBO) is now established at AIIMS, New Delhi, with the sole aim to facilitate organ donation that would help save or improve the quality of life of the awaiting organt transplant recipients. A National Organ and Tissue Transplant Organization (NOTTO) is being set up at Safdurjung Hospital, New Delhi, and is expected to be functional by April 2013.

CLINICAL PEARLS

- Ethics in organ transplantation has gained the rightful significance that protects donor's autonomy, generates a just organ allocation system, brings down the awkward commercial implications related to organ transplantation, settles unnatural conflict of interest(s), paves way for the future research, and most importantly, it builds a socio-scientific bridge that hinges on mutual trust and cooperation.

REFERENCES

1. Theodore M I. Surgery and life: The extraordinary career of Alexis Carrel. Harcourt, 1979.
2. Childress JF. The failure to give: Reducing barriers to organ donation. Kennedy Institute of Ethics Journal, 2001;11:1-16.
3. Beauchamp TL, Childress JF. Principles of Biomedical Ethics. 4th edn, Oxford, Oxford University Press, 1994.
4. Ethical Guidelines for Biomedical research on Human Participants. Indian Council of Medical Research, New Delhi, 2006: pp.7.
5. Fortin MC, Dion-Labrie M, Hébert M-J, Doucet H. The enigmatic nature of altruism in organ transplantation: a cross-cultural study of transplant physicians' views on altruism. BMC Research Notes, 2010;3:216.
6. Dossetor JB, Manickavel V. Ethics in organ donation: contrasts in two cultures. Transplant Proc, 1991;23(5):2508-11.
7. Epstein RA. The human and economic dimensions of altruism: The case of organ transplantation. The Law School, The University of Chicago, January 2008.
8. Daar AS. Paid organ donation--the grey basket concept. J Med Ethics, 1998;24(6):365-368.
9. Daar AS, Land W, Yahya TM, et al. Living donor renal transplantation: evidence-based justification for an ethical opinion. Transpl Rev, 1997;11:95.
10. Sells RA. Toward an affordable ethic. Transplant Proc, 1992:24:2095.
11. Douglas DD. Should everyone have equal access to organ transplantation? An argument in favor. Arch Intern Med, 2003;163:1883-85.
12. Truog RD. Consent for organ donations-Balancing conflicting ethical obligations. New Engl J Med, 2008;358:1209-11.
13. Mossialos E, Costa-Font J, Rudisill C. Does organ donation legislation affect individuals' willingness to donate their own or their relative's organs? Evidence from European Union survey data, BMC Health Services Research, 2008;8:48.
14. Minnesota Medical Association website. http://www.mnmed.org/News/fullstory.cfm? rec Num=2777.
15. Childress JF. Putting patient first in organ allocation: An ethical analysis of the US debate. Cambridge Quarterly of Healthcare Ethics, 2001;10:365-76.
16. Benjamin M. Medical ethics and economics of organ transplantation. Health Progress, 1998;69:47-52.
17. Neuberger J. Should liver transplantation be made available to everyone? The case against. Arch Intern Med, 2003;163:1881-3.
18. Veatch RM. Transplantation Ethics. Washington DC, Georgetown UP, 2000:pp.277-413.
19. Adams PL, Cohen DJ, Danovitch DM, et al. The non-directed live-kidney donor: Ethical considerations and practice guidelines: A National Conference Report. Transplantation, 2002;74:582-89.
20. UNOS website. www.unos.org.
21. Kahn J. "Where have all the organs gone?" http://www.cnn.com/2001/HEALTH/04/30/ethics.matters/. [CNN Ethics Matters website].
22. Ubel PA, Arnold RM, Caplan AL. "Rationing Failure": The Ethical Lessons of the retransplantation of scarce vital organs. In: Caplan AL, Coelho DH (eds). The Ethics of Organ Transplants. Amhurst, New York, Prometheus Books, 1998:260-73.
23. Ubel PA, Jepson C, Baron J, et. Al. Allocation of transplantable organs: Do people want to punish patients for causing their illness? Liver Transplant, 2001;7:600-7.

24. Kluge EH. Drawing the ethical line between organ transplantation and lifestyle abuse. Can Med Assoc J, 1994;150:745-46.
25. The Transplantation Society, Council of. Commercialization in Transplantation. The problems and some guidance for practice. Lancet, 1985;2:715-6.
26. Cohen CB. Public policy and the sale of human organs. Kennedy Institute of Ethics Journal, 2002;12:47-64.
27. Dossetor JB. Rewarded gifting: Is it ever ethically acceptable? Transplantation Proceedings, 1992;24:2092-94.
28. Reiss MJ. The ethics of xenotransplantation. J Appl Philosophy, 2000;17:253-62.
29. Purdy L. The risks of animal-human transplants: Why they may be a bad idea. Free Inquiry, 1999;19:38-41.
30. Singer P. Animal liberation. Random House, New York, 1975.
31. Regan T. The case for animal rights. University of California Press, 1983.
32. Gift of Life Donor Program website. http://www.donors1.org/donation/history.html.
33. World Health Organization. Guiding principles on human organ transplantation. Lancet, 1991;337:1470-71.

3 CHAPTER

Brain Death

Manish Gupta, Subhash Gupta

INTRODUCTION

The study of death is as old as human existence. For ages death has affected the human psyche socially, emotionally and spiritually. Ancient civilizations namely Greek, Roman, Egyptian, Indian and many others, had rituals and myths associated with the death of their dear ones. There was a strong belief amongst these civilizations regarding the presence of a life energy, loss of which meant the death of the individual. Indians called this life energy as **'Prana'**, Chinese called it **'Chi'**. The belief of this Life Energy had a very strong influence on the day-to-day rituals as well as on the medical practices of these civilizations. Since those times death was associated or rather is still associated with permanent cessation of respiration and heartbeat as far as a common man is concerned. However, for modern medical community it all changed in 1950s when Bjorn Isben of Denmark[1] invented artificial respirator, as breathing and heartbeat could be continued for a long time with the person in deep coma, or rather (brain) dead. This was just the beginning of a long debate, and issues that became more complicated by the introduction and refinements in the technique of organ transplantation later. The quest still goes on.

CONCEPT OF BRAIN DEATH

Lofstedt and Von Reis[2] in 1956 first described about six mechanically ventilated patients with lethal brain injuries who were unarousable, unresponsive, flaccid, areflexic and had no spontaneous respiratory effort. Cerebral angiography demonstrated no blood flow to the brain of these patients. In 1959, Wertheimer et al[3] described such cases as the death of the nervous system. The description of brain death was first given by two French physicians Mollaret and Goulon[4] who described it as 'coma depasse'. They differentiated this condition from the prolonged coma now termed as persistent vegetative state. In 1968 an adhoc committee of Harvard Medical School[5] defined the term ***'brain-death'*** as, "a person who is unreceptive and unresponsive, has absent reflexes and no spontaneous effort is present on disconnection from the ventilator for a period of 3 minutes". The same day 22nd World Medical Assembly at Sydney[6] (Australia) it was declared that Life "lies not in the preservation of isolated cells but in the fate of the person." The assembly did not recommend any clinical criteria for the diagnosis but stressed the need for diagnosis of death by two physicians other than the transplant team, in case organ donation is planned after death. This was done in view of ethical considerations after the first heart transplant in 1967. In 1971 Mohandas and Chou[7] described damage to the brainstem as a critical component of severe brain damage. In 1976 a conference of Royal colleges passed a memorandum which specified that brainstem death is equivalent to brain death and a person should be declared brain dead only with proved irreversible structural brain damage with exclusion of conditions that may cause or contribute to coma. A second memorandum was issued in 1979 which stated that brainstem death means the death of the person, therefore a person can be declared dead if the diagnosis of the brainstem death is confirmed. In 1980 ***Uniform Determination of Death Act***[8,9] ***(UDDA)*** was passed by the National Commissioners on Uniform State Law along with American Medical Association, American Bar Association and Presidents Commission on Medical Ethics. This Act was gradually accepted by most of the states in USA although some modifications were made which varied from state-to-state in accordance to ethical, cultural and social issues, e.g. a repeat examination by a second physician or a mandatory investigation to confirm brain death.

In 1987, guidelines for the determination of brain death in children was released by the American Academy of Pediatric Task Force[10] for brain death in children which stressed the determination of brain death by various confirmatory tests as clinical neurological examination can be misleading in pediatric cases.

In 1995 the American Academy of Neurology[1,11] published guidelines for determining brain death, which stated that the diagnosis of brain death should be preceded by the following findings—'Demonstration of coma and the cause for coma, with the absence of confounding factors like hypothermia, drugs, electrolyte and endocrine imbalance along with absent brainstem, motor reflexes and respiration. A repeat examination should be done after about 6 hours, although this time limit can be varied as per the circumstances. Confirmatory laboratory investigations are required only if specific components of the clinical testing cannot be relied upon.'

These guidelines were adapted by many countries and were modified as per their social and legal customs. Most of the countries throughout the world now have their own laws related to brain death and organ donation.[12]

MECHANISM OF BRAIN DEATH

Human brain is a very delicate organ, which is provided protection by the skull. In spite of the fact that skull surrounds the brain and protects it from various injuries, this protection becomes a major contributing factor for the destruction of the brain itself in case of acute brain injury. Although brain injury has a number of causes ranging from trauma to hypoxia all these lead to a single outcome, i.e. **cerebral edema**.[12] This cerebral edema results in the disturbance of cellular osmoregulation and further increases the entry of water in brain parenchyma.

This cerebral edema may remain restricted to a localized area initially but gradually spreads to the entire brain. Since, the brain is confined to the boundaries of the rigid bony skull this edema leads to the rise in the intracranial pressure (ICP). This continuous rise of the ICP may lead to the decrease of cerebral perfusion pressure and eventually exceeds arterial blood pressure resulting in further brain injury. This increase of ICP leads to cerebral circulatory arrest and necrosis of the brain ensues. The brain gradually turns to a liquefied mass, a condition known as ***'respirator brain'***. The entire brain infarct gradually sets in, including the brainstem. Cranial nerve functions are lost and brain death ensues. The spinal cord is the only part of the central nervous system which remains alive as it lies outside the skull and starts working independently.

The brain death usually spreads in a rostral to caudal direction and sometimes medulla oblongata[13] is the only part of the brainstem which survives while the midbrain and pons do not exhibit signs of activity. In such cases patient is comatose but his blood pressure is normal, cough response is present after tracheal suctioning and tachycardia is seen after the administration of 1mg of atropine. It may take several hours to days for the complete loss of function of the brainstem. The rest of the body may survive for many days to years if proper support is maintained.[14]

PREREQUISITES FOR BRAIN DEATH

The diagnosis of brain death is strongly suspected if a patient exhibits the following signs.

Coma

A patient exhibiting irreversible coma not responding to visual/auditory/sensory (painful) stimuli after excluding the effects of any CNS suppressing drugs/toxins/neuromuscular blockers has a strong possibility of brain death. Barbiturates, tricyclic antidepressants poisons like organophosphates, carbamates, snake bites and sedatives like fentanyl are being implicated for the misdiagnosis of brain death in the past. Alcohol intoxication and opioid poisoning may be the confounding factors along with head injury. It is recommended to measure the concentrations of a known sedative/toxin prior to suspecting brain death but in cases where such a test is not possible, it is recommended that the time more than four times (sometimes quoted five times) the half-life of that particular substance should be allowed to pass before suspecting brain death. The concentration of the CNS suppressant drug need not be zero but the levels should not be expected to interfere with the consciousness. If neuromuscular blocking agents have been used, there should be evidence of neuromuscular transmission, i.e. deep tendon reflexes[15] or other clinical muscle functions. Train of four can be useful in such cases. Any acid-base, electrolyte, metabolic disturbances and hypothermia should be ruled out and corrected, if present. Hypothermia causes a temporary loss of brainstem reflexes and pupillary dilatation at temperature of 28–32°C. All the brainstem reflexes disappear at a temperature below 28°C. These deficits are potentially reversible even after extreme hypothermia. Any neurological disease that can mimic brain death should be excluded.

The cause of coma should be clearly demonstrable and should be irreversible for making a diagnosis of brain death.

Absent Motor Response

Flaccid tone and absence of spontaneous or induced movements is seen in brain dead patients. Cough and gag reflexes are absent on tracheal and oral suction respectively. Some patients do exhibit spontaneous movements such as sudden shoulder or limb movement or turning of head to one side or sudden abdominal movement. Such occasional movements are usually due to spinal cord reflexes and should not be confused with spontaneous motor activity. These movements may occur in response to painful stimulus, at the time of organ retrieval or at the time of apnea testing and should not be regarded as purposeful movements as in case of live subjects because these are usually spinal cord reflexes. These movements can be sudden and jerky in nature or they may be continuous or intermittent like fasciculations.[16] Sometimes facial twitchings are described in the texts which may be due to local muscular irritation and should not be confused with the residual function of the brain stem or facial nerve. These movements are called **Lazarus[17] movements**.

Absence of Cardiovascular Collapse

The circulatory system is controlled by the centers present in the pons and medulla oblongata namely nucleus tractus solitarius which get their feedback from the carotid and aortic sinuses. Activation of these centers causes systemic hypertension and bradycardia in response to the rise in intracranial pressure as a result of sympathetic and vagal stimulation in cases of head injury and intracranial bleeding. This combination of hypertension and bradycardia is known as **Cushing's phenomenon**. Further rise in the intracranial pressure leads to ischemia of the entire brainstem which also involves vagal cardiomotor nucleus. This leads to tachycardia along with hypertension in place of bradycardia which is seen earlier. This is due to unopposed sympathetic stimulation and resulting high catecholamine levels in the blood, often referred as **'autonomic storm'** in the texts. This autonomic storm is followed by sudden hypotension due to sudden interruption of the vasomotor output. This marks the sign of cerebellar tonsillar herniation which results in sudden cessation of sympathetic outflow from the vasomotor and cardioaccelerator neurons. This hypotension may further reduce the cerebral perfusion and may result in early false positive diagnosis of brain death, particularly on EEG testing. A vasopressor therapy is thus indicated so as to achieve normotension prior to confirming brain death. This vasopressor therapy is also considered especially important in case of potential organ donor.

Heart rate variability[18] is lost in brain dead persons as cardiovascular autonomic control is lost due to brainstem lesions. Freitas et al has suggested the use of heart rate variability as one of the diagnostic methods for confirming brain death. No change of heart rate in response to vagolytic drugs is also seen in brain dead patients (there is no increase in heart rate in response to injection atropine) due to absent vagal activity.

Absence of Bronchial Secretions

Bronchial secretion activity is predominantly dependent upon the preganglionic vagal efferent fibres that originate from the dorsal motor nucleus of the brainstem, which in turn innervates the laryngeal and tracheobronchial parasympathetic ganglia. Cholinergic stimulation of these neurons increase exocytosis and perhaps the ciliary beat. Brainstem injury with edema and/or ischemia thus results in the reduction of bronchial secretions. Pina et al[19] found a significant decrease in the number of tracheal suctions done in the brain dead patients in comparison to alive patients on ventilator, in a retrospective study conducted in ICU patients over four years.

The diagnosis of brain death is mainly established on the basis of clinical findings and a strong suspicion of brain death is necessary prior to starting a neurological examination as this proceeding can have a change of attitude of the treating team towards the patient and can affect the care of an already critical patient.

CLINICAL TESTS FOR DETERMINING BRAIN DEATH

A number of tests[12] are employed clinically to confirm brain death.

Pupils

The normal human pupil size varies from 4 to 6 mm. Brainstem death results in the dilatation of pupil to more than 6 mm and a loss of pupillary constriction in response to light. Pupillary reflex is mediated by optic nerve as an afferent and oculomotor nerve as its efferent. Thus this reflex can get affected by lesions involving either or both these nerves. The shape of the pupils is usually round or oval but may be irregular if there is synechiae formation due to adhesions formed by the iris on the cornea anteriorly. Sometimes these adhesions are quite strong enough and do not break even by the dilatation caused by the absent motor activity of the oculomotor nerve and results in the false diagnosis of non-dilatation of pupils in spite of absent brainstem function. On the contrary, pupillary dilatation can occur due to variety of other causes such as the effect of mydriatics, sympathetic stimulation and hyperthermia in live subjects. Thus one should rule out these possibilities before considering the pupillary sign for diagnosing brain death.

In case of adults, brainstem death results in the increase of the pupillary size. However the same finding may not be an indication of brainstem death in case of infants of less than two months of age, thus making it mandatory to correlate other clinical findings and laboratory investigations for the confirmation of brain death in case of infants, (as dilated pupils can be a normal finding in such small infants).

Vestibulo Ocular Reflex (Doll's Eye Sign)

In a normal living person the eye muscles move the eyeball in the direction opposite to the movement of the head to one side while keeping the gaze fixed at an object. This ability is lost in case of injury to the brainstem and the eyes move like a toy doll. They do not move in accordance to the movement and remain mid position. This is known as absent or negative doll's eye sign which signifies injury to the brainstem or to oculomotor and/or abducent cranial nerves.

This sign is not reliable in case of conscious persons as they can modify their response voluntarily but is a frequent finding in patients having cerebellar or brainstem lesions.

A variant of this sign is sometimes seen where the conjugate movement of the eye is lost. In such cases one eye moves laterally/medially and the other one remains in the midline. The reason for such a response is metabolic coma or raised intracranial pressure locally which might be an indicator of impending brainstem injury.

This reflex involves the movement of the neck hence it should not be performed on patients suspected of or with proven cervical spine injury.

Caloric Test

This test is performed by irrigating patient's ears with 50 mL of cold and hot water air one by one after raising the patient's head at 30° to the horizontal so as to make the lateral semicircular canal horizontal. Irrigation is done to both the ears one by one for over 30 seconds at a gap of at least 2 minutes (5 minutes as per AAN guidelines) and eye movements are observed for a minimum duration of 1 minute.

Warm Caloric Test

Irrigation of the ear by hot water or air (temperature > 44°C or 7°C more than the body temperature) causes the endolymph inside the ipsilateral semicircular canal to rise resulting in turning of the eye to the ipsilateral side.

Cold Caloric Test

Irrigation of the ear by cold water or air (temperature <30°C or 7°C less than the body temperature, ice cold water may be used in case of no response) causes the endolymph inside the semicircular canal to fall turning the eye to the opposite side.

In comatose patients with cerebral damage, the initial fast phase of the eye movement is absent as this is controlled by the cerebrum. The eyes turn to the opposite side on cold irrigation in that case. If there is no movement of the eyes then it indicates brainstem damage (can also be indicative of vestibular damage alone). Some authorities advocate performing of cold caloric test only.

This test should not be performed in patients with trauma to the ears/perforated tympanic membrane or if cerumen (wax) or pus in the ear canal is present. Basal fractures of the petrous bone may abolish the caloric response unilaterally. Thus a thorough examination of the external ear is mandatory prior to performing this test. The help of an ENT specialist may be required sometimes.

Motor Responses

Corneal Reflex

A normal corneal reflex is blinking of both the eyes in response to touch at the conjunctiva or cornea at one side and movement of the eyeball in upward direction (Bell's phenomenon). Brainstem injury results in the loss of this blinking and upward movement in response to touch. However a recent instillation of local anesthetic agents, local dryness, conjunctival trauma or lesions of the oculomotor, trigeminal or facial nerve should be ruled out.

Jaw Reflex

Tapping of the jaw should not produce any response in a case of brain death. The American Neurology Association does not include this test amongst the mandatory clinical tests for the determination of brain death.

Response to Pain

A patient with brainstem injury does not exhibit any response to the painful stimulus such as pressure over the nail bed, supraorbital ridge (lesions involving trigeminal and facial nerve to be ruled out) or temporomandibular joint. Occasional movements may occur due to reflex spinal activity in response to painful stimulus or spontaneously in the distribution of the spinal cord. These movements are known as LAZARUS movements and should not be confused with purposeful motor response.

Pharyngeal Reflexes

There is no gag reflex in response to the stimulation of the posterior pharyngeal wall in a brain dead patient. Recent instillation of any local anesthetic agent should be excluded. This reflex may be present till the medulla oblongata is spared from injury. Glossopharyngeal and vagal nerve pathways should be intact for testing.

Tracheal Response

There is no cough reflex in response to the tracheal suctioning in brain dead patients.

Sucking and Rooting Reflex

These reflexes are particularly important in the case of infants as cranial nerve functions are not fully developed at this age, although absence of these reflexes alone does not constitute a diagnosis of brain death.

Apnea Test

Apnea test[20–23] is usually performed to confirm the diagnosis of brain death clinically. This test is performed after other clinical tests have ruled out any chances of brainstem survival since this test can precipitate a sudden catastrophic event. A positive result almost confirms the diagnosis of brain death. One must ensure a core temperature of more than 36.5°C or higher, a systolic blood pressure of more than 90 mm Hg or more and a positive fluid balance for more than 6 hours prior to conducting this test.

- The patient is pre-oxygenated by 100% oxygen for at least 10 minutes so as to raise the PaO_2 to a level of 200 mm Hg or more and a $PaCO_2$ of 40 mm Hg or more. Patient should remain connected to a pulse oximeter and blood pressure monitoring should continue.
- Disconnect the ventilator and start oxygenating the patient by delivering 100% oxygen @ 6l/m preferably by a cannula placed at carina.
- Patient is monitored for any respiratory movement (chest or abdominal movement). An $EtCO_2$ monitor can be helpful but may be misleading as strong cardiac contractions may appear like spontaneous breaths.
- If the SpO_2 and blood pressure remain within normal limits this observation is continued for about 8 minutes and then arterial blood gas analysis is performed and ventilator is reconnected.
- If the $PaCO_2$ is $\geq$ 60 mm Hg or 20 mm Hg more than the baseline value while patient does not show any respiratory movements the test is considered positive, i.e. brain death is almost certain.
- The test is terminated in between if the patient starts having respiratory movements or develops arrhythmias or there is a significant fall in the oxygen saturation and/ or blood pressure. In such cases the result of the test is considered to be inconclusive and other confirmatory tests are recommended.

The completion time of positive apnea test is considered as the time of death for documentation.[22, 23]

Apnea test is contraindicated in patients with significant lung injury, hemodynamic instability and high spinal cord injury.

DIFFERENTIAL DIAGNOSIS OF BRAIN DEATH

Brain death is usually diagnosed on the basis of clinical criteria but needs to be differentiated from conditions that can mimic brain death.[24]

Locked in Syndrome

This is a condition caused by focal injury to the ventral pons which results in anarthria and quadriplegia but the patient is conscious and aware of his surroundings. These patients usually respond by blinking their eyes or vertical eye movements. In cases of total locked in syndrome even these eye movements are also lost. Such a condition may result because of injuries to midbrain and rostral pons. The diagnosis can be confirmed by an EEG.

Guillain Barré Syndrome

It is an acute inflammatory demyelinating polyneuropathy characterized by ascending paralysis. A severe form can mimic brain death as it may involve the autonomic nervous system and cranial nerves; paralysis can be in descending order. A proper detailed history gives a fair idea about the diagnosis and is usually confirmed by CSF examination and nerve conduction velocity studies.

Vegetative State[1]

These patients demonstrate a lack of awareness to the surroundings despite showing signs of arousal. Neither these patients interact in any meaningful way nor do they follow commands. Spontaneous eye opening is present but the gaze does not follow any movement or object in particular. Variable amount of cortical activation has been demonstrated on neuroimaging and electrophysiological studies despite extensive cortical damage but with relative sparing of the brainstem.

Minimally Conscious State

This is a condition which is associated with lesser degree of cortical damage as compared to the vegetative state. The patients usually show signs of occasional and inconsistent awareness to the surroundings. They might follow commands, recognize the objects and persons, initiate speech but the inconsistency of such behavior is always there. Generally such patients recover gradually over time to a varying degree.

Endocrine Disorders

There are many hormonal disorders that can give rise to coma and these should be excluded in order to be sure about the diagnosis of brain death. These include diabetic coma, ketoacidosis, hypoglycemia, myxedema coma and adrenal crisis. These conditions may not be directly responsible but can significantly contribute to comatose state. All these causes should be specifically looked for and should be ruled out prior to declaring a person brain dead.

Electrolyte and Acid-Base Imbalance

Various electrolyte disorders such as hyponatremia, hypernatremia, hypokalemia and severe hypophosphatemia may mimic or contribute to conditions like coma and should be corrected if present. Extremes of pH or severe hypotension due to any cause may be the reason for unresponsiveness or may act as a contributing factor to the diagnosis of brain death.

Pharmacologically Induced Coma

Many anesthetic agents, neuroparalytic drugs, MAO inhibitors and certain poisons may not only induce coma but they can also abolish cranial nerve reflexes completely. A thorough clinical history is mandatory to exclude the possibility of such substances. This should include the proper checking of case files and nursing records. Declaration of brain death should not take place if the patient is admitted to the hospital a few hours back. The only exception to this case may be that the patient is shifted from some other hospital with complete details of the drugs administered in the last few days.

Others

Conditions which can give rise to coma such as uremia and hepatic encephalopathy should be ruled out.

INVESTIGATIONS

Confirmatory tests are optional in adults but recommended in children younger than one year of age. In several European, Central and South American and Asian countries confirmatory testing is required as per law. Certain countries (e.g. Sweden, Norway) require only cerebral angiography. In India the choice of tests is left to the discretion of the physician and is not mandatory. These confirmatory tests are especially indicated if there is a doubt regarding the result of the clinical findings.

A variety of clinical investigations are advocated for confirming brain death but they are broadly divided into three major categories.

Tests Determining Cerebral Blood Flow

Cerebral Angiography

Cerebral Angiography[25] is one of the most commonly used methods for the diagnosis of brainstem death. It is more popular method of diagnosing brain death in the European countries than in the United States, where EEG is a more popular method. It is mandatory to perform Cerebral Angiography in case organ donation is planned as per the law in some countries, e.g. Norway, Sweden.

Cerebral Angiography is performed by injecting an iodinated contrast dye into the aortic arch or directly to the cerebral vessels by passing a catheter from the femoral artery. Brain death is diagnosed if the blood flow is obstructed in the internal carotid arteries and vertebral arteries due to raised intracranial pressure.

The **four vessel cerebral angiography** gives a fair idea of the blood flow in the cerebrum as well as the posterior fossa but this method is too expensive and invasive for the patient. The patient needs to be shifted to the area where the facility of imaging is available. This poses an additional risk of hemodynamic instability for the concerned patient. The toxic contrast dye may also have a deleterious effect on the organs in case of potential organ donor. Wijdicks[11] et al suggest that the contrast should be injected in both the anterior and posterior circulation with pressure (although some authorities consider that injection with pressure may result in intracerebral filling which is otherwise not present). No intracerebral filling should be detected at the level of the internal carotid or the vertebral artery. The external carotid circulation should be patent.

Vatne et al compared **digital subtraction angiography (DSA)**[26] with conventional angiography and found it to be equally sensitive. They proposed its use in place of conventional angiography as it is easier to perform, less time consuming and can be performed by less experienced persons. It requires less contrast medium concentrations and is thus beneficial for organ procurement, being less toxic. The perfusion of the organs which have to be retrieved can be examined in advance by this method. In comparison to the conventional angiography DSA is less expensive. Injections into the inferior vena cava and ascending aorta (in case of

DSA) provide a more physiological circulation than selective injections in the common carotid and vertebral arteries (in conventional angiography), because the injections in the latter examination may raise the pressure in the arteries for a short time pushing the contrast medium high in the neck and the caudal parts of the intracranial arteries. This gives a false impression of intracranial blood circulation if conventional angiography is chosen for diagnosing brain death over DSA.

Radionuclide Studies

Radionuclide angiography[27] is performed using an intravenous bolus of radioactive material into the circulation. Brain dead patients exhibit absence of blood flow in the cerebral arterial system. In cases where partial blood flow is present it gives a fair idea about the activity of the brain by assessment of the perfusion. Venous sinuses are usually visualized, but not in the case of brain death. Sometimes these venous sinuses are visualized because of the venous return from the scalp. Application of a tourniquet over the scalp may prevent this but should be avoided in case of head trauma. Radionuclide Angiography can detect blood flow in patients with coma due to drug intoxication. The major disadvantage of this procedure is its inability to evaluate posterior fossa circulation. There can be occasional procedure failures due to insufficient quantity of radioactive substance bolus.

Planar cerebral perfusion scan[28] (CPS) involves uptake of radioactive material by the brain tissue selectively. A static planar image is taken up by a scintillation camera after the intravenous injection of a radioactive material. A large bolus of radioactive material is not required while performing CPS as compared to radionuclide angiography. This method also has the advantage of direct visualization of the perfusion of cerebral cortex and brainstem along with the blood flow assessment. This procedure is also considered superior to radionuclide angiography as it provides direct visualization of the posterior fossa, but increased cost is a major constraint. The American College of Radiology and Society of Nuclear Medicine both recommend anterior view but only the latter considers lateral view mandatory for the diagnosis of brain death, whereas the former considers it optional. Joffe et al[27] reported a case of brain death where a 9 month old girl which had respiration for 20 minutes after extubation despite the anterior, dynamic views taken during ethyl cysteinate dimer (ECD) radionuclide study which showed complete absence of brain stem blood flow earlier. No lateral view was taken in this case.

A **single photon emission computed tomographic scintillation scan[27,28] (SPECT)** is used to obtain images in great detail as compared to other methods. Several Tc –labeled agents are in use for this investigation but brain specific tracers **HMPAO** and **Tc-ECD** are more commonly used. In brain dead patients no concentration of radioactivity could be demonstrated in the brain substance. Although considerable diagnostic detail can be elicited using this method but evidence of any significant advantage is still lacking. This procedure is three to four times costlier than simple radionuclide angiography which is a major deterrent to its use.

Hot nose sign[29]—This sign denotes increased nasopharyngeal perfusion in comparison to the rest of the brain in cases of brain death. In normal persons the radionuclide activity is normally not appreciated with normal cerebral perfusion, or is seen only in venous phase. This sign may be present in cases of transient ischemic attack, cerebrovascular accident, subdural hematoma, hepatic encephalopathy and in cases of internal carotid artery obstruction due to any reason. It lacks sensitivity and specificity as this sign is present in about 52% of brain death cases only and radionuclide studies are not preferred investigation of choice for diagnosing brain death.[15]

In recent years **computed tomography (CT)[30]** and **positron emission tomography scan (PET)** are in use with or without angiography and have quite good results, but are not universally accepted.

Transcranial Color Doppler (TCD)

Early diagnosis of brain death is very important for organ procurement, for the availability of ventilators for patients in need and for ethical reasons (as it is wrong to ventilate a dead person while the relatives are financially burdened more and more as the time goes by). So the clinical tests employed for the detection of brain death should be able to detect it at an early stage, should be easy to perform, preferably at bedside whenever required and should be of low cost and transcranial color doppler is one such test.

Transcranial color doppler sonography[31] was introduced into clinical practice by Rune Aaslid in 1982. It is used as a non-invasive method for studying internal carotid and basal artery blood flow velocity at the patient's bedside. Extensive ischemia, cerebral edema, intracranial bleeding causes a rise in the intracranial pressure. When the ICP rises to a very high level it obstructs the cerebral microcirculation. At this point of time systemic systolic blood pressure leads to the expansion of the distal arterial tree but is unable to push the blood into the cerebral microcirculation. During the diastole there is backflow of the blood. This reverse flow of blood is detected by the transcranial color doppler and a diagnosis of brain death is established.

Transient reversal of blood flow is reported in cases of acute rise of ICP in patients not fulfilling the brain death criteria. Such situations are quite short lasting and are at a stage where brain death can be prevented by taking measures to reduce the ICP. Thus it is also a very significant tool for monitoring the onset and prevention of brain death. But whenever TCD is used for the diagnosis of brain death, patient should satisfy the clinical criteria of brain death and the examination should be repeated after 30 minute interval. A repeat examination is very much essential to rule out false positive diagnosis of brain death.

There are case reports where cerebral blood flow was present partially or completely on examination by TCD or cerebral angiography despite patient satisfying all clinical criteria of brain death. Such a situation may occur where cerebral perfusion is established a little late after the critical brain damage has already occurred and rest of the areas are having adequate blood supply. In such cases other diagnostic tests should be performed to confirm the diagnosis of the brain death, such as cerebral scintillography.

Hassler et al correlated and compared transcranial doppler[32] patterns with cerebral circulatory arrest by angiographic criteria and found it to be an effective method for the diagnosis of brain death. Azevedo[33] et al reported 90.9% sensitivity and 100% specificity with TCD for the diagnosis of brain death. Wijdicks[11, 12] et al suggested that to confirm brain death bilateral insonation should be present, as cranial bones can obscure the TCD view. A good view may be obtained from temporal (thin bones) and orbital areas along with suboccipital area. Absence of blood flow alone should not be considered a diagnosis of brain death, but the reverberating flow or small systolic peaks in early systole should be considered confirmatory. There are case reports where partial cessation of blood flow is present in some areas of the brain resulting in a false positive diagnosis. Litscher et al reported a case where **Transorbital Doppler**[34] was able to detect the cerebral blood flow whereas conventional TCD was unable to do so and suggested it to be a useful adjunct to the conventional TCD. Trauma of the head may sometimes cause difficulty or even inability to perform this test. TCD may be less reliable in patients with prior craniotomy.

Limitations of Cerebral Blood Flow Studies[35]

Insufficient Rise of ICP

Cerebral blood flow tests are unable to demonstrate complete absence of blood flow to the brain if the rise in ICP has not reached a stage where it becomes equal to the systemic arterial pressure. In such a case a repeat examination may be able to demonstrate complete circulatory arrest of the brain if such a stage is reached. Berquist and Bergstrom[25] have documented progressive circulatory arrest with the help of serial angiographies.

Ineffective Deep Brain Flow

Sometimes blood flow is present in some parts of the brain, e.g. the superior sagittal sinus. This finding is usually present because of the venous return from the scalp and particularly seen during the XeCT and radionuclide angiography. This may give a false impression of cerebral blood flow when it is actually not there.

Reperfusion of the Brain

In cases of hypotension accompanying brain death, use of vasopressors can restore the cerebral blood flow by increasing the systemic blood pressure. This may also occur if the intracranial pressure is restored to normal levels by taking various measures to reduce the ICP, e.g. continuous CSF drainage.

Decompressing Fractures of the Skull

Large bony defects of the skull, due to fractures and after craniotomy inhibit the rise of ICP by providing the brain enough space to expand in response to cerebral edema. This in turn maintains the cerebral perfusion pressure despite enough brain parenchymal injury sufficient to cause brain death.

Ventricular Shunts and Drains

These devices are used to reduce the rise in the ICP and prevent brain death. The delay in the instalment of these devices may lead to a decrease in the ICP only after the occurrence of brain death and subsequent restoration of cerebral blood flow may result in a false negative result.

Infant Skull Expansion

An infant skull is different from adult skull in that it can provide extra space to the traumatized brain due to its increased elasticity and non-fusion of the fontanels. That is the reason why an infant can withstand minor head trauma like falling from bed better than the adults. There are case reports where infants with complete electrocerebral silence on EEG along with all clinical signs suggesting brain death having near normal cerebral blood flows. Some clinicians advise not to use a cerebral blood flow measurement technique for determination of brain death in infants for the same reason.

Jugular Reflux

It has been documented that jugular reflux can cause persistent venous sinus activity on cerebral blood flow studies as this can cause a retrograde filling of the venous sinuses.

Extracranial Herniation of Intracranial Vessels

There have been case reports of blood flow in the vertebral arteries after the herniation of the brain as the proximal part of these arteries remained outside the skull even after the herniation of the brain.

Excessive Pressure of Contrast Injection

It has been shown that direct injection of the contrast material in the cerebral arteries by excessive pressure can result into the filling of cerebral arteries which is otherwise absent.

Brain Death with Persistent Blood Flow

There are cases on record where the brain death has occurred due to some reason but where cerebral blood flow is not affected at all, e.g. hypoxia. In such cases brain death is due to injury at cellular level and cerebral blood flows are found to be completely normal (radionuclide studies may be helpful in such cases where delayed films can demonstrate no tracer uptake in the brain cells).

Tests Determining Brain Function

Electroencephalogram (EEG)

The EEG is one of the most common investigations performed for the diagnosis of brain death. It is not considered a mandatory investigation in many countries but has got a high confirmatory value. In some countries it is mandatory to do EEG prior to declaring a person brain dead. Hans Berger a German physiologist and psychiatrist recorded the first human EEG in 1924 since then this investigation has gained acceptance in a wide variety of neurological disorders and brain death in particular.

The EEG is the recording of the spontaneous electrical activity along the scalp and is produced by the firing of the neurons in the brain. It is usually performed for a period of about 20 to 40 minutes. Since it can get affected by the surrounding electrical charges it has to be performed outside the intensive care unit.

The EEG recording is done by the electrodes placed over the scalp preferably at specified locations as per the international 10–20 system and usually more than 12 electrodes are used at a time. Additional electrodes can be added or reduced depending upon the scalp area available. The American Academy of Neurology[11] recommends that minimum 8 electrodes should be placed at a distance of at least 10 cm and interelectrode impedence should be at least 100 to 10000 Ω and the sensitivity should be increased to 2μV for at least 30 minutes with inclusion of appropriate calibration prior to the procedure. Integrity of the entire recording system should be tested prior to performing this test on the patient. High frequency filter setting should not be below 30 Hz and low frequency setting should not be above 1 Hz.

An isoelectric EEG usually confirms the diagnosis of brain death but instrument malfunction and presence of any sedatives, e.g. barbiturates should be strictly ruled out before concluding the diagnosis of brain death. Generalized epileptiform discharges or suppression burst pattern usually predict poor neurological outcome but is not conclusive of brain death. In such cases a repeat EEG after 12 to 24 hours later may be able to clinch the diagnosis. In a recent study by Rundgren and Westhall[36] **continuous amplitude integrated EEG (aEEG)** was studied after cardiac arrest in 95 patients who were treated with hypothermia. Out of these 57 patients regained consciousness including 3 flat aEEG patients at normothermia, 38 died without regaining consciousness. None of the patients with suppression burst at any point of time survived or ever regained consciousness. Out of these 38 only 3 were declared brain dead. Initial flat aEEG has no prognostic value as per this study and should be considered different from isoelectric EEG which establishes the diagnosis of brain death.

The EEG should demonstrate a lack of reactivity to intense somatosensory and audiovisual stimuli, failure to do so may be considered as a lack of evidence for the diagnosis of brain death.

The EEG is considered to be a very useful test but it has several limitations. The foremost is the effect of surrounding currents or artefacts, e.g. blinking of the eyes, cardiac artefacts. Poor grounding of the electrodes can cause significant artefacts. The skull, cerebrospinal fluid and meninges obscure the electric signal. EEG is not reproducible as the signals keep on varying (it is mathematically impossible to reconstruct a unique intracranial current as some currents produce potentials, that cancel each other).

Hockaday et al[37] and Schwab and co-workers[38] classified EEG abnormalities in five grades determining final outcome in head injury patients. Grade 1 had a favorable outcome. Grade 2 and 3 required repeat EEGs which could turn into a favorable outcome on day 2 or 3 or may get worsen. Grade 4 and 5 had a bad prognosis. Grade 5b had no EEG (isoelectric) at all, which represented brain death.

Paolin[39] and co-workers reported cases of clinical brain death where persistent EEG activity was present.

Bispectral index (BIS) is a computer processed electro-encephalographic value that is used for monitoring the depth of anesthesia during surgeries. Vivien et al[40] and later Dunham et al[41] studied bispectral index in brain dead patients and found 100% sensitivity and negative predictive value but a positive predictive value of 84%. A continuous BIS monitoring can help in timely evaluations of brain death as a value of 20 or less is considered as an indicator of brain death in the absence of sedation. The easiness and anesthetist's familiarity of this tool can make it one of the most favoured methods for monitoring in suspected patients and those who are prone to become brain dead.

Evoked Potentials

Evoked potentials[42] are one of the newer methods of ascertaining brain death. Evoked potentials are the action potentials produced by the nervous system of a living organism in response to a stimulus. These potentials can be recorded from cerebral cortex, brain stem, spinal cord or peripheral nerves. Evoked potentials are named depending upon the type of stimulus provided to the nervous system from which the response is elicited, e.g. sensory, somatosensory, auditory, visual and motor.

These sites of stimulation make these potentials specific for the diagnosis of activity of the concerned area of the brain. While evaluating brain death the demonstration of these evoked potentials gives a fair idea of the activity of different brain areas but a single such test can provide a misleading result if there is inactivity of the concerned area of the brain, e.g. Auditory evoked potentials can be absent in cases of cochlear ischemia and can give a false positive result of brain death.

Amplitude and latency of the evoked potentials are the two most important features. Amongst the evoked potentials tested so far somatosensory potentials of short latency in the cervical region give quite a fair idea of brain death as they provide information regarding the brainstem. Facco et al reported that P13, N13 are two very important such points which give an idea of activity of the caudal region of the brainstem and upper spinal cord respectively. As per American Academy of Neurology guidelines absent bilateral cortical SSEPs, i.e. N20 response within one to three days is considered a good evidence of brain death.[43]

Biochemical and Genetic Markers

Brain releases a few substances in the blood and CSF in response to brain injury[44]. It is postulated that the levels of these biomarkers correspond directly to the severity of brain injury. Many biomarkers are studied for predicting the outcome of traumatic brain injury but their role in the diagnosis of brain death is yet to be established. A few of the important ones are enumerated here.

Neuron Specific Enolase (NSE) Serum

This enzyme is a gamma isomer of enolase and is particularly present in neurons and neuroectodermal cells. The level of this marker is usually low in patients treated with hypothermia. A post CPR level of more than 33μg is considered a good level of evidence for a poor prognostic outcome as per American Academy of Neurology[43] guidelines.

Serum S100 Creatine Kinase Brain (CKBB) Isoenzyme

It is an astroglial protein that binds with calcium and is found in neurons and astrocytes. The raised CSF levels of this marker are considered a poor prognostic factor in patients resuscitated from cardiac arrest. As per American Academy of Neurology[43] guidelines it is a poor predictor for the determination of brain death as there is insufficient data to support this investigation.

Brain Tissue Oxygenation ($PbtO_2$)

This method is recently[45, 46] used for determination of brain death but is difficult to perform in clinical setting and is more often used in surgical cases. The advantage of this method is that it can be used in cases where cerebral blood flow is normal but brain death has occurred, e.g. hypoxia. $PbtO_2$ predicts brain death very accurately, as there is no brain tissue oxygenation if the value of $PbtO_2$ falls to zero. This is not a very reliable method if probe is placed inside a blood clot or outside the brain parenchyma. It is also important to place the probe correctly to get the reliable information but focal nature of the method renders this method free from erroneous readings and especially in cases where it is necessary to ascertain the condition of the entire brain. Further studies are required to determine the exact role of this method in diagnosing brain death.

Apolipoprotein E

Brain injuries of same severity and same location in two different individuals with similar treatment strategies may result in different outcomes. This may be due to the difference in the genetic constitution of these two persons. Several genetic markers have been implicated for different outcomes in different disease states. Apolipoprotein E and C are specific brain injury markers.[44] Out of these Apolipoprotein E is mainly studied till now. This is one of the few genetic markers[47] which was thought to offer some breakthrough initially in traumatic brain injured[48] patients but no clear cut result was obtained from further studies. Interleukin -1 is also studied as a predictor for the outcome of traumatic brain injury. Although these genetic markers may be the ultimate predictors for brain injury prognosis but they still do not offer any help in the diagnosis of brain death as of now.

DETERMINING BRAIN DEATH IN CHILDREN

The clinical examination to determine brain death in children[10] follows the same principles as that in adults. However, many children have hypothermia when they become comatose after a severe brain injury or hypothermia is induced after resuscitation from cardiac arrest. Several of the cranial nerve responses are not fully developed in preterm and full-term neonates, and it is difficult to perform a complete neurologic examination in an infant who is inside an incubator. Because of the limitations on the clinical examination of neonates, an observation period of 24 to 48 hours is recommended, as well as a confirmatory test, such as electroencephalography or a study of cerebral blood flow has to be performed before the declaration of brain death. In elder children an observation period of 12 hours is considered sufficient. However, clinical examination should not be performed for brain death declaration immediately after cardiopulmonary resuscitation or other severe acute brain injury. An observation period of 24 to 48 hours should pass this acute event.[49] No particular test is completely reliable but non-invasive methods are usually preferred because of the feasibility to perform them. Some physicians advice against cerebral blood flow measurement methods as the infantile skull has great potential to expand in response to cerebral edema because of the elasticity of the skull and non-fusion of the fontanels, thus persistence of blood flow may be there despite brain death. EEG is usually the investigation of choice but there are case reports on record which demonstrated the presence of EEG activity despite the absence of cerebral blood flow and reappearance of activity after a period of isoelectric EEG.

BRAIN DEATH AND LAW

Brain death has been recognized by the Indian law in 1994 along with **The Transplantation of Human Organs Act**.[50] As per this act the brainstem death should be certified by a Board of medical experts consisting of the following.

- The registered medical practitioner in charge of the hospital in which brainstem death has occurred.
- An independent registered medical practitioner, being a specialist, to be nominated by the registered medical practitioner in charge of the hospital from the panel of the names approved by the appropriate authority.
- A neurologist or a neurosurgeon to be nominated by registered medical practitioner in charge of the hospital, from the panel of the names approved by the appropriate authority.
- The registered medical practitioner treating the person whose brainstem death has occurred.

The Transplantation of Human Organs (Amendment) Act, 2009 however made the following changes to the principal Act.[50,51]

"Provided that where a neurologist or a neurosurgeon is not available, the registered medical practitioner may nominate an independent registered medical practitioner, being a surgeon or a physician and an anesthetist or intensivist subject to the condition that they are not members of the transplantation team for the concerned recipient and to such conditions as may be prescribed."

This act does not define any guidelines or diagnostic criteria for the diagnosis of brainstem death.

MEDICAL RECORD DOCUMENTATION

The American Academy of Neurology[23] recommends a proper documentation of all the clinical tests and investigations mentioning all details so that it can be used as a reference for future examinations and studies, as well as for legal purposes later on. Greer et al[1] studied the differences in practice of brain death declaration in 50 different hospitals in USA and found that many physicians were overlooking the guidelines regarding the pre-conditions that needs to be excluded prior to the diagnosis of brain death. They also found the differing investigation protocols followed by different hospitals in order to confirm brain death. Hence, it becomes very important to document every detail so that nothing goes unnoticed. This becomes especially important if the brain dead patient turns out to be an organ donor. In Indian scenario where involvement of four different physicians is mandatory for declaring a person brain-dead it becomes very important as all the procedures cannot be repeated again and again and it is very difficult for all four physicians to be present at the time of clinical tests and investigations.

The time of death should be clearly mentioned in the records. Time of death is the time when arterial pCO_2 is reached the critical level or when the ancillary test has been interpreted officially.

CONTROVERSIES RELATED TO BRAIN DEATH

Brain death has remained a controversial issue since the time of its initial reporting to the present era amongst the physicians, ethics groups, lawyers and general public.

There have been debates regarding which part of the brain is actually responsible for sustaining life since the time of Sydney declaration and Harvard guidelines. Countries are still divided in two groups, one considering brain stem responsible for this (e.g. United Kingdom) while the other group advocates that the death of the whole brain should be considered as brain death (e.g. USA).[22] The debate still goes on but most of the authorities consider ensuring the death of the whole brain in order to be absolutely sure.

The other controversy that remains unresolved till date is performing the apnea test.[23] Although this test is very important in declaring a person brain dead but it can also cause sudden deterioration of the hemodynamic condition of an already critical patient. This test can suddenly precipitate bradycardia, arrhythmias, hypercarbia, hypoxia, acidosis, hypotension and even cardiac arrest. There are arguments whether we are ethically justified to conduct such a test, but the other group[20, 21] advocates performing apnoea test if proper preoxygenation is performed and test is done properly as patient can be connected to the ventilator whenever required. There are differences of opinion regarding the exact time after which a person can be declared brain dead or how much rise of carbon-dioxide levels should be allowed before a decision can be made. A safe method is needed for the same which can reduce the risk.

The determination of exact time of death[52] or brain death is one of the major necessities in view of anticipated organ retrieval and a better transplant outcome. No method or ancillary test has so far been able to pinpoint the exact time of death. Differences of opinion are present over this issue and some researchers even say that death is a process which is dynamic and continuous in nature and no exact timing of death can be exactly defined. Nevertheless, the issue of organ retrieval is so important that it is very much desired to determine the death as early as possible in order to recover the organs as early as possible after death. The determination of time of death is also important to settle insurance claims, property disputes and execution of will posthumously.

The time interval between two clinical examinations has remained a debatable issue for long.[23] Some authorities suggest that there is no need for a repeat test if sufficient time has passed after the initial injury and there are no possible chances of recovery. This argument is also favored by some in order to decrease the harmful effects suffered by the organs which are going to be retrieved if there is a delay in the declaration of brain death. The others however want to be absolutely sure as it is a matter of life and death for the patient and human as well as judgmental errors can happen in case of single examination. This holds true especially for pediatric age group. There have been a recent report where an adult patient showed signs of activity after being pronounced brain dead twice with an interval of 6 hours and despite strictly following the guidelines by American Academy of Neurology.[53] There may be few such instances but none of these patients ever survived till date. This reinforces the fact that a 24 hour period should be the minimum time interval between the two examinations. But a common agreement is far from reach.

The choice of ancillary test which can diagnose brain death in time, is cost effective and easy to use, with sensitivity and specificity of 100% is still far from reach. The institution and country policies regarding this matter are usually followed as a matter of fact but till date no method is considered to be completely safe as there is no room for judgmental error.

And last but the most important issue is brain death itself. There are many philosophical, religious and social views which do not consider brain death as a valid entity at all. As per them the organism is constituted by the coordination of brain and body both and they should not be considered separately, especially when the matter is as important as death. Many physicians[54] social and religious organizations and even law makers are not convinced with the idea of brain death or are misquoting[55] brain death. The confusion gets more and more as medical community itself confuses brain death with persistent vegetative state. The diagnostic protocol and high chances of misdiagnosis and errors make the concept a bitter pill even to those who are practising it and this all gets more complicated with the involvement of organ retrieval process which makes the situation worse. This is one of the most important reason due to which many physicians try to avoid making such a diagnosis and allow the time to take its own course. Let us hope for a future where we can decide brain death at a click of a button and the demand for organ transplant is fulfilled by artificially synthesized organs which can reduce the pressure from the mind of the physician making such a diagnosis.

THE FUTURE

Death has no future or will it lead us back to a better life remains to be seen. In the light of the technological advances[44] that are taking place day-by-day the gap between a live brain and brain that is dead is decreasing continuously. The future probably belongs to methods which can be applied soon after the brain injury and are able to monitor the progress in a continuous manner. This will not only aid in the management of a severely traumatized brain but as well help in pinpointing the exact time at which a person can be declared brain dead. Apnea test which is considered a gold standard till date in deciding brain death may be replaced by these more reliable and safe methods. The present tests which are used to determine brain death are subjected to the high standards of evidence based criteria lately, but further studies and research are needed to establish the exact role of these methods. The improvisation of the imaging techniques is leading to an added advantage of studying the dynamic aspect of the events that takes place during brain injury. Combination of two or more imaging techniques, e.g. PET-CT and angiography is leading to better results than before. The strict laws and policy changes may be the need of the hour but increasing scrutiny and detailed analysis on individual and institutional levels is going to contribute more significantly than the former. The media may act as an important tool in popularizing the concept of brain death to the masses but it also has a great potential to harm in case of slight carelessness. The situation may be much more complicated in our country when brain death will be seen as a part and parcel of organ procurement program, in comparison to the present state when it is a rarely known and poorly understood entity. A better understanding of brain death is definitely needed by the human brain.

CLINICAL PEARLS

- Brain death has remained controversial since its inception as a clinical entity and still remains the same after so many years.
- A strong clinical suspicion is required to diagnose brain death despite several investigations being available for the confirmation.
- A detailed history, thorough clinical examination and strict adherence to the protocol are a must for preventing a wrong diagnosis.[56]
- It should be always be remembered that a slight laziness in obtaining proper history, hastiness during checking of the nursing records, a small mistake during the clinical examination or a mild error of judgement can convert a sincere, knowledgeable doctor of a good conscience to a murderer in no time.

REFERENCES

1. Steven Laureys, Joseph J. Fins Are we equal in death? Avoiding diagnostic error in brain death, Neurology, 2008;70.
2. Lofstedt, von Reis G. Intracranial lesions with abolished passage of X-ray contrast throughout the internal carotid arteries Opuscula Medica (abstracted) 1956:Vol. 8:199-202.
3. Wertheimer P, Jouvet M, Descotes J. A propos du diagnostic de la mort du systeme neroeux dans les comasavec arret respiratoire traits par respiration artificielle Presse Med (abstracted), 1959; 6787-88.
4. Mollaret P, Goulon M, Le coma depasse memoire preliminaire Rev Neurol Paris (abstracted), 1959;1013-15.
5. Adhoc committee of the Harvard Medical School: A definition of irreversible coma. Report of the adhoc committee of the Harvard School to examine the definition of brain death, Journal of American Medical Association, 1968;Vol. 205,337-340.
6. Machado C, Korein J, Ferrer Y, Portela L, Garcia M de la C, Chinchilla M, et al. The declaration of Sydney on human death Journal of Medical Ethics, 2007;Vol. 33 699-703.
7. Mohandas A, Chou SN. Brain death: A clinical and pathological study Journal of Neurosurgery 1971;Vol. 35 No. 2 211-218.
8. Uniform determination of death act (UDDA) 1980, National conference of commissioners on uniform state law with American Medical Association with American Bar Association and President's commission on medical ethics. 12 Uniform laws Annotated (ULA) 589 (West 1993 and West Supp 1997).
9. James L Bernat, Alexander M Capron, Thomas P Bleck, Sandralee Blosser, Susan L Bratton, James F Childress, et al. White The circulatory-respiratory determination of death in organ donation, Critical Care Medicine, 2010;Vol. 38:963-970.
10. American Academy of Paediatric Task Force on brain death in children: Guidelines for the determination of brain death in children, Paediatrics, 1987;280-298. (abstracted)
11. Wijdicks EFM. The diagnosis of brain death, New England Journal of Medicine, 2001; Vol. 344, no. 16, 1215-1221.
12. Kenjiro Mori, Koh Shingu, Shinichi Nakao Brain Death, Chapter 98 Miller's Textbook of Anaesthesia 7th Edition, 3003-19.
13. Eelco FM Wijdicks, Atkinson JLD, Okazaki H. Isolated medulla oblongata function after severe traumatic brain injury Journal of Neurology, Neurosurgery and Psychiatry, 2001;Vol. 70,127-9.
14. Alan Shewmon D. Chronic "Brain death" Meta-analysis and conceptual consequences, Neurology, 1998;Vol. 51:1538-1545.
15. New York State Department of Health: Guidelines for determining Brain Death, December 2005.
16. Yesim Yetimalar Beckmann, Yeliz Ciftci, Yaprak Secil, Solen Eren Fasciculations in brain death Critical Care Medicine, 2010;Vol. 38, No. 12 2377-8.
17. Hornby K, Hornby L, Sam D. Shemie Lazarus phenomenon, autoresuscitation and non-heart beating organ donation Critical Care Medicine. 2010;Vol. 38, No. 8,1757-1758.
18. Freitas J, Azevedo E, Teixeira J, Carvalho MJ, Costa O, Falcao de Freitas A. Heart rate variability as an assessment of brain death. Transplantation Proceedings, 2000;32;2584-85.
19. Pina J, Martins M, Morujao N. Absence of bronchial secretions in brainstem death. Transplantation Proceedings, 2000;Vol. 32:2582-83.
20. Rupa Sreedhar, Sanjeev V. Thomas brain death and apnoea test, Annals of Indian Academy of Neurology, 2009;Vol. 12:201.
21. Calixto Machado, Jesus Perez, Claudio Scherle, Alejandro Pando Brain death diagnosis and apnoea test safety, Annals of Indian Academy of Neurology, 2009;Vol. 12:197-200.
22. Anne J. Sutcliffe Current issues in the diagnosis of brain stem death, Indian Journal of Critical Care Medicine, July-September 2004;Vol. 8 Issue 3:185-9.
23. Eelco FM Wijdicks, Panayiotis N Varelas, Gary S Gronseth, David M Greer. Evidence based guideline update: Determining brain death in adults: Report of the quality Standards Subcommittee of the American Academy of Neurology. Neurology. June 2010;Vol. 74, Issue 23:1911-18.

24. Robert D Stevens, Paul A Nyquist. Types of brain dysfunction in critical illness Neurologic Clinics, 2008;Vol. 26:469-86.
25. Bergquist E, Bergstrom K. Angiographic documentation of the development of the cerebral circulatory arrest. Acta Radiol Diagn, 1972;Vol. 12:7-11.
26. Vatne K, Nakstad P, Lundar T. Digital subtraction angiography (DSA) in the evaluation of brain death. Neuroradiology, 1985;Vol. 27:155-7.
27. Ari R Joffe, Laurance Lequire, Dominic Cave. Specificity of Radionuclide Brain Blood Flow Testing in Brain Death: Case Report and Review, Journal of Intensive Care Medicine, 2010;Vol. 25(1):53-64.
28. Society of Nuclear Medicine procedure guideline for brain death Scintigraphy version 1.0 February 25,2003.
29. Govind B Chavhan, Manohar M Shroff Twenty classic signs in neuroradiology: A pictorial essay. Indian Journal of Radiology & Imaging, May 2009;Vol. 19, Issue 2, 135-45.
30. Bohatyrewics R, Sawicki M, Walecka A, Walecki J, Rowinski O, Bohatyrewicz A, et al. Computed tomographic angiography and perfusion in the diagnosis of brain death. Transplant Proceedings, 2010;Dec 42 (10):3941-6.
31. Aaslid R, Markwalder TM, Nornesh Non-invasive Transcranial Doppler ultrasound recording of flow velocity in basal cerebral arteries Journal of Neurosurgery, 1982;Vol. 57:769-774.
32. Maher Saqqur, David Zygun, Andrew Demchuk Role of transcranial Doppler in neurocritical care, Critical Care Medicine, 2007; Vol. 35 (suppl):S216-S23.
33. Azevedo E, Teixeira J, Neves JC, Vaz R. Transcranial Doppler and Brain Death, Transplant Proceedings, 2000;2579-81.
34. Gerhard Litscher Orbital Doppler Sonography and documentation of brain death. The Internet Journal of Neuromonitoring ISSN: 1531-300X.
35. Flowers jr W Mel, Bharti R Patel, Ms Jackson Persistence of cerebral blood flow after brain death. Southern Medical Journal Apr, 2000;Vol. 93 no. 4:364-370.
36. Malin Rundgren, Erik Westhall, Tobias Cronberg, Ingmar Rosen, Hans Friberg. Continuous amplitude integrated electroencephalogram predicts outcome in hypothermia-treated cardiac arrest patients, Critical Care Medicine, 2010;Vol. 38:1838-44.
37. Hockaday JM, Potts F, Epstein E, et al. Electroencephalographic changes in acute cerebral anoxia from cardiac or respiratory arrest Electroencephalogr. Clin. Neurophysiology (abstracted) 1965; Vol. 18:575.
38. Schwab RS, Potts F, Bonazzi A. EEG as aid in determining death in the presence of cardiac activity (ethical, legal and medical aspects) Electroencephalogr. Clin. Neurophysiology (abstracted) 1962;Vol. 15:147.
39. Paolin A, Manuali A, Paola FD, et al. Reliability in diagnosis of brain death Intensive Care Medicine 1995;Vol. 21:657.
40. Vivien B, Paqueron X, Le Cosquer P, et al. Detection of brain death onset using the bispectral index in severely comatose patients Intensive care medicine, 2002;Vol. 28:419-425.
41. Michael Dunham C, Alisa Katradis D, Mark D. Williams Bispectral index, a useful adjunct for the timely diagnosis of brain death in the comatose trauma patient. The American Journal of Surgery, 2009;Vol. 198:846-51.
42. Facco E, Casertelli Liviero M, Munari M, Toffoletto F, Baretto F, Giron GP. Short latency evoked potentials: New criteria for brain death. Journal of Neurology, Neurosurgery and Psychiatry, 1990;Vol. 53:351-53.
43. Eelco FM Wijdicks, Hijdra A, Young GB, Bassetti CL, Wiebe S. Practice Parameter: Prediction of outcome in comatose survivors after cardiopulmonary resuscitation (an evidence-based review): Report of the quality standards subcommittee of the American Academy of Neurology Neurology 2006;Vol. 67:203-21.
44. Sunil Kothari, Steven R Flanagan, Christina Kwasnica, Allen W Brown, Elie P Elovic Congenital and acquired brain injury: Emerging concepts in prognostication, Evaluation and treatment Archives of Physical and medical Rehabilitation, 2008;Vol. 89(3 Suppl 1):S27-S31.
45. Van H Santbrink, Mass A, Avezaat C. Continuous monitoring of partial pressure of brain tissue oxygen in patients with severe head injury, Neurosurgery, 1996;Vol. 38:21-31.
46. Sylvain Palmer, Mary Kay Bader. Brain tissue oxygenation in brain death Neurocritical care, 2005;Vol. 2:17-22.
47. Michael Souter, Gail Van Norman. Ethical controversies at end of life after traumatic brain injury; Defining death and organ donation, Critical Care Medicine, 2010;Vol. 38(Suppl.): S502-S9.
48. Berger R.P. The use of serum biomarkers to predict outcome after traumatic brain injury in adults and children Journal of Head Trauma Rehabilitation (abstracted) 2006;Vol. 21:315-33.
49. Nakagawa TA, et al. Guideline for the determination of brain death in infants and children: An update of the 1987 Task Force recommendations. Critical Care Medicine. 2011 Sep;39(9):2139-55.
50. Transplantation of Human organs Act, 1994.
51. Transplantation of Human Organs (Amendment) Act, 2009.
52. Karlis Purins, Amir Sedigh, Christian Molnar, Leif Jansson, Olle Korsgren, Tomas Lorant, et al. Standardized experimental brain death model for studies of intracranial dynamics, organ preservation and organ transplantation in pig, Critical Care Medicine, 2011;Vol. 39:512-7.
53. Webb AC, Samuel OB. Reversible brain death after cardiopulmonary arrest and induced hypothermia Critical Care Medicine, June 2011;Vol. 39 (6):1538-1542.
54. Brian J Murray. Brain death by thousand hypoxic cuts in sleep American Journal of Respiratory and Critical Care Medicine, 2007; Vol. 175:528-29.
55. Eelco FM Wijdicks. Intellectual death is not brain death American Journal of Respiratory and Critical Care Medicine 2007;Vol. 176: 625-26.
56. James F Bartscher, Panayiotis N Varelas. Determining brain death-No room for error, Virtual Mentor, Nov. 2010;Vol. 12, No. 11:879-84.

4 CHAPTER

Deceased Organ Donation

Manish Gupta, Subhash Gupta

HISTORY

Death is the most mysterious phenomenon that has scared humanity for ages. For centuries people have tried to evade death and to regenerate new body and body parts. Different cultures have stories, myths, philosophies and historical records related to organ regeneration, donation and transplantation. The history of organ donation goes hand in hand with the advances in the technology related to transplantation.

Indian mythology has some famous stories related to transplant of body parts. Lord Ganesha got a head transplant, when his father lord Shiva transplanted an elephant's head on him, but even he had great difficulty in finding a suitable donor for him. In another instance Daksha Prajapati was implanted a goat's head after being beheaded by lord Shiva. Another story related to organ donation was of Saint Dadhichi, who was requested by Indra the king of heaven to donate his bones for killing demons. He obliged Indra by sacrificing his life. There may be other instances of sacrifice in Hindu culture but stories of wilful organ donations are rare.

Hindu text from 2500 BC provide the details of skin grafting and reconstruction surgeries performed in persons having punishment injuries such as cutting of nose, in order to reconstruct the mutilating nose.[1] In Greek mythology there are description of Gods, heroes and beasts with chimeric anatomy. Egyptians used to preserve the bodies of their king 'Pharaos' by the process of mummification with the belief that they will need these bodies in future. These mummies are still kept in different museums throughout the world and provide us the information regarding organ preservation in that era.

PATHOPHYSIOLOGY OF BRAIN DEATH

Brain is a delicate organ which is protected by the bony skull in order to prevent it from external injuries. In case of intracranial bleeding due to trauma, stroke or fast expanding space occupying lesions or sudden increase in external pressure as in case of skull bone fractures the brain tissue gets compressed, surrounding the area of injury. This leads to local edema which gradually spreads to the entire brain tissue. The skull surrounding the brain resists this expansion and allows the expansion to take place in the only available direction, which is the foramen magnum. This leads to the pushing of brain structures attached to the spinal cord through the foramen magnum, a process which is known as herniation of brain. The compression of brain progresses from midbrain to pons to medulla in cephalic to caudal direction and affects the centers responsible for control of different brain activities in a similar manner. Thus loss of pupillary light reflex (midbrain function) is followed by loss of corneal, oculocephalic and oculovestibular reflexes (pontine function), and gag, cough reflex and respiration (medullary function) are last to disappear.[2,3]

In human subjects this sequence is not very well defined as it depends on the rapidity of onset of brain death and the distribution of cerebral edema while the herniation of brain is taking place.

The compression of nerves at the nucleus tractus solitarius and center controlling vagus nerve leads to sympathetic stimulation and increased vagal tone characterized by bradycardia and hypertension and is popularly known as **'cushing phenomenon'** after American neurosurgeon Harvey Cushing who first described it in 1902.[4] The onset of Cushing's phenomenon denotes the onset of brain death. This is the time up to which active measures taken to reduce the intracranial pressure may help to halt the ongoing process of brain death. As the entire brainstem becomes ischemic there is a brief phase of unopposed sympathetic activity due to loss of function of vagal cardiomotor nucleus characterized by hypertension,[5] tachycardia and increased blood catecholamine levels up to 200 to 1000 times (including norepinephrine and dopamine) and is also known as **'autonomic storm'**.[6] Finally as the tonsillar herniation takes place the entire vasomotor and cardioaccelarator activity is lost and there is sudden hypotension. This sudden drop of arterial blood pressure marks the completion of brain death.

All these events observed during the process of brain death are not very well defined in cases of sudden cardiac arrest or hypoxic brain damage. In such cases the oxygen gets consumed within a few seconds whereas the stores of glucose and ATP get depleted within 5 minutes.[7] This eventually manifests into the loss of transmembrane potential and leads to failure of axonal conduction. As the synaptic transmission fails the neurotransmitter glutamate is released and intracellular calcium starts accumulating. This calcium influx leads to release of enzymes like protease, lipase and endonuclease. All these processes lead to excitotoxic cell death. Apoptosis and neuronal necrosis both contribute to this excitotoxic cell death, but their exact contribution to the brain injury is unclear. A fast resuscitation may restore the blood supply but may lead to further neuronal damage due to reperfusion and reoxygenation injury. Reoxygenation results in the release of oxygen free radicals and leucocyte infiltration which lead to further tissue destruction. This injury is further contributed by cerebral edema, hypotension, hypoxia and impaired cerebral autoregulation.[7] All the organs of the body face this self-destructive injury from the start of the sympathetic surge. Intense vasoconstriction leads to decreased organ blood flow despite increased perfusion pressures. This results in various brain death associated systemic problems which are summarized in Table 4.1.

Catecholamine Release and Vasopressor Therapy

There is a sharp rise in the blood catecholamine levels at the start of herniation which is marked by the **autonomic storm**. This autonomic storm leads to peripheral vasoconstriction and results in hypertension as this is body's last attempt to maintain cerebral perfusion. In controlled animal studies this phase takes about 5–15 minutes and lasts about an hour but may take up to 6–24 hours in hospital setup as far as human beings are concerned. Shivalkar et al demonstrated that the rapidity of the process of herniation has a direct relation to the rise in haemodynamic parameters, i.e. hypertension and tachycardia.[8] The more rapid the onset of herniation the higher is the haemodynamic derangement. Unopposed sympathetic activity is responsible for this sudden rise of heart rate and blood pressure. A slower rate of herniation leads to more stable haemodynamic parameters. This sympathetic activity may cause myocardial ischemia and significant cardiac tissue damage and may even lead to pulmonary edema. Novitzky et al studied the histopathological changes in the heart that took place 24 hours after the onset of brain death in baboons and described these changes as **contraction bands, focal myocardial cell necrosis, interstitial edema and mononuclear cell infiltrates around myocytes.**[9] These changes were quite similar to the changes seen in cases having acute graft rejection postoperatively and in ischemic reperfusion injury. In their study on dogs Shivalkar et al clearly demonstrated that these changes were more marked in cases of sudden brain death as compared to gradual brain death and weaning from bypass was easier in case of cardiac transplant recipient from donors having gradual brain death.[8] Once the whole brainstem herniation takes place there is complete loss of sympathetic over-activity and a sharp drop of blood pressure is observed. The hypotension is manifested due to the following reasons[5, 10]

Table 4.1: Systemic problems associated with brain death[5]

- Cardiovascular: Hypotension, arrhythmias, cardiac arrest
- Respiratory: Hypoxia, pulmonary edema
- Fluid and electrolytes: Hypoklaemia, hypernatremia, acidosis, hypomagnesemia
- Endocrine: Diabetes insipidus, hyperglycemia
- CNS: Seizures, lazarus movements
- Others: Hypothermia, DIC

Modified from Fitzgerald[5]

1. Peripheral loss of resistance due to abolition of vasomotor control as a result of neurogenic shock (similar to spinal cord shock seen after transection of cord)
2. Hypovolemia secondary to diabetes insipidus, diuretic therapy (to decrease the ICP), fluid restriction (for the treatment of cerebral edema), diuresis (due to hyperglycaemia & induced hypothermia).
3. Myocardial dysfunction secondary to increased sympathetic activity earlier.[11] The contribution of this factor is more in cases of sudden brain death and in cases of subarachnoid haemorrhage. Hypoperfusion secondary to ischemia, electrolyte imbalance, hypoxia and hypothermia are other contributing factors.[5]

This sudden vasodilatation leads to hypotension, hypothermia, arrhythmias, electrolyte and endocrine abnormalities which lead to further reperfusion injury to the peripheral organs (Table 4.1). High energy stores get depleted and calcium ion influx takes place. Accumulation of oxygen free radicals and activation of inflammatory mediators like complement system, thromboxanes result in further tissue injury (especially endothelial) which diminishes the blood supply to the organs further and result in further organ damage. As the time progresses, subsequent macrophages and other leucocytic infiltration damage the organ, as well as increase its immunogenicity. There is a measurable increase in the inflammatory compounds such as intercellular adhesion molecule-1, vascular adhesion molecule-1, interleukins, interferons, tumor necrosis factor α and numerous others which not only contribute to the reperfusion injury but also have profound effect on graft survival in the recipient later.[12] Most of the earlier studies have been performed on animal models as controlled human trials were not possible, but as more and more information is getting available from countries where organ donation from brain dead and non-heart beating donors are the major contributors of organ donation, these changes are studied in enormous detail and remediable measures are applied to correct them. There are several studies which clearly demonstrate the performance of organs from brain dead donors to be inferior in comparison to the live donors even in cases where HLA matching is better in former.[13] Increased concentrations of inflammatory mediators like interleukin-6 and tissue necrosis factor α in brain dead donors are directly associated with inadequate fluid resuscitation and results in lower recipient six month hospital free survival.[12]

Perez Lopez et al studied the catecholamine levels and histological changes in heart tissues (in brain dead human patients where organ donation was not possible or refused) and found out apoptosis to be the main process for tissue damage after brain death.[14] Contraction bands in subepicardiac and sub-endocardiac area were present in 54% of the cases studied after brain death. Cardiomyocyte necrosis was seen in isolation or groups showing cytoplasmic hypereosinophilia, nuclear picnosis and loss of striations. They concluded these changes to be due to varying degree of acute hypoxia but the total area affected was not more than 3–5% of the total cardiac tissue, although may be responsible for reduced cardiac contractility after brain death and poor cardiac graft function after transplant.

The sudden surge of sympathetic activity and then a complete loss of it lead to multitude of hemodynamic variations that affect the potential organs to be donated. In order to reduce the effect of these changes multiple therapies are recommended in brain dead and non-heart beating donors which will be discussed later.

Wijdicks et al studied the blood pressure changes taken place in brain dead subjects who were chosen for organ donation and found that vasopressor support was required in 77% and 26% required three or more inotropes to achieve adequate blood pressure levels. Increased inotropic support (dose or number) was required by 22% of the subjects in order to maintain stable hemodynamics, although 30% had stable hemodynamic parameters without any increase in vasopressor requirement. A small group of about 7% subjects required antihypertensive agents after initial need for vasopressors and 2% required the reverse therapy, i.e. antihypertensive first and vasopressor later. They implicated hypertension to be a response similar to early autonomic dysreflexia commonly encountered in acute spinal cord injury or an early peripheral α-adrenoceptor hyperresponsiveness or lingering function of caudal medullary pressor areas. None of these mechanism has been proven so far and more research is required to pinpoint exact mechanism for the same.[15]

A sudden fall in blood pressure is counteracted by starting vasopressor infusions such as Dopamine, Dobutamine, Norepinephrine, Epinephrine or a combination of these. Dopamine is usually the drug of choice as it has a renal protective mechanism at doses lower than 10 µg/kg/min. At higher doses especially more than 20 µg/kg/min vasoconstriction takes place which may lead to decrease organ perfusion and subsequent poor graft outcome. Thus dobutamine, norepinephrine and/or epinephrine is usually combined when dopamine requirements exceeds more than 10 µg/kg/min. Norepinephrine is not a preferred agent now a days because of its peripheral vasoconstrictive action although it is still used worldwide.[16] Lung transplant teams usually prefer norepinephrine as it helps in reducing the accumulation of fluid in alveoli by β stimulation.[17] Schnuelle et al demonstrated that donor pre-treatment with dopamine leads to adverse liver and heart transplant outcome, but the renal graft survival is increased with low dose dopamine treatment of the donors.[18]

Hormone Replacement Therapy

During the previous century the studies conducted on animals suggested that there is a drop in the circulating pituitary hormones after induction of brain death in a controlled laboratory environment. Although these findings could not be confirmed in human subjects because of lack of controlled induction of brain death, time course and coexisting diseases in human beings, but there were enough indirect evidences to confirm the drop in the pituitary hormone levels after the brain death. It was quite difficult to get a human subject with known hormone levels before the onset of brain death if not impossible and to get the changes in the hormone levels post brain death. The studies conducted on human brain dead patients showed variable results as far as pituitary hormone levels were concerned.[10]

Diabetes insipidus is one of the most common endocrine abnormalities seen in brain dead patients. It is diagnosed if urine output is more than 5 mL/kg/hr, specific gravity of urine less than 1005, serum osmolality more than urine osmolality and blood sodium levels more than 155 mmol/L.[5, 19] Diabetes insipidus can cause electrolyte abnormalities such as hypokalemia, hypocalcemia and hypomagnesemia. Delay in the treatment can result in loss of renal medullary concentration gradient and reduced responsiveness to vasopressin therapy and subsequently may contribute to the ischemic injury of the transplantable organs. At times there is increased urine output despite normal levels of vasopressin. The causes for this are diuretic therapy given before the confirmation of brain death in order to protect the brain, hyperglycemia and diuresis due to induced hypothermia or contrast dye injected for angiography. All these reasons should be considered before starting vasopressin therapy although they are unlikely to increase the urine output to this much extent.

Hyperglycemia is another frequent finding in case of brain dead subjects. The cause for this is not the pancreatic dysfunction but resistance to insulin as seen in cases of major trauma. Infusion of dextrose containing fluids for correction of diabetes insipidus and associated vasopressor therapy are other contributing factors. Most of the ICUs nowadays prefer to treat this hyperglycemia in a manner similar to what is done in case of live persons as it results in better transplant outcome.[20] Barklin et al demonstrated that infusion of insulin in brain dead donors has an anti-inflammatory effect on the donor organs.[21]

Although vasopressin therapy is an accepted measure taken for correction of diabetes insipidus (induced by decreased posterior pituitary function after brain death) but hormone replacement therapy for anterior pituitary hormones remained quite controversial for a long time. This may be due to the fact that blood supply of the pituitary is spared in most cases of brain death and the normal anterior pituitary hormone levels can be detected even a week after the brain death. Small areas of active tissue seen on biopsy of anterior pituitary confirm the finding that anterior pituitary function is not entirely lost after brain death, but there are reports which suggest the normal levels of these hormones could be found despite proven damage to the pituitary, suggesting a source of these hormones other than the pituitary.[10] Kooper et al reported improved post-transplant renal function in controlled animal studies after hormone replacement therapy by triiodothyronine, cortisol and insulin.[22] Wheeldon et al reported improved cardiac function after the transplant in patients who were judged unacceptable earlier for donation of heart but were considered suitable after treatment with methylprednisolone, insulin, vasopressin and thyroid hormone.[23] Both of these studies also demonstrated a reduction of vasopressor therapy after starting hormone replacement therapy in addition to control of hormone levels. Novitzky et al reported a reduction of dopamine infusion to as much as 20 μg/kg/min after giving T_3 boluses and Wheeldon et al in the range of about 0–40%.[22, 23] Ali et al also confirmed these findings by administration of hormone levothyroxine in hemodynamically unstable brain dead subjects.[24] But there are documented animal studies which showed deleterious effect of thyroid hormone supplementation on donor liver (especially steatotic livers) due to increased concentration of reduced glutathione levels as a consequence of this therapy.[25] Goarin et al showed that triiodothyronine administration does not improve myocardial function and hemodynamic status.[26] They recommended the use of thyroid hormone replacement should be restricted to only hemodynamically unstable subjects. Choi et al also recommend the use of thyroid hormone replacement in brain dead subjects who require norepinephrine infusion of more than 0.05 μg/kg/min for maintenance of hemodynamic stability.[27]

Adrenal insufficiency is seen in about 80% of brain dead subjects. However, this is a matter of debate whether this occurs due to brain death itself, as it is quite commonly observed in critically ill patients also. The total cortisol levels correlate very well with free cortisol levels in these subjects, even despite the associated lower levels of circulating binding proteins.[28] Robin et al recommended better hemodynamic stability in brain dead subjects who received hydrocortisone infusion while getting prepared for organ donation.[29]

The last century remained an era of many controversies but as the evidence accumulated in favor of hormone replacement therapy more and more researchers started using it for favorable transplant outcomes. A multidisciplinary consensus conference of transplant physicians, organ procurement organizations and United Network of Organ Sharing (UNOS) issued guidelines regarding hormone replacement therapy in March 2001 held at Crystal City, USA.[30] As per their recommendations patient is considered a suitable heart donor if left ventricular ejection fraction of more than 45% is seen on echocardiography. If patient does not have this much ejection fraction then patient should be optimized with the help of vasopressors and hormone replacement therapy. Fluid therapy and vasopressor doses should be adjusted with the help of pulmonary artery catheterization. If the patient still does not get optimized then he/she should not be considered for donation of heart for transplantation but may still be considered suitable for donation of other organs. Since, then the hormone replacement therapy is practiced worldwide

Table 4.2: Hormone replacement therapy[10,31]

	Bolus	*Infusion*	*Comments*
Triiodothyronine/ levothyroxine	4.0 μg (T3) 20 μg (T4)	3.0 μg/h (T3), 10 μg/h (T4)	Inotropic effects, hyperkalemia with bolus
	+		
Methylprednisolone	15 mg/kg	Repeat every 24 hours	Anti-inflammatory
	+		
Vasopressin	1 unit	0.5–6.0 units/h	Titrate as per BP, urine output, Na^+ levels
	+		
Insulin (+50% dextrose+KCl)	Maintain blood sugar 80–150 mg/dL	1unit/h	Maintain euglycemia

but exact protocols differ from country to country and even from hospital to hospital. The standard doses of hormone replacement therapy are summarized in the Table 4.2.

Hypothermia and it's Effects

Brain dead patients exhibit a loss of temperature control mechanism due to damage of the thermoregulatory center in the hypothalamus.[5] These patients do not develop fever despite of severe infection or application of warmers. Massive fluid replacements for treatment of diabetes insipidus and depressed metabolism also contribute to hypothermia. Although controversies exist regarding the therapeutic effect of hypothermia, some centers still practice induction of therapeutic hypothermia for cerebral protection after the cardiac arrest. The role of therapeutic hypothermia is quite well established after documented ventricular fibrillation but it remains of uncertain benefit after asystole or pulseless cardiac activity and in cases where cardiac arrest is due to noncardiac reasons, e.g. drug intoxication and hypoxia.[32] Therapeutic hypothermia is induced by lowering the body temperature to 32°C to 34°C in order to reduce the neurological damage. The process of induction of hypothermia for the above mentioned purpose may take several hours to achieve the desired temperature and the patient may be kept under the effect of hypothermia for 12 to 48 hours, sometimes extended up to 72 hours. Additional doses of sedation and muscle relaxants may be required to prevent shivering which might take extra time to get metabolized at the time of rewarming and can cause a delay in the diagnosis of brain death. Shivering usually occurs at temperatures between 34 to 35.5°C and may be misinterpreted as a sign of life at the time of neurological examination. Temperatures below 31°C are usually avoided as they may precipitate cardiac arrhythmias. Therapeutic hypothermia is considered to reduce the morbidity and mortality and improves the neurological outcome but it is believed to increase the inotropic requirement as well as the chances of neutropenia and thrombocytopenia. All these issues have to be tackled if the patient is considered as prospective donor. Various techniques are available for induction of hypothermia which include cool air blankets, administration of cold intravenous fluids, nasopharyngeal cooling by evaporation of a perfluorochemical administered via nasal prongs and recently pharmacologically induced hypothermia by drug administration such as cannabinoid receptor agonists.[33]

Hypothermia causes a reduction in the cerebral metabolism which causes a reduction in the oxygen requirement and ATP consumption. It also reduces the release of glutamate, dopamine and brain derived neurotrophic factor. Lipid peroxidation and release of free radicals is also reduced. Reduction of calcium overload and glutamate levels result in inhibition of apoptosis and induction of antiapoptotic Bcl-2 which suppresses further inflammatory response and cerebral injury.

Hypothermia not only poses a major problem in the diagnosis of brain death but may also result in decreased organ perfusion as a result of peripheral vasoconstriction and can lead to myocardial depression and cardiovascular instability. It can also lead to tissue anoxia and coagulopathy by a leftward shift of oxygen dissociation curve. Renal tubular concentration gradient gets decreased by cold diuresis. Metabolic disturbances like hypokalemia, hypomagnesemia, hypophosphatemia can get manifested during the induced hypothermia.[34]

Brain dead subjects need to be kept warm by the administration of warm fluids, application of hot air blankets till the time of aortic cross clamping or cardiac arrest. All rewarming methods should be immediately terminated once the circulatory arrest takes place in order to prevent warm ischemic injury to the organs.

Coagulation Abnormalities

Brain dead subjects develop a number of coagulation disorders which need to be taken care of at the time of organ procurement.[5] The coagulation system of the body gets shifted to a procoagulant state after brain death. The Von Willebrand Factor (VWF) levels are increased 1.5 times whereas the VWF cleaving protease (ADAMTS13) is significantly decreased in the brain dead donors. An imbalance in the VWF/ADAMTS13 ratio results in the increased chances of unregulated platelet thrombus formation. Plasma levels of glycocalicin (a fragment of the platelet membrane glycoprotein which is shed upon platelet activation) is also increased 1.5 times whereas the levels of D-dimers are also found to be increased in brain dead subjects. The elevated levels of TNF α and IL6 also contribute to the derangement of coagulation cascade. This procoagulant state leads to increased platelet aggregation and fibrin deposits in transplantable organs and results in the formation of microthrombi. These thrombi not only hampers the supply of blood and preservative fluid to these organs but also lead to poor transplant outcome by their direct toxic effects.[35] Along with the increased microthrombi formation brain death is also associated with increased clot lysis time, despite the high levels of D-dimer. This signifies that the body's anticoagulant mechanisms are ineffective in dissolving these microthrombi. It seems very unlikely that the anticoagulant therapy given just prior to circulatory arrest is able to take care of the damage that has already been done by these microthrombi. It remains to be seen in future whether better anticoagulant strategies can help prevent the formation of microthrombi or not. Simultaneously a platelet count below 50,000/dL is corrected by platelet transfusion as a very low platelet level may result in sudden hemorrhage resulting in hypotension and early circulatory arrest. Use of aminocaproic acid is not recommended as it is known to increase the formation of microthrombi in donor organs.[5]

In the case of DCD (donation after circulatory death) donors similar findings are noted and the formation of microthrombi is enhanced with the prolongation of warm ischemia time. However, pretreatment of the controlled DCD donors with heparin reduce the chances of thrombus formation but is unable to completely abolish it. These microthrombi result in delayed graft function and primary graft failure but usually do not affect the long-term graft outcome, probably because the recipient's coagulation system takes care of that.

TYPES OF DECEASED ORGAN DONATION

Deceased organ donation has been in practice for long but the increased demand of the organs always exceeds the supply. Apart from living organ donation various methods have been derived to increase the supply of organs from the cadavers in order to stop organ trafficking. The deceased organ donors are broadly divided into the following categories.

1. Brain dead donors-already described earlier.
2. Non heart beating donors-a non heart beating donor (NHBD) or donor after circulatory death (DCD) is one whose organs are retrieved only after a documented cardiocirculatory arrest and who are not revived[19] till a certain predefined time (which varies as per the laws of the concerned country and decided as per the time of autoresuscitation) after the cardiac arrest (unlike brain dead donors whose heart keeps on beating during the process of organ retrieval till the heart is stopped by a cardioplegic solution). These type of donors were introduced in practice quite early but were not given much importance till 1994 when during Maastricht conference at Netherland, four major categories were identified in an effort to fulfil the growing demand for organ donation as both the living and brain dead donors were unable to meet the demand of organs.
   - Category 1–patient dead on arrival to the hospital
   - Category 2–unsuccessful resuscitation at the hospital or in ambulance
   - Category 3–patient waiting for cardiac death in ward/ICU
   - Category 4–cardiac death in brain dead donor.

However, these categories broadly include all donors for major organ donation, the donors can be divided into two different groups on the basis whether the death was in controlled environment or as a result of uncontrolled cardiac arrest. Such donors are called **controlled non heart beating donors** (Maastricht category 3 and 4) and **uncontrolled non heart beating donors** (Maastricht category 1 and 2) respectively.

It is quite obvious from the above categories that a brain dead person can become a non heart beating donor while waiting for the organ retrieval process to start but there is also another group of patients who are having extensive neurological injuries but do not fulfil brain death criteria. The certainty of poor prognosis and unfavorable neurological outcome prompts the physician to discuss the issue with the family members. If an affirmation is obtained from the kin, patient is extubated in a controlled environment by a group of physicians who are usually neither the part of the treating team nor the part of organ retrieval team. Extubation results in a sudden deterioration of the patient's condition and cardiac arrest follows after sometime. Once this group declares the patient dead, the organ procurement team takes the charge and starts the retrieval process. If however cardiac arrest is not observed for quite sometime, patient is reconnected to the ventilator.

The process of non heart beating organ donation is not as simple as it seems from the above statement. There are legal, ethical, moral and technological issues which need to be addressed before making a policy decision at a hospital or at a ministry level. A decision maker is always troubled with the question whether it is appropriate to decide the withdrawal of ventilatory support in the presence of brainstem reflexes. There are high chances of misuse or wrong decision making on the part of the physician since non controversial guidelines are not present. Autoresuscitation is another debatable issue which troubles the physician who declares death after cardiac arrest. **Autoresuscitation** is the phenomenon that is characterized by spontaneous resumption of cardiac rhythm after the onset of cardiac arrest. There are differences of opinion regarding how much time should be considered enough to rule out the possibility of autoresuscitation. The time limit varies from 3 to 7 minutes but 5 minutes are generally agreed upon. The issue still remains debatable as from the point of view of transplant team a warm ischemia time of even 5 minutes is very crucial for the anatomical and functional performance of these vital organs once they are transplanted. Certainly the extension of the donor pool cannot be considered a valid reason for a wrong decision and so this much time is allowed to elapse before the declaration of death. Another big hurdle regarding such a donation is the ischemic insult suffered by the end organs, the chances of which are quite high as compared to the living or brain dead donors where the perfusion of the organ remains maintained till the organ is retrieved or heart is stopped by the cardioplegic solution. Transplant teams often face this dilemma of subjecting a critically ill recipient to a major surgical procedure with a compromised organ to offer for transplant. Many transplant surgeons are of the opinion that recipients with better hemodynamics should be chosen to yield good results while transplanting organs from the non heart beating donors, but most of the times one is unable to select a recipient due to time constraints. Nonetheless, non heart beating donors are quite useful in increasing the donor pool particularly in countries like Japan where religious and legal restrictions downsize the brain dead donor pool to a large extent.[36] Utilization of this donor pool also excludes the ethical, legal and religious issues associated with brain dead organ donation. Category 1 and 2 of this pool can be utilized for organ donation which can be retrieved late after death such as cornea and kidneys.[37] Some physicians argue regarding retrieval of heart for transplant purpose in case of non-heart beating donors as the dead donor rule clearly states that the person should be declared dead only after irreversible loss of cardiac function. If the heart can still be revived later for transplant it means that the loss of cardiac function was reversible. According to them the only condition where heart transplant can take place in a non-heart beating donor is refusal of resuscitation by the deceased family or deceased himself when alive.[38]

PROCUREMENT OF ORGANS

A successful organ procurement process involves preparation at various levels and a whole team effort is needed to accomplish the task. The first and foremost of these is identifying a potential donor by the ICU or ward personnel. It involves high level of suspicion and action in order to start the ball rolling in advance. Once such a case is identified the organ transplant team is informed so that they can assess the donor for potential problems and contraindications. If such a patient is considered suitable for transplant then a battery of tests are ordered to ascertain the suitability of donation. Any comorbidity which can pose a problem at the time of organ procurement should be taken care of, from this point of time only. Simultaneously a neurologist or neurosurgeon examines the patient for confirmation of brain death. In the absence of neurologist or neurosurgeon a physician or an anesthetist can also do the needful (as per Human Organ Act Amendment, 2009 in India along with three other physicians as described earlier, such practice may vary from country to country) and transplant coordinator should talk to the family to mentally prepare them regarding the poor outcome as well as persuading them for organ donation. The job of transplant coordinator is very crucial as the patient's relatives should not feel offended and simultaneously should be given time to come to terms with the prevailing situation of their loved one. In countries like USA once such a case is identified it is informed to **OPO (organ procurement organization)** which coordinates the process of consent and procurement of organs and tissues as per the federal laws for a given region. All these processes should go hand in hand so that once brain death is confirmed no time is lost for organ retrieval. A team of four doctors is required to declare a person brain dead in Indian scenario, which may take a lot of time and may prolong the decision making time taken by the family.

Once brain death is confirmed the legal formalities has to be taken care of as they might take a long time. This includes taking an informed valid consent from the family. A decision of not donating the organs should not be taken as an offence and their decision should be respected. Sometimes the family might take decision of donation a little late or on repeated persuasion. As most of these cases are trauma victims medicolegal clearance is required from the concerned police station. In such cases all the findings at the time of organ retrieval should be noted and a copy of this record should be sent to the police station where it can be of great help at the time of autopsy.

Preparation of the Donor

Once brain death is confirmed the emphasis of the care shifts from cerebral protection to haemodynamic stability and maintaining adequate organ perfusion. This alteration of care may be considered from the point of suspicion of brain death as the confirmation of brain death and preparation of donor should go hand in hand and no additional time is wasted but the patient care should not be stopped till the time brain death is confirmed. This is important as the condition of the organs may deteriorate with time. The efforts done for the preparation at this stage not only results in better graft outcome initially but also results in prolonged graft survival later. This not only increases the trust of those who are benefited by the process but also reduces the demand for the organs by these patients in future.

General Care

Infection control, maintenance of hemodynamic parameters are the main aims of the nursing care once the patient is diagnosed as brain dead.

Infection Control

All measures are taken to avoid any infection as this is the most important and frequently encountered contraindication for organ donation. There have been instances of transmission of infection from the deceased donor to the recipient via the transplanted organs. Major life threatening infections to the recipients are rare as they usually manifest in the donor itself. Chronic infections like hepatitis B and C may not only effect the recipient (if active viremia is present in the blood of the donor) in the long run but may also have profound effect on the graft outcome of liver transplant recipient even during the period when the disease is still confined to the liver only. The chances of transmission in recipient depend on the stage of hepatitis infection in the donor's body. Once the donor is diagnosed as brain dead on initial examination the number of investigations send include the tests for surface and core antigens as well as the antibody titres. Nonetheless, final decision regarding choosing a donor who is found to be positive is taken considering the chances of mortality of the recipient in near future and after assessing the risk and benefit of transplanting such an organ in this recipient. The organ which is to be transplanted in such cases is important, as liver graft has maximum potential for transmission of such infection as compared to kidney or heart. Long term antiviral therapy should be considered along with the use of immunoglobulin prophylaxis for recipient when the donor is hepatitis B positive but this treatment is of unpredictable value in case of hepatitis C positive donor. It is usually not advisable to transplant a hepatitis C positive liver to a hepatitis C positive recipient as it may lead to faster recurrence of disease in the recipient.[39]

Infection of cytomegalovirus from the donor not only can infect the recipient but may even lead to increased morbidity in the form of decreased graft survival. The presence of this virus may also predispose the donor to other opportunistic infections like fungal infections. The procurement of organs is still not considered a contraindication from such donors despite the above facts because of the high prevalence of this disease in general population. Antiviral therapy in the form of valacyclovir is considered to benefit such patients.[39]

Epstein-Barr Virus positive donors pose more threat to seronegative recipients as compared to seropositive recipients. The risk of developing post transplant lymphoproliferative disease depends on the choice of immunosuppressive agent and the dose given. Antiviral agents like acyclovir and ganciclovir have shown good results for prevention of disease in the seronegative recipients.[39]

Bacterial infections like *Staphylococcus*, *Streptococcus*, *Pseudomonas*, *E coli*, *Klebsiella* and *Enterobacter* can get transmitted from donor to the recipient but are generally not considered a contraindication to transplant, unless leading to frank septicemia, as they can be controlled by prophylactic broad spectrum antibiotics. Chronic bacterial infections like syphilis and tuberculosis also have been reported to get transmitted from donor but are generally not considered a reason for organ rejection. However, multidrug resistant tuberculosis may pose a dilemma for the transplant team.

There are reports of transmission of fungal and parasitic infections from donor but can be taken care of post transplant.[39] The final decision regarding transplantation of infected organs is taken at the time of procurement of organs. Pathological examination in the form of biopsy or microscopic examination from the concerned organ may be taken, if considered necessary and analyzed simultaneously while retrieval process is on.

A broad spectrum antibiotic is generally administered to the donor after confirmation of brain death.

Nursing Care

It includes frequent posture changes for prevention of bed sores, regular dressing changes and skin care. Intravenous and urinary catheters are taken care of and should be changed if required. Regular oropharyngeal and endotracheal suctioning should be done as per the requirement only (in order to prevent any aspiration) as these patients usually do not have excessive secretions and repeated suctioning at regular intervals can increase the chances of infection. A nasogastric tube is placed to decompress the stomach in order to prevent regurgitation and aspiration. Cultures of blood and urine should be sent and appropriate antibiotics are started to prevent any infection as per the ICU protocols or on the basis of culture reports (if available), if they are not started already. A central venous line and arterial line should be placed if not done already as these are not only required in the hemodynamic management of the deceased in the intensive care unit but also during the organ retrieval process in the operation theatre. A swan-ganz catheter might be of great help if hemodynamic instability is present or if lung donation is planned in order to decide regarding the fluid management or the heart is having ejection fraction of less than 45%.[10]

Ventilatory Support

A brain dead person is kept on ventilator till the time organs are removed. Ventilator settings are usually adjusted as per the requirement decided by the transplant team in coordination with the intensivist. The general rule is to avoid hyperventilation and excessive airway pressures. Hyperventilation causes hypocapnia which results in vasoconstriction and consequent reduced blood supply to the organs. High airway pressures lead to decrease in cardiac output and organ perfusion, as well as barotrauma to the lungs. Thus the tidal volumes are usually kept at around 6–8 mL/kg body weight and $FiO_2 \leq 60\%$ but these settings can be changed as per the need. The ventilator strategy is also influenced by the decision regarding the retrieval of lungs for transplant. Lung recruitment maneuvers, bronchial toileting should be used for improving lung transplant outcome.[10] In such cases excessive endotracheal cuff pressures are to be avoided to prevent mucosal injury of trachea as this is the site of tracheal anastomosis in the recipient. Generally a cuff pressure of less than 25 mm of water is recommended. Once cross clamping of the aorta is done endotracheal tube is removed after gentle suction.[5]

Informed Consent

The preparation of the deceased person as well as taking care of legal formalities go on simultaneously in these subjects as the each passing minute results in deterioration of the condition of organs to be procured. Although some research groups argue that an informed consent is not required as the donor is already dead but it is important to inform the relatives in order to make them believe in the organ donation system and to prevent any public outrage as well.[40] The relatives of the deceased should be explained in detail regarding the process of organ retrieval as this is quite a sensitive issue for them especially when they are already facing the trauma of the death of their dear one. They must get answers to all their queries regarding the process, condition of the body after the organ retrieval and the benefits of the procedure if any. The hospital/district authorization committee should be informed and their approval is taken. In medicolegal cases the concerned police station should be informed.

Maintenance of Organ Perfusion

Once a person becomes brain dead the body undergoes into a generalized inflammatory kind of state as this is the start of the body's decaying process. Active measures are required to maintain adequate organ perfusion and oxygenation at this point of time. Hemodynamic parameters are maintained by fluid resuscitation and vasopressor therapy if required. Blood transfusion may be required in order to maintain hemodynamic stability, especially if hemoglobin levels are below 7g/dL. But it should be remembered to obtain blood serology and tissue typing samples before transfusion as it can interfere with these. Vasopressin is usually the drug of choice if diabetes insipidus is present with hemodynamic instability but DDAVP is useful if only maintenance of urine output is required. Many transplant centers prefer to use dopamine as the first line of treatment because of its ability to increase the renal and splanchnic circulation at a dose of 2–5 μg/kg/min. At doses more than 5 μg/kg/min it increases cardiac output without increasing the myocardial oxygen consumption but at doses higher than 10 μg/kg/min it can cause vasoconstriction by α-adrenergic stimulation and that is the reason why higher doses of dopamine are avoided. A combination of dobutamine and epinephrine is added if higher doses of vasopressors are required. Norepinephrine is usually not preferred as the peripheral vasoconstriction may lead to decrease in organ perfusion. However, the final decision regarding vasopressors is usually governed by individual preferences or hospital protocols despite the above mentioned generalizations. No special preferences are present as far as the type of the fluid is concerned. Both crystalloids and colloids have been used in the past for resuscitation but high molecular weight colloids are usually avoided because of their deleterious effect on donor kidneys. Some centers prefer relatively low molecular weight colloids as it facilitates plasma volume expansion and improve micro circulation of organs by mild hemodilution.[5] Low sodium containing crystalloids are generally administered in order to avoid hypernatremia. This is especially true if ADH replacement has been started to take care of diabetes insipidus. Fluid therapy is usually guided by CVP monitoring with the target central venous saturation >70 mm Hg, but pulmonary artery catheterization can be used in hemodynamically unstable patients. The pulmonary artery wedge pressure (PAWP) 6–12 mm Hg and cardiac index of >2.4 l/min/m^2 should be achieved, especially if cardiac procurement is also planned. Hormone therapy should be considered if left ventricular ejection fraction (LVEF) <40% on echocardiography. Some researchers advocate the use of stroke volume variation as a better guide for fluid resuscitation.[41] Judicious use of diuretics may be necessary if oliguria is present. Phenoxybenzamine 100 mg and chlorpromazine 50 mg have been used in the past to improve kidneys' tolerance to warm ischemia. A high dose of intravenous heparin 10,000 mg is given in the operation theater 30 minutes prior to the removal of organs in case of DCD donors to prevent any thromboembolic phenomenon in the concerned organs.

Organ Procurement at Remote Location

Sometimes the organ transplant team receives the call for organ donation from a hospital where transplant surgeries are not being performed. In those circumstances the transplant team may have to travel far distances for collection of organs. A detailed patient history is elicited in order to gather information regarding the condition of the organs to be procured, as well as to ascertain the cause of death which may have a direct effect on the entire transplant process, e.g. malignancy, infection or poisoning. Details regarding the clinical course in the hospital should be elicited and any investigation reports should be collected. The medications received by the patient during the ICU stay may have a direct impact over the outcome of this entire exercise. The present condition of the deceased person is ascertained at this point of time and optimization of the organs is started. Telephonic conversations can help the transplant team before departure and can help in the optimization of organs as well as saving the time of transplant team on arrival. One can go at great length about the optimization of deceased donor but it should be remembered that the clock is ticking continuously.

Anesthetic Management

The anesthesiologist is often faced with multitasking in the operation theater. This fact is especially applicable to organ retrieval from a cadaver. The coordination between various surgical teams revolve around the anesthesiologist and due to small number of deceased organ donation in our country one may come face-to-face with this kind of situation quite unexpectedly. The preparation of the donor starts in the ICU itself which is already described earlier and continues during transport to the operation theater and inside the operation theater.

Transport

The confirmation of the donor's body is a must before shifting to the operation theater as nobody from the transplant team might have seen this person before. A copy of brain death check list, consent and authorization form should be taken along with. If blood or blood products are arranged for intraoperative use checked units and appropriate documents should be sent along the cadaver to the operation theater.

During the transport of the donor there are high chances of hemodynamic deterioration and even collapse. One must prepare for any untoward incidence during this phase. The inotropic infusions are continued along with continuous monitoring of the vital parameters. It is advisable to keep the donor's body warm as far as possible with the help of warm blankets and fluids. Emergency drugs like epinephrine should be kept ready in case cardiac arrest (as it can occur in 10% of all brain dead persons[5]) takes place during the transit even if donor is receiving epinephrine infusion. Barotrauma to the lungs should be avoided if patient is ventilated manually.

In case if cardiac arrest takes place external cardiac massage is initiated and rewarming is stopped immediately as there are high chances that this brain dead donor may get converted to a DCD donor. Cold preservative solution of choice can be infused immediately in order to reduce warm ischemia of the organs. A large bolus dose of heparin is also administered at this time so as to reduce the chances of thrombus formation. Donor is shifted to the operation theater as soon as possible and surgical retrieval of organs is initiated. All this should be done in a manner so that it does not appear offensive to the donor's relatives as most of the times they are accompanying the body during this journey.

Organ Retrieval

Once inside the operation theater CVP and arterial cannulation should be done (if not done previously) preferably on the upper part of the body (internal jugular/subclavian for CVP and radial/ulnar artery for IBP) in order to avoid any false readings due to aortic manipulation and clamping of the major vessels by the surgeon while preparing the abdominal organs for retrieval. The preferred site for arterial cannulation is the left radial artery as it allows access to the brachiocephalic artery which is divided at the time of lung retrieval. Femoral cannulation is usually avoided as ligation of the iliac arteries and/or distal aorta can be performed for perfusion of the liver. Similarly internal jugular cannulation is preferred as the CVP line needs to be withdrawn at the time of superior vena cava ligation and it would be difficult to do so under the drapes if subclavian route is chosen.

The body is positioned supine but the arms can be hyper-extended and taped above the head as no fear of damage to the axillary structures by traction is present. This provides a direct access to the arterial line and also facilitates the surgeons' job in case the donor is obese or too many surgical teams want to share the area simultaneously. Care should be taken at this time to ensure that there is no compression of the brachial artery which may result in false blood pressure readings.

A long or intermediate acting muscle relaxant is usually administered to prevent any spinal reflex movements (Lazarus movements) which can trigger panic among the operating room teams as these may be perceived as a sign of life especially in response to the incision. Vecuronium, or even pancuronium can be used as its use does not result in tachycardia. Neuromuscular blockers are also helpful in providing adequate abdominal relaxation for better surgical exposure of the organs. A large midline incision is given to open the whole abdomen or sometimes both chest and abdomen are opened simultaneously. Such a large incision may result in sudden loss of blood and reflex tachycardia, which should not be taken as a response to incision as this could be spinally mediated in a manner similar to that seen in case of quadriplegic patients.[42] There could be sudden hypotension due to blood loss which should be corrected at the earliest by administration of fluids. Sternotomy may still be required even if heart and lungs are not procured for the exposure of suprahepatic vena cava. Use of inhalational anesthetic agents is controversial but some researchers prefer them to maintain better organ perfusion.[43] The use of inhalational agents also help prevent the catecholamine release in response to spinal reflex stimulation (Fentanyl is unable to prevent it completely).

The gastrointestinal surgery and urology team examines the abdomen for any active infection and malignancy. Liver, pancreas and kidneys are mobilized and portal vein and iliac arteries are cannulated and IVC is clamped when allowed by cardiothoracic team. Biopsies of the internal organs can be taken at this time for assessment. Ascending aorta is generally cannulated by cardiothoracic team for administration of cardioplegic solution after opening the pericardium. An additional bolus of muscle relaxant can be required at this time as diaphragmatic twitching can take place in response to cautery. Bronchoscopy may be performed sometimes at this point of time if lungs are to be procured, which may require the sharing of the same space by Chest physician (Sudden hemodynamic derangement can occur during this period). Placement of an additional cannula is performed in pulmonary artery, if lung procurement is planned. Anesthetist is usually asked to give a large bolus dose of heparin (25,000-30,000 units IV) before aortic cross clamping. Some centers prefer administration of chlorpromazine along with heparin due to its alpha blocking property which increases renal blood flow. However, a prostacyclin infusion suffices its requirement if lung retreival is also planned along with.

Once the aorta is cross clamped CVP/PAP line is gently withdrawn to ligate the superior vena cava and cold cardioplegic solution is run. Cold preservative solution is also run in the portal venous and iliac artery cannula and IVC clamp is opened to flush out the venous blood. The abdominal field is filled with cold ice slush prepared from preservative solution in order to bring the temperature of the organs down. This time marks the onset of circulatory arrest and should be noted for the beginning of cold ischemia time. It should be kept in mind that any delay in lowering of temperature may lead to warm ischemic injury to the organs, so the whole process should take the least amount of time possible. The ventilator and monitors are generally switched off and endotracheal tube is withdrawn after gentle suction. The organs are generally procured in the following manner

Heart → Lungs → Liver → Pancreas → Kidneys → Small Intestine → Blood Vessels→ Corneas

The idea is to keep all the organs viable for transplant and retrieved in accordance to their ability to withstand ischemia. The abdomen is closed in the usual manner and body is send to the mortuary after removal of all lines and cleaning. Hospital records are maintained in a usual manner. The copy of detailed surgical procedure and findings is send along with the organs (fully labelled) if organs are sent to a remote location for transplant. The person carrying the organs should carry all the necessary documents. A copy of intraoperative findings and procedure is also send to concerned police station in medicolegal cases which might be required at the time of autopsy.

The past century has witnessed many technological advances during the later years which enabled the improvement in management and outcomes of these donors. Earlier an ideal donor had to fit into a wide range of criteria, which was very difficult to achieve in any given setting regardless of the efforts made, but slowly more and more such criteria were relaxed due to successful outcomes with the donors who were rendered unfit earlier and also in order to increase the donor pool as the demand for the organs kept growing.

- Age less than 55 years and more than 1 year of age
- No major uncontrolled systemic or organ specific illness
- Absence of major chest wall and abdominal trauma
- Non smoker or smoking < 20 pack years
- No history of addiction
- No active infection or sepsis
- No extracerebral malignancy
- Normal laboratory values.

Procured tissue is processed for storage or may be immediately transplanted. If storage of the tissue or organ is planned then the following steps come into role.

Disinfection

Sometimes the organs and tissues are procured from an unidentified body or the cause of death is not determined before carrying out the transplantation. The fear of deterioration of condition of organs and the resulting haste makes infection control a secondary issue in such cases. It is very important to disinfect the graft before applying it to a suitable recipient. Initial lab results can be falsely negative for any infections and error in lab testing is also a possibility. This is particularly important for viable allografts such as heart valve and vessels, cornea, articular cartilage, skin and stem cells procured from cadavers as these can be disinfected but cannot be completely sterilized as the sterilizing agents can cause damage to these tissues. Various organisms have been found to infect the recipients in the past. This is not only true for major organs but is also true for tissues which may be transplanted late.

Sterilization

This process is mostly applied to nonviable tissue like bones, cartilage, ear ossicles, fascia, tendons.

Sterile Packaging and Storage

An organ or tissue is put in a sterile package or container if the suitable recipient is not available then and there. Sometimes procured tissue or organ has to be transported a long distance away from the site of retrieval. In such cases it is mandatory to keep it sterile during the transport. Temperatures have to be kept low, preferably ice cold in order to decrease the cellular metabolism and prevent further tissue damage. Various preservative solutions are used to store these organs in order to maintain the cellular integrity. Machine perfusion may be employed for better organ preservation.

Organ Preservation

A preservative solution is often used to protect the organs from damage due to ischemia after the cessation of circulation. Most of the preservative solutions which are used commercially have three main ingredients which are colloids, buffers, and antioxidants (Table 4.3). These three components are added to minimize cellular edema, acidosis

Table 4.3: Properties of organ preservation solutions

Components	*Function*	*Commonly used components*
Colloids	Prevents cellular edema	Hydroxyethyl starch (HES), Polyethylene glycol (PEG)
Buffers	Maintains pH	Phosphate, citrate, histidine
Antioxidants	Prevents ROS formation or helps as scavengers	Allopurinol, glutathione, mannitol, tryptophan
Electrolytes	Maintains cellular integrity	Na+, K+, Mg+, Ca++, Cl-
Impermeants	Prevent cellular water intake	Glucose, mannitol, raffinose, lactobionate, sucrose
Membrane stabilizers	Prevent cell membrane damage	Dexamethasone, magnesium sulfate
Additives	Energy substrates	Adenosine, glutamic acid, ketoglutarate

and production of reactive oxygen species respectively. These solutions are very helpful in maintaining the cellular volume and integrity as well as the physiological pH during the long transport timings. Energy providing nutritional substrate is usually added to take care of the energy requirement by providing the necessary ATPs. In addition to these, calcium antagonists, complement regulators and antiplatelet agents have been used in the past. A preservative solution is often administered at very low temperatures so as to reduce the metabolism of the concerned organ and prevention of subsequent cellular damage. However, some recent studies have demonstrated the deleterious effect of this hypothermia by inhibition of ATPase leading to subsequent cellular edema, especially during prolonged periods of ischemia.[44]

University of Wisconsin (UW) Solution

This solution was developed at the University of Wisconsin by Belzer et al in 1986 and is named so. The solution is highly viscous due to addition of 5% hydroxyethyl starch and has to be injected with pressure in order to achieve adequate organ perfusion. The viscosity of solution increases with the drop in temperature and increases to three times that of water at 4°C. The solution has high potassium and low sodium content which mimics intracellular environment. Allopurinol and glutathione act as free radical scavengers while KH_2PO_4 acts as a buffer. Raffinose and lactobionate are osmotically active ingredients which help in preventing cellular edema. Adenosine is present as a precursor of ATP. The solution has high cost as compared to other solutions but is still considered to be gold standard amongst various preservative solutions available.

Histidine Tryptophan Ketoglutarate (HTK) Solution

The HTK solution was introduced as a cardioplegic solution in open heart surgery but was used for organ preservation later as it was found to be useful during transplantation. The solution contains histidine as buffer which prevents the pH drop during subsequent cold ischemia. It contains tryptophan and ketogluterate which are amino acids, acts as free radical scavenger and as a substrate for anaerobic metabolism during preservation respectively. It is an extracellular preservation solution with high sodium and low potassium content. The electrolyte composition helps in organ recovery by facilitating the removal of blood faster as compared to UW solution.

The main advantage of using this solution as compared to UW solution is its low viscosity which results in faster and better organ perfusion, although large volume of the solution is usually required to achieve this task. However, recent studies have shown that even smaller volumes can be as effective as large volumes. Most of the single center studies have not found any significant difference between HTK and UW solutions as far as deceased donor transplant is concerned but recent multicenter long-term UNOS data has shown that use of HTK may result in increased delayed graft function and poor graft survival.[45-47]

Euro-collins

This solution was prepared after modifications from the original collins solution. It has high concentration of potassium. Glucose is replaced by mannitol in order to decrease viscosity and improve osmotic properties. This solution was found to be associated with delayed graft function in kidney transplant cases when compared to UW and HTK solutions in multicenter trials.[48]

Celsior Solution

This solution acts as a cardioplegic solution and often used for preservation of organs, particularly heart. It has high sodium and low potassium content similar to extracellular fluid environment. Mannitol and lactobionate provide osmotic properties to the solution while histidine and reduced glutathione act as ROS. Glutamate present in the solution work as energy substrate.[49]

The advances taken place in the present era has not only resulted in better survival of the procured organs due to better donor management but also due to refinements taking place in the preservation of these organs till the time they are transplanted in recipients. The worldwide practice of the use of static cold preservation is slowly giving way to better machine perfusion techniques. Machine perfusion not only reduces the risk of delayed graft function but is also associated with better long-term graft outcome.[50,51] Freezed preservative solutions have dominated the scene worldwide till date but recently introduction of glycoproteins with antifreezing properties is presumed to change the scenario worldwide. These glycoproteins are derived from organisms found in natural environments having subzero temperatures and help them survive by preventing ice formation in vivo. It has been found that the ice crystals present in the preservative solutions cause cell damage and makes the organs unsuitable for transplantation. These glycoproteins prevent ice formation and simultaneously allow the solutions to be cooled at subzero temperatures.[52]

INDIVIDUAL ORGAN DONATION

Corneal Transplantation

Corneal transplant is probably the first successful transplant in the history of mankind. But the long-term survival of corneal transplant remains low despite the fact that first successful full thickness corneal allograft was performed by Dr E Zirm as early as 1905.[53] A good 1 year survival (90%) of this treatment modality is attributed mainly to the fact that the cornea is a relatively avascular tissue. But the 5 year and 10 year survival (75% and 64% repectively) remains low and even comparable to other organs like heart, liver and kidneys even in the developed nations. Corneal transplant is the most common form of transplant done in India. It is probably by far the most publicised form of transplantation in this country. The contributing factors may be the low cost of the procedure, ease of corneal tissue storage, increased public awareness and access of services to a common man. Lately scleral graft and ocular stem cells have also been used with variable success.

The process of corneal transplant starts from a successful retrieval of cornea. The eye banks throughout the world are engaged in procurement, storage and distribution of suitable corneas for transplantation. Simultaneously these eye banks are also engaged in screening of potential donors, establishing the suitability of procured corneas by performing laboratory tests, meticulous record keeping and fair and equal distribution of these corneas amongst the patients belonging to various socioeconomic and cultural backgrounds.[54]

Donor Selection

The donor selection is an integral part of an eye bank and is influenced by a number of factors.

Age

Although age of the donor does not constitute a strict criteria for contraindication but young donor's corneas are generally considered healthy as compared to the older donors. The reason for this is the higher endothelial cell count in the younger age group which is responsible for maintaining the corneal epithelium generation and transparency of the cornea. Corneal endothelial cell count is around 5000 to 6000/cu mm at birth.[55] It gets reduced to about 2700/cu mm at 10 years of age and keep on decreasing every year by about 0.22% to 0.6% throughout the adult life.[56] The regenerative capacity of this endothelial cell layer in vivo is very limited even in the donor himself, thus having very small chances of recovery in the recipient eye.

This decrease in endothelial cell count is further affected by trauma, refractive and intraocular eye surgeries and some genetic defects. This leads to inability of these cells to effectively pump out fluid from the stroma which further results in stromal edema, corneal clouding and opacification. Many donor corneas are rejected worldwide due to decreased endothelial cell count. Generally there is no age limit bar for corneal donation but infantile corneas are rejected due to their small size and corneas from donor age more than eighty years due to reduced endothelial cell count.[57] Although most of the researchers advocate for younger corneas (excluding infantile corneas) due to good endothelial cell count,[58] but a few differ and find that corneal grafts from donors more than 80 years of age to be having better graft survival if the endothelial cell counts of these corneas are adequate in number.[59]

Infections and Malignancy

Transmission of various infectious diseases namely bacterial, viral and fungal, as well as malignancies which can be transmitted from donor cornea to the recipient are of paramount importance despite the cornea being a tissue with relatively less vascularization. There have been numerous reports of transmission of various infections (Hepatitis B,[60] Rabies,[61] Creuzfeldt Jakob disease[62]) in the past which prompted the eye banks to obtain the patient's history in detail. But even after taking all due precautions some infections may go undetected. This is particularly important in country like India where regular health checkups are not carried out on all the suitable donors or the cornea is obtained from an unidentified body. These details are usually available if multi organ donation is planned in a brain dead person but usually not available if death takes place at home or in a hospital ward where patient is shifted just prior to death. Nevertheless, all due precautions are taken to prevent the spread of infection through the donor cornea. There are reports of nontransmission of HIV from an infected donor cornea to a recipient but it is advisable not to transplant a HIV infected cornea to a recipient who is not HIV positive previously.[63] There had been reports of transmission of retinoblastoma and adenocarcinoma[64] through the corneal transplant but other malignancies like leukemia and lymphoproliferative disorders[65] are also considered absolute contraindications.

Intrinsic Eye Disease and Surgeries

Disorders of cornea which may affect the outcome of keratoplasty such as large pterygium or keratoconus are generally considered contraindication for the procurement of donor cornea. A previous anterior segment surgery such as cataract surgery is no longer considered a contraindication to eye donation if the endothelial cell count and morphology are found appropriate on specular examination. Refractive surgeries like LASIK renders most of the corneas unsuitable for transplant purpose due to reduced thickness of the cornea, but final decision for transplanting such corneas depend on slit lamp microscopy and specular examination findings.

Preparation

In case if willingness to donation is informed in advance an ophthalmologist usually examines the patient to obtain the history of any previous surgery, eye trauma in the past or any medical disease that may affect the outcome. The condition of cornea is especially noted for any scars, pterygium, and presence of folds or foreign body that might hinder the view of the recipient. A suitable antibiotic eye drop may be advised despite the fact that the patient may be on systemic antibiotics as the chances of systemic antibiotic reaching the relatively avascular corneal tissue are quite minimal, especially if the time constraint is also there. In addition to antibiotic cover eye drops to keep the corneal surface moist are also added to the treatment. Exposure of corneal surface by inadvertent eye opening is to be avoided.

Once the donation of cornea is confirmed after brain death or cardiocirculatory arrest instructions are given to avoid any trauma, exposure, bacterial infection and maintenance of low eye temperature is started. Instillation of lubricant and antibiotic drop is followed by taping of eyes to prevent exposure keratopathy. Head is elevated to prevent any dependent edema by placing a pillow or elevating the head of the bed. Excessive flexion of the head should be avoided in order to maintain the venous drainage from the head in a brain dead subject. Ice packs are placed over the eyes in order to cool the temperature to 0°C approximately but not lower than this. Direct cooling by ice should not be done as it can cause trauma to the lid and underlying structures and also if the eyelid opens up below the melting ice as it can wet the tapes applied to keep the lids closed. The other reason for not keeping the ice directly over the eyes is to prevent the temperature of eyes falling below 0°C which can freeze the fluids inside the eyeball and will cause irreversible damage to the cornea. Surgical gloves can be filled with ice and kept over the lids for the same purpose. It should be ensured that ice packs put a very light pressure over the eyes as heavy pressure can damage the corneal tissue. The tapes should be checked intermittently for opening of eyelids as moisture may accumulate as a result of condensation of water present in the surrounding air. Ice prepared from other sources like dry ice (made from carbon dioxide) should not be used for cooling as their temperature is quite low to 0°C. All these measures are taken to retard the effect of metabolic byproducts released after brain death or circulatory arrest.

Retrieval Process

Russian ophthalmologist Vladimir Filatov used the cornea obtained from a deceased donor for the first time in 1937. In the past retrieval of cornea was considered to be done by a trained and qualified surgeon but now cornea can be retrieved by a trained technician alone (as per the Human Organ Transplant Act, Amendment 2009), in India as compared to other organs which can only be retrieved by the surgeons. One of the most important consideration at the time of corneal retrieval is the consent from the family members. The consent papers should be thoroughly checked in order to ascertain how much tissue can be removed from the eye (whether it is whole of the eyeball or only the corneal button). The person who is retrieving the cornea should ensure that the appearance of the eyes after the retrieval process should not be appalling to the relatives of the deceased. The removal of the tissue should be done with strict aseptic precautions as the body's immune system is no longer going to help in the prevention of infection. It is important to remember while decontaminating the eye that the disinfectant should not affect the graft viability adversely and simultaneously minimizes the possibility of any infection as the eyes can get infected or contaminated by the bacteria present in the vicinity like eyelids soon after death. These are generally gram positive cocci, but sometimes gram negative bacteria from the gut are also found from the cultures. Some ophthalmologists prefer to use decontaminating agents which are less toxic to the corneal graft and reserve strong

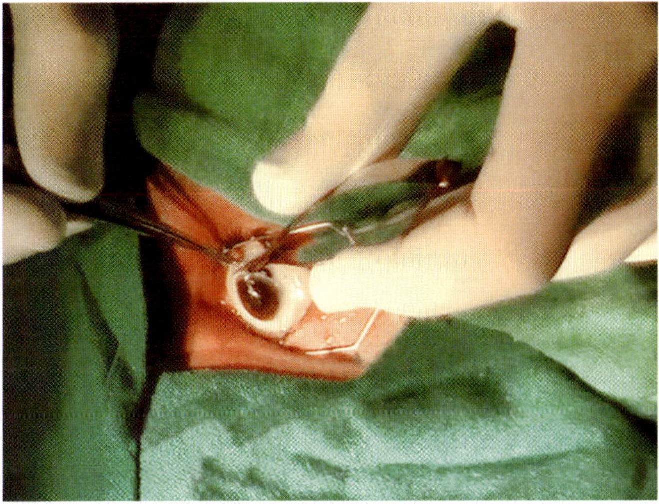

Fig. 4.1: Extraction of corneal button from a brain dead person

antibiotics for the recipient (in case endophthalmitis develops after the keratoplasty). The standard approach is to irrigate the cornea with 1% povidine-iodine solution for less than 2 minutes. Concentrated solutions of povidine-iodine solution for prolonged period can adversely affect graft viability by dehydrating the graft.[66] This is followed by rinsing the whole area by normal saline solution.[67] The blood samples of the deceased should be collected simultaneously for cultures and lab investigations.

The procurement of cornea can be done by two methods which are described in the following text. Authorities around the globe have different reasons to prefer either of the method but none of them is considered to be superior than the other universally. Most of the times the method chosen is influenced by the consent, the place of retrieval, the experience of the person who is procuring the cornea and the practice guidelines of the concerned eye bank.

Corneal Button

Along with the surrounding conjunctiva is retrieved in most of the cases especially when the process is carried out in a hospital setup or at a place from where the procured tissue can be transported to the eye bank in a very short period of time. This method also maintains the cosmetic appearance of the eye better than the complete removal of the eyeball (as a prosthesis is put to simulate the donor cornea after the retrieval).

Enucleation Process

Complete eyeball is sometimes removed especially when the procurement is done at an area remote from the eye bank or when the condition of eyeball structures is suspected to put the transplant process in jeopardy such as having endophthalmitis. Complete enucleation of the eyeball is usually discouraged nowadays as this results in a bad cosmetic appearance of the deceased donor. Eye banks usually advocate the proper closure of the eyelids after placing a cotton ball in the eye socket after the enucleation process is complete.

Storage and Transportation

The cornea or the eyeball should be stored aseptically at appropriate temperature in a suitable organ preservative medium. The person carrying such material should be in possession of all the relevant documents to prove his/her identity and association with the particular eye bank so as to avoid any legal hassles during the transportation process. Corneal tissue should be accompanied by a sample of blood of the deceased in order to carry out a battery of tests mentioned earlier (Table 4.4). The preserved tissue should be properly labelled with all the relevant details whenever transportation of it is done, whether after the procurement or from the eye bank to the place of transplantation (Table 4.5).

Table 4.4: Investigations required with corneal graft

Tests	*Requirement*
Microbiological culture	Mandatory
HIV screening	Mandatory
Hepatitis B screening	Mandatory
Hepatitis C screening	Mandatory
Syphilis screening	Not Mandatory
HLA testing	Not Mandatory
Slit lamp report	Mandatory
Specular microscopy	Mandatory

If whole eyeball is enucleated earlier, it is examined carefully under the microscope and any significant findings are noted once it reaches the eye bank. Later the corneal button is removed aseptically if the cornea is found suitable for transplant and preserved appropriately.

The quality of the cornea obtained is ascertained by various laboratory investigations. Apart from investigations for infections[67] like HIV, HBsAg, HCV and VDRL which are done for any other organ transplant the corneal tissue is also examined for any structural abnormalities by slit lamp and specular examination.[68] Cultures of the procured cornea are done to rule out any infection that might be hazardous for the recipient. It should be kept in mind that any transfusion of blood or blood products to the donor in the recent past may

Table 4.5: Label accompanying corneal graft

<table>
<tr><td>1. Name and age of donor</td><td rowspan="9">Name of the Eye Bank with Address and Phone number</td></tr>
<tr><td>2. Identification number</td></tr>
<tr><td>3. Type of specimen</td></tr>
<tr><td>4. Date and time of donor death (cause of death)</td></tr>
<tr><td>5. Date and time of the specimen procured</td></tr>
<tr><td>6. Time of start of cooling</td></tr>
<tr><td>7. Expiry date</td></tr>
<tr><td>8. Tested for
HIV
HBsAg
HCV
VDRL</td></tr>
<tr><td>9. Type of preservation medium and antibiotics</td></tr>
</table>

affect the serological findings of the tests mentioned above thus a history of any such event should be reported to the eye bank along with the procured cornea.

Slit lamp microscopy and specular examination should be performed only after the specimen is allowed to reach room temperature as this not only prevents the condensation of the droplets over the media vial but also gives a good view of the cell morphology, which may be misleading if examined at subnormal temperatures.

Corneas are usually stored in hypothermic environment at 4–6°C using a suitable storage media like M-K media[69] or Optisol solution.[70] This provides a storage time of about 4–10 days without a significant endothelial cell loss. Various other storage media are also available which are advantageous in different conditions but at our centre we are using M-K media as it provides sufficient time for the corneal examination and transplantation process. A suitable antibiotic combination is also added to the storage medium to prevent the graft infection.

Record Keeping

The eye bank should not only keep the records of the donor but also of the recipient in order to contact them in case of any new information related to the donor graft is obtained. This is also essential in view of any legal suites later on. Slit lamp microscopy and specular examination is performed at the eye bank and findings are clearly noted especially for endothelial cell count, cell morphology[46] and any significant structural defects. A minimal endothelial cell count of about 2,000 to 2,500/cu mm is generally considered necessary for successful keratoplasty.[71] Endothelial counts below this number is usually seen in corneas from donors older than 80 years of age or those who have undergone any refractive eye surgery in the past or have used contact lenses for a prolonged period of time and is one of the most common reason for discarding a cornea even if it fulfils all other mandatory criteria,[72] as a repeat keratoplasty has a worse prognosis than a primary procedure. Some eye banks recommend a second examination before the corneal transplant,[55] but most of them leave it to the discretion of ophthalmologist who is going to carry out the transplant, as the standard examination methods employed by the eye banks have their own limitations and can overestimate the number of endothelial cells[71] as these methods cannot predict precisely how many of these cells are viable at the time of transplant[73] and how many of these will remain viable after the transplant due to various recipient related factors.[74]

Corneal transplant is a useful modality for those who suffer from blindness due to corneal structure abnormality but it has to go a long way to achieve the goals for which it has evolved.

Deceased Kidney Transplant

First kidney transplant from a brain dead donor was performed in 1963 by a Belgian surgeon named Alexandre.[4] This was the time when the concept of brain death was not universally accepted, so it led to a lot of criticism worldwide. Slowly brain death became an established fact all over the world and became one of the most popular methods of organ donation. One of the main reasons for the progress of deceased donor kidney transplant program is that a deceased donor is usually able to benefit two recipients as compared to one in case of living donor. In the recent past the encouraging results from DCD donors have also contributed significantly to the increase of donor pool.

The last century witnessed a gradual progress in the deceased transplant outcomes by better donor preparation and the discovery of powerful immunosuppressants. But most of these donations were restricted to a group now known as standard criteria donors (SCD). These donors were otherwise healthy persons having no systemic illness and were generally young trauma victims who became brain dead due to road traffic accidents. The only disadvantage with the organs recovered from these patients was the deleterious effect of brain death resulting in poorer graft outcomes despite a better HLA matching as compared to live donors, and kidney was no exception to it.[13] Even with the donors belonging to same age group the live donors scored better in terms of graft survival in the long run.[13] The transplant centers all over the world faced the shortage of transplant organs despite making all the possible efforts for organ retrieval from the deceased donors. The transplant surgeons were thus forced to compromise on the quality of organs available and other alternatives such as live donors or transplantation of two suboptimal kidneys in one recipient were explored.

A complete change of scenario took place over the last two decades as far as deceased donors are concerned. There had been an increase in the use of expanded criteria donors (ECD) to provide organs to the growing population of people who require transplant. The term ECD was first used by Kaufman in 1997 for those donors who were utilized for organ donation despite failing the criteria of a standard donor. The young trauma victims which used to form the large proportion of brain dead donor pool got reduced to almost half by the addition of older donors having cerebrovascular accidents. Transplantation of two suboptimal kidneys in one recipient was also tried to increase the functioning nephron mass with variable success.[75] This approach is especially helpful in cases where donors are more than 60 years or less than 5 years of age or the nephron mass is reduced due to diseases such as diabetes, hypertension.[76] This group of suboptimal donors posed an increased risk to the recipient in the form of higher chances of primary non function or delayed function of the graft and lower graft survival in the long run. Kidney grafts obtained through ECD usually have a 10–15% lesser graft survival as compared to the standard criteria donor at 5 year interval after the transplant.[77] Although this phenomenon has led to increase in the recovery of large number of organs but the quality of organs has gone down despite the advancement in technology of organ preservation, reduction of cold ischemia time and improved organ allocation system.[4] The compromise is resulting in the decrease of overall graft function and subsequently lead to the rise in the number of patients in need of a kidney again. However, at present these expanded criteria donors are contributing successfully to make those patients survive who are on the transplant waiting list for long and undergoing dialysis. It has been observed at present that these suboptimal organs reduce the cost of living in these recipients. It remains to be seen in the future whether the use of expanded criteria donors get merged with the standard criteria donors due to technological advancements or they remain as a second choice for the transplant for ever. At present a deceased donor graft which offers 70% chances of graft survival outcome as compared to a standard criteria donor is accepted as ECD. The change in the present organ allocation policies may also result in diminishing the divide between these two groups.[78]

Lately it has been proposed to replace the existing definitions of "standard criteria" and "expanded criteria" donors with the Kidney Donor Profile Index (KDPI). KDPI is a clinical assessment of the given kidney offered to a recipient which gives an idea that for how much time the graft is likely to continue its function once transplanted. This index rates the graft as per the different risk factors associated with it, rather than considering individual donor risk factors separately. Estimated Post-transplant Survival (EPTS) is an estimate that how much a recipient would benefit from a kidney transplant in terms of number of years by a given donor.[79]

Another important change that became evident during the past decade was the decreasing significance of immunologic factors that affect the long-term graft outcome as compared to non immunologic methods such as the effect of brain death. This may be attributed to improvements in the immunosuppressive therapy. Su et al analyzed the data of 33,443 renal transplant recipients from deceased donors and found 78.6% graft survival in non HLA matched donors at 3 year post transplant as compared to 80.7% from HLA matched transplants for the same duration. Many donor factors have been attributed to influence the final transplant outcome, a few of them are discussed below.[80]

Age

Donor age is an independent factor influencing renal graft function. Renal grafts from donors more than 50 years of age show a survival rate of about 50% as compared to 70% from those of age 19 to 45 years. The kidneys from donors younger than 19 years and more than 50 years are more vulnerable at the time of procurement, during preservation and at the time of immunosuppressive therapy later after the transplant as they have poor functional reserves.[81] A kidney obtained from a dead donor whose age is less than 10 years has poor chances of survival as a rejection episode is not tolerated by this kidney in comparison to an adult kidney.[82] It is advisable to transplant such kidneys en block, i.e. both the kidneys are transplanted in a single recipient. The actual long-term renal graft survival is also decreased from the kidneys procured from old donors and transplanted in younger recipients.[83] The young donors (along with female gender and black race) are shown to have smaller glomerular size which gradually increases as the age advances.[84] Larger glomerular size of the donor kidney allograft leads to chronic allograft dysfunction. Some of the transplant centers recommend a biopsy from a renal donor graft from an old donor in order to ascertain the glomerular size before transplantation. This is the reason why it is recommended that the transplantation of kidneys from elderly donors should be done to elderly recipients. The older recipients require lesser amount of immunosuppressants in comparison to younger ones which is helpful in improving long-term outcome of these grafts and more kidneys from the expanded donor pool can be utilized in this manner.

Ramos et al recommends that creatinine clearance should be more than 60cc/min if the kidney donor belongs to elderly age group and a wedge biopsy should be performed on the graft (a minimum of 70 glomeruli should be inspected).[81] If the degree of glomerular sclerosis is found to be more than 15%, it should not be transplanted as a single kidney and should be totally discarded if moderate interstitial fibrosis and arteriolar hyalinosis are present additionally. But Perico et al differ and recommend a suitable donor age up to 65 years of age with a creatinine clearance of up to 90cc/min and donor serum creatinine levels as high as 3.0 mg/dL.[76] In their view a glomerular sclerosis of up to 20% is acceptable.[85] United States Renal Data System from 1988 to 1998 shows that the graft survival is affected by both donor and recipient age but more from the donor age as compared to the recipient.[76] Although age is one of the most important factors but other donor and recipient specific variables also affect the graft outcome in an individual case. In nutshell only donor age cannot be regarded as a definite predictor of graft outcome, although old donors may adversely affect prolonged graft survival.

Diabetes

Abouna et al published a case of successful kidney transplant from an insulin dependent diabetic donor. Both the recipients were non diabetic and regained a good renal function. Renal biopsy specimens taken 7 months after the transplant demonstrated complete resolution of diabetic nephropathy from these allografts.[76] Similar findings were demonstrated by Orlowski et al later.[81] There are reports available in literature about good outcome of a renal transplant from a diabetic donor to a diabetic recipient as well, provided the recipient had a good diabetic control after the transplant.[86] The UNOS data is also suggestive of the fact that diabetes mellitus in a donor is no longer a risk factor even if the duration is more than 10 years, but the severity of the disease along with biopsy findings should be taken into consideration before using this graft for transplant. Pretransplant renal function gives a fair idea about the status of the graft but the choice of a suitable recipient should be made and ischemia times should be kept to a minimum as far as possible.

Hypertension

Unlike diabetes, hypertensive deceased donors are still considered a significant risk factor for the renal allograft outcome.[82] Various studies have demonstrated the lower survival of the transplanted renal graft taken from hypertensive donors who had a history of hypertension for more than 10 years after the onset of disease. In a study by Madden et al they demonstrated that posttransplant 5 year survival was less in recipients who received kidney from hypertensive donors but the difference was not statistically significant, although the difference was significant if the hypertensive donor's age was more than 50 years. In another study the incidence of acute tubular necrosis was found to be comparable between the hypertensive and normotensive deceased donor groups but the incidence of rejection was found to be more in the hypertensive donor group 1 year after the transplant. Most of these earlier studies had their limitations because of small number of hypertensive in comparison to large number of normotensive donors. Carter et al and Ojo et al in two different retrospective studies analyzed multicenter data from UNOS which included about 33595 and 25039 deceased renal transplant recipients respectively and demonstrated similar findings. Older donors with a history of hypertension more than 10 years led to worst transplant outcomes if the creatnine clearance was <80 mL/min.[87, 88]

Cause of Donor Death

The kidney graft procured from a trauma victim generally has a better initial outcome as compared to those taken from patients having CVA.[82] This difference is not only restricted to brain dead donors but is also evident in case of DCD renal grafts.[37] Brain death related immune response as well as hemodynamic variations also affect the graft outcome. If the graft is obtained from a donor after cardiocirculatory death the increased warm ischemia time also affects the graft adversely. In case of DCD grafts initial poor performance of the grafts are usually seen when compared to brain dead donors but long-term outcome is usually comparable. Renal grafts have been transplanted successfully from patients died due to DIC (disseminated intravascular coagulopathy) and poisoning, provided the poison has been removed from the body or is considered to be in amount which cannot harm the recipient.[89, 90]

Poor Renal Function and Surgical Anomalies

A small number of donor kidneys which have a poor function during the lifetime of a donor may pose problems for the transplant team once they are grafted in the recipient. A preharvesting serum creatinine of more than 1.7 mg/dL or a creatinine clearance of <80 mL/min is considered as a significant predictor of poor outcome.[76, 87] However, such kidneys are not an absolute contraindication for transplant as these kidneys may undergo changes which result in improved function postoperatively. Kidneys with surgical anomalies like multiple arteries or partial ureteropelvic junction obstructions may pose problems to the surgery team but have been used successfully in the past. Polycystic kidneys, although debatable have been grafted in the past and worked well for years. Disappearence of renal cysts have also been reported in some cases.[91] Kidneys having a creatinine clearance of <80 mL/min or kidneys received from donors less than 5 years of age are transplanted en-bloc. Microscopic hematuria and proteinuria in donor also results in worse graft outcomes. Presence of renal arteriosclerosis also results in unfavorable graft outcome.[92]

Ischemia Time and Organ Preservation

Kidneys are better tolerant organ of the ischemic process as compared to the organs like heart and liver. Many studies have shown that a cold ischemia time of less than 24 hours results in reduced incidence of delayed graft function after the transplant and improved post-transplant long-term outcome as compared to those having cold ischemia times longer than this.[95] The long-term graft survival can be improved if pulsatile machine perfusion is used rather than static cold preservation[96] but even then a cold ischemia time of more than 36 hours results in a worse outcome.[85] The prognosis gets worse when prolonged ischemia times are accompanied with marginal donors.[76, 97] In case of DCD donors a warm ischemia time of more than 45 minutes is generally considered a bad predictor for renal transplant.

Various preservative solutions have been used for preservation of deceased renal graft, e.g. Celsior solution, University of Wisconsin solution, HTK solution. None of these solutions is considered superior to other and they are mostly used as per institutional guidelines and availability. However, most of the researchers prefer to use HTK solution for deceased donor organ protection due to its low potassium content but recent multicenter analysis of UNOS data suggest that use of University of Wisconsin solution results in more favorable outcomes as compared to HTK solution.[45] Machine perfusion is usually preferred as compared to static cold perfusion in case of brain dead donors due to decreased chances of delayed or non-function of the graft. It also results in improved graft survival duration.[50] Similar findings are also reported from DCD donors.[96]

Intraoperative Considerations

Apart from preoperative considerations mentioned above intraoperative deceased donor management has got great impact on the renal graft outcome. Intraoperative fluid therapy is probably the most important factor apart from maintainence of renal perfusion by taking care of patient's hemodynamics as far as kidney transplant is concerned. There is no universal opinion regarding the choice of fluid, but crystalloids are usually preferred. Cittanova et al reported the adverse transplant outcome after renal graft when hydroxyethyl starch was used in brain dead donors prior to the procurement of kidneys. They reported impairment of immediate graft function after the use of hydroxyethyl starch for volume expansion when compared to the use of gelatin.[93] Another important aspect is the maintanance of electrolyte imbalance in these donors. Kazemeyni et al reported a poor renal allograft outcome from deceased donors who had hypernatremia and polyuria after brain death.[94] It is a usual practice to maintain a urine output of around 100 mL/hr and serum sodium levels below 155 mmol/liter. A CVP of more than 8 cm of water is preferred but such an arrangement may not be appreciated by the lung transplant team who prefer to have a lower CVP. Continuation of low dose dopamine infusion is considered beneficial in the intraoperative period but the use of vasopressin or norepinephrine is controversial as they may adversely affect the graft outcome. However, it is very difficult to avoid their use most of the times in order to maintain adequate perfusion pressures. It should be remembered that the intraoperative use of any catecholamine may adversely affect the heart if cardiac transplant is to be carried out simultaneously.

Anticoagulation

Development of microthrombi at the time of procurement and transplant has remained a problem for long and is associated with delayed graft function as well as rejection. Apart from high doses of heparin anticoagulation with various agents have been tried in the past with variable results. Most of the studies done so far have been performed on laboratory animals and their use in human beings is still questionable. Melagatran is one such anticoagulant which inhibits fibrin deposition and has shown good results in pigs for prevention of microthrombi formation. In a pig model it has been shown that donors treated with Melagatran prior to the infusion of University of Wisconsin solution results in improved graft function and survival but human trials are still awaited.[85]

Renal Changes After Brain Death

The brain death induced catecholamine rise may result in decreased renal blood flow to as much as 2.4 times the normal. This leads to decreased renal perfusion and subsequent ischemic damage. Once the tonsillar herniation takes place the resulting hypotension adds to this injury by reducing the renal blood flow further. The more this phase is prolonged the more is the damage. Higher rates of tubular necrosis are seen in cases of prolonged brain death.[4] The decreased levels of anti-diuretic hormones due to posterior pituitary dysfunction results in cerebral injury related diabetes insipidus. The massive fluid loss and resultant electrolyte imbalance has a detrimental effect on renal allograft outcome. Stress induced hyperglycemia adds to the renal injury in a manner similar to that seen in diabetes mellitus in live subjects and many ICUs prefer to treat it in a similar manner as done in live patients. A tight glycemic control is thus advisable in brain dead donors, for a better transplant outcome.[4] Nagareda et al studied the histological changes in the kidneys of brain dead subjects and found vacuolar degeneration along with atrophy and necrosis of both the proximal as well as distal convoluted tubules, but these changes were more extensive in the latter. The arterial intimal proliferation also increased gradually after brain death from 7% to 42–85% in these subjects during a period of 15 days. Glomerular hyperemia also started decreasing gradually after 3 days of brain death and remained almost up to 10% in 7 to 14 days post brain death as compared to 92% initially at day 0. Fibrosis and inflammation around the glomeruli showed an increase from 16% to 92% and from 4% to 65% respectively from brain death to 15–48 days post brain death. Urinary sodium output gradually increased in these subjects while the serum levels of sodium gradually declined with time. This is probably seen due to sympathetic denervation of the kidneys and partly because the subjects were given continuous infusions of vasopressin during this study.[98] Similarly potassium output was also increased after brain death probably due to depletion of ATP which results in opening of potassium channels in these kidneys.[4] Brush border enzymes like alkaline phosphatase and lysosomal enzymes like N-acetyl-b-D-glucosaminidase are also found in the urine of brain dead patients in very high concentrations signifying the injury to the tubular epithelium. The concentration of Kidney Injury Molecule -1 is also increased in urine which can be used for predicting the viability of kidney after the transplant.[99]

Increased concentrations of cytokines, chemokines, and adhesion molecules as a result of brain death induced immune response results in a chemotactic gradient that promotes the influx of leucocytes to the kidney. Koo et al demonstrated that after the reperfusion, neutrophilic infiltration is seen in almost half of the brain dead donor kidneys in comparison to none of the living donor kidneys.[100] This neutrophylic infiltration can be directly correlated with long cold ischemia time and delayed graft function as well as high creatinine levels after the transplant.[101] Increased levels of cytokines like TNF-α and IL-6 are seen to be present in huge quantities in brain dead donor renal grafts. The renal dendritic cells have been demonstrated to release large quantity of TNF-α in response to renal reperfusion injury.[102] Proximal tubular increases of intercellular adhesion molecule-1, vascular cell adhesion molecule-1 and human leucocyte antigen-DR are also very much evident in case of deceased donors, but this difference became very minimal when biopsies were analyzed after the cold storage. Among the deceased donors, expression of these molecules was seen more in case of brain death due to trauma as compared to other causes, as well as those who were on ventilator support for more than 3 days or had infection during the ICU stay. E-selectin expression was also high in the intertubular capillaries of the deceased donor kidneys, whereas P-selectin expression was comparable in both deceased as well as living donors. The peak expression of E-selectin is seen around 6 hours following cytokine stimulation of endothelial cells whereas ICAM-1 and VCAM-1 levels peak after 24 hours. This is the reason why leucocytic infiltration peaks 24 hours after the transplantation and may affect the graft adversely in the form of acute rejection or chronic graft dysfunction. The events occurring at reperfusion contribute further to the ischemic injury and results in gradual adherence of leukocytes to the vascular endothelium and subsequent graft infiltration.[103] Thus it is advisable to counteract the immune reaction induced by the brain death. Two different methods are available to antagonize the effects of this immune response. Some researchers prefer the hemodynamic stabilization more,[104] while others recommend the use of glucocorticoids or the induction of protective proteins (e.g. hemoxygenase-1) instead of this.[105] The simultaneous application of both these methods is slowly emerging concept. Apart from the brain death induced immune mediated inflammatory changes these grafts are also affected by antibody presensitization of the recipient which may influence the outcome in the absence of significant preoperative screening due to lack of time and available technology.[106] Kunzendorf et al demonstrated that more the duration after brain death, better is the long-term graft survival, probably due to induction of these protective proteins.[107] Other modalities like pretreatment of brain dead donors with dopamine or norepinephrine have also shown encouraging results as per the analysis of eurotransplant database.[105] Dopamine treatment causes HO-1 induction and also inhibits the P-selectin expression. This results in rapid fall of creatinine levels and also improves the long-term renal graft survival.[108] Low-dose dopamine treatment is shown to decrease the production of various other inflammatory mediators and improve renal transplantation outcome of the brain dead donor,[105] but it can have adverse effects on the donor heart if cardiac transplant is also planned along with as it can precipitate tachyarrythmias and chances of myocardial ischemia are high.[4,109] It is also believed to induce ischemic injury to the intestines.[109] Norepinephrine is quite useful in donors having septic shock as it optimizes renal blood flow and renal vascular resistance effectively but the peripheral vasoconstrictive effects of this drug make it controversial as far as other organs are concerned, although it is still used worldwide. Other substances like carbamylated erythropoietin and carbon monoxide inhalation has shown benefits during initial studies but long-term results are yet to be ascertained as no human studies are there to support this evidence.[105] There has been previous reports of successful kidney transplantation from the person dying due to carbon monoxide poisoning.[90]

Renal Transplant from DCD Grafts

For the last two decades DCD donors are used successfully in many parts of the world as a means of renal transplant. This mode of renal transplant is still not used in India due to lack of adequate laws and ethical issues involved with the practice of euthanasia. In other countries particularly Netherland and Japan DCD donors are used as the main source for kidney transplant as it is quite difficult to obtain a brain dead donor in these countries because of legal considerations. DCD grafts are usually considered as an inferior graft because of initial warm ischemia time after cardiac arrest which is quite minimal in cases of brain dead or live donors and prolonged cold ischemia times because of lack of instant availability of a recipient. Cho et al analyzed multicenter UNOS data and concluded that DCD kidneys had a higher chances of primary non function (4% vs. 1%) when compared to brain dead donor renal grafts. These grafts were associated with increased hemodialysis requirement during first week after the transplant (48% vs. 22%) as compared to those obtained from brain dead donors. Despite of initial poor graft function these grafts had comparable long-term results with the grafts obtained from brain dead donors.[37] In a Canadian study by Alejandro et al there was delayed graft function in 86% of cases but 1 year follow-up showed an estimated mean creatinine clearance of 64 mL/min.[110] A long-term follow-up of these cases was performed by Weber et al for 10 years and they found a graft survival of 76.7% when compared to donors with heartbeat who had the graft survival of 78.8% for the same period.[111] Snoeijs et al compared DCD kidney transplant with the patients on hemodialysis awaiting transplant and concluded that the patients who received a DCD renal transplant got additional 2.4 month of average life benefit.[112] However most of these results are encouraging but are restricted to DCD donors from Maastrict category III, i.e. patients who are waiting for cardiac arrest and not to Maastrict category I or II where patients were either dead on arrival or could not be resuscitated after cardiac arrest in the hospital.[113] Although a retrospective analysis by Hoogland et al concluded that uncontrolled cardiac dead donor grafts had similar results when compared to those who had controlled cardiac death.[114] Steegh et al compared the renal biopsy findings between live, DBD and DCD donors and concluded that peritubular capillary loss occurring during the first 3 months after the transplant was associated with the severity of interstitial fibrosis and tubular atrophy and had a direct correlation to the renal function at 1 year after the transplant. The maximum peritubular capillary loss was noted in DCD donor biopsies.[115] This study also demonstrated the importance of serial renal biopsies in predicting the long-term transplant outcome. Recently the use of ECMO has been introduced to maintain oxygenation and reduce the warm ischemic injury for procurement of kidneys from donors after cardiocirculatory death and the improved function was comparable to the grafts obtained from brain dead donors.[116] ECMO provides oxygenation to the tissues in the absence of cardiac activity and there was an anticipated increase of donor pool by 33% by its use. However, all these advances have made DCD donors a very useful option for renal transplant but careful selection of donors and reduction of ischemia times to a minimum is very much required.

The improvement in renal deceased transplant outcome is expected to increase the number of donors available for transplant in the coming years. A simultaneous improvement in the dialysis technology may reduce the number of patients requiring renal transplant in future. The judicious use of both these techniques may lead us to an era where a successful treatment for end stage renal disease is available to all the mankind.

Deceased Liver Transplantation

History

Although living donor liver transplant (LDLT) is the more common method of transplantation in most of the Asian countries excluding China, deceased liver transplant rates are also showing a rising trend during the last decade. The first deceased liver transplant was performed by Dr Thomas Starzl at Denver as early as 1963, but long-term success in terms of survival could not be achieved by him till 1967. The success of these deceased transplants led to the better understanding of surgical techniques, immunosuppression methods and the postoperative care which resulted in first LDLT in 1987 by Dr Raia at Brazil. Later on LDLT became the most common method for liver transplant in this part of the world as it is very difficult to find a deceased donor due to various reasons but deceased liver transplant remains the most common form of liver transplant in most of the North American and European countries so far. First Non Heart Beating Donor (NHBD) liver transplant was performed by Dr Nakayama in Japan as early as 1964 but its true potential as a method of liver transplant has yet to emerge.[117]

Liver transplant from a dead donor is quite commonly performed method for the treatment of acute and chronic liver failure caused due to various reasons. Few countries of North American continent as well as many european nations are catering about 90% of their transplant needs through this type of organ donation, but requirement of more donors is still there to take care of increasing demand. The better understanding of pathophysiology of diseases and improved surgical outcomes has encouraged the surgeons to perform surgeries on patients who were thought to be inoperable earlier. Although deceased donors are taking care of most of the transplant needs in these countries, but the use of more and more grafts from extended criteria donors or suboptimal donors are leading to poor transplant outcomes in the form of primary non function of graft, delayed or poor graft function and also biliary complications later on. Nevertheless, better donor management, improved surgical techniques and preservation methods are compensating these pitfalls to a large extent and resulting in better utilization of these grafts. This has also generated interest in non-heart beating donation of organs worldwide due to short supply of organs available for transplant.

Post Death Liver Changes

Generally brain death is quite well tolerated by the liver graft but if hemodynamic derangements persist central venous congestion takes place which leads to piecemeal and periportal necrosis.[103] However, in usual clinical settings the liver is taken up for transplantation before these changes occur. The main feature of deceased transplant is the Ischemic reperfusion injury caused by brain death itself as well as later by the cold ischemia (after the explantation of liver from the donor) followed by a brief period of warm ischemia (at the time of reimplantation) which again cause ischemic - reperfusion injury to the liver graft. Although all the three mechanisms are quite interrelated and cannot be distinguished entirely from one another, during the present discussion the latter two will be discussed in detail as the former has already been discussed earlier during this chapter.

Cold ischemia is induced just prior to the explantation of the organs by infusion of a cold preservative solution like UW or HTK at a temperature of 0°C to 4°C through the descending aorta. If heart and lungs are also taken out and/or if the liver graft is to be transported to another hospital it takes a lot of time which adds up to the prolongation of cold ischemia time. A significant period of warm ischemia time also gets added to it if the donation is made after circulatory arrest (as in NHBD donor). This temperature drop of the liver graft which is meant to reduce the metabolic activity of the liver sharply, not only causes injury to liver cells (which is proportional to the rapidity of temperature drop), but is also unable to stop the metabolism completely despite a 1.5 to 2 fold drop in the metabolism for every 10°C drop in the temperature. Once the Kupffer cells are exposed to ischemia they release reactive oxygen species and inflammatory mediators like cytokines and oxidants into the circulation which starts acting on the hepatocytes as well as the endothelial lining of the vessels supplying the liver. This leads to reduction in intracellular glutathione levels which is responsible for protection of these cells against oxidative injury secondary to ischemia and results in cholangiocyte apoptosis. Glutathione reduction also contributes to impaired bile flow and formation of biliary clumps which results in obstruction of the free flow of bile in the bile canalicular system even as late as 3 months after the transplant and may lead to rehospitalization, endoscopic intervention, repeat surgery and sometimes retransplantation also. Hepatocytes are more susceptible to ischemic injury associated with anoxia and ATP depletion, whereas cholangiocytes are more prone to reperfusion injury once the circulation is established again as they have less glutathione reserve to protect themselves against reactive oxygen species and other inflammatory mediators.[118] The biliary duct cells of rat are shown to withstand a period of ischemia of 120 minutes safely after which alterations in the plasma membranes and disappearance of interdigitation processes along with apical microvilli starts.[119] A prolonged ischemia time more than this has a detrimental effect on the biliary canaliculi structure throughout the liver. Impairment of bile secretion from the bile ducts lead to further hepatocyte and cholangiocyte injury. The bicarbonate secretion from the cholangiocytes is also reduced which results in further hepatocellular damage. The other important reason for biliary complications is its sole blood supply from the hepatic artery. Any decrease in the hepatic arterial supply whether due to thrombosis or anastomotic leak results in damage to the biliary ducts. Apart from circulatory causes immune causes such as ABO incompatible graft transplant or direct injection of chemotherapeutic agents into the anastomosed hepatic artery for treatment of HCC can also give rise to such a situation. The peribiliary capillary plexus is quite susceptible to microvascular injury in the long run which is quite evident in cases of chronic rejection.[120] Low perfusion state after cardiac arrest or hypotension in case of deceased donors lead to formation of microthrombi that plug the capillaries and diminish the perfusion, further contributing to ischemic injury. To clear the hepatic circulation from these microthrombi adequate amount (at least 3 liters) of flushing is required with the cold preservation fluid at pressures as high as 150 mm Hg. Inadequate flushing will result in suboptimal cold preservation and further ischemic reperfusion injury. Accumulation of these bile salts and a low phospholipid/bile salt ratio results in poor graft function after the transplant as hydrophobic type of bile salts are quite cytotoxic, especially to the cholangiocytes. The transcystic placement of T tube in liver allograft helps prevention of bile duct closure and detection of biliary leak at different postoperative intervals with radiological follow up. It is important to check the patency and hepatic arterial blood flow before making any diagnosis.

Prolonged cold and warm ischemia times are a major cause of concern with DCD liver grafts as these lead to sinusoidal and hepatocyte injury respectively in these livers which is much more in comparison to living or brain dead donor even if the death has occurred in a controlled manner. More cholestatic complications are seen in these livers in the form of biliary strictures both at the site of anastomosis as well as elsewhere in the biliary tree, once they are transplanted. These strictures may be focal or diffuse in nature and may be intra or extrahepatic. Various studies have quoted such complications ranging from 13.8% to 66% while these complications are seen in less than 5% of brain dead donors.[121] Although this complication can be reduced to a minimum by a variety of measures such as allowing the death in a controlled environment and employing various methods like induction of hypothermia as early as possible once the donor is declared dead. But sudden induction of cold ischemia may itself lead to sinusoidal injury despite a sharp drop in the metabolic activity of the liver. Combination of these two types of insults results in significant liver injury in comparison to what is seen in live or brain dead donation. Various studies have reported variable results when long-term survival of liver allograft is compared in these patients to brain dead donors. Abt et al reported a lower survival of hepatic graft in NHBD (Non heart beating donor) grafts as compared to HBD (Heart beating donor) grafts at 1 year (70.2% vs. 80.4%) and 3 year (63.3% vs. 72.1%) in liver transplants done in USA from year 1993 to 2001. Early graft failure was more for NHBD liver grafts within a period of first 60 days, which was 18.1% vs. 11.7% in HBD liver grafts. This study also showed an increasing trend of NHBD grafts from 0.26% in 1993 to 1.1% in 2001 when compared to HBD liver grafts.[122] Although the grafts from controlled as well as uncontrolled groups had similar graft survival (72.3% vs. 68.2% respectively at 1 year) but the small number of uncontrolled group (n = 11) compared to the controlled group (n = 117) makes the conclusion from this study limited. The length of cold ischemia time of more than 8 hours and patients receiving life support (on ventilator and inotropic support) prior to transplant were the only predictors of poor outcome, whereas donor age below 60 years and length of warm ischemia time of less than 30 minutes did not had much effect on graft loss. More research and selection of hemodynamically stable recipients was advised to get better results from NHBD livers. In another study by Detry et al at the University of Liege, Belgium 13 patients of Maastricht category III were transplanted NHBD liver graft with 100% survival rate for 1year with mean time from cardiac arrest to arterial flushing of 7.7 minutes, mean cold ischemia time of 295 minutes and mean warm suture ischemia time of 38 minutes. Only 2 patients developed main bile duct stenosis which was taken care of by endoscopic intervention.[123] Foley et al evaluated long-term outcome in 87 DCD liver graft recipients and found significantly lower survival rates when compared to brain dead donors at 1, 5, 10, 15 years posttransplant (DCD: 84%, 68%, 54%, 54% vs. DBD 91%, 81%, 67%, 58% respectively). Biliary complications (DCD 47% vs. DBD 26%) as well as ischemic cholangiopathy rates were found to be higher in case of DCD liver grafts (DCD 34% vs. DBD 1%).[124] Sibulesky et al reported a higher incidence of retransplantation in DCD liver grafts (14.8%) when compared to DBD liver grafts (9.3%) at the same center due to biliary complications.[121] Similar results were found by Skaro et al with a high rate of ischemic cholangiopathy and retransplantation.[125] Maheshwari et al even demonstrated a high mortality rate among these patients.[126] Retransplantation due to biliary complication is one of the most common causes of liver transplant in China. Improvement strategies in organ preservation, cell protection and better markers to predict postoperative graft function are required to improve the outcomes from these donors. Another strategy may be using these grafts in pediatric patients, despite ABO incompatibility which can be present in such transplants due to time constraints.[127]

List of Factors that cause Ischemic Type Biliary Lesions (ITBL)

- Increased donor age> 40 years
- Donor BMI > 25 and Donor weight > 100 kg
- Small liver graft size
- Type of graft donation DCDLT > DBDLT > LDLT
- Prolonged use of dopamine infusion in the donor
- Prolonged warm ischemia time > 30 minutes
- Prolonged cold ischemia time > 8 hours
- High viscosity of cold preservative solution (UW)
- Graft steatosis
- Hepatic artery thrombosis (HAT)

- Microemboli induced microvascular injury in liver graft
- Prolonged warm ischemia at reimplantation
- Reperfusion injury
- Decrease in hydrophilic bile salts
- Increase in hydrophobic bile salts causing cytotoxicity
- Accumulation of bile in cholangiocytes
- Inadequate flushing of bile from the ducts at the time of transplant
- ABO incompatibility
- Acute or chronic liver graft rejection
- Long-term immune mechanisms

Measures taken for Better Graft Outcome

There are many factors which can not be controlled by the transplant team such as donor age and graft size but the transplant team can choose a young recipient with minimal and no ventilator and inotropic support as far as possible. This mode of liver transplant is more suitable for patients who have MELD scores > 18 and have higher chances of tolerating inferior graft function. The initial warm ischemia time should be kept to a minimum in case of DCD donors (preferably less than 3 minutes once the patient is declared dead). Some centres advocate establishing femoral artery cannulation prior to extubation in these patients which can be used to induce cold ischemia as soon as the death is declared. In case of brain dead donors the field of all the organs should be prepared before flushing of the cold preservative solution through the aorta before their explantation. This helps in minimizing cold ischemia time for each individual organ. Adequate flushing of the cold preservative fluid preferably UW (University of Wisconsin) solution should be done at pressure around 150 mm Hg as lower pressures will result in inadequate flushing of hepatic vasculature and will lead to biliary strictures whereas higher pressures will result in more intimal damage. UW solution is preferred nowadays as there are some reports regarding poor performance of HTK solution for liver transplant especially if cold ischemia time is more than 8 hours.[46] An ideal solution would be the one which can minimize cellular changes and can provide adequate flush in minimum possible time. It has been hypothesized to use a combination of these two solutions instead of one.

Heparin (20,000 to 30,000 units) should be administered to prevent formation of microthrombi prior to cardiac arrest in deceased donors. Some centres advocate administration of another 10,000 units of heparin as portal flush at the time of bench dissection.[121] Some centers use other thrombolytics like streptokinase, urokinase or recombinant tissue plasminogen in addition to heparin along with the preservative solutions. Amongst this recombinant tissue plasminogen has shown the best results in the form of least chances of biliary stricture development. Some centers suggest injection of tissue plasminogen activator (tPA) directly to the hepatic artery after portal venous reperfusion for maximum enzymatic activity.[124] The graft should be flushed clear of these thrombolytics at the time of graft anastomosis because high dose of these can still be present inside the graft tissue and may lead to stroke in a recipient who is already having deranged coagulation. In some centers N-Acetylcystein is administered to both donor as well as recipient to prevent reperfusion injury.[128] NAC acts as a reducing agent, free radical scavenger and helps in improving glutathione levels. It is found to be especially useful in case of suboptimal grafts donated by DCD donors. The patients receiving NAC show fast improvements in factor V levels and low peak alanine transaminase levels, signifying decreased graft injury.[121] Phentolamine (10–20 mg) is used at some centers to prevent vasospasm and facilitates flushing.

Deceased liver transplant is an important method to take care of increasing organ demand in developing countries like India. But the complications related to this method of transplantation may require more postoperative monitoring, increased chances of rehospitalization thereby leading to more transplant costs. Despite so many strategies available for making deceased liver transplantation a viable option, it has to go a long way in order to stand close to LDLT.

Other individual organs like deceased heart and lung transplant are discussed in the separate chapters given in this book.

LEGAL ASPECT

The Human Organ Transplant Act 1994 and its amendment in 2009 accept brain death as a means of mode of death and a useful resource for organ donation in India. To prevent misdiagnosis on the part of treating physician this act makes it mandatory to diagnose brain death by four doctors but lacks on the detailed guidelines for the diagnosis of brain death and the policy for distribution of organs amongst various available recipients.[129] Two examinations are usually done 6 hours apart although second examination is not considered mandatory by law and even by few researchers as it can negatively affect the outcome of organs procured.[130] This fact remains debatable as few organs may show improved function as a result of delay after brain death provided the hemodynamic stability is maintained throughout this period.[107] The details of the Human Organ Transplant Act 1994 and its amendment are discussed in a separate chapter in the present book, only few issues important to deceased organ donation are dealt here.

The deceased donors are the main source of organs in most of the developed countries and are expected to be one in India soon. The technology involved in the process of deceased donor transplant has improved a lot during the last many years but still these organs can not be equated to the organs procured from live donors. The major risks involved with the deceased donor organs should be informed to the recipient and donor's family (at the time of getting informed consent) prior to the transplantation. The family should be informed regarding the number of organs and tissues going to be removed and whether any part of the body is going to be used for purpose other than transplant, especially if the whole body is donated for educational purpose also.[131]

Infection

High risk of infections such as HIV, hepatitis B, hepatitis C etc. is present to the recipient as these infections may occur despite initial negative results. There have been reported cases where all the organ recipients from a single deceased donor got infected from HIV despite of initial negative test,[132] or died due to donor being infected with rabies.[61] This issue usually poses a dilemma as donor's behavioral history is usually not available to the transplant team. The behavioral risk factors associated with the donors are history of alcoholism, drug addiction or substance abuse, history of repeated blood transfusions, illicit sexual relations, etc. It is highly unlikely to get a history suggestive of such life threatening infections from the donor's relatives due to social taboos involved, especially in Indian scenario. The highly virulent infections are usually detected but chronic infections may go unnoticed if the tests conducted are false negative. The results also depend on the method of testing used to confirm these infections, as time consuming methods cannot be used. The information regarding the possibility of these infections should be informed to the recipient in advance.[39]

Quality of Organs

The organs obtained from either the brain dead donors or donors after circulatory death are poorer as compared to those obtained from live donors. Although the technological advancements have decreased this gap to a large extent but is unable to completely abolish it. However, these organs are certainly helpful for those who are unable to find a suitable live donor, but the knowledge of this fact should be given to the recipient so that they can take decision accordingly. This becomes especially important when an expanded criteria donor is used for organ retrieval.

Ownership of Organs

Another important issue with the deceased organ donation is that whether the family of the deceased owns any right over the organs donated. It is widely debated if any benefits should be given to them in order to increase the donation of organs. The usual practice is to obtain an informed consent that they will not claim any benefits once the organs are wilfully donated.[133] The recipient's family should not have any information regarding the donor and similarly no information about the recipients should be given to the donor's family. This practice reduces the chances of any underhand financial gains to the donor's family and thus will be helpful in reducing the organ trade practices prevalent. Simultaneously it will increase public belief in the organ donation system.

INDIAN SCENARIO

The deceased organ transplantation in India is still in its infantile form as many superstitions, beliefs amongst the masses result in very poor donation rate. In one study by Seth et al it is estimated that India has an estimated deceased organ donation rate of 0.05 per million as compared to 33 per million in Spain which has the highest deceased organ donation rate in the world.[134] There may be many reasons for such a low conversion rate in the second most populated country of the world but a few common ones are as follows:

- Lack of public awareness regarding the concept of brain death and organ donation from a person with a beating heart is the most important of all. This fact remains unaltered despite various campaigns from the media and medical community. The public awareness programs are mostly limited to corneal donation which is usually performed hours after stopping of the heartbeat.
- The confusion regarding the diagnosis of brain death amongst the medical community is also a contributing factor. There are very few ICUs in the country which confirm the diagnosis of brain death despite suspicion and a very few amongst them give the family of the deceased the option of organ donation. The reluctance of the medical staff is probably due to the legal formalities involved and the taboo of getting the blame of involvement in the racket of organ trade from the deceased person's family.[135]

The family of the deceased have many reasons for refusal of organ donation the foremost being that most of the times they are not in a mental position to decide such an issue with a very limited period of time in hand. Seth et al described these reasons in order of prevalence.[134]

- Difference in opinion of family members towards consent
- Fear of criticism by society
- Concerns with quality of patient care
- Brain death concept is not understood
- Fear of mutilation
- Negative publicity of organ trade
- Hope for a miracle
- Many superstitions also form the basis of denial from the family members of the deceased person. The dead person will not have the organ in the next life which is lost in this life.

Mohan Foundation is a NGO involved in promoting deceased organ donation in India but still a lot of effort is required for improvement of various aspects related to brain death and deceased organ donation. The negative publicity of the organ trade related scandals by the media has proved to be a detrimental factor in the diminished response by the educated section of the society for deceased organ donation. The absence of any organ allocation policy by the government makes the picture shady in the eyes of general public.

WORLD SCENARIO

India and China may be the most populated countries over the globe but western countries particularly European countries are the world leaders as far as organ donation is concerned. The underdeveloped countries like African nations are far behind and at some places organ donation is yet to take off.

Europe—The European nations particularly Spain, Belgium and France are countries having highest organ donation around the globe. Spain leads the list with organ donation of around 35 PPM (Population per million) and is followed by Belgium and Austria at around 28.15 and 25 PPM. The Spanish legislation and organization is often cited as a gold standard to achieve the maximum number of organ donation. Spain is the only country in the world which is able to achieve a gradual decrease in the waiting list for renal transplant and living donation of less than 1% of the total number of transplants.[136] One of the main reasons for achieving such high rate of organ donation is the concept of **presumed consent** prevalent in these countries. Presumed consent puts the responsibility on the population to express and inform their denial for organ donation in advance otherwise the organs will be procured if the deceased person is found to be a suitable donor.[137] This practice is in sharp contrast to the practice of informed consent where a positive affirmation is necessary from the relatives after the death of their loved one. Presumed consent is also practiced in Austria, Bulgaria, Croatia, Czech republic, Estonia, Finland, Greece, Hungary, Italy, Latvia, Luxembourg, Norway, Poland, Portugal, Sweden, Greece and Ukraine but is mainly limited to the European continent only. Informed consent is still practiced in United Kingdom, Ireland, Germany and Switzerland.[138] The other reasons for high donation rate in these countries are increased public awareness,[139] fast communication at various levels, good transport network across the country, media support and willingness of the government machinery to improve the results at various levels.[139,136,138,140]

Principles of the Spanish Model of Organ Donation

1. Countrywide transplant network (ONT)
2. Transplant coordination at all three levels (National, regional, transplant coordinator)
3. Continuous audit of brain deaths in hospitals throughout the country
4. Audit of outcome of donations at ICUs in transplant procurement hospitals
5. Regular quality improvement program at various levels
6. Central office of ONT as an agency in support of all the process of donation
7. Great emphasis on transplant related medical training
8. Reduction of health budget by hospital reimbursement for transplants
9. Advertisements for increased public awareness and media support
10. Support from government and Church.

Asia—Asian countries lag far behind as compared to their European counterparts as far as deceased organ donation is concerned. The rates of organ donation are quite low even in advanced countries like Japan and Korea where the annual deceased organ procurement rate is still around 5 pmp.[141] The low rate of organ donation is mainly attributed to religious beliefs, legal hurdles and lack of adequate coordination between different teams of transplant network. In Japan till the year 2002 most of the deceased donation comprised of non heart beating donors and only a very small fraction from brain dead donors. The transplant law in japan clearly states that the donor's desire to donate their organs while they are alive should be respected.[36] Recent changes in the law related to organ donation after brain death is likely to increase the number of organs obtained by donation after brain death.[142] In China the deceased organ donation has developed in an unregulated manner due to lack of proper laws and control of the process by the ministry of health. In 2007 the ministry of health has laid down certain rules in order to maintain the standards by the transplant organizations. It has been made mandatory for these centers to be certified by the ministry in order to carry out transplant procedures. To curb transplant tourism Chinese citizens are preferred for receiving organs instead of foreigners. Informed consent is also made a mandatory requirement whereas no such rule existed before. China has been blamed for using the organs of their prisoners who get life sentence in the past but Chinese government has always denied it.[143] As per the Chinese registry 92% of the liver transplants (total no. 11888) belong to DCD category while a meagre 0.7% belong to brain dead donors from the year 1993 to 2008, but any significant analysis of this large data is not yet available for research purpose.[144] Korea has seen a gradual rise in the number of deceased donor transplants over the past one decade but now more and more ECD and DCD donors are getting utilized than before.[136] Singapore and Israel are the only Asian countries where presumed consent is legalized, but practised in Singapore only.[145] Informed consent is usually practised in Israel despite the permission by the law to practice presumed consent. Israel is one country in the world where a recipient gets priority over the other if he agrees to donate his organs posthumously (have a donor card for more than 3 years at the time of transplant). Patients are still given priority depending upon the severity of their condition but if two such patients get the chance for transplant the one who has registered as an organ donor is preferred or if one of his first degree relative has donated earlier, is preferred over the other recipient. A person whose age is less than 18 years or is not eligible to sign a donor card, and a mentally challenged gets equal priority for transplant. A previous live donor also gets preference if he has not donated for any particular individual.[146]

Africa—Transplant program is in a very poor state in most of the African countries. The countries like South Africa where many transplant surgeries were performed during the infancy of transplant era are still performing a good number of transplants but many underdeveloped African nations are yet to start a proper transplant program.

America—The transplant program of many North American countries is running quite successfully and lot of research is going on in countries particularly Canada and USA. USA has a United Network for Organ Sharing (UNOS) which collects the nationwide data from various organ procurement organizations (OPO) spread across the country. It has an online database system to collect, store, analyze and publish data regarding patient waiting list, organ matching, transplant and related outcome. This data is then analyzed for developing strategies to improve transplant outcomes and increase organ donation.[147] The deceased transplant rates in USA are around 25 pmp/year. This retrospective data analysis from hospitals with different transplant practices gives an insight about the possible future guidelines as controlled human studies are not possible in this field of medicine. Establishment of organ donation collaborative breakthrough (ODBC) in October 2005 which involved high organ donor potential OPOs, large organ donor potential hospitals and transplant centers has led to substantial increase in organ donation around the country.[138] Canada also has a very well developed transplant program with well documented guidelines for deceased organ procurement from brain dead[148] and DCD donors.[149]

South American countries also have well established transplant program of their own and are steadily making progress in the field of deceased transplants. The annual pmp rates vary from 5 to 20 amongst various countries. Presumed consent is practiced in some countries like Argentina, Colombia, Costa Rica and Peru.[138]

Australia—The deceased donor transplants are increasing in Australia over the years but have remained more or less the same in New Zealand although the donor age is steadily increasing in both the countries. This fact may be due to low population of this country. Both the countries have legislation and transplant guidelines available.

In May 2004, the Fifty seventh world assembly of WHO in its resolution advised the director general to continue monitoring the safety, quality, efficacy and epidemiology of transplant related practices throughout the world and to promote cooperation between the health authorities of member countries in order to improve these practices and to reduce organ trafficking. They also advised to promote live donor transplant as most of the active members are having well established deceased donor transplant program in place already.[150]

In May 2008 the international summit on transplant tourism and organ trafficking held at Istanbul which was organized by the transplantation society (TTS) and International Society of Nephrology (ISN) a consensus was made to promote the recovery of organs from the deceased donors and their equal distribution to the recipients in need. This includes the development and implementation of legislation, increasing of transparency and safety of transplant procedures, maintaining of national/regional registry, increasing public education and awareness, allocation of organs to suitable recipients without regard to gender, religion, and ethnicity, social or financial status. The same practice was advocated for live donors also. This consensus is popularly known as "**The declaration of Istanbul.**"[138,151]

Deceased organ transplant is emerging as an extremely useful method for the treatment of end organ diseases and is expected to benefit mankind till the artificial organs or culture grown organs replace them completely. The identification, preparation and improvisation of surgical techniques for the deceased donor along with better organ allocation policies will lead to optimization of these organs and help in decreasing the need for live organ donation.

REFERENCES

1. Linden PK. History of solid organ transplantation and organ donation. Crit Care Clin, 2009;25:165-84.
2. Braunfeld MY. Cadaveric donors. Anaesth Clin N Am, 2004;22:615-31.
3. Sreedhar R, Thomas SV. Brain death and apnea test. Annals of Indian Academy of Neurology, 2009;12:201.
4. Bos EM, Leuvenink HGD, H van Goor, Ploeg RJ. Kidney grafts from brain dead donors: Inferior quality or opportunity for improvement? Kidney International, 2007;72:797-805.
5. Fitzgerald RD. Management of the brain dead organ donor. Saudi Journal of Kidney Diseases and Transplantation, 1997;8(1):21-31.
6. McKeown DW, Bonser RS, Kellum JA. Management of the heart-beating brain-dead organ donor. Br J Anaesth, 2012;108(S1): i96-i107.
7. Holzer M. Targeted temperature management for comatose survivors of cardiac arrest. N Engl J Med, 2010;363:1256-64.
8. Shivalkar B, Vanloon J, Wieland W, Tjandra-Maga TB, Borgers M, Plets C, et al. Variable effects of explosive or gradual increase of intracranial pressure on myocardial structure and function. Circulation, 1993;87(1):230-9.
9. Novitzky D, Wicomb WN, Cooper DKC, Rose AG, Fraser C, Barnard CN. Electrocardiographic, haemodynamic and endocrine changes occurring during experimental brain death in chacma baboon. Journal of Heart Transplant, 1984;4(1):63-8. (abstracted)
10. Wood KE, McCartney J. Management of the potential organ donor. Transplantation Reviews, 2007;21:204-18.
11. Darracott-Cankovic S, Stovin PGI, Wheeldon D, Wallwork J, Wells F, English TAH. Effect of donor heart damage on survival after transplantation. Eur J Cardio-thorac Surg, 1989;3:525-32.
12. Murugan R, Venkataraman R, Wahed AS, Elder M, Hergenroeder G, Carter M, et al. Increased plasma interleukin-6 in donors is associated with lower recipient hospital-free survival after deceased organ transplantation. Crit Care Med, 2008;36:1810-16.
13. Terasaki PI, Cecka JM, Gjertson DW, et al. High survival rates of kidney transplants from spousal and living unrelated donors. N Engl J Med, 1995;333:333-36.
14. López SP, Hernández JO, Moreno NV, Augusto DE, Menéndez FA, González AA. Brain death effects on catecholamine levels and subsequent cardiac damage assessed in organ donors. Journal of Heart and Lung Transplant, 2009;28:815-20.
15. Wijdicks EFM, Fugate JE, Rabinstein AA. Blood pressure patterns after brain death. Neurology, 2011;77:399-401.
16. Ueno T, Zhi-Li C, Itoh T. Unique circulatory responses to exogenous catecholamines after brain death. Transplantation, 2000;70:436-44.
17. Dark JH. More and better donors for cardiac transplantation. European Heart Journal, doi:10.1093/eurheartj/ehp215.
18. Schnuelle P, Berger S, Jan De Boer, Persijn G, Van Der Woude FJ. Effects of catecholamine application to brain-dead donors on graft survival in solid organ transplantation. Transplantation, 2001;72:455-63.
19. O'Connor KJ, Wood KE, Lord K. Intensive management of organ donors to maximize transplantation. Crit Care Nurse, 2006;26:94-100.
20. Nicolas-Robin A, Amour J, Ibanez-Esteve C, Coriat P, Riou B, Langeron O. Effect of glucose-insulin-potassium in severe acute heart failure after brain death. Crit Care Med, 2008;36:2740-45.
21. Barklin A. Systemic inflammation in the brain dead organ donor. Acta Anaesth Scand, 2009;53:425-35.
22. Cooper DKC, Novitzky D, Wicomb WN. The pathophysiological effects of brain death on potential donor organs, with particular reference to the heart. Annals of the royal college of surgeons of England, 1989;71:261-66.
23. Wheeldon DR, Potter CDO, Jonas M, Wallwork J, Large SR. Using "unsuitable" hearts for transplantation. Eur J Cardio-thorac Surg, 1994;8:7-10.
24. Salim A, Vassiliu P, Velmahos GC, Sava J, Murray JA, Belzberg H, et al. The role of thyroid hormone administration in potential organ donors. Arch Surg, 2001;136:1377-80.
25. Imberti R, Vairetti M. Thyroid hormone therapy in organ donors. CMAJ, 2007;176(12):1737.
26. Goarin JP, Cohen S, Riou B, Jacuens Y, Guesde R, Francoise Le Bret, et al. The effects of triiodothyronine on haemodynamic status and cardiac function in potential heart donors. Anesth Analg, 1996;83:41-7.
27. Choi YS, Na S, Kang SY, Koh SO. Hormonal changes of the brain dead organ donors: A 3-year experience. South Korean journal of Crit Care Med, 2008;23:30-35.
28. Nicolas-Robin A, Barouk JD, Darnal E, Riou B, Langeron O. Free cortisol and accuracy of total cortisol measurements in the diagnosis of adrenal insufficiency in brain-dead patients. Anesthesiology, 2011;115:568-74.
29. Nicolas-Robin A, Barouk JD, Amour J, Coriat P, Riou B, Langeron O. Hydrocortisone Supplementation Enhances Hemodynamic Stability in Brain-dead Patients. Anesthesiology, 2010;112:1204-10.
30. Zaroff JG, Rosengard BR, Armstrong WF, Babcock WD, D'Alessandro A, Dec GW, et al. Consensus conference report maximizing use of organs recovered from the cadaver donor: cardiac recommendations. March, 2001;28-29. Crystal City, Va. Circulation, 2002;106:836-41.
31. Frontera JA, Kalb T. How I Manage the adult potential organ donor: Donation After Neurological Death (Part 1). Neurocrit Care, 2010;12:103-10.
32. 2010 American Heart Association Guidelines for Cardiopulmonary Resuscitation and Emergency Cardiovascular Care. Circulation, 2010;122:S639.
33. Sun S, Tang W, Song F, Chung SP, Weng Y, Yu T, et al. Pharmacologically induced hypothermia with cannabinoid agonist WIN55, 212-2 after cardiopulmonary resuscitation. Crit Care Med, 2010;38(12):2282-86.
34. Polderman KH, Peerdeman SM, Girbes ARJ. Hypophosphatemia and hypomagnesemia induced by cooling in patients with severe head injury. J Neurosurg, 2001;94:697-705.

35. Lisman T, Leuvenink HGD, Porte RJ, Ploeg RJ. Activation of hemostasis in brain dead organ donors: an observational study. J Thromb Haemost, 2011;9:1959-65.
36. Ishida H, Toma H. Organ donation problems in Japan and Countermeasures. Saudi J Kidney Dis Transplant, 2004;15(2):125-28.
37. Cho YW, Terasaki PI, Cecka JM, Gjertson DW. Transplantation of kidneys from donors whose hearts have stopped beating. N Engl J Med, 1998;338:221-5.
38. Veatch RM. Donating hearts after cardiac death: Reversing the Irreversible. N Engl J Med, 2008;359(7):672-73.
39. Rao YG, Mirza DF. Infections transmitted from donors to recipients following organ transplantation. Nat Med J India, 2005;18(4):189-94.
40. Rey MM, Ware LB, Matthay MA, Bernard GR, Mcguire AL, Caplan AL, et al. Informed consent in research to improve the number and quality of deceased donor organs. Crit Care Med, 2011;39:280-83.
41. Murugan R, Venkataraman R, Wahed AS, Elder M, Carter M, Madden NJ, et al. Preload responsiveness is associated with increased interleukin-6 and lower organ yield from brain-dead donors. Crit Care Med, 2009;37(8):2387-93.
42. Wetzel RC, Setzer N, Stiff JL, Rogers MC. Haemodynamic responses in brain dead organ donor patients. Anesth Analg, 1985;64:125-28.
43. Elkins LJ. Inhalational anesthesia for organ procurement: potential indications for administering inhalational anesthesia in the brain-dead organ donor. AANA Journal, 2010;78(4):293-99.
44. Ahmad N, Hostert L, Pratt JR, Billar KJ, Potts DJ, Lodge JPA. A pathophysiologic study of the kidney tubule to optimize organ preservation solutions. Kidney International, 2004;66:77-90.
45. Stewart ZA, Lonze BE, Warren DS, Dagher NN, Singer AL, Montgomery RA, Segev DL. Histidine-Tryptophan-Ketoglutarate (HTK) Is Associated with Reduced Graft Survival of Deceased Donor Kidney Transplants. Am J Transplantation, 2009;9:1048-54.
46. Stewart ZA, Cameron AM, Singer AL, Montgomery RA, Segev DL. Histidine-tryptophan-ketoglutarate (htk) is associated with reduced graft survival in deceased donor livers, especially those donated after cardiac death. Am J Transplantation, 2009; 9:286-93.
47. Fridell JA, Mangus RS, Powelson JA. Histidine-tryptophan-ketoglutarate for pancreas allograft preservation: The Indiana university experience. Am J Transplantation, 2010;10:1284-89.
48. O'Callaghan JM, Knight SR, Morgan RD, Morris PJ. Preservation solutions for static cold storage of kidney allografts: a systematic review and meta-analysis. Am J Transplantation, 2012;12:896-906.
49. Remadi JP, Baron O, Roussel JC, Oussana Al Habash, Treilhaud M, Despins P, et al. Myocardial preservation using celsior solution in cardiac transplantation: early results and 5-year follow-up of a multicenter prospective study of 70 cardiac transplantations. Ann Thorac Surg, 2002;73:1495-99.
50. Treckmann J, Moers C, Smits JM, Gallinat A, Maathuis MHJ, Margitta van Kasterop-Kutz, et al. Machine perfusion versus cold storage for preservation of kidneys from expanded criteria donors after brain death. Transplant International, 2011;24:548-54.
51. Moers C, Pirenne J, Paul A, Ploeg RJ. Machine perfusion or cold storage in deceased-donor kidney transplantation. N Engl J Med, 2012;366(8):770-1.
52. Amir G, Rubinsky B, Horowitz L, Millerd L, Leor J, Kassif Y, et al. Prolonged 24-hour subzero preservation of heterotopically transplanted rat hearts using antifreeze proteins derived from arctic fish. Ann Thorac Surg, 2004;77:1648-55.
53. Peh GSL, Beuerman RW, Colman A, Tan DT, Mehta JS. Human corneal endothelial cell expansion for corneal endothelium transplantation: An Overview. Transplantation, 2011;91:811-19.
54. Pollock G. Eye Banking-A Practical Guide In Rasik B Vajpayee Corneal Transplantation. Jaypee Brothers Medical Publishers Pvt. Ltd. First Edition 2002.
55. Bourne WM. Biology of the corneal endothelium in health and disease. Eye, 2003;17:912-18.
56. McCarey BE, Edelhauser HF, Lynn MJ. Review of corneal endothelial specular microscopy for fda clinical trials of refractive procedures, Surgical Devices and New Intraocular Drugs and Solutions. Cornea, 2008;27(1):1-16.
57. Gal RL, Dontchev M, Beck RW, Mannis MJ, Holland EJ, Kollman C, et al. The effect of donor age on corneal transplantation outcome: Results of the Cornea Donor Study. Ophthalmology, 2008;115:620-6.
58. Miyata K, Drake J, Osakabe Y, Hosokawa Y, Hwang D, Soya K, et al. Effect of donor age on morphologic variation of cultured human corneal endothelial cells. Cornea, 2001;20(1):59-63.
59. Borderie VM, Scheer S, Touzeau O, Vedie F, Carvajal-Gonzalez S, Laroche L. Donor organ cultured corneal tissue selection before penetrating keratoplasty. Br J Ophthalmol, 1998;82:382-8.
60. Khalil A, Ayoub M, El-Din Abdel-Wahab KS, El-Salakawy A. Assessment of the infectivity of corneal buttons taken from hepatitis B surface antigen seropositive donors. Br J Ophthal, 1995;79:6-9.
61. Srinivasan A, Burton EC, Kuehnert MJ, Rupprecht C, Sutker WL, Ksiazek TG, et al. Transmission of rabies virus from an organ donor to four transplant recipients. N Engl J Med, 2005;352:1103-11.
62. Heckmann JG, Lang CJG, Petruch F, Druschky A, Erb C, Brown P, et al. Transmission of Creutzfeldt-Jakob disease via a corneal transplant. Journal of Neurology, Neurosurgery, and Psychiatry, 1997;63:388-90.
63. Simonds RJ, Holmberg SD, Hurwitz RL, Coleman TR, Bottenfield S, Conley LJ, et al. Transmission of human immunodeficiency virus type1 from a seronegative organ and tissue donor. N Engl J Med, 1992;326:726-32.
64. McGeorge AJ, Vote BJ, Elliot DA, Polkinghorne PJ. Papillary Adenocarcinoma of the iris transmitted by corneal transplantation. Arch Ophthalmol, 2002;120:1379-83.
65. Salahuddin SZ, Palestine AG, Heck E, Ablashi D, Luckenbach M, McCulley JP, et al. Isolation of the human T-cell leukemia/ lymphotropic virus type III from the cornea. Am J Ophthalmol, 1986;101(2):149-52 (abstracted).
66. Pels E, Vrensen GFJM. Microbial decontamination of human donor eyes with povidone-iodine: penetration, toxicity, and effectiveness. Br J Ophthalmol, 1999;83:1019-26.
67. Badenoch PR, Alfrich SJ, Wedding TR, Coster DJ. Effectiveness of a decontamination method for donor corneas. Br J Ophthalmol, 1988;72:225-27.
68. Sturrock GD, Sherrard ES, Rice NSC. Specular microscopy of the corneal endothelium. Br J Ophthalmol, 1978;62:809-14.
69. Lindstrom RL, Doughman DJ, Skelnik DL, Mindrup EA. Corneal preservation at 4°C with chondroitin sulfate containing medium. Tr Am Ophthal Soc, 1987;85:332-49.
70. Raeder S, Utheim TP, Utheim ØA, Nicolaissen B, Roald B, Cai Y, et al. Effects of organ culture and optisol-gs storage on structural integrity, phenotypes, and apoptosis in cultured corneal epithelium. Thalmol Vis Sci, 2007;48:5484-93.
71. Pipparelli A, Thuret G, Toubeau D, He Z, Piselli S, Lefe`vre S, et al. Pan-corneal endothelial viability assessment: Application to endothelial grafts predissected by eye banks. Invest Ophthalmol Vis Sci, 2011;52:6018-25.
72. Kalevar V. Preservation and suitability of donor human corneas for keratoplasty. Ind J Ophthalmol, 1966;14(2):75-82.

73. Armitage WJ. Assessment of corneal quality by eye banks. J Ophthal & Vision Research, 2011;6(1):3-4.
74. Bourne WM, O'Fallon WM. Endothelial cell loss during penetrating keratoplasty. Am J Ophthalmol. 1978;85(6):760-6. (Abstracted)
75. Modi P, Rizvi J, Pal B, Trivedi H, Shah V, Modi M, et al. Dual kidney transplantation from expanded criteria deceased donor: Initial experience from single centre. Ind J Urol, 2011;27:30-33.
76. Perico N, Ruggenenti P, Scalamogna M, Remuzzi G. Tackling the shortage of donor kidneys: how to use the best that we have. Am J Nephrol, 2003;23:245-59.
77. Ojo AO. Expanded criteria donors: process and outcomes. Seminars in dialysis, 2005;18(6):463-68.
78. Geddes CC, Rodger RSC. Kidneys for transplant radical changes should mean we get more of them, better allocated. Br Med J, 2006;332:1105-06.
79. Baskin-Bey ES, Nyberg SL. Matching graft to recipient by predicted survival: can this be an acceptable strategy to improve utilization of deceased donor kidneys? Transplantation Reviews, 2008;22:167-70.
80. Su X, Zenios SA, Chakkera H, Milford EL, Chertow GM. Diminishing significance of HLA matching in kidney transplantation. Am J Transplantation, 2004;4:1501-08.
81. Ramos E, Aoun S, Harmon WE. Expanding the donor pool: Effect on graft outcome. J Am Soc Nephrol, 2002;13:2590-99.
82. Vergoulas G. Patient and graft survival after renal transplantation. Hippokratia, 2004;8(2):51-56.
83. Waiser J, Schreiber M, Budde K, Fritsche L, Bohler T, Hauser I, et al. Age matching in renal transplantation. Nephrol Dial Transplant, 2000;15:696-700.
84. Abdi R, Slakey D, Kittur D, Burdick J, Racusen L. Baseline glomerular size as a predictor of function in human renal transplantation. Transplantation, 1998;66:329-33.
85. Siedlecki A, Irish W, Brennan DC. Delayed graft function in the Kidney Transplant. Am J Transplant, 2011;11(11):2279-96.
86. Mieghem AV, Fonck C, Coosemans W, Vandeleene B, Vanrenterghem Y, Squifflet JP, et al. Outcome of cadaver kidney transplantation in 23 patients with type 2 diabetes mellitus. Nephrol Dial Transplant, 2001;16:1686-91.
87. Jonathan CT, Lee CM, Rebecca WJ, Amy LD, Donald DC, Edward AJ. Evaluation of the older deceased kidney donor: the impact of donor hypertension and creatinine clearance on graft performance and survival. Transplantation, 2000;70(5):765-71(abstracted).
88. Ojo A, Leichtman AB, Punch JD, et al. Impact of pre-existing donor hypertension and diabetes mellitus on deceased renal transplant outcome. Am J Kidney Dis, 2000;36:153-58 (abstracted).
89. Pastural M, Barrou B, Delcourt A, Marc-Olivier Bitker, Ourahma S, Richard F. Successful kidney transplantation using organs from a donor with disseminated intravascular coagulation and impaired renal function: case report and review of literature. Nephrol Dial Transplant, 2001;16:412-15.
90. Marie-Josée Hébert, Boucher A, Beaucage G, Girard R, Dandavino R. Transplantation of kidneys from a donor with carbon monoxide poisoning. N Engl J Med, 1992;326(23):1571.
91. Yan-Shen Shan, Po-Chang Lee, Sy ED, Chung-Jye Hung, Yih-Jyh Lin. Polycystic kidney patient as a deceased donor: is it appropriate? Nephrol Dial Transplant, 2001;16:410-11.
92. Pokorna E, Vitko S, Chadimova M, Schuck O. Adverse effect of donor arteriosclerosis on graft outcome after renal transplantation. Nephrol Dial Transplant, 2000;15:705-10.
93. Cittanova ML, Leblanc I, Legendre Ch, Mouquet C, Riou B, Coriat P. Effect of hydroxyethyl starch in brain-dead kidney donors on renal function in kidney-transplant recipients. Lancet, 1996;348:1620-22.
94. Kazemeyni SM, Esfahani F. Influence of hypernatremia and polyuria of brain-dead donors before organ procurement on kidney allograft function. Urology J, 2008;5:173-7.
95. Cheung CY, Chan HW, Chan YH, Chau KF, Li CS. Impact of delayed graft function on renal function and graft survival in deceased kidney transplantation. Hong Kong Med J, 2010;16:378-82.
96. Moers C, Smits JM, Mark-Hugo J. Maathuis, Treckmann J, Frank van Gelder, Napieralski BP, et al. Machine perfusion or cold storage in deceased-donor kidney transplantation. N Engl J Med, 2009;360:7-19.
97. Michelon T, Piovesan F, Santos P, Santos A, Keitel E, Bittar A, et al. Impact of using marginal cadaver donors and long cold ischemia time in renal transplant survival. Transplantation Proceedings, 2000;32:2586-88.
98. Nagareda T, Kinoshita Y, Tanaka A, Takeda M, Sakano T, Yawata K, et al. Clinicopathology of kidneys from brain-dead patients treated with vasopressin and epinephrine. Kidney International, 1993;43:1363-70.
99. Nijboer WN, Schuursa TA, Damman J H van Goor, Vaidya VS, JJ Homan van der Heide, et al. Kidney Injury Molecule-1 is an Early Noninvasive Indicator for Donor Brain Death-Induced Injury Prior to Kidney Transplantation. Am J Transplant, 2009;9(8):1752-59.
100. Koo DDH, Welsh KI, McLaren AJ, Roake JA, Morris PJ, Fuggle SV. Cadaver versus living donor kidneys: Impact of donor factors on antigen induction before transplantation. Kidney International, 1999;56:1551-59.
101. Koo DDH, Welsh KI, McLaren AJ, Roake JA, Morris PJ, Susan V, et al. Ischemia/Reperfusion Injury in Human Kidney Transplantation An Immunohistochemical Analysis of Changes after Reperfusion. Am J Path, 1998;153:557-66.
102. Dong X, Swaminathan S, Bachman LA, Croatt AJ, Nath KA, Griffin MD. Resident dendritic cells are the predominant TNF-secreting cell in early renal ischemia–reperfusion injury. Kidney International, 2007;71:619-28.
103. Pratschke J, Wilhelm MJ, Kusaka M, Basker M, Cooper DKC, Hancock WW, et al. Brain death and its influence on donor organ quality and outcome after transplantation. Transplantation Overview, 1999;67:343-48.
104. Joost AB, Hoeven VD, Molema G, Ter Horst GJ, Freund RL, Wiersema J, et al. Relationship between duration of brain death and hemodynamic (in) stability on progressive dysfunction and increased immunologic activation of donor kidneys. Kidney International, 2003;64:1874-82.
105. Vergoulas G, Boura P, Efstratiadis G. Brain dead donor kidneys are immunologically active: is intervention justified? Hippokratia, 2009;13(4):205-10.
106. Muro M, Llorente S, Marı´n L, Moya-Quiles MR, Gonzalez-Soriano MJ, Prieto A, et al. Acute vascular rejection mediated by HLA antibodies in a deceased kidney recipient: discrepancies between FlowPRATM, ELISA and CDC vs luminex screening. Nephrol Dial Transplant, 2005;20:223-26.
107. Kunzendorf U, Hohenstein B, Oberbarnscheid M, et al. Duration of donor brain death and its influence on kidney graft function. Am J Transplant, 2002;2:292-94.
108. Schnuelle P, Lorenz D, Mueller A, et al. Donor catecholamine use reduces acute allograft rejection and improves graft survival after deceased renal transplantation. Kidney International, 1999;56: 738-46
109. Jacob R. Acute renal failure Indian Journal of Anaesthesia, 2003;47(5):367-72.
110. Hernandez-Alejandro R, Caumartin Y, Marotta PJ, Ghent C, Levstik MA, Quan D, et al. Kidney and liver transplants from donors after cardiac death: initial experience at the London Health Sciences Centre. Can J Surg, 2010;53(2):93-102.

111. Weber M, Dindo D, Demartines N, Ambühl PM, Pierre-Alain Clavien. Kidney transplantation from donors without a heartbeat. N Engl J Med, 2002;347:248-55.
112. Snoeijs MG, Schaubel DE, Hené R, Hoitsma AJ, Mirza MI, Ijzermans, et al. Ernest van Heurn Kidneys from donors after cardiac death provide survival benefit. J Am Nephrol, 2010;21:1015-21.
113. Miguel Á, Frutos-Sanz, Francisco Guerrero-Gómez, Domingo Daga-Ruiz, Mercedes Cabello-Díaz, Miguel Lebrón-Gallardo, et al. Kidney transplantation with grafts from type III Maastricht death cardiac donors. Nefrologia, 2012;32(6):760-6.
114. Hoogland ERP, Snoeijs MGJ, Winkens B, Christaans MHL, L. WE van Heurn. Kidney Transplantation from donors after cardiac death: Uncontrolled versus controlled donation. Am J Transplantation, 2011;11:1427-34.
115. Steegh FMEG, Gelens MACJ, Nieman FHM, Johannes P. van Hooff, Cleutjens JPM, Robert Jan van Suylen, et al. Early Loss of peritubular capillaries after kidney transplantation. J Am Soc Nephrol, 2011;22:1024-29.
116. Lee JH, Hong SY, Chang-Kwon Oh, Hong YS, Yim H. Kidney transplantation from a donor following cardiac death supported with extracorporeal membrane oxygenation. J Korean Med Sci, 2012;27:115-19.
117. Abbasoglu O. Liver transplantation: Yesterday, today and tomorrow. World J Gastroenterol, 2008;14(20):3117-22.
118. Cursio R, Gugenheim J. Ischemia-reperfusion injury and ischemic-type biliary lesions following liver transplantation. Journal of Transplantation, 2012, Article ID 164329,17 pages.
119. Doctor BR, Dahl RH, Salter KD, Fitz JG. Reorganization of cholangiocyte membrane domains represents an early event in rat liver ischemia. Hepatology, 1999;29(5):1364-74.
120. Murase AJDN, Delaney CP, Woan M, Fung JJ, Starzl TE. The liver allograft, chronic (ductopenic) rejection, and microchimerism: what can they teach us? Transplantation Proceedings, 1995;27(1):67-70.
121. Sibulesky L, Nguyen JH. Update on biliary strictures in liver transplants. Transplantation Proceedings, 2011;43:1760-64.
122. Abt PL, Desai NM, Crawford MD, Forman LM, Markmann JW, Olthoff KM, et al.. Survival following liver transplantation from non-heart-beating donors. Ann Surg, 2004;239(1):87-92.
123. Detry O, Seydel B, Delbouille MH, Monard J, Hans MF, A. De Roover, et al. Liver transplant donation after cardiac death: experience at the university of liege. Transplantation Proceedings, 2009;41:582-84.
124. Foley DP, Fernandez LA, Leverson G, Anderson M, Mezrich J, Sollinger HW, et al. Biliary complications after liver transplantation from donation after cardiac death donors: an analysis of risk factors and long term outcomes from a single center. Ann Surg, 2011;253(4):817-25.
125. Skaro AI, Jay CL, Baker TB, Wang E, Pasricha S, Feinglass JM, et al. The impact of ischemic cholangiopathy following donation after cardiac death liver transplantation–the untold story. Surgery, 2009;146(4):543-53.
126. Maheshwari A, Maley W, Li Z, Thuluvath PJ. Biliary complications and outcomes of liver transplantation from donors after cardiac death. Liver Transplantation, 2007;13:1645-53.
127. Heffron T, Welch D, Pillen T, Asolati M, Smallwood G, Hagedorn P, et al. Successful ABO-incompatible pediatric liver transplantation utilizing standard immunosuppression with selective postoperative plasmapheresis. Liver Transplantation, 2006;12:972-78.
128. Fusai, Glantzounis GK, Hafez T, Yang W, Quaglia A, Sheth H, et al. N-Acetylcysteine ameliorates the late phase of liver ischaemia/reperfusion injury in the rabbit with hepatic steatosis. Clinical Science, 2005;109:465-73.
129. Shroff S. Legal and ethical aspects of organ donation and transplantation. Indian J Urol, 2009;25:348-55.
130. Lustbader D, O' Hara D, Wijdicks EFM, Maclean L, Tajik W, Ying A, Berg E, et al. Second brain death examination may negatively affect organ donation. Neurology, 2011;76:119-24.
131. P J van Diest, Cardoso NWJL, Niesing J. Cadaveric tissue donation: a pathologist's perspective. J Med Ethics, 2003;29:135-36.
132. Halpern SD, Shaked A, Hasz RD, Caplan AL. Informing Candidates for solid-organ transplantation about donor risk factors. N Engl J Med, 2008;358(26):2832-37.
133. Glantz L, Roche P, Annas GJ. Rules for donations to tissue banks —What Next? N Engl J Med, 2008;358(3):298-303.
134. Seth AK, Nambiar P, Joshi A, Ramprasad R, Choubey R, Puri P, et al. First prospective study on brainstem death and attitudes towards organ donation in India. Liver Transplantation, 2009;15:1443-47.
135. Kumar M, Shengdge P, Kumar V, Trivedi V, Waghela J, Rajpal D. Our experience with deceased organ donor maintenance. Ind J Crit Care Med, 2007;11(2):49-53.
136. Matesanz R. A decade of continuous improvement in deceased organ donation: the Spanish model Nefrología, 2001;21(5):59-67.
137. HILL DJ, Palmer TC, Evans DW. Presumed consent. BMJ, 1999;318:1490.
138. Rhee J, Kern B, Cooper J, Freeman RB. Organ donation. Seminars in Liver Disease, 2009;29:19-39.
139. Scandroglio B, Domı´nguez-Gil B, Lo´ pez JS, Valentı´n MO, Martı´n MJ, Coll E, et al. Analysis of the attitudes and motivations of the Spanish population towards organ donation after death. Transplant International, 2011;24:158-66.
140. Miranda B, Lucas MF, C de Felipe, Naya M, González-Posada JM, Matesanz R. Organ donation in Spain. Nephrol Dial Transplant, 1999;14(Suppl3):15-21.
141. Min SI, Kim SY, Park YJ, Seung-Kee Min, Kim YS, Ahn C, et al. Trends in deceased organ donation and utilization in korea: 2000-2009. J Korean Med Sci, 2010;25:1122-27.
142. Aikawa A. Organ donation from brain-dead donors and the role of the japan organ transplant network. JMAJ, 2011;54(6):357-62.
143. Caplan AL, Danovitch G, Shapiro M, Lavee J, Epstein M. Time for a boycott of Chinese science and medicine pertaining to organ transplantation. Lancet, 2011;378:1218.
144. Asian Pacific Association for the Study of the Liver 2010. transplant course: The art of liver transplantation. Hepatol Int, 2010;4(Suppl 1):S86-S93.
145. Vathsala A, Chow KY. Renal Transplantation in Singapore. Ann Acad Med Singapore, 2009;38:291-9.
146. Lavee J, Ashkenazi T, Gurman G, Steinberg D. A new law for allocation of donor organs in Israel. Lancet, 2010;375:1131-33.
147. Sheehy E, Conrad SL, Brigham LE, Luskin R, Weber P, Eakin M, et al. Estimating the number of potential organ donors in the United States. N Engl J Med, 2003;349:667-74.
148. Shemie SD, Doig C, Dickens B, Byrne P, Wheelock B, Rocker G, et al. On behalf of the pediatric reference group and the neonatal reference group brain arrest: the neurological determination of death and organ donor management in canada severe brain injury to neurological determination of death: canadian forum recommendations. CMAJ, 2006;174(6):S1-S12.
149. Shemie SD, Baker AJ, Knoll G, Wall W, Rocker G, Howes D, et al. National recommendations for donation after cardiocirculatory death in Canada Donation after cardiocirculatory death in Canada. CMAJ, 2006;175(8):S1-S24.
150. http://www.who.int/gb/ebwha/pdf_files/WHA57/A57_R18-en.pdf
151. The Declaration of Istanbul on Organ Trafficking and Transplant Tourism. Clin J Am Soc Nephrol, 2008;3:1227-31.

5 CHAPTER Immunology and Immunosuppressants in Transplantation

Rahul Bhayana, Anil Jain

INTRODUCTION

Nature has provided an elaborate and effective mechanism to combat foreign agents in the form of "Immune System." However, the same mechanism also acts as the most formidable barrier to the transplanted organs, which are recognized by this system as "foreign." But for the immune system, organ transplantation could have been the final and the most reliable solution to the malfunction of any organ system, be it the pancreas, liver, kidney or heart. An insight into the details of this mechanism is therefore the understanding of the process of "transplant rejection." It is also a guide for developing strategies to minimize the same so as to ensure a smooth acceptance of the graft.

The success of transplant is determined by the extent of immune response triggered by the graft which depends upon the degree of genetic disparity between the donor and the recipient. That is why autologous transplantations (from one site to another of the same individual, e.g. skin graft) do not undergo rejection because of the same genetic source. The transplantation between monozygotic twins is also unlikely to undergo rejection as the two individuals are genetically identical. Xenografts on the other hand (between different species) are most likely to attract a vigorous immune response and undergo rejection. Allografts, which are the most common form of transplants, lie in between. They are carried out between genetically separate individuals belonging to same species.

The strategies for the downregulation of immune system using immunosuppressant agents have traditionally been the favourite of physicians and researchers dealing in 'transplantation.' However few researchers have shifted their interest to 'immune modulation' through the development of "tolerance" to the transplanted organ so as to nullify (or minimize) the use of immunosuppressant drugs thereby avoiding their unwanted effects. The subject is still under study and may have some promising results in future.[1]

Evolution of Transplant Immunology

One of the first clinically relevant observations pertaining to transplantation immunology was made by Dr Earl Padgett in 1920s. He noted that skin grafts survived longer when skin from a close relative was used. Ten years later, Dr Barrett Brown, a fellow American plastic surgeon, extended these observations when he transplanted a skin graft from an identical twin of the patient and achieved permanent survival of the graft. In 1944, Medawar showed that skin allograft rejection is a host versus graft response. Mitchison later demonstrated the cell mediated features of this response. Sir Joseph E Murray performed the first successful identical twin transplant of kidney in 1954.[2] This was followed by first liver transplant by Dr Thomas E Starzl in 1967, first heart transplant in 1967 by Dr Christian Barnard and first successful bone marrow transplant by E Donnall Thomas in 1968. The era of immunosuppressive drug treatment was initiated in 1959 when Schwartz and Daneshek showed that 6-mercaptopurine was immunosuppressive in rats. Since then many new and progressively more selective immunosuppressive agents have been developed. The concept of immune tolerance, though born as early as 1940s, is yet to attain an adequate stature in clinical practice.[3]

The Phenomenon of Rejection

Types of Rejection

"Hyperacute rejection" occurs within minutes to three days after transplantation. This is a humorally mediated phenomenon and occurs due to prior host sensitization thereby leading to the presence of pre-exiting antibodies in the host body. The prior sensitization can be induced by prior blood transfusions, multiple pregnancies, prior transplantation or xenografts against which humans already have antibodies. The antigen-antibody complexes activate the complement system, causing massive thrombosis in capillaries, which leads to an ischemic damage to the graft. The kidney is most susceptible to hyperacute rejection; while the liver is relatively resistant, possibly because of its dual blood supply.[4]

"Acute rejection" may occur within 4–5 days of transplantation, but most commonly occurs in the 2nd to 3rd postoperative week. Acute rejection is a critical condition, but responds well to immunosuppressant drug therapy. Activated lymphocytes are primarily responsible for the cascade ending up in acute rejections although humoral immunity also has an important role to play.

"Chronic rejection" develops within months to years.[5] These are triggered by both humoral and cell mediated immunity and are characterized by development of severe vessel changes. Chronic rejection is seen more commonly in cases of initial delayed graft function, reperfusion injury, post-transplantation infection (e.g. CMV), graft taken from elderly or hypertensive individual, inadequate immunosuppression or previous episodes of acute rejection. Uncontrolled diabetes mellitus and hypertension in the recipient also add to the risk of chronic graft rejection. Once triggered they are not easily manageable even by high-dose immunosuppressants thereby resulting in a low graft survival rate.

The Human Leukocyte Antigen (HLA) System

The "histocompatibility antigens," which are mainly responsible for igniting the immune reaction leading to graft rejection are coded by a special set of genes called the "major histocompatibility complex (MHC)." In humans this is called the human leukocyte antigen (HLA) system and is located on the short arm of chromosome 6. An individual inherits two half sets of these genes from each parent. Therefore every individual has 25% probability of being HLA identical to his or her sibling. The HLA parity or closeness between two individuals determines to a great extent the probability of graft survival. Every organ transplantation must therefore be preceded by an elaborate HLA typing.[6]

The Mechanisms of Rejection

The immune response to a transplanted organ consists of both cellular (lymphocyte mediated) and humoral (antibody mediated) mechanisms. Although other cell types are also involved, the T cells are pivotal in rejection of grafts.[7] The T lymphocytes recognize an antigen only when presented in a complex with an MHC molecule.[8] The class I MHC molecules may be present on all nucleated cells whereas the class II molecules are expressed only on the professional antigen-presenting cell (APCs) such as dendritic cells, activated macrophages and β-cells. The class I molecules are responsible for presenting antigenic peptides from within the cells, i.e. self antigens to CD 8 T cells while class II molecules present extra cellular antigens such as extra cellular bacteria to CD 4 T cells. This is of prime importance in the process of transplant rejection. The mechanism of rejection has been divided into two stages; the sensitization stage and the effector stage.[9]

'The sensitization' of CD 4 and CD 8 cells can occur as a result of two signals. The first one is the result of interaction of T cell receptor with the antigen MHC complex. This is followed by another signal via the interaction of co-stimulatory receptor (usually CD 28) on T cell with a corresponding ligand (usually B7-1 and B7-2) on the surface of antigen presenting cells (APC).[10] If the second signal from the co-stimulatory ligand via CD 28 is absent, the activation of T cells remains incomplete and does not reach the effector stage. This condition is called 'anergy' and has been exploited in the phenomenon of immune tolerance.[11]

The transplanted organ carries a variable number of APLs which have a high density of MHC molecules. The host T-cells recognize these allo-MHC molecule + allo-peptide complexes as foreign. This results in exorbitant proliferation of T cells thereby leading to acute allorejection.

Some alloantigens that are immunologically silent initially may undergo changes and are presented as "processed" alloantigen by self APCs thereby leading to T cell proliferative response. Such secondary responses may occur in late acute or chronic rejection.[12]

An inflammatory injury or ischemia to the transplanted organ may contribute to this secondary response.

Once sensitized, CD 4 T cells initiate a series of immune reactions.[10] These include initiation of macrophage-mediated delayed type hypersensitivity (DTH) response, providing help to B cell for antibody production, production and upregulation of cytokines (IL-2 and IFN-r) and chemokines, TNF-d, inducible nitric oxide synthatase (iNOS) and growth factors. These lead to the production of more T cells thereby leading to a self proliferating cascade which ultimately leads to cytotoxicity and apoptosis in the graft tissues. The CD 8 cells also act as cytotoxic agents by releasing cytotoxic granules containing perforin and granzymes. These granules fuse with the effector cell membrane and empty their contents into its cytoplasm therapy hastening the process of cell death. They have been shown to play a significant role in acute, though not chronic, allograft rejection. The natural killer (NK) cells through their profound cytotoxic properties on the other hand, have a role in both acute as well as chronic rejection.[12] In addition their response is more resistant to immunosuppressive therapy.[13]

In chronic rejection the growth factors, including TGF-B and endothelin cause smooth muscle proliferation, intimal thickening, fibrosis and scarring. However the specific histopathological picture varies with different organs. It may manifest as accelerated coronary artery atherosclerosis in heart, bronchiolitis obliterans in lungs, vanishing bile duct syndrome in liver and glomerulosclerosis in kidney.[14]

The Remedy of Rejection

Immunosuppression in Transplantation

As is known, there is a huge mismatch between the demand and supply of transplantable organs. Primary reasons accounting for this are non-availability of donors, problems due to inappropriate HLA/ABO matching and legal and ethical issues. Graft rejection, in the given scenario, makes the problem even worse and adds to the burden of disease. It negates the entire essence of phenomenon of transplantation. Researchers have, therefore, always been for finding new and better modalities to minimize it.

The foremost step in this is an accurate and detailed cross-matching between the donor and the recipient. Three types of cross matches are usually done in this regard. Out of these, first is the ABO blood group cross match. Any incompatibility between the blood groups of the two shall turn out to be a cause of hyperacute rejection.[15] The second is HLA typing wherein the priority of HLA compatibility is sequenced as DR-B-A-C. Although a "full house-match" occurs only in 20% of cases, it is important that cross testing of donor cells with recipient's serum should turn out negative. In the lymphocytotoxicity assay, patient's serum is tested for reactivity with donor lymphocyte. Others tests available are panel reactive antibody (PRA) assay wherein a patient's serum is screened for lymphocytic antibodies against a random cell panel and mixed lymphocyte reaction (MLA) that can assess the degree of major histocompatibility complex (MHC) class I and II compatibility.

Therapeutic modalities form the second step in this direction.[16] Although radiation and other non-selective therapies have been tried in the past, immunonosuppressant drugs have been the main stay of treatment in this regard for many decades.[17] 6-mercaptopurine was introduced in the late 1950s followed by azathioprine in the 1960s. Steroids have always been an important component of the regimen, either alone or in combination with other drugs. However, the side effects of these drugs have always been a cause of concern. Steroid induced diabetes had always been a barrier in the success of renal transplantation prior to the introduction of cyclosporine. Although the search for the least toxic agent is still on, many other drugs with lesser side effects and greater efficacy have since been developed.[18] Some of the most commonly used agents have been explained here.

Immunosuppressant Drugs

These drugs have been classified into following categories[19,20]

1. Glucocorticoids–prednisolone
2. Calcineurin inhibitors–cyclosporine and tacrolimus
3. Antiproliferative drugs–sirolimus, azathioprine, cyclophosphamide, methotrexate, chlorambucil, mycophenolate mofetil (MMF)
4. Antibodies muromonab CD3, antithymocyte globulin (ATG), Rho(D) immunoglobulin

I. Adrenocortical Steroids

The introduction of glucortocorticoids as immunosuppressants in 1960s played a key role in making organ transplantation possible. Prednisone, prednisolone and other glucocorticoids are used alone and in combination with other drugs for prophylaxis and treatment of transplant rejection.[21]

Glucocorticoids inhibit MHC expression and IL–1, IL–2 and IL –6 production which prevent the activation of helper T cells and cause a rapid, transient decrease in peripheral blood lymphocyte count. Neutrophils and monocytes also display poor chemotaxis and decrease lysosomal enzyme release in their presence. Therefore glucocorticoids have broad anti-inflammatory effects on multiple components of cellular immunity. In contrast, they have relatively little effect on humoral minority.

Extensive use of glucocorticoids is associated with severe adverse effects and disabilities. The greatest risk stands of hyperglycemia and risk of infection in transplantation and more so in diabetics. Other effects include growth retardation in children, avascular necrosis of bone, osteopenia, poor wound healing, cataract and hypertension. The advent of combined use of glucocorticoid and cyclosporine therapy has allowed reduced doses of steroids thereby making renal transplantation in diabetics successful. But despite all means, steroid induced morbidity still remains a major problem in many transplant patients.

II. Calcineurin Inhibitors

Cyclosporine and tacrolimus are the most widely used immunosuppressive agents in transplant rejection. These block a calcineurin mediated intracellular response resulting from T-cell activation.[18]

a. **Cyclosporin A** was introduced in 1977 and has been the mainstay of therapy since then. It is a cyclic polypeptide consisting of laminoacids and is produced by a fungus called "Beauveria nivea."

Cyclosporin preferentially inhibits antigen—triggered signal transduction in T-lymphocytes thereby blunting expression of many lymphokines including IL-2 and TGF-β. It forms a complex with cyclophilin, a cytoplasmic receptor protein present in target cells.

This complex binds to calcineurin which leads to the inhibition of Ca^{++} mediated dephosphorylation of the cytosolic component of nuclear factor of activated T cells (NFAT).

The dephosphorylation of NFAT is otherwise essential for its entry into the nucleus where it activates the gene transcription responsible for the entire response of T-lymphocyte to antigenic stimulation. Thus cycloporin has profound effects on cell mediated immunity.

Cyclosporine can be administered intravenously or orally. Oral cyclosporine is absorbed slowly with 20% to 50% bioavailability. It is recommended to shift to oral formulations as early as possible because IV formulations are generally associated with greater incidence of adverse effects.

It is given usually in combination with other agents, especially glucocorticoids and either azathioprine or mycophenolate mofetil and more recently, sirolimus. The dose of cyclosporine varies, depending on the organ transplanted and other drugs used in the regimen.

The major limitation to the use of cyclosporine is nephrotoxicity. This occurs in majority of patients and is the major indication for cessation or modification of therapy. Therefore therapeutic algorithms have been developed especially for renal transplant patients which delay the cyclosporine introduction until a threshold renal function is attained. However it is important to differentiate renal-toxicity from graft rejection. USG guided allograft biopsy is helpful in this. Other adverse reactions include tremors, hirsutism, hypertension, hyperlipidemia, gum hyperplasia and hyperuricemia leading to worsening of gout.

b. **Tacrolimus** is indicated for the prophylaxis of solid-organ allograft rejection in a manner similar to cyclosporine and as a rescue therapy in patients with rejection episodes despite "therapeutic" levels of cyclosporine. It is macrolide antibiotic produced by *Streptomyces tsukubaensis.*

Like cyclosporine, tacrolimus inhibits T-cell activation by inhibiting calcineurin. It is however 100 times more potent than cyclosporine and binds to a different cytoplasmic protein labelled "FKBP." However the subsequent steps are same, i.e. inhibition of calcineurin thereby preventing the dephosphorylation and nuclear translocation of NFAT. Due to its potency it is more suitable for use in a setting of acute rejection.

Tacrolimus is available for oral administration as capsules (0.5, 1 and 5 mg) and as potential formulation for injection (5mg/mL). The recommended starting dose for injection is 0.03 to 0.05 mg/kg/day as a continuous infusion and that of oral is 0.15 to 0.20 mg/kg/day for adult kidney transplant patients. These doses are intended to achieve typical blood trough levels in the 5 to 15 mg/mL range. It has a half life of about 12 hours and is extensively metabolized in liver and bulk of excretion is in the faeces.

Tacrolimus causes nephrotoxicity, neurotoxicity (tremors, headache, motor disturbances, seizure), GI complaints, hypertension (less common than with cyclosporin) and hyperkalemia. It has a negative effect on pancreatic islet beta cells–glucose intolerance and diabetes mellitus are therefore well recognized complications of tacrolimus based immunosuppression. As with other immunosuppressants there is an increased risk of secondary tumors and opportunistic infections.

Because of its potential for nephrotoxicity, tacrolimus blood levels and renal functions should be monitored. Whole blood rather than plasma is the most appropriate sampling compartment evaluating for tacrolimus concentration. Coadministration with cyclosporin or other nephrotoxic drugs may lead to additive effects on kidney, therefore a delay of at least 24 hours is required when switching a patient from cyclosporin to tacrolimus.

III. Anti-proliferative and Antimetabolic Drugs

a. **Sirolimus** is a macro cyclic antibiotic produced by fermentation of streptomycin hygroscopicus. It inhibits T-lymphocyte activation and proliferation downstream of IL-2 and other T-cell growth factor receptors. It forms a complex with FKBP-12 and inhibits a protein kinase, the designated mammalian target of rapamycin (mTOR) which is a key enzyme in IL-2 mediated signal transduction and cell cycle progression. This results in T and B cell cycle arrest in G1-s phase.[22]

Sirolimus is mainly indicated for prophylaxis of organ transplant rejection in combination with a calcineurin inhibitor. However, in patients at high risk for calcineurin inhibitor associated nephrotoxicity, it has been used with glucocorticoids and mycophenolate mofetil. In animal models sirolimus not only inhibits transplant rejection graft versus host disease and a variety of autoimmune diseases, but its effect also lasts several months after discontinuing therapy, suggesting a tolerating effect. Another use of sirolimus is for incorporation into stents to inhibit local cell proliferation and blood vessel occlusion.

The initial dosage in patients 13 years or older should be adjusted based on body surface area (1 mg/m^2 per day) with a loading dose of 3 mg/m^2. After oral administration, sirolimus is absorbed rapidly and reaches a peak blood concentration in 1 to 2 hours. A high meal causes a reduction in peak concentration by as much as 34%. It has a high plasma protein (albumin) binding. It is extensively metabolized by CY P3A4 leading to multiple metabolites which are excreted mainly in faeces. It is recommended that maintenance dose be reduced by one third in patients with hepatic impairment. The blood half life after multiple doses in stable renal transplant patients is 62 hours.

Although sirolimus per se is not nephrotoxic, it accentuates the renal impairment caused by cyclosporin (as against combination with azathioprine or placebo). Renal function therefore must be monitored closely when it is used in combination with calcineurin inhibitor. It also causes leukopenia, thrombocytopenia, anemia and increased incidence of neoplasms or opportunistic infections especially pneumocystis carinii or cytomegalovirus. Another notable adverse effect of its use is clinically significant hypercholesterolemia and hypertriglyceridemia. It has also been associated with delayed wound healing, lymphocele formation, pneumonitis and prolonged delayed graft function.

Evarolimus (40-0[2-hydroxy]ethyl-rapamycin) is another mTOR inhibitor which is clinically and chemically close to sirolimus. It has similar mechanism of action, dosage and toxicity as sirolimus but differs in having a shorter half life and a shorter time to achieve a steady state concentration. Like sirolimus it also enhances the nephrotoxic effect of calcineurin inhibitors.

b. **Azathioprine** is an antiproliferative agent which is a purine antimetabolite, a derivative of 6 mercaptopurine. The basic mechanism of action of these drugs is by the inhibition of DNA replication thereby suppressing T cell proliferation. This is achieved by the cleavage of azathioprine to 6-mercaptopurine which along with other metabolites inhibit the de novo purine synthesis and formation of frandulent nucleotides which get incorporated into the DNA.

There is an important place for azathioprine in transplant for prevention of renal and other allografts rejection, though it is less effective than cyclosporin. It is generally given in combination with calcineurin inhibitors or used as an alternative in patients developing cyclosporin toxicity. It is also used in severe rheumatoid arthritis, although in lesser doses. For prophylaxis of organ rejection, it is used in a starting dose of 3 to 5 mg/kg per day. Orally it is absorbed well and reaches maximum blood levels within 1 to 2 hours after administration.

Azathioprine itself has a short half life of about 1 hour but it is extensively metabolized into active components (like 6-mercaptopurine) which have a half-life of upto 5 hours. Both azathioprine and mercaptopurine are moderately bound to plasma proteins and partially dialyzable. Renal clearance has little impact on biological effectiveness or toxicity but the dose should be reduced in patients with renal failure. The major side effect of azathioprine is bone marrow suppression. It causes most commonly leucopenia but also can cause thrombocytopenia or anemia. It is recommended, therefore to monitor complete blood count in patients on azathioprine. Monitoring of liver functions is also recommended since it causes hepatotoxicity. Other side effects include GI toxicity, alopecia, increased susceptibility to infections (especially varicella and herpes simplex viruses), pancreatitis and increased risk of neoplasms. The side effects of azathioprine are increased upon concurrent usage with allopurinol and ACE inhibitors.

c. **Mycophenolate mofetil (MMF):** It is a relatively new immunosuppressant which, through its active metabolite myocophenolic acid, selectively inhibits the T and B lymphocyte proliferation and subsequent antibody production and cell mediated immunity. MMF is often used as an "add on" therapy and has been found as good or even superior to azathioprine.

After oral or intravenous administration, mycophenolate mofetil undergoes rapid and complete metabolism to mycophenolic acid (MPA) which is a selective, non competitive and reversible inhibitor of enzyme ionosine monophosphate dehydrogenase (IMPDH). This enzyme is essential for de novo synthesis of guanosine nucleotides in the T and B cells. As these cells, unlike others, do not have the Purina salvage pathway, their proliferation is selectively inhibited in presence of MPA. After administration, MMF is cleared within minutes from the blood while MPA has a half life of about 16 hours.

Mycophenolate mofetil is used as an adjuvant, for

prophylaxis of transplant rejection, in combination with glucocorticoids and calcineurin inhibitors (cyclosporine), but not with azathioprine. Combined treatment with sirolimus is possible, but necessitates the monitoring of drug levels.[22] It helps to reduce the dosage of cyclosporin and thereby its toxicity. For renal transplants 1g is administered orally or intravenously (over 2 hours) twice daily (2 g per day). A higher dose of 3g per day is recommended for cardiac transplant patients.

The principle toxicities of MMF are gastrointestinal and hematologic. These include leucopenia, diarrhea and vomiting. There is also an increased incidence of some infections, especially sepsis associated with cytomegalo virus. Tacrolimus in combination with mycophenolate mofetil has been associated with devastating viral infection including polyoma nephritis.

Tacrolimis also enhances the GI toxicity of mycophenolate mofetil by impairing its elimination.

d. **Other Antiproliferative Drugs,** Many of the cytotoxic and antimetabolic agents used in cancer chemotherapy are immunosuppressive due to their action on lymphocytes and other cells of immune system. They have therefore been tried in prophylaxis for organ transplant rejection with varying success. The most notable among these are cyclophosphamide and methotrexate.

   Cyclophosphamide is a cytotoxic agent with more marked effect on B cell and humoral immunity compared to T cells and cell medicated immunity.

   Traditionally, it is widely used in treatment of vasculitis syndromes like systemic lupus erythematosus and Wegner's granulomatosis as an adjuvant in rheumatoid arthritis and in treatment of variety of malignancies. For the purpose of graft rejection, it has been particularly utilized in bone marrow transplantation in which a short course with high dose is generally given.

   Methotrexate is a folate antagonist which has a marked immunosuppressant effect on cytokine production and cellular immunity. It has been used in graft versus host disease. Its main indications are autoimmune diseases like rapidly progressing rheumatoid arthritis, pemphigus, myasthenia gravis, uveitis and chronic active hepatitis.

IV. Immunosuppressant Antibodies

Antibodies against lymphocyte cell surface antigens have an important role in prevention and treatment of organ transplant rejection. These may be either polyclonal or monoclonal. Polyclonal antibodies have a wide variation in efficacy and toxicity and are generated by repeated injections of human lymphocytes or thymocytes into animals such as horses, rabbits, sheep or goats. On the contrary, monoclonal antibodies are target specific and are generated by a single antibody.[8]

a. **Antithymocyte globulin (ATG):** It is a polyclonal antibody prepared from human thymocytes and is targeted against T-lymphocytes. It is a potent immunosuppressant and has been used primarily to suppress acute allograft rejection episodes, specially in steroid resistant cases. Being polyclonal in nature it can elicit major side effects including fever and chills, hypotension, serum sickness and rarely anaphylaxis.

b. **Muromonab CD3:** This is a murine monoclonal antibody which binds to a glycoprotein (CD3) receptor located on the surface of helper T cells. CD 3 receptor is involved in antigen—recognition which is hampered following association with muromonab CD 3 thereby preventing subsequent cell proliferation and generation of other mediators. Administration of this antibody leads to a rapid disappearance of T lymphocytes from the circulation.

   Muromonab CD3 has been used with considerable efficacy for prevention of acute organ transplant rejection since past three decades although the use has now declined owing to its toxicity and availability of better alternatives. It has been used as an induction therapy together with corticosteroids and azathioprine with delayed use of cyclosporin in "sequential regimen." This serves to postpone the potential nephro and hepatotoxicity of cyclosporin. Muromonab-CD3 has also been found to be useful in steroid resistant rejection episodes.

   The major limitation of its usage is the "cytokine release syndrome" which occurs after the initial dose of this antibody. This is characterized by symptoms such as fever with chills and rigor, headache, tremor, nausea/vomiting, abdominal pain, malaise and generalized weakness. The syndrome has been attributed to the release of cytokines by the activated T cells and can sometimes be fatal leading to pulmonary edema, acute respiratory distress syndrome, arrhythmias, cardiovascular collapse and arrest. It can be prevented by prior administration of glucocorticoids.

Immune Tolerance?–The Future of Transplant Immunology

In 1945, Dr Ray Owen discovered that most dizygotic-twin cattle fetuses had placental anastomosis with each other and shared their blood supply in utero. The cattle maintained a stable mixture of each other's red cells throughout their lives. He noted that, despite having distinctly different blood groups, transfusion between these twins did not cause any transfusion reaction which otherwise does occur between non-twin cattle of different blood groups. This observation opened the gate for a new concept which can have promising implications in transplant immunology—the concept of 'immune tolerance'.[1,11] His observation was furthered by Bellingham and Medawar in 1949 who postulated that the 'age' of the animal at the time of first encounter of the foreign body was the critical factor in determining its responsiveness and hence its recognition of non self antigens. These two researchers along with Medawar's postgraduate student, Leslie Brent, went a step further to show that immune tolerance can be "artificially" induced. They proved that if living cells from the mouse strain CBA were injected into an adult mouse of strain A, some immunologic process destroyed the CBA cells and the A line mouse that received them quickly destroyed any subsequent graft from the same donor strain.

However if CBA cells were injected into A line fetus or new born who was still immunologically immature, the cells and any future graft from the strain A donor was subsequently accepted as well. The three doctors shared the Nobel Prize for this remarkable work.

Immunologic tolerance is a state of immune unresponsiveness specific to a particular antigen or set of antigens induced by previous exposure to that antigen or set. Induction of tolerance is now a primary area of study in transplant immunology.[23] It is being looked upon as a major tool in hands of researchers for achieving the ultimate goal of indefinite graft survival without the need for life long immunosuppressant therapy. Three mechanisms have been postulated for the accomplishment of tolerance:[24]

a. **Clonal Deletion:** The chief mechanism of T-cell tolerance is the deletion of auto-reactive T-cells in thymus gland so that the organism is rendered tolerant to self.[12] Immature T-cells migrate from the bone marrow to the thymus, where they encounter peptides derived from endogenous proteins bound to MHC molecules on thymic epithelial cells. In other words T-cells undergo "education" in thymus so that they do not act against the self antigens in later life.
b. **Clonal Anergy:** As has been stated previously, T-cells require 2 signals to become activated—first by direct stimulation and second by costimulatory molecule via CD 28 and lack of second signal makes them unresponsive. Studies have experimented on the exploitation of this fact for artificial induction of tolerance in animal models by using anti-CD28 antibodies.[11]
c. **Regulatory T-cells:** Over the past 10 years, the approach of the scientific community for achieving the goal of induction of immune tolerance has evolved from that focused on inhibition of T-effector cells to one that involves primarily the promotion of regulatory T-cell (TREG), i.e. the ones with immunosuppressive properties. Although several such types of T-cells have been identified, but fox P3+ regulatory T cells have emerged as dominant ones in this category. They are of prime importance in induction and maintenance of tolerance. It is now believed that the balance between alloantigen-reactive TREG cells and T-effector cells ultimately determines the acceptance or rejection of the graft. Promoting the development and maintenance of regulatory responses via TREG cells, therefore, represents a promising approach for the induction of transplantation tolerance. Although the existence of TREG cells is now undisputable, harnessing them for therapeutic purposes is not a simple process. For example, the local micro-environment in which TREG cells reside can have considerable influence on their functional status. Certain inflammatory cytokines can also render them ineffective. In certain conditions their source can also undergo "reprogramming" thereby converting them into effector T-cells which will on the contrary aid in tissue destruction.

Partial Tolerance

Although researchers have not yet successfully harnessed the benefit of immune tolerance, they have been able to exploit the phenomenon of partial tolerance with reasonable success. This enables a combined use of tolerance mechanism and drug therapy to achieve the goal of adequate immunosuppression without inviting excessive adverse effects of immunosuppressant drugs. Alemtuzumab (campath 1H) in combination with low dose cyclosporine or sirolimus, with O_2 without steroid therapy has been successfully tried in various studies. Long-term results in relation to graft rejection have been found similar to full immunosuppression group.

CLINICAL PEARLS

- Immune system is the primary mechanism responsible for the rejection of any organ transplantation. This can occur within hours or may be after many years. Cell mediated immunity via T-lymphocytes is mainly responsible for graft failure, though other immune mechanisms too have a role to play. The Histocompatibility antigen (HLA) and blood group closeness between the donor and the recipient is a major determinant of graft survival. The HLA system has a major role to play in the phenomenon of rejection through the MHC type I and II complexes. These aid in the sensitization of the CD4 and CD8 cells by the graft antigens. Once sensitized, they initiate a cascade of immune reactions involving proliferation of T-cells, release of mediators such as cytokines, etc. and activation of compliment system. If not timely controlled, these reactions ultimately end up in ischemia and rejection of graft. Humoral immunity mainly acts in acute rejections.

It is therefore of prime importance to suppress this cascade for allowing the acceptance of graft by the host. Various modalities including immunosuppressant drugs are used for achieving this aim. Corticosteroids, cyclosporine, azathioprine, methotrexate, mycophenolate mofetil and antibodies are most notable amongst them. These are used in various combinations and doses but have considerable side effects. Recently the phenominon of immune tolerance has gained much popularity for this purpose. Although its complete exploitation for this purpose is still under research, partial tolerance has been used with considerable success.

REFERENCES

1. Wood KJ. Transplantation tolerance. Curr Opin Immunol, 1991; 3:710-4.
2. Nonovitch GM. Handbook of Kidney Transplantation 2nd edn. Philadelphia, Pa: Lippincott Williams and Wilkins; 1996.
3. Paul WE ed. Fundamental Immunology, 4th edn. Lippincott-Raven, Philadelphia, 1999;586-98.
4. Pattison Jm, Sibley RK, Krenskey AM. Mechanisms of allograft rejection. In Immunologic Renal Disease. (Neilson EG, and Couser WG eds) Lippincot-Raven. Philadelphia, 1997:331-54.
5. Monaco AP, Burke JF Jr, Ferguson RM, Halloran PF, Kahan BD, Light JA, et al. Current thinking on chronic renal allograft rejection: issues, concerns, and recommendations from a 1997 roundtable discussion. Am J Kidney Dis, 1999;33:150-60.
6. Klein J, Sato A. The HLA system. First of two parts. N Engl J Med, 2000;343:702-9.
7. Sayegh MH, Turka LA. The role of T-cell contimulatory activation pathways in transplant rejection. N Engl J Med, 1998;338:1813-21.
8. Steinman L. Immune therapy for autoimmune diseases. Science, 2004;305:212-6.
9. Sathia Thiru, Herman Waldmann. Pathology and immunology of transplantation and rejection. N Engl J Med, 2001;344:1953-4.
10. Rocha PN, Plumb TJ, Crowley SD, Coffman TM. Effector mechanisms in transplant rejection. Immunol Rev, 2003;196:51-64.
11. Clarkson MR, Sayegh MH. T-cell costimulatory pathways in allograft rejection and tolerance. Transplantation, 2008;80:555-13.
12. Jukes JP, Wood KJ, Jones ND. Natural killer Tcells: a bridge to tolerance or pathways to rejection ? Transplantation, 2007;84 (6):679-81.
13. Loupy A, Hill GS, Suberbielle C, Charron D, Anglicheau D, Zuber J, et al. Significance of C4d Banff scores in early protocol biopsies of kidney transplant recipients with preformed donor-specific antibodies (DSA). Am J Transplant, 2011;11:56-65.
14. Clayberger C, Krensky AM. Mechanisms of allograft rejection. In Immunologic Renal Diseases. Neirson EG, Cuser WG (eds.) Lippincot-Raven, Philadelphia, 2001.
15. Denton MD, Magee CC, Sayegh MH. Immunosuppressive strategies in transplantation. Lancet, 1999;353:1083-91.
16. Alloway RR, Isaacs R, Lake K, Hoyer P, First R, Helderman H, et al. Report of the American Society of Transplantation conference on immunosuppressive drugs and the use of generic immunosuppressants. Am J Transplant, 2003;3:1211-5.
17. Jordan SC, Tyan D, Czer L, Toyoda M. Immunomodulatory actions of intravenous immunoglobulin (IVIG): potential applications in solid organ transplant recipients. Pediatr Transplant, 1998;2:92-105.
18. Hardinger KL, Koch MJ, Brenmnan DC. Current and future immunosuppressive strategies in renal transplantation. Pharmacotherapy, 2004;24:1159-76.
19. Krensky AM, Vincenti F, Bennett WM. Immunosuppressants, tilerogens and immunosti mulants. Goodman and Gilman's. The Pharmacological basis of therapeutics 11th edn. McGraw Hill Medical Publishing Division, July 2005:1405-31.
20. Tripathi KD. Immunosuppressants, gene therapy. Essentials of Medical Pharmacology 5th edn. Jaypee Brothers Medical Publishers, 2003:785-92.
21. Hong JC, Kahan BD. Immunosuppressive agents in organ transplantation: past, present, and future. Semin Nephrol, 2000;20: 108-25.
22. Kreis H, Cisterne JM, Land W, Wramner L, Squifflet JP, Abramowicz D, et al. Sirolimus in association with mycophenolate mofetil induction for the prevention of acute graft rejection in renal allograft recipients. Transplantation, 2000;69:1252-60.
23. LaRosa DF, Rahman AH, Turka LA. The innate immune system in llograft rejection and tolerance. J Immunol, 2007;178:7503-9.
24. Starzl Te, Zinkernagel RM. Transplantation tolerance form a historical perspective. Net Rex Immunol, 2001;1:233-9.

6 CHAPTER

Pharmacokinetics and Pharmacodynamics in Transplant Surgery

Raminder Sehgal, Dinesh Gautam

INTRODUCTION

Pharmacokinetics (PK), derived from the Greek word *pharmakon* "drug" and *kinetikos* "to do with motion", is a branch of pharmacology dedicated to the determination of the fate of drugs or substances administered to a living organism. Pharmacokinetics explores what the body does to a specific drug after administration. It includes the study of the mechanisms of absorption and distribution of an administered drug, the rate at which a drug action begins, the duration of the effect, the chemical changes of the substance in the body and routes of excretion of the metabolites of the drug. Pharmacokinetics is often studied in conjunction with pharmacodynamics (PD), which explores what a drug does to the body. It determines the relationship between the drug concentration and drug effect. Together, they aid in establishing patient-specific medication regimens that optimize efficacy and minimize toxicities.

Pharmacokinetics is divided into several areas which include the extent and rate of **A**bsorption, **D**istribution, **M**etabolism and **E**xcretion. This is commonly referred to as the ADME scheme. However, recent understanding about the drug-body interactions brought about the inclusion of new term **L**iberation. Now Pharmacokinetics can be better described as **LADME**.[1]

- **L**iberation, the process of release of drug from the formulation.
- **A**bsorption, the process of a substance entering the blood circulation.
- **D**istribution, dispersion or dissemination of substances throughout the fluids and tissues of the body.
- **M**etabolism, irreversible transformation of parent compounds into daughter metabolites.
- **E**xcretion, the elimination of the substances from the body. In rare cases, some drugs irreversibly accumulate in a tissue in the body.

Since most drugs do not act in the blood, computerized pharmacokinetic and pharmacodynamic models are constructed to describe drug behavior. These models express the relationship between drug dose and concentration (pharmacokinetics) and drug concentration and effect (pharmacodynamics). It is necessary to combine pharmacokinetic and pharmacodynamic models so that plasma concentration can be linked to the effect site concentration and thus drug effect.

Population pharmacokinetics is the study of variability in drug concentrations among individuals receiving clinically relevant doses of a drug. Patient demographic or pathophysiological features such as body weight, excretory and metabolic functions, and concomitant drug therapy, can alter dose-concentration relationships. For example, steady-state concentrations of drugs eliminated mostly by the kidney are usually greater in patients suffering from renal failure than they are in patients with normal renal function receiving the same drug dosage.

Pharmacokinetic properties of drugs may be affected by elements such as the site of administration, the dose and the concentration in which the drug is administered. Moreover, there is inter-individual variability in drug response. Pharmacokinetics is also affected by end stage renal and hepatic disease which alter the bioavailability, volume of distribution, protein binding and clearance of drugs. In addition, the effect of anesthetic drugs on the hepatico-renal and peripheral circulation and fluid shifts during surgery alter the drug disposition and response.

PHARMACOTHERAPEUTIC IMPLICATIONS OF KIDNEY FAILURE

Chronic kidney disease (CKD) influences drug disposition through changes in several pharmacokinetic parameters which are both drug and patient specific and cannot be easily assessed. It is further complicated by polypharmacy required to treat the related comorbidities, making these

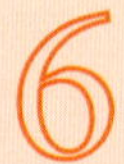

patients prone to drug toxicity and drug interactions. It is important to understand the alterations in pharmacokinetic and pharmacodynamic parameters in patients with kidney failure, so that appropriate selection of the medication and its dosing is ensured for optimal patient outcome.

Absorption

The bioavailability of orally administered drugs may be influenced by several physiologic changes in the gastrointestinal tract, which are commonly seen in the CKD population.[2] These changes include:

- *Gastroparesis*, which may prolong the time to reach maximum drug concentration, although this delay does not affect the overall absorption.
- *Increased gastric pH* is a common manifestation of CKD, and it results from ammonia formation in the gut, secondary to conversion of salivary urea by urease enzyme. In addition, these patients are often given phosphate binders, oral antacids, H_2 receptor antagonists and proton pump inhibitors which also alter the gastric pH. Thus with increase in gastric pH, the bioavailability of drugs which are best absorbed in acidic pH (frusemide, ferrous sulfate) is decreased, and that of weakly acid molecules (glipizide, tolbutamide) is increased.[3]
- *Bowel wall edema* has also been cited as a potential cause of diminished oral absorption in CKD patients.
- *Decreased activity of cytochrome P-450 (CYP450) and P-glycoprotein* in the intestines reduces intestinal metabolism of drugs and increases their systemic concentration. As higher quantity of drug reaches the portal circulation from the gut, a larger percentage undergoes first-pass biotransformation in the liver.

Distribution

Plasma drug concentration is a representation of volume of distribution as well as protein and tissue binding.

Volume of distribution (V_d) quantifies the drug distribution in blood and different body tissues. It is a function of total volume of the tissues into which the drug distributes and their average affinity for that drug. CKD-induced changes in body composition, such as increased total body water and adipose tissue, and decreased muscle mass can have profound effect on the distribution of drugs. Excessive fluid retention, manifesting as increased extracellular fluid volume or ascites, increases the V_d of hydrophilic drugs (morphine, codeine) thereby reducing their serum concentration. On the contrary, muscle wasting and increased adipose tissue may reduce V_d and increase serum concentration of hydrophilic medications.

Alteration in protein binding in patients with CKD occurs due to low serum albumin, predominantly due to hypoalbuminemia. Acidic drugs (phenytoin, frusemide, salicylates) are bound to albumin and their serum concentration is likely to be high after a normal dose. Alkaline drugs (propranolol, morphine, oxazepam) are bound to alpha 1-acid glycoprotein whose plasma concentration is often elevated in CKD.[4] The serum concentration of these drugs may be reduced or may remain unchanged. Altered tissue binding may also affect the V_d especially in the case of digoxin where the V_d is reduced by half in stage-5 CKD.

Metabolism

Renal dysfunction significantly alters biotransformation of drugs.[2] Phase I hydrolysis and reduction reactions are slowed and CYP450 mediated oxidative reactions are altered.[5] Phase II reactions are also altered and therefore acetylation (procainamide, hydralazine), glucuronidation (morphine, lorazepam, oxazepam), sulfation (dopamine, acetaminophen) and methylation (dobutamine, dopamine) are all slowed in patients with CKD. Slowed phase I and II reactions result in increased serum drug concentrations.[2]

Kidney also serves as a site for drug metabolism with most of the metabolic enzymes located in the renal cortex. It has approximately 15% of metabolic function of the liver.[2] Drugs metabolized in the kidney include acetaminophen, insulin, morphine, meperidine, oxytocin, salicylic acid and vasopressin. Reduction in the overall metabolic rate in CKD also increases the drug concentration.

Elimination

Renal excretion of drugs depends upon the glomerular filtration rate (GFR), renal tubular secretion and reabsorption. In CKD, the medication eliminated by glomerular filtration is decreased, resulting in prolonged free drug elimination half life. Normally there is increased renal tubular secretion of protein bound drugs, but this is also decreased in CKD as is the reabsorption from the distal portion of the nephrons. Biological and toxic metabolites of the medications which are excreted by the kidneys are also affected. Active metabolites of midazolam and pethidine accumulate in patients with CKD.[2]

Generally, higher the contribution of kidney to the drug elimination, greater will be the effect of CRF on the drug elimination. For most medications, when kidney clearance accounts for less than 30% of total body clearance, kidney dysfunction has negligible effect on total body clearance. For others, renal dysfunction may induce an overexposure after a single administration and accumulation after repeated administrations. Use of too small a dose may result in suboptimal pharmacodynamic reponse and ultimately treatment failure.

PHARMACODYNAMICS IN RENAL FAILURE

Patients with end stage renal disease show sensitivity to nonsteroidal anti-inflammatory drugs (NSAIDs) probably due to inhibition of permissive prostaglandin dependent renal function. They also show greater toxicity to aminoglycosides.[6] Induction dose of propofol needed to achieve a BIS of 50 is reported to be 40–60% higher in patients with end stage renal disease (ESRD).[7] These patients also show increased sensitivity to vecuronium.[8]

DRUG DOSING IN END STAGE KIDNEY DISEASE

Drugs are usually administered in a dose adequate to achieve therapeutic serum drug concentration. However, in patients with ESRD it is difficult to predict the effect of a given dose due to changes in pharmacokinetics and pharmacodynamics. Normally recommended dose may result in higher drug concentrations with potential for toxicities. Therefore, in these patients the dose of the drugs should be adjusted to achieve an appropriate free drug concentration. The following rules should be considered while administering drugs to a patient with renal disease:

Adjust the Dose only When Required

Dose adjustment should only be considered when at least 70% of the drug is excreted by kidney, either unchanged or as an active metabolite. It is also required when it has a narrow therapeutic window or is metabolized by the kidney.

Estimate the Glomerular Filtration Rate

Dose adjustment is generally based on the presumption that only the renal clearance is changed and other factors like absorption, protein binding and pharmacodynamics are unaltered. Glomerular filteration rate generally correlates with the renal elimination of most medications. A rapid assessment of the GFR may be possible using plasma clearance of creatinine. However, calculations should not be based on plasma concentration of creatinine as its relationship with GFR is not linear.

Choose An Adequate Dosing Strategy

Loading dose is usually administered as a bolus or short infusion at the beginning of treatment to obtain rapid therapeutic concentration. Its duration of action depends upon redistribution and not elimination. Therefore, if the steady state V_d and the bioavailability are unchanged, the loading dose in CKD patients is same as in healthy individuals. However, the dose may need to be increased if the V_d is increased, as in patients with ascites and edema, or decreased in dehydrated patients.[2] The loading dose can be omitted if immediate pharmacological activity is not urgently required.

Maintenance dose is administered by a repeat dose or prolonged infusion to achieve steady state plasma concentration after the loading dose, or when pharmacological activity is not urgent. The duration of action of the maintenance dose depends upon elimination by the kidney and therefore needs to be reduced in ESRD. Two methods can be used to administer maintenance dose in patients with renal dysfunction: reducing the dose or increasing the dosing interval.

- *The dose reduction method* involves reducing the individual dose while maintaining normal dose intervals. This method achieves more constant drug concentration but is associated with higher risk of adverse events. It is appropriate when the dosing interval is less than the elimination half life and the drug has low therapeutic index and has time dependant activity.
- *The expanded interval method* involves giving the standard dose but at an increased interval, to account for the CKD induced delay in drug excretion. This method is useful when the drug has concentration dependent activity, broad therapeutic window and long half life.

When using any of these methods, the risks of subtherapeutic serum concentration must be weighed against the risk of adverse events. Combining the two approaches may be necessary to optimize medication efficacy.

Monitor Concentration of Drugs

In case a drug has a narrow therapeutic index, the plasma concentration of the drugs may need to be monitored at regular intervals especially when the renal disease is progressing, there is an adverse event or a therapeutic failure occurs. This increases the cost of treatment and the patient needs to be hospitalized for frequent blood sampling.

Drug Dosing in Patients on Hemodialysis (HD)

The impact of hemodialysis on drug removal depends on the drug characteristics, dialysis filter used and the constitution of the dialysis fluid. The mechanism of drug removal involves diffusion or convection. Drugs which are water soluble, are not highly protein bound, have a small V_d and low molecular weight are more likely to be removed by hemodialysis.[9] Increasing the hydrostatic pressure gradient across the dialysis membrane and using a more permeable dialysis filter maximizes drug removal by HD.

PHARMACOTHERAPEUTIC IMPLICATIONS OF LIVER DISEASE

Liver is a key organ for drug disposition and elimination because it receives all parenterally as well as the orally administered drugs via the systemic or the portal system. These drugs undergo enzymatic degradation for ultimate excretion by the kidney. The impact of liver disease on drug disposition depends upon the severity of the hepatic dysfunction. Drug elimination is more affected by parenchymal dysfunction than by biliary obstructive disease.

Absorption

Orally ingested drugs which are well absorbed from the gut and are extensively metabolized in the liver have low availability due to high first-pass effect. With liver disease, their extraction and metabolism is compromised resulting in drug accumulation in the plasma.

Distribution

Volume of distribution is increased in end stage liver disease due to fluid retention and the presence of ascites, thereby altering the serum drug concentration.

Protein binding of drugs is also altered in liver disease through its synthesis of drug binding proteins. Thus the systemic availability of most oral or parenterally administered drugs is affected. In liver disease, the serum albumin levels are low and there is decrease in binding affinity for albumin, thereby shifting the dose-response curve to the left. As a result there is increased availability of acidic drugs. On the other hand the $alpha_1$ glycoprotein levels increase, thereby enhancing the binding of basic drugs and reducing their bioavailability.

Metabolism

The liver is an important site for drug metabolism. Both phase 1 and phase 2 reactions alter the drug in such a manner that its elimination by renal or biliary mechanism is facilitated. Phase 1 reactions involve P-450 isoenzyme and are more affected by the liver disease than phase 2 reactions.[6] Thus oxidation is impaired in hepatic disease whereas glucuronidation is relatively spared, probably due to extrahepatic glucuronidation and glucuronidating reserves. Therefore, glucuronides are preferred in patients with liver disease. However, with severe hepatic dysfunction, all detoxifying mechanisms are impaired.

In patients undergoing liver transplant, perioperative drug metabolism depends upon the pre, intra and post transplant liver functions, the amount of blood loss, hemodynamic stability and the anesthetic agents that are used. Intraoperative metabolism is also affected by the surgical phase, i.e. the prehepatic, the anhepatic and the posthepatic phase. It is also important to know if the patient is undergoing transplant for chronic liver disease or fulminant hepatic failure.

The Preanhepatic Phase

Drug metabolism in preanhepatic phase is affected by the preexisting liver dysfunction and the effects of anesthesia. The intraoperative drug metabolism and clearance is affected directly by the anesthetic drugs or indirectly by hypotension or hypoxia.[6] Surgical manipulation of the bowel and liver also decrease the blood supply to the liver. Reduced blood supply affects the clearance of high extraction (flow dependent) drugs. The low extraction, flow-independent drugs are also affected, as reduced blood flow causes hepatic hypoxia which in turn affects oxidative metabolism. Halothane impairs hepatic function, blood flow and oxygen supply more than any other inhalational anesthetic and therefore is not used for transplant anesthesia. Compared to other anesthetics, isoflurane and fentanyl are the preferred drugs during liver transplant as they minimize hepatic ischemic injury and optimize hepatic oxygen supply and demand. It is also important to remember that a large amount of drug is lost due to heavy blood loss and this is difficult to quantitate. Usually, the initial or the top up dose of the medication needs to be individualized based on hemodynamic and other parameters. Deranged renal functions also necessitate dosage adjusments.

The Anhepatic Phase

No hepatic metabolism occurs during the anhepatic phase but some metabolism does occur at the extrahepatic sites. Though not clinically important, metabolites of midazolam, morphine and propofol have been found during this phase.[10,11] The oxygen consumption also decreases during this period, to increase once reperfusion takes place. If any drug is administered during this period, the dose should be reduced as liver contains only 15% of the normal blood volume.

The Postanhepatic Phase

In this phase, there is reperfusion of the transplanted liver and the metabolism of drugs will depend upon the function of new liver. The metabolic enzymes are sensitive to hypoxia and sensitivity of an individual enzyme to low oxygen varies. The normal liver oxygen level is only 2–3 times the KmO_2 (the concentration of oxygen at which the activity of the enzyme is half normal).[6] Even moderate hypoxia due to hemodynamic instability prior to liver harvesting, the quality and duration of organ preservation and the quality of donor and recipient surgery is likely to affect the function of oxidative enzymes. Oxidative reactions are more likely to be affected, probably because oxidation reactions occur mostly in pericentral areas which tend to be more hypoxic. The conjugation reactions and sulfation is more resistant than glucuronidation.

Drug Elimination

Clearance of drugs by the liver depends on the hepatic blood flow, the intrinsic ability of the liver to extract the drug from the blood and the protein binding. The *intrinsic clearance* reflects the fraction of drug load that is metabolized or extracted during a single pass through the liver. The high clearance drugs like lignocaine are metabolized so efficiently that their hepatic clearance is determined by the liver blood flow (flow dependent). The low clearance drugs like diazepam are independent of the blood flow and depend upon the metabolizing capacity of liver for elimination (capacity dependent).[12] Liver disease decreases the intrinsic clearance of most drugs and prolongs their half life. In other words even high clearance drugs behave like low clearance drugs.

In hepatic disease, the drugs eliminated by the liver accumulate over time. Their dosage should be reduced to avoid drug accumulation and possible toxicity. For the drugs removed via the bile without prior biotransformation, the excretion will by governed by the degree of intrahepatic cholestasis. A normally functioning kidney is important to excrete drugs after biotransformation in the liver and may serve as a safety valve when the liver function is compromised. Total body clearance and the renal clearance are relatively easy to measure, but there are no predictive tests available for hepatic drug clearance. It can be measured indirectly as the difference in total and renal clearance.

PHARMACODYNAMICS IN LIVER DISEASE

In addition to altered pharmacokinetics, the patients with hepatic disease also have altered pharmacodynamics. They exhibit greater end-organ sensitivity to various drugs, especially those affecting the central nervous system, independent of altered pharmacokinetics. The cerebral uptake of benzodiazepines increases significantly probably due to a leaky blood-brain barrier. At equal plasma concentration of diazepam, the EEG changes are more pronounced in patients with liver disease than in healthy individuals. Sedatives and analgesics are also known to precipitate encephalopathy in patients with hepatic failure.[13] The mechanism of this sensitivity is not known but may be due to sensitization of the γ-aminobutyric acid (GABA) supramolecular complex to endogenous benzodiazepine like compounds.[14] Another explanation may be the summation of subliminal sedative influences.[6] Nonsteroidal anti-inflammatory analgesic induced renal failure and resistance to loop diuretics has also been reported in patients with liver failure and ascites.[15]

DRUG DOSING IN HEPATIC FAILURE

Drug dosing in hepatic failure is particularly challenging because there is no simple test to quantify liver function. Tests to detect hepatocellular damage or the synthetic function do not reflect the ability of liver to metabolize drugs. Drugs having high hepatic extraction have increased bioavailability and decreased clearance and for those having low hepatic extraction, bioavailability is unaltered but clearance is decreased. Drugs that are metabolized by oxidation (diazepam, alprazolam) have reduced clearance and are likely to accumulate, whereas those which are glucoronidated are better metabolized.

When developing a dose plan for patients with liver failure, it is best to choose agents which are not metabolized by the liver (cisatracurium rather than vecuronium) or have shorter duration of action (lorazepam rather than diazepam). Lower dose of midazolam should be used preoperatively as increased free drug fraction resulting from decreased protein binding and decreased clearance will increase its cerebral effects. Drugs that have high hepatic extraction and are administered orally, the initial and maintenance dose should be reduced. When these drugs are administered intravenously, only the maintenance dose should be reduced. It is unnecessary to adjust initial doses of drugs that have low hepatic extraction regardless of the route of administration, but the maintenace dose should be reduced, generally to 50% of the recommended.[16]

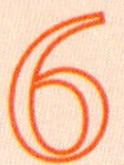

POST-TRANSPLANT PHARMACOKINETIC CONSIDERATIONS

Metabolism and excretion of the drugs after kidney or liver transplant depends upon the function of the transplanted organ. Both oxidative and conjugative drug-metabolizing abilities of the transplanted liver are similar to normal controls in stable patients. Ischemia, infection or rejection of the transplanted liver will impair drug metabolism. Although most drugs do not interact with cyclosporine or tacrolimus, certain drugs like dexamethasone and phenobarbitone may induce cyclosporine oxidase to decrease the blood levels of cyclosporine and thus have the potential to reduce immunosuppression and increase the risk of organ rejection.[6] On the other hand ketoconazole and diltiazem inhibit the enzyme and increase cyclosporine levels and thus have the potential to cause nephrotoxicity.

PHARMACOKINETICS OF INDIVIDUAL DRUGS

Induction Agents

Barbiturates: Both thiopentone and methohexitone are metabolized in the liver to water soluble, inactive metabolites which are excreted by the kidneys. They are highly bound to albumin and their blood concentration is elevated due to decreased albumin in chronic liver and kidney disease.[17] Moreover, the unionized fraction increases in acidosis leading to larger amount reaching the brain. It has a small hepatic extraction ratio, therefore its elimination half life is unchanged. In patients with cirrhosis of liver, clearance from plasma was no different from that in normal patients and therefore a single dose is unlikely to have a prolonged effect.[18] Lower initial dose may be needed if there is hypoalbuminemia. On the other hand higher dose may be required if the volume of distribution is increased due to edema and ascites associated with chronic kidney and liver disease. Therefore, in clinical use the induction dose should be reduced and the amount titrated based on hemodynamics and other clinical parameters.

Propofol is rapidly metabolized in the liver by cytochrome P-450 to water soluble metabolites which are excreted by the kidneys. However, kinetic studies after induction and maintenance with propofol have shown no major alteration in terminal half-life or clearance in cirrhosis or chronic renal failure patients.[19, 20] The plasma protein binding of propofol is not significantly affected by end-stage renal disease.[21] An increase in the induction dose of propofol has been observed in patients with end-stage renal disease, which has been attributed to increased cardiac output accompanying the anemia seen in renal failure.[8] Infusions of propofol have also been used for maintenance of anesthesia for renal transplantation prolonged infusions of propofol may cause excretion of green urine because of the presence of phenols in the urine, but this discoloration does not affect renal function. In patients with cirrhosis, the volume of distribution for propofol is reported to increase but the clearance is not reduced significantly and its elimination half life is also not prolonged.[22] Extra-hepatic elimination of propofol is reported to occur during the anhepatic phase of liver transplantation.[20]

Ketamine has a high hepatic extraction ratio and alterations in hepatic blood flow may influence its clearance rate. It is metabolized in the liver and its water soluble metabolites are excreted by the kidneys. Elimination of the metabolites of ketamine, especially the active norketamine and glucuronide conjugates is reduced in patients with ESRD.[23] It causes increase in heart rate and blood pressure, which may be deleterious in a patient with pre-existing hypertension or coronary artery disease, commonly associated with patients with end-stage renal disease. Therefore it is best avoided for induction of anesthesia for transplantation.

Etomidate has moderate lipid solubility and exists as a weak base (pK 4.2). It is 76% bound to albumin and therefore decrease in plasma albumin concentration as seen in hepatic and renal disease will dramatically increase the unbound, pharmacologically active fraction in the plasma. It has a high hepatic extraction ratio and in patients with cirrhosis, its volume of distribution is doubled but the clearance is normal, resulting in elimination half life being twice normal.[24] Its cardiostable action is useful in patients who are hypovolemic or hypertensive. It causes adrenocortical suppression but this effect is short lived and is of no consequence in transplant patients receiving hydrocortisone for immunosuppression.

Neuromuscular Blocking Drugs

Neuromuscular blockers are ionized, water soluble drugs and their kinetics and dynamics are significantly altered in end stage renal and hepatic disease, either due to decreased elimination of the drug or its metabolites by these organs or by decreased activity of cholinesterase. Most of them are <50% protein bound and therefore the decrease in serum albumin seen in end stage kidney and liver disease does not affect the drug availability. However, higher initial dose may be required due to increased volume of distribution seen in end stage kidney and liver disease. In uremic patients undergoing transplant surgery, the neuromuscular block may also be potentiated by hypokalemia, hypocalcemia and hypermagnesemia.

The duration of action of *depolarizing neuromuscular blocking drug, succinylcholine*, is prolonged due to decrease in the level as well as decrease in the activity of pseudocholinesterase, both in ESRD and in liver failure. However this prolongation is not clinically significant unless large dose of the drug is given by prolonged infusion. The pseudocholinesterase levels return to normal with adequate allograft function. Another problem with the use of succinylcholine in ESRD is related to increase in serum potassium concentrations. Succinylcholine causes a rapid but transient increase of 0.5 mEq/L in the serum potassium concentration. However, the increase in potassium levels in patients on hemodialysis has been found to be comparable with that seen in normal healthy subjects.[25] Succinylcholine can be safely used as long as the patient is on hemodialysis and the serum potassium is less than 5.5 mmol/L.[26] Pretreatment with nondepolarizing neuromuscular blocking drugs prevents the muscle fasciculations but not the increase in serum potassium.[27] Repeated doses or infusion of succinylcholine should be avoided in patients with chronic kidney disease. For a rapid-sequence intubation in renal transplant recipients, succinylcholine remains the drug of choice in the absence of hyperkalemia. However, in patients with hyperkalemia rocuronium offers an alternative.

The choice of *non-depolarizing neuromuscular blocking drug* for kidney or liver transplant will largely depend on the extent of their elimination from these organs. Amongst the older drugs, *d-tubocurarine, gallamine, pancuronium* and amongst the newer drugs *pipecuronium* and *doxacurium* are excreted unchanged by the kidneys to a large extent. They show significant alteration in their dynamics in renal disease with prolonged duration of action, and therefore are not recommended for patients undergoing renal transplant.

Vecuronium depends more on the liver rather than the kidney for its elimination and therefore its clearance is decreased and elimination half life is increased in hepatic disease. The duration of effect from injection to 50% recovery is reported to increase by 100%.[28] Renal failure also causes prolongation of its effect probably due to accumulation of the parent drug as well as its desacetyl metabolites which have 80% potency of the parent drug.[29] Therefore complete reversal of neuromuscular paralysis should be ensured if multiple increments or an infusion of vecuronium has been used in patients undergoing renal or hepatic transplant. Patients with renal failure also demonstrate tolerance to vecuronium and atracurium as they have higher plasma concentration at 25% and 75% recovery.[30]

Rocuronium is a steroid molecule and is primarily metabolized in the liver and only 10% of the unchanged drug is recovered from the urine. Therefore, its onset and duration of action and recovery is prolonged in patients with hepatic failure but is not much affected in patients undergoing renal transplant.[31] It can safely be used as an alternative to succinylcholine for rapid-sequence intubation and for maintenance of neuromuscular block in patients with impaired renal functions.

Rapacuronium is another steroidal muscle relaxant with rapid onset and short duration of action. In a dose of 1.5–2.5 mg/kg, complete block occurs in 60–90 seconds with 25% recovery of first ‘train of four’ twitch occurring at 13–25 minutes. Its duration of action can be prolonged in renal disease probably due to accumulation of active metabolites.[32]

Atracurium and *cisatracurium* have organ independent mode of elimination and therefore their clearance is not affected by end stage renal or hepatic disease. Hofmann elimination and ester hydrolysis account for 50% of atracurium and 70% of cisatracurium clearance. Laudanosine, the principal metabolite of atracurium, depends upon hepatic function for elimination and can accumulate in hepatic and renal failure, but the concentration is not significant in clinical settings.[33] *Mivacurium*, a short acting muscle relaxant is also metabolized by the plasma esterases as well as in the liver. Its kinetics are not much altered in renal or hepatic disease.[34]

Anticholinesterases

Pharmacokinetics of anticholinesterases is affected by renal failure as they are excreted through kidney by glomerular filtration and tubular secretion. Renal excretion accounts for 50% of excretion of *neostigmine* and 75% of that of *pyridostigmine* and *edrophonium* and is delayed in ESRD.[35] As the reduction in plasma clearance of anticholinesterases exceeds that of long acting neuromuscular blocking drugs, there is no risk of recurarization in patients undergoing renal transplant.

Anticholinergic Drugs

About 20 to 50 percent of *atropine* and *glycopyrrolate* are eliminated by the kidneys in the unchanged form or in the form of active metabolites.[36] As these agents are usually administered only as single doses, accumulation with toxic side effects is unlikely. Only one-tenth as much scopolamine is recovered from urine as atropine. However, because of its untoward central nervous system effects, scopolamine should not be substituted for atropine or glycopyrrolate when large or repeated doses of an antimuscarinic agent are required. Single dose of scopolamine is satisfactory as a premedicant for patients with renal failure.

Benzodiazepines

Benzodiazepines are extensively metabolized in the liver before excretion by the kidney and their kinetics and dynamics are altered in patients with acute liver or renal failure. They are extensively protein bound and due to low serum albumin the free unbound fraction of the drug increases. *Diazepam* and *alprazolam* which are metabolized by oxidation have reduced clearance and are likely to accumulate in liver failure. On the other hand *lorazepam* and *temazepam* which are glucoronidated are metabolized better in these patients. The free unbound drug fraction of diazepam increases from 1.4% to 7.9% in renal failure, and due to this the apparent volume of distribution and systemic clearance is increased.[37]

Midazolam is metabolized by phase I oxidation and then by phase II conjugation. Due to decrease in oxidative metabolism in liver disease it has decreased clearance and prolonged elimination.[6] The free unbound fraction of midazolam increases in liver and renal failure but there is no difference in the unbound drug kinetics and the elimination half-life. In patients with impaired renal function, there is no correlation between onset time of midazolam sedation and the free drug fraction, probably due to inherent alterations in drug sensitivity in the uremic patients.[27] Because the increased free fraction of unbound drug is rapidly distributed to the richly vascularized tissues, it is probably advisable to give intravenous midazolam slowly, titrating dose to effect. Patients with liver failure also show increased sensitivity to midazolam and therefore its dose should be reduced during anesthesia.[6]

Opioids

All opioids are metabolized in the liver and are excreted by the kidney, either unchanged or through their metabolites. In addition, upto 40% of *morphine* is also metabolized in the kidney by conjugation. It undergoes glucuronidation to morphine-3-glucuronide and the morphine-6-glucuronide which accumulate in patients with renal failure and cause severe respiratory and cardiovascular depression.[38] The pharmacokinetics of *pethidine* is also altered in hepatic and renal failure. It is mainly metabolized in the liver with only 1 to 5% excreted unchanged in the urine. When repeated doses of pethidine are given to patients in chronic renal failure, its N-methylated metabolite, norpethidine accumulates. It has half the analgesic activity of the parent drug but its central nervous system excitatory effects may cause convulsions.[39] In patients with hepatic failure, all narcotics can precipitate hepatic encephalopathy irrespective of their pharmacokinetics. Therefore, their dose should be reduced if given by oral or parenteral route.[6]

The clinical pharmacology of *fentanyl, alfentanil and sufentanil* is not grossly altered by hepatic or renal failure. Although they are extensively metabolized in the liver, only a small fraction of each of these three phenylpiperidine derivatives is excreted unchanged, and their metabolites are inactive. They have the advantage of causing little change in hemodynamics, hepatic blood flow and oxygenation. There is wide variability in the clearance of these drugs due to variable loss of synthetic and detoxifying function of the liver in patients awaiting transplant.[6] They are given in usual dose during induction and later titrated to the effect. An increased clinical effect is likely with alfentanil in renal failure because of a decreased initial volume of distribution and an increased free fraction of alfentanil.[40] However, recovery is not delayed after alfentanil administration.

Remifentanil is a piperidine derivative which does not depend on liver and kidneys for its metabolism or elimination, but rather on plasma and tissue nonspecific esterase hydrolysis. Thus, neither the pharmacokinetics nor the pharmacodynamics of remifentanil are altered by impaired hepatic or renal functions.[41, 42] Its kinetics do not change even during the anhepatic phase of liver transplant.[43] Although the renal elimination of its principal metabolite is reduced, it is of no clinical significance.[42]

Inhalational Anesthetic Agents

Volatile anesthetic agents affect the liver and the kidney functions by reducing the cardiac output and blood flow or by producing toxic metabolites.[27] *Halothane* is not recommended for organ transplant as it is associated with 'halothane hepatitis'.[44] The incidence of liver injury with other inhaled anesthetic agents is in the order, *enflurane* > *isoflurane* > *desflurane*, and correlates with the extent of their oxidative metabolism.[45] Both *isoflurane* and *desflurane* are used for liver transplant as they are minimally metabolized (0.2% and 0.01% respectively). *Sevoflurane* does not metabolize to form acetyl halide and therefore does not produce immune-mediated hepatotoxicity or causes cross sensitivity in patients exposed to halothane.[46] Moreover its metabolites are less reactive and therefore less injurious to the liver. Both isoflurane and sevoflurane preserve hepatic circulation and oxygen delivery whereas desflurane reduces it to some extent.

All inhalational anesthetics produce dose related reduction in GFR, renal blood flow, and urine output, probably due to their effect on the systemic blood pressure and cardiac output. Post transplant renal functions are not influenced by inhalational anesthetics.[47] *Sevoflurane* produces inorganic fluorides and compound A associated with nephrotoxicity. However, no nephrotoxicity is seen in clinical practice probably because it has low blood gas solubility and is eliminated rapidly from the body.[27] Fresh gas flow is an important determinant of compound 'A' levels in clinical practice. The key factor for nephrotoxicity produced by sevoflurane is the total exposure to the drug rather than its concentration. Even though the renal changes seen are transient, it is not recommended in patients with preexisting renal disease.

Desflurane is highly stable and does not undergo breakdown either by the liver or by contact with sodalime. The safety of desflurane has been confirmed in patients with renal failure.[48] There is no absolute contraindication to the use of *nitrous oxide* in transplant anesthesia, but it may cause bowel distension in prolonged procedures. This is important in children undergoing renal transplant with adult size kidney.[27]

Analgesics

Nonsteroidal anti-inflammatory analgesics (NSAIDs) are not recommended for use in patients undergoing hepatic or renal transplant as they cause worsening of volume status, hyperkalemia and hyponatremia.[6, 27] They cause hepatic toxicity and precipitate reversible renal failure. Their effect on the kidney is caused by the action of NSAIDs on the prostaglandin synthesis, which is important for renal blood flow and glomerular filtration rate autoregulation. Inhibition of prostaglandin can lead to excessive vasoconstriction and decrease in the renal blood flow.[49] Few drugs in this group (*salicylates, naproxen*) are highly bound to plasma albumin and therefore will present more unbound drug for action on target organ in end stage liver and kidney disease. They are extensively metabolized in the liver and only small percentage of NSAIDs are excreted unchanged by the kidney. However there is evidence of reduced clearance of *ketoprofen* and *naproxen* in renal failure.[27] They also promote gastrointestinal bleeding and this can be detrimental in patients with underlying portal hypertension.

Acetaminophen is recommended in patients with renal and mild to moderate liver disease as it is metabolized by conjugation with very minor oxidation. In severe hepatic failure where conjugation is also affected and where there has been chronic ethanol intake, there is formation of toxic metabolites.[6] COX-2 inhibitors have similar renal effects as conventional NSAIDs.[2]

Antacids and Prokinetic Drugs

The H_2-receptor antagonists, such as *cimetidine* and *ranitidine* are primarily excreted by the kidneys and with well compensated cirrhosis, their elimination remains unchanged. However, with severe liver or kidney damage, there is decreased elimination of these drugs and their dose should be reduced in these patients. Their accumulation though well tolerated, may cause central nervous system irritability in patients with severe liver damage.[6] Proton-pump inhibitors, such as *omeprazole*, *lansaprazole* and *rabeprazole*, are metabolized in the liver through cytochrome P-450 enzyme and their removal is significantly reduced in liver damage but is largely unaltered in end-stage renal disease.[6, 27]

Metoclopramide is eliminated via the kidneys, 20% in the unchanged form and rest as metabolites. The elimination half-life after intravenous or oral administration is dose-dependent. In patients with end-stage renal disease, there is a significant reduction in its clearance, and there is prolongation of its terminal half-life from 2.8 hours to 13.9 hours.[50] In patients maintained on hemodialysis, altered kinetics of metoclopramide after single doses of 10 mg, produced significant side effects like drowsiness, restlessness, and diarrhea.[51] Hemodialysis does not affect metoclopramide elimination from the body, and clearance of the drug after dialysis is unaltered.

CLINICAL PEARLS

Most drugs used in the perioperative period are metabolized in the liver to active or inactive water soluble metabolites, to be excreted via bile or the urine. End stage liver or the renal disease alters the pharmacokinetics of drugs by increasing the volume of distribution, decreasing protein binding and decreasing enzymes for metabolism of drugs. In addition pharmacodynamics also get altered independent of pharmacokinetics. Solid organ transplant, especially liver transplant are complex surgical procedures which significantly influence the pharmacokinetics and pharmacodynamics of various drugs by altering body internal environment. The changes in the blood volume due to losses and fluid therapy, the effect of organ failure and finally the function of the transplanted organ affects drug dosing and their effect. Anesthesiologists should be familiar with the unique PK and PD changes that occur in patients undergoing renal or liver transplant to achieve effective drug concentration at the site of action while minimizing undesirable side effects.

REFERENCES

1. Retrieved from "http://en.wikipedia.org/wiki/Pharmacokinetics" last modified on 30 June 2010 at 06:21.
2. Gabardi S, Abramson S. Drug dosing in chronic kidney disease. Med Clin N Am, 2005;89:649-87.

3. Gugler R, Allgayer H. Effect of antacids on the clinical pharmacokinetics of drugs: an update. Clin Pharmacokinet, 1990;18:210-9.
4. Lam YW, Banerji S, Hatfield C, Talbert RL. Principles of drug administration in renal insufficiency. Clin Pharmacokinet, 1997; 32:30-57.
5. Swan SK, Bennett WM. Drug dosing guidelines in patients with renal failure. West J Med, 1992;156:633-8.
6. Speeg KV, Halff GA, Schenker S. Metabolism of drugs before and after liver transplantation. In: Maddrey WC, Schiff ER, Sorrel MF. (eds). Transplantation of the Liver. 3rd edn. Lippincott William and Wilkins. Philadelphia, 2001;12:177-97.
7. Goyal P, Puri GD, Pandey CK, Srivastva S. Evaluation of induction doses of propofol: comparison between end-stage renal disease and normal renal function patients. Anaesth Intensive Care, 2002;30:584-7.
8. Sakamoto H, Takita K, Kemmotsu O, Morimoto Y, Mayumi T. Increased sensitivity to vecuronium and prolonged duration of its action in patients with end-stage renal failure. J Clin Anesth, 2001;13:193-97.
9. Bugge JF. Influence of renal replacement therapy on pharmacokinetics in critically ill patients. Best Pract Res Clin Anaesthesiol, 2004;18:175-87.
10. Bodenham A, Quinn K, Park G. Extrahepatic morphine metabolism in man during the anhepatic phase of orthoptic liver transplant. Br J Anaesth, 1989;63:380-4.
11. Veroli P, O'Kelly B, Bertrand F, Trouvin JH, Farinotti R, Ecoffey C. Extra-hepatic metabolism of propofol in man during the anhepatic phase of orthoptic liver transplantation. Br J Anaesth, 1992;68:183-6.
12. Sear JW, Hutton P, The Liver. In: Hutton P, Cooper GM, James FM, Butterworth J, (editors). Fundamental Principles and practice of Anaesthesia. Martin Dunitz Ltd. London, 2002;28:525-40.
13. Rodighiero V. Effects of liver disease on pharmacokinetics: an update. Clin Pharmacokinet, 1998;37:399-431.
14. Bakti G, Fisch HU, Karlaganis G, Minder C, Bircher J. Mechanisms of the excessive sedative response of cirrhotics to benzodiazepines: model experiments with triazolam. Hepatology, 1987;7:629-38.
15. Delcò F, Tchambaz L, Schlienger R, Drewe J, Krähenbühl S. Dose adjustments in patients with liver disease. Drug Saf, 2005; 28:529-45.
16. Devlin JW, Barletta JF. Principles of drug dosing in critically ill patients. In: Parrilo JE, Dellinger RP. (eds.) Critical Care Medicine: Principles of Diagnosis and Management in the Adult. 3rd edn. Mosby Elsevier, Philadelphia, 2008;343-76.
17. Burch PG, Stanski DR. Decreased protein binding and thiopental kinetics. Clin Pharmacol Ther, 1982;32:212.
18. Pandele G, Chaux F, Salvadori C, Farinotti M, Duvaldestin P. Thiopental pharmacokinetics in patients with cirrhosis. Anesthesiology, 1983;59:123-6.
19. Ickx B, Cockshott ID, Barvais L, Byttebier G, De Pauw L, Vandesteene A, et al. Propofol infusion for induction and maintenance of anaesthesia in patients with end-stage renal disease. Br J Anaesth, 1998;81(6):854-60.
20. Stoelting RK, Hillier SC. Nonbarbiturate intravenous anesthetics. In: Stoelting RK, Hillier SC (eds). Pharmacology and Physiology in Anesthetic Practice. 4th edn. Lippincott Williams & Wilkins. Philadelphia, 2006;6:155-78.
21. Costela JL, Jiménez R, Calvo R, Suárez E, Carlos R. Serum protein binding of propofol in patients with renal failure or hepatic cirrhosis. Acta Anaesthesiol Scand, 1996;40(6):741-5.
22. Servin F, Cockshott ID, Farinotti R, Haberer JP, Winckler C, Desmonts JM. Pharmacokinetics of the propofol infusions in patients with cirrhosis. Br J Anaesth, 1990;65(2):177-83.
23. Grant IS, Nimmo WS, Clements JA. Pharmacokinetics and analgesic effects of ketamine in man. Br J Anaesth, 1981;53:805-10.
24. Van Beem H, Manger FW, Van Boxtel C, Van Bentem N. Etomidate anaesthesia in patients with cirrhosis of the liver: Pharmacokinetic data. Anaesthesia, 1983;38(Suppl):61-61.
25. Miller RD, Way WL, Hamilton WK, Layzer RB. Succinyl-induced hyperkalemia in patients with renal failure? Anesthesiology, 1972;36:138-41.
26. Thapa S, Brull SJ. Succinylcholine-induced hyperkalemia in patients with renal failure: an old question revisited. Anesth Analg, 2000;9(1):237-41.
27. Sear JW. Anesthesia for patients undergoing renal transplant. In: Morris PJ (eds). Kidney Transplantation–Principles and Practice. 5th edn. 2001;13:184-206.
28. Lebrault C, Berger JL, D'Hollander AA, Gomeni R, Henzel D, Duvaldestin P. Pharmacokinetics and pharmacodynamics of vecuronium (ORG NC 45) in patients with cirrhosis. Anesthesiology, 1985;62(5):601-5.
29. Segredo V, Caldwell JE, Matthay MA, Sharma ML, Gruenke LD, Miller RD. Persistent paralysis in critically ill patients after long-term administration of vecuronium. N Engl J Med, 1992; 327:524-8.
30. Hunter JM, JonesRS, Utting JE. Comparison of vecuronium, atracurium and tubocurarine in normal patients and in patients with no renal function. Br J Anaesth, 1984;56:941-50.
31. Khuenl- Brady KS, Pomaroli A, Puhringer F, Mitterschiffthalr G, Koller J. The use of rocuronium (ORG 9426) in patients with chronic renal failure. Anaesthesia, 1993;48:873-5.
32. Schiere S, Proost JH, Schuriga M, Wierda JMKH. Pharmacokinetics and pharmacokinetic-dynamic relationship between rapacuronium (Org 9487) and its 3-desacetyl metabolite (Org 9488). Anesth Analg, 1999;88:640-7.
33. Hunter JM. Atracurium and laudanosine pharmacokinetics in acute renal failure. Intensive Care Med, 1993;19 Suppl 2:S91-3.
34. Cook DR, Freeman JA, Lai AA, Kang Y, Stiller RL, Aggarwal S, et al. Pharmacokinetics of mivacurium in normal patients and in those with hepatic or renal failure. Br J Anaesth, 1992;69: 580-5.
35. Cronnelly R, Morris RB. Antagonism of neuromuscular blockade. Br J Anaesth, 1982;54(2):183-94.
36. Kirvela M, Ali-Melkkila T, Kaila T, Iisalo E, Lindgren L. Pharmacokinetics of glycopyrronium in uraemic patients. Br J Anaesth, 1993;71(3):437-9.
37. Ochs HR, Greenblatt DJ, Kaschell HJ, Klehr U, Divoll M, Abernethy DR. Diazepam kinetics in patients with renal insufficiency or hyperthyroidism. Br J Clin Pharmacol, 1981;12:829.
38. Davies G, Kingswood C, Street M. Pharmacokinetics of opioids in renal dysfunction. Clin Pharmacokinet, 1996;31:410-22.
39. Schochet RB, Murray GB. Neuropsychiatric toxicity of mepiridine. J Intensive Care Med, 1988;3:246-52.
40. Bower S, Sear JW. Disposition of alfentanil in patients receiving a renal transplant. J Pharm Pharmacol, 1989;41:654-7.
41. Dershwitz M, Hoke JF, Rosow CE, Michałowski P, Connors PM, Muir KT, et al. Pharmacokinetics and pharmacodynamics of Remifentanil in volunteer subjects with severe liver disease. Anesthesiology, 1996;84:812-20.
42. Hoke JF, Shlugman D, Dershwitz M, Michałowski P, Malthouse-Dufore S, Connors PM, et al. Pharmacokinetics and pharma-

codynamics of remifentanil in persons with renal failure compared with healthy volunteers. Anesthesiology, 1997;87(3):533-41.
43. Navapurkar VU, Archer S, Frazer NM, et al, Pharmacokinetics of remifentanil during hepatic transplantation. Anesthesiology, 1995; 83:A382.
44. Elliott RH, Strunin L. Hepatotoxicity of volatile anesthetics. Br J Anaesth, 1993;70:339-48.
45. Njoku D, Laster MJ, Gong DH, Eger EI 2nd, Reed GF, Martin JL. Biotransformation of halothane, enflurane, isoflurane, and desflurane to trifluoroacetylated liver proteins: association between protein acylation and hepatic injury. Anesth Analg, 1997; 84:173-8.
46. Stoelting RK, Hillier SC. Inhaled Anesthetics. In: Stoelting RK, Hillier SC (eds). Pharmacology and Physiology in Anesthesia Practise. 4th edn. Lippincott Williams & Wilkins. Philadelphia, 2006;2:42-86.
47. Cronnelly R, Salvatierra O, Fedusca NJ. Renal allograft function following halothane, enflurane, or isoflurane anesthesia. Anesth Analg, 1984;63:202.
48. Weiskopf RB, Eger EI 2nd, Ionescu P, Yasuda N, Cahalan MK, Freire B, et al. Desflurane does not produce hepatic or renal injury in human volunteers. Anesth Analg, 1992;74:570-4.
49. Bennett WM, Henrich WL, Stoff JS. The renal effects of nonsteroidal anti-inflammatory drugs: summary and recommendations. Am J Kidney Dis, 1996;28(Suppl 1):S56-62.
50. Bateman DN, Gokal R. Metoclopramide in renal failure. Lancet, 1980;1(8175):982.
51. Lehmann CR, Heironimus JD, Collins CB, O'Neil TJ, Pierson WP, Crowe JT, et al. Metoclopramide kinetics in patients with impaired renal function, and clearance by hemodialysis. Clin Pharmacol Ther, 1985;37:284.

7 CHAPTER Kidney Transplantation

Natural History of Kidney Disease

Rachna Bhutani

INTRODUCTION

Kidney disease is recognized as a major health problem affecting a large group of the population. It can be broadly classified into two major categories-acute kidney injury (AKI) and chronic kidney disease (CKD). Understanding the natural history of kidney disease helps us to identify the risk factors, diagnose the disease and reduce its progression to end stage. Early detection and timely management reduces the complications of renal disease.

The mortality of several surgical procedures is substantially increased in the presence of chronic kidney disease, therefore detecting and treating patients with CKD is extremely important.

ANATOMY AND PHYSIOLOGY

The structural and functional unit of the kidney is the nephron. Each nephron comprises of a glomerulus and a tubular system. The glomerulus consists of capillary endothelium, glomerular basement membrane, visceral and parietal epithelium and mesangium. The afferent arteriole feeds the glomerular tuft which is made up of highly convoluted capillary loops which in turn drains into the efferent arteriole. The glomerulus invaginates the Bowman's capsule which is the blind parietal epithelial sac of the renal tubule.

Formation of the Glomerular Ultrafiltrate

Glomerular ultrafiltration is governed by the balance of Starling forces regulating fluid flux across the filtration barrier.[1] The filtration barrier consists of endothelial fenestrations, the glomerular basement membrane and the epithelial slit diaphragm. This barrier is both size and charge selective. Molecules like hemoglobin and albumin which are larger than 3.6 nm are not filtered. Anions between 1.8 and 3.6 nm are not filtered however cations of the same size are filtered. Molecules less than 1.8 nm are freely filtered (e.g. water, glucose, sodium, urea, inulin), but in disease like glomerulonephritis the negatively charged glycoproteins are destroyed causing the polyanionic proteins to be filtered resulting in proteinuria.

Glomerular filtration rate (GFR) depends on[2]

- Permeability of the filtration barrier
- Hydrostatic forces—pushing fluid into the Bowman's space (which lies between visceral and parietal layers of the Bowman's capsule)
- Osmotic force—keeping fluid in the plasma

The Juxtaglomerular Apparatus

The chemoreceptors in the macula densa cells of the juxtaglomerular apparatus sense the concentration of tubular sodium chloride. The adjacent segment of arterioles which contain granular cells produces renin responsible for catalyzing the formation of angiotensin, the regulator of the GFR by altering the tone of afferent and efferent arteriole.

A primary determinant of the GFR is the glomerular filtration pressure which depends on renal artery perfusion pressure and balance between the afferent and efferent arteriolar tone.

Filtration fraction (FF) = Glomerular filtration rate (GFR)/ renal plasma flow (RPF).

Under normal circumstances the GFR is maintained via tubuloglomerular feedback (Flow chart 7.1) and renal autoregulation.[2]

Renal autoregulation enables the kidneys to maintain solute and water regulation through an arterial pressure range of 80 to 180 mm Hg.

Physiologic and Metabolic Functions of the Kidney

- Maintenance of normal electrolyte balance and fluid volumes of the body
- Regulation of the blood pressure
- Regulation of several endocrine functions
- Excretion of waste products.

CLASSIFICATION OF KIDNEY DISEASE

These can be broadly grouped into two major categories

- Acute kidney injury
- Chronic kidney disease.

ACUTE KIDNEY INJURY (AKI)[3,4]

The AKI is defined as rapid reduction in renal function, characterized by progressive azotemia (best measured clinically by serum creatinine) which may or may not be accompanied by oliguria. It can be diagnosed with certainty when the patient's prior renal function is known.

Classification of AKI[4]

- Pre-renal
  - Volume depletion
  - Cardiac causes (decreased cardiac output)
  - Redistribution of extracellular fluid
- Intrinsic renal
  - Acute glomerulonephritis (AGN)
  - Acute interstitial nephritis (ATN)
- Post-renal
  - Obstruction of the urinary tract

Flow chart 7.1: Tubuloglomerular feedback[1]

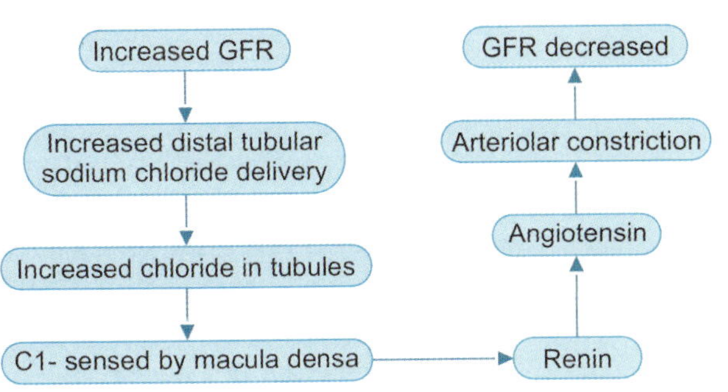

CHRONIC KIDNEY DISEASE (CKD)

- Kidney damage for ≥3 months, as defined by structural or functional abnormalities of the kidney, with or without decreased glomerular filtration rate (GFR), manifests as either:
  - Pathological abnormalities
  - Abnormalities in composition of blood or urine, or abnormalities in imaging tests (markers of kidney damage)
- GFR <60 mL/min/1.73 m^2 <1.00 mL/s) for ≥3 months, with or without kidney damage
- Proteinuria is the earliest marker of kidney damage in diabetes, hypertension and glomerular disease

Criteria for chronic kidney disease is described in Table 7.1.

Epidemiology

The prevalence of CKD is estimated at approximately 11% of the adult USA population.[6] Approximately 20 million[4] individuals in the USA have CKD (National Kidney Foundation 2002) out of which 8 million are suffering from CKD, stage III or IV (Table 7.2). The increase in the number of patients with ESRD in the USA has the features of an epidemic, since more than 40% of these patients require renal replacement therapy (RRT).

The exact prevalence of CKD in India is not clear. Few studies have been conducted according to which there is approximately 1% prevalence of CKD in India (0.79% to 1.39%).[7,8]

Table 7.1: Criteria for the definition of chronic kidney disease[5]

Structural or functional abnormalities of the kidneys for at least 3 months, as manifested by either:
▪ Renal damage, with or without ↓ GFR, as seen by: • Pathologic abnormalities • Markers of renal damage—abnormalities in ♦ Urine (proteinuria) ♦ Blood (renal tubular syndromes) ♦ Imaging abnormalities ♦ Renal transplantation • Renal transplant recipients ▪ (2) GFR < 60mL/min/1.73m^2, with or without kidney damage

Table 7.2: Classification of CKD[10]

Stage	GFR (mL/min/1.73 m^2)	Description	Actions
1	≥90	Normal or ↑ GFR	Diagnosis and treatment of comorbid conditions
2	60–89	↓ GFR	Estimate the progression
3	30–59	Moderately ↓ GFR	Complication evaluation and management
4	15–29	Severely ↓ GFR	Preparation for renal replacement therapy (RRT)
5	<15	Renal failure	RRT (if uremia present)

Classification of CKD

Chronic kidney disease is classified into five stages depending upon the GFR and renal damage as described in Table 7.2.[9]

EVALUATION OF RENAL FUNCTION

Clinical Markers of Renal Function - Urine Output

Perioperative oliguria is defined as urine flow rates less than 0.5 mL/kg/hr.

Perioperative oliguria is almost always prerenal and it implies acute renal failure.

Acute renal injury (ARI) may be defined as persistent elevation of serum creatinine to above 2 mg/dL (177 umol/L) on two consecutive occasions despite correction of any abnormal hemodynamic or mechanical factors.

Laboratory Assessment of Renal Function

Although serum creatinine is widely used as an index of renal function, the measured value is affected by factors other than GFR.

- GFR can be measured by using parenteral insulin, iohexol or iothalamate but the technique is not widely applied clinically
- In clinical practice GFR is estimated by
  - Creatinine clearance—estimation will depend on age, bodymass, nutritional status and laboratory measurement of creatinine.
  - Steps for creatinine clearance include
    - 24 hours urine collection
    - Creatinine measured in blood and urine[11]
    - GFR calculated by MDRD (Modification of Diet in Renal Disease) equation, explained in detail below
  - Urea clearance and cystatin C clearance

The MDRD equation predicts the GFR by incorporating serum creatinine concentration, demographic characteristics (age, gender and ethnicity), serum urea and albumin which is better than previous Cockcraft Gault formula.[12]

People at high-risk should have urine analysis, including micro-albumin testing and imaging studies for evaluating structural abnormalities.

RISK FACTORS FOR DEVELOPMENT OF CKD[13]

- Underlying disease
  - Diabetes mellitus[14]
  - Hypertension[14]
  - Dyslipidemia
- Lifestyle factors
  - Tobacco
  - Inactivity
  - Obesity
- Family history of CKD
- Prenatal factors
  - Maternal diabetes mellitus
  - Low birth weight
  - Small-for-gestational-age status
- Exposure to nephrotoxic drugs
- Recovery from acute kidney injury
- Reduction in kidney mass[15]
- Autoimmune diseases
- Systemic infections
- Urinary tract infections
- Sociodemographic factors
  - Older age
  - Racial predisposition[16]
  - Exposure to certain chemicals and environmental conditions
  - Low income/education

The natural history of CKD begins with an individual's susceptibility to kidney damage, family history of CKD, older age group and lower income or racial predisposition. However these factors can be aggravated by direct kidney damage which takes place in diseases like hypertension, diabetes mellitus, autoimmune diseases (e.g. glomerulonephritis), systemic and urinary tract infections, kidney stones or lower urinary tract obstruction and certain drug toxicities (e.g. aminoglycosides). Further progression of kidney damage and declining function is caused by poorly controlled diseases as mentioned above, for example higher level of proteinuria, inadequately controlled hypertension, smoking and uncontrolled diabetes. Finally the end stage factors which cause the damaged kidney to reach the point of no return are lower dialysis dose, temporary vascular access, anemia and low serum albumin level.[17,18]

CAUSES OF CKD[19]

- Hypertensive nephrosclerosis
- Diabetic glomerulosclerosis
- Glomerular disease
  - Glomerulonephritis
  - Amyloidosis
  - Systemic lupus erythematosus, Wegener's granulomatosis
- Tubulointerstitial disease
  - Chronic pyelonephritis
  - Analgesic nephropathy
  - Obstructive nephropathy
  - Myeloma kidney
- Vascular disease
  - Atheroembolic renal disease
  - Renovascular renal failure
  - Scleroderma
  - Vasculitis
- Cystic disease
  - Medullary cystic kidney disease
  - Autosomal dominant polycystic kidney disease.

SIGNS AND SYMPTOMS OF KIDNEY DISEASE

Patients with chronic renal failure (CRF) are often asymptomatic with little evidence of disease other than laboratory abnormalities until late in the course of kidney disease.

- Anemia—presents as easy fatigability
- Elevation in parathyroid hormone—presents as bone pains, ruptured tendons or disorders of soft tissue structures
- Moderate to severe renal failure—leads to electrolyte abnormalities, e.g. hyperkalemia which present as arrhythmias, heart block and muscle weakness
- Metabolic acidosis—causes fatigue, weight loss
- Retention of uremic toxins—leads to weight loss
- Moderate to severe renal failure—presents in the form of sexual dysfunction, reduced libido, reduced fertility
- Severe renal failure—leads to uremic syndrome which manifests as
  - Decreased appetite
  - Nausea, vomiting
  - Changes in sleep patterns

However, even with severe renal failure many patients feel surprisingly well.

Consequences of Impaired Renal Function[19]

- Hyponatremia, hyperkalemia, hypokalemia, hypocalcemia, hyperphosphatemia and decreased tolerance to electrolyte or mineral loading
- Hypertension, cardiovascular disease
- Anemia (low erythropoietin), hypertension (renin system activation), bone disease (secondary hyperparathyroidism, prolonged half life of insulin)
- Anorexia, nausea, soft tissue deposition of oxalates and phosphates, neurologic dysfunction, loss of muscle protein

CLINICAL AND LABORATORY ABNORMALITIES IN CKD[20]

- Anemia
- Hyponatremia and hypernatremia
- Hyperkalemia
- Metabolic acidosis
- Abnormal divalent ion metabolism
- Volume overload
- Hypertension.

During progression of CKD, various abnormalities are seen in clinical and laboratory parameters. In stage 3, when the GFR is less than 60 mL/min, a patient shows signs and symptoms of hypertension and anemia. Electrolyte disturbances in the form of hyponatremia, hypernatremia, hyperkalemia, hyperphosphatemia or metabolic acidosis are seen in stage 4 of CKD when the GFR falls to less than 30 mL/min. Uremic symptoms are present in the form of nausea, vomiting or disturbances in sleep, when the GFR falls further to less than 15 mL/min in stage 5 of CKD.

PATHOPHYSIOLOGY AND NATURAL HISTORY OF CKD[21]

1. Systemic hypertension, intraglomerular hypertension and glomerular hypertrophy.
   - Glomerular hypertension results from systemic hypertension

- Activation of renin angiotensin—aldosterone system produces glomerular hypertension and activates fibrosis
- Due to the loss of nephrons, mesangial cells produce cytokines and extracellular matrix which causes expansion of mesangium and glomerular sclerosis.

2. Proteinuria is both a marker and contributor to renal injury; and excretion of urinary proteins is directly proportional to severity of renal injury.
3. Hyperglycemia causes glomerular hyperfiltration due to increased cell growth and expansion in kidney which leads to increased GFR.
   - Long standing hyperglycemia causes mesangial expansion, this expansion is mediated by TGF-P (transforming growth factor). Later fibrosis is caused by collagen and fibronectin.
   - Glucose bound to proteins forms AGEs (advanced glycosylation end products) which cause damage by growth and fibrotic factors.
   - Proteinuria also accompanies diabetic nephropathy (DN)
   - Tubulointerstitial fibrosis seen in advanced DN is a better predictor of renal failure than glomerular sclerosis
   - Angiotension II contributes to progression of DN, therefore control of hypertension can decrease progression of DN
4. Tubulointerstitial disease
   - Causes atrophy of tubules and obstruction, destroying individual nephrons
   - Progressive scarring
5. Hyperlipidemia
   - Promotes progression of renal failure
   - Mesangial lipid deposition
6. Calcium phosphate deposition
   - Precipitation of calcium phosphate in renal interstitium causes inflammatory response
7. Prostaglandin production
   - Increased prostanoids produce vasodilatation and augment progression of disease
8. Metabolic acidosis
   - In response to acidosis, ammonia production is increased which induces tubular interstitial damage.

MANAGEMENT OF CKD

- General measures for CKD:
  - Adjust drug doses
  - Avoid nephrotoxic agents
  - Nephrology consultation
  - Patient education.
- Modalities that are specific to the underlying disorder, e.g. systemic lupus erythematosus, immune mediated or inflammatory disease benefit with steroids and immunosuppressive agents.
- Modalities which are used to treat all patients with CRF
  - Preventing and delaying progression of renal failure
  - Alleviating the electrolyte and hormonal abnormalities that can lead to symptoms or complications of the disease.

Recommendations and Goals for Management of CKD

- Anemia is to be corrected with erythropoietin and iron to maintain hemoglobin levels between 11 and 12 gm/dL
- Administration of diuretics to control hypertension and volume overload
- Blood pressure should be controlled with drugs to less than or equal to 130/80 mm of Hg
- Recommended daily intake of proteins is 0.6 to 0.8 gm/Kg bodyweight so that there is slow progression of renal disease and protein depletion is prevented
- Urine protein excretion should be less than 1 gm per day by administering angiotensin converting enzyme inhibitors or angiotensin receptor blockers or both
- Maintain serum potassium levels at less than 5.0 mEq/L by dietary restrictions and diuretics
- Maintain 25 hydroxycalciferol levels at 30 ng/mL by administration of ergocalciferol
- Administration of vitamin D or calcium to prevent hyperparathyroidism so that parathormone levels are below 150 pg/mL
- Serum phosphates should be kept below 4.5 mg/dL with dietary restrictions and phosphate binders
- Metabolic acidosis is controlled by administration of sodium citrate so that serum bicarbonate levels are kept more than 20 mEq/L

INTERVENTIONS TO REDUCE RATE OF PROGRESSION OF CKD[22]

1. Control of systemic and intraglomerular hypertension
2. Protein restriction
3. Treatment of underlying risk factors
   - Decreasing low density lipoprotein and control of cholesterol to < 100 mg/dL with statins
   - Decreasing glycosylated hemoglobin (HbA_1C) to <7.5%[9,23]

4. Lifestyle changes
   - Smoking cessation
   - Exercise reduces proteinuria

COMPLICATIONS OF CKD AND THEIR MANAGEMENT[24]

A. Bone and mineral disorders[25]

Elevation of phosphorus occurs due to reduced creatinine clearance which triggers diminished vitamin D production which in turn causes hypocalcemia. The above mechanism causes secondary hyperparathyroidism which produces metabolic bone disease termed as renal osteodystrophy (ROD). ROD includes abnormalities in bone turnover, bone density and bone architecture.

Treatment

1. Nonpharmacologic—avoid high phosphorus foods, e.g. chocolates, colas and dairy products. Dietary phosphate restriction to 800 to 1000 mg/day.
2. Pharmacologic-phosphate binders[26] with meals to minimize phosphate absorption and retention
   - Aluminium containing binders
   - Calcium containing binders
   - Polymeric binders-sevolamer which is preferable
   - Lanthanum containing binders-introduced recently, so long-term effects are not known

B. Anemia[9,25] National Kidney Foundation (NKF) guidelines indicate workup should be initiated for patients with CKD when

Hb < 12 gm/dL in adult males and post menopausal females

Hb < 11 gm /dL in premenopausal females

Treatment of Anemia

- Improves ischemic and structural heart disease
- Improves cognitive function
- Improves quality of life
- Decreases overall morbidity

Anemia Caused by CRF Results From

- Insufficient erythropoietin production
- Shortened red blood cell survival
- Iron deficiency
- Gastrointestinal bleed due to decreased platelet function

Workup for Anemia Includes

- Measurement of hemoglobin for hematocrit
- Red blood cell indices
- Reticulocyte count
- Iron studies
  - Serum iron
  - Total iron binding capacity
  - Transferrin saturation
  - Serum ferritin
- Other causes of anemia to be excluded

Complications of Anemia

- Left ventricular hypertrophy or failure
- Poor quality of life
- Impaired intellectual functioning

Recommendations to Treat Anemia/Pharmacologic Therapy

- To replete iron stores
- Supplement erythropoietin

National Kidney Foundation (NKF) Guidelines

- Recombinant human erythropoietin should be given initially at a dose of 80–120 units/kg/week, administered subcutaneously
- To achieve transferrin saturation 20% and serum ferritin ~ 100 ng/mL, parenteral iron is used

C. Proteinuria[25]

Proteinuria is defined as urinary protein excretion of >150 mg/day. It may be

- Low grade < 1 to 2 g/day
- High grade (> 3 to 3.5 g/day)

Proteinuria can be detected on urine dipstick or urinalysis which are sensitive to urinary albumin, but they are not accurate for quantifying proteinuria.

Methods for Quantifying Proteinuria

- Spot urine to creatinine ratio—less accurate but it is rapid and patient convenience is better.
- 24 hours urine protein collection—more accurate but compliance is poor.

Management of Proteinuria

- Associated with significant morbidity and mortality
- An independent risk factor for progressive renal failure and ESRD as well as both cardiovascular and non-cardiovascular disease related mortality
- Treatment of proteinuria results in significant reduction in progression of renal failure
- Reduction of proteinuria is a desirable goal in the treatment of CKD

Non-pharmacological Therapy

- Salt restriction in diet
- Losing weight if overweight or obese
- Cessation of smoking
- Dietary protein restriction

Pharmacological Therapy

- Control of blood pressure—benefit is maximum with low BP goal (125/75 mm Hg) than the usual BP goal (140/85 mm Hg)
- Suppression of renin—angiotensin system with ACE inhibitors and/or angiotensin receptor blockers is more effective
- Addition of aldosterone antagonist results in greater anti-proteinuric effects.

D. Cardiovascular disease[27]

CKD is associated with increased risk for cardiovascular disease (CVD). Risk factors are

- Anemia
- Hypertension
- Glucose intolerance
- Dyslipidemia
- Vascular calcification
- Endothelial dysfunction
- Elevated levels of homocysteine, C-reactive protein

E. Metabolic acidosis

- Metabolic acidosis has normal or high anion gap
- Plasma bicarbonate level is 12 to 22 mEq/L (mmol/L). There is inability to enhance bicarbonate generation with acid load. The probable reasons are
    - Impaired renal acidification process
    - Impaired ammonia genesis
    - Impaired excretion of titratable acid
    - Loss of nephron mass
- **Treatment includes**
    - Supplemental sodium bicarbonate to maintain serum bicarbonate level at 22mEq/L (mmol/L)

F. Malnutrition[28]

- Potential mechanisms include: anorexia, imposed dietary restrictions, accelerated protein catabolism and chronic inflammation
- **Complications includes**
    - Hypoalbuminemia, hypocholesterolemia
    - Erythropoietin hyporesponsiveness
    - Growth retardation in children
    - Progressive muscle weakness, poor exercise tolerance, debilitation and increased mortality
- **Treatment**
    - Nutritional assessment to include dietary history, serum albumin, pre-albumin, vitamin B_{12}, trans-ferain, 25-hydroxy vitamin D, and 24-hour urine for urea nitrogen excretion
    - Protein intake 0.6 g/kg/d for CKD stages 4 to 5, 0.75 g/kg/d for earlier stage CKD
    - Energy intake of 30 kcal/kg/d for CKD stages 4 to 5, higher for earlier stage CKD

G. Infection

- Potential mechanisms of increased infection include:
    - Nutritional deficiency including vitamin D
    - Decreased B-cell, T-cell, and macrophage function due to uremic toxins
    - Diminished mucocutaneous barrier due to dry skin, gastrointestinal ulcerations, poor mucus clearance from airways
- It is the second most common cause of death in CKD patients
- **Treatment**
    - Attention to personal and personnel hygiene
    - Enhance nutritional status
    - Aggressive vaccination including routine hepatitis B, *Pneumococcus*, and influenza vaccination and booster, which results in lower rates of hospitalization and death
    - Vaccination for hepatitis A, tetanus, varicella and *Haemophilus influenzae* also considered.

H. Volume overload

- Salt retention is an important component for development of hypertension and volume overload
- Diuretic administration is usually necessary
- Thiazides used in normal renal function
- When GFR falls to ≤ 30% of normal then loop diuretics, e.g., furosemide or combined loop and proximal tubule diuretic e.g. metolozone is indicated.

CLINICAL PEARLS

- Normal kidney function is important for maintaining fluid volume, electrolytes, blood pressure, excretion of waste products and drugs.
- Derangement of kidney function leads to fluid and electrolyte imbalance, anemia, hypertension and hormonal imbalance.

- Risk factors for kidney disease should be identified and if possible, eliminated.
- Once disease is established then its progression should be controlled.
- Kidney disease should be managed with supportive measures and timely complications should be diagnosed and managed.
- Patients with kidney disease pose challenges for anesthesiologists when posted for transplant or other surgeries. These patients should be optimized before surgery.

REFERENCES

1. Robert N Sladen. Renal Physiology. In: Ronald D Miller, Lars Eriksson, Lee A Fleisher, Jeanine P Wiener-Kronish, William L Young (Eds). Miller's Anesthesia 7th edn. Churchill Livingstone/ Elsevier, 2010.
2. Robert Thomas, Abbas Kanso, John R Sedor. Chronic Kidney disease and its complications. Prim Care Clin Office Pract, 2008;35:329-44.
3. Walsh TJ, Krieger IN. Urologic aspects of AIDS and HIV infection. In W Scott McDougal, Alan J Wein, Louis R Kavoussi, Andrew C Novick, Alan W Partin, Craig A Peters, Parvati Ramchandani (eds). Campbell-Walsh Urology, 10th edn.
4. Devid A goldford, Emitio D Poggio, Scott McDougal, Alan J Wein, Louid R Kavoussi, Andrew C Novick, et al. Campbell-Walsh Urology, 10 edn.
5. Levey AS, Eckardt KU, Tsukamoto Y, et al. Definition and classification of chronic kidney disease: a position statement from kidney disease: Improving Global Outcomes (KDIGO). Kidney Int, 2005;67(6):2089-100.
6. Coresh J, Astor BC, Greene T, Eknoyan G, Levey AS. Prevalence of chronic kidney disease and decreased kidney function in the adult US population: Third National Health and Nutrition Examination Survey. Am J Kidney Dis, 2003 Jan;41(1):1-12.
7. Prabahar MR, Chandrasekaran V, Soundararajan P. Epidemic of chronic kidney disease in India -what can be done? Saudi J Kidney Dis Transpl, 2008;19(5):847-53.
8. Dash SC, Agarwal SK. Incidence of chronic kidney disease in India. Nephrol Dial Transplant, 2006;21(1):232-3.
9. K/DOQI. Clinical practice guideline for chronic kidney disease: Evaluation, classification and stratification. Am J Kidney Dis, and Clinical Practice Recommendations for Anemia in Chronic Kidney Disease 2007 update of hemoglobin Target.
10. Johnson CA, Levey AS, Coresh J, Levin A, Lau J, Eknoyan G. Clinical practice guidelines for chronic kidney disease in adults: part I. definition, disease stages, evaluation, treatment, and risk factors. Am Fam Physician, 2004:70:1091-7.
11. Eleanor L, Rosemary O. Chronic kidney disease. American Journal of Kidney Diseases, Vol 49, No 1 (January), 2007:pp 162-171.
12. Poggio ED, Wang X, Greene T, Lente FV, Hall PM. Performance of the modification of diet in renal disease and cockcrogy-gault equations in the estimation of GFR in health and in chronic kidney disease. J Am Soc Nephrol, 2005;16:459-66.
13. Vassalotti J, Stevens L, Levey A. Testing for chronic kidney disease: a position statement from the National Kidney Foundation. Am J Kidney Diseas, 2007;50:169-180.
14. Maura Ravera, Giuseppe Noberasco, Michela Re, Alessandro Filippi, Anna Maria Gallina, Ursula Weiss, et al. Chronic kidney disease and cardiovascular risk in hypertensive type 2 diabetics: a primary care perspective. Nephrol Dial. Transplant, 2009;24:1528-33.
15. Wendy E Hoy, Michael D Hughson, John F Bertram, Rebecca Douglas-Denton, Kerstin Amann. Nephron number hypertension, renal disease and renal failure. J J Am Soc Nephrol, 2005;16:2557-64.
16. Meguid El Nahas, Adeera Levin. Chronic kidney disease: a practical guide to understanding and management (Oxford Clinical Nephrology). Oxford University Press 2009.
17. National kidney foundation. K/DOQI Clinical practice guideline from chronic kidney disease. Am J Kidney Dis, 2002;39:55-266.
18. Brenner and Rector's the kidney-Vdn I section III chapter 18. Frainewark for natural history classification of CKD.
19. William E Mitch. Chronic kidney disease. Colman Crcil Medicine, 24 edition.
20. Kraut JA. Chronic renal failure. Bope, Kellerman (eds), Conn's Current Therapy, 2012, (PP. 883-889). Elsevier Saunders.
21. Butt S, Hall P, Nurko S. Diabetic nephropathy, cleveland clinic: Current Clinical Medicine, 2nd edn. Section 9 Nephrology, Page 830-5.
22. Smogorzewski MJ, Rude RK, Yu ASL. Disorders of calcium, magnesium, and phosphate balance. In Taal: Brenner and Rector's The Kidney, 9th edn. Taal MW, Chertow GM, Marsden PA; Skorecki K, (eds). Elsevier Sauders 689-725.
23. Executive Summary. KDOQI, Clinical practice guidelines and clinical practice recommendations for diabetes and chronic kidney disease. American Journal of Kidney Diseases, Vol 49, No 2, Suppl2 (February), 2007: pp S13-S19.
24. Robert Thomas, Primary Care: Clinics in office practice, chronic kidney disease and its complication, 2008.
25. Lam A, Shah S, Paparello J. Outpatient management of chronic kidnet disease: proteinuria anemia and bone disease as therapeutic targets. Disease-a-month, 2010;56(4).
26. Fridman EA. An introduction to prosphate binding for the treatment of hyperthosphatemia in patients with chronic kidney disease. Kidney Int Supply 2005;S2-S6.
27. Ketteler M, Gross ML, Ritz E. Calcification and cardiovascular problem in renal failure. Kidney Int Supply, 2005;(94):S120-7.
28. Jassal SV. Clinical presentation of renal failure in the aged: chronic renal failure. Clin Geriatr Med, 2009 Aug; 25(3):359-72.

Preoperative Assessment and Management of Donor and Recipient for Renal Transplantation

Nitin Sethi, Jayashree Sood

INTRODUCTION

The five year survival rate after renal transplant is approximately 70% compared to a five year survival rate of 30% for a similar group of patients receiving dialysis.

In recent times there has been an increase in the number of patients awaiting renal transplant, however, the gap between the organ supply and demand has increased. A shortage of cadaveric organ donation has made living donors a potential source for organs for transplantation at an earlier stage of the disease with minimal delay. The graft survival rate is higher in living related allograft recipients as compared to recipients of cadaveric donor grafts.[1-4]

ASSESSMENT OF THE LIVING KIDNEY DONOR

Donor protection is the most important criteria to be taken into account during the selection and assessment of a living donor. For living organ donation, the benefits to both donor and recipient must outweigh the risks associated with donation and transplantation. The assessment of a potential donor includes the following issues:[5]

- The donation is made freely and with the donor's consent. The donor should not have any underlying cognitive or emotional disorder and should be intelligent enough to understand the risk and benefits of donation.
- The donor should have normally functioning kidneys with a low risk of developing kidney disease in the future.
- The donor should not have any disease that increases the surgical or anesthesia risk, or which can be transmitted to the recipient such as cancer or infections.
- Recipients accepted for transplantation should have a good prognosis after living donor kidney transplant.

A thorough medical, surgical and psychosocial evaluation is essential. The overall purpose is to ensure that the potential donor is in good health, has normal kidney function and structure and is not a risk to the recipient.

MEDICAL EVALUATION

The initial donor evaluation begins with the estimation of the donor and recipient blood group and HLA typing. In some centers HLA typing is not performed for most donors because of the current availability of improved immunosuppressive regimens and outcomes. The following are important points for preoperative evaluation of a living kidney donor:

Age

Most centers report a minimum age of 18 years for kidney donation. Older donors were previously not considered suitable for donation. However, such donors are acceptable if their renal function is adequate and the individual is in good physical and mental condition. An upper age limit of 75 years has been reported from 5% of the centers in the United States, with almost 60% of the centers having no upper age limit for a kidney donor.[6]

Diabetes Mellitus and the Metabolic Syndrome

Potential donors with a family history of diabetes mellitus, elevated fasting glucose and a history of gestational diabetes should be evaluated for this disorder. Fasting blood glucose values >126 mg% on two occasions, or non fasting blood glucose or blood glucose level two hours after oral glucose tolerance test (OGTT) >200 mg% is an absolute contraindication to donation. Previous history of gestational diabetes is also a contraindication to donation, given the high rate of developing diabetes later in life. Blood glucose levels 140–199 mg%, 2 hours after OGTT are relative contraindications and must be assessed individually.[7] Severe obesity (BMI > 35 kg/m^2) is a contraindication to donation as it is associated with a greater surgical risk and greater risk of developing chronic renal disease in the long run.[8] The baseline laboratory tests that need to be done are blood sugar levels, HbAIc and lipid profile.

Cardiovascular Assessment

The blood pressure should be <140/90 mm Hg with an average measurement of <135/85 mm Hg during the day and <120/75 mm Hg during sleep. According to a meta-analysis, donation has been associated with a 5 mm Hg increase in blood pressure. However in the general non-diabetic population the risk of chronic renal disease secondary to mild high blood pressure is low in the long-term.[9, 10]

Potential donors with mild or moderate high blood pressure with no other cardiovascular risk and who have good renal function can donate, if the following criteria[5] are met: (A) They are over 50 years old; (B) They are not Afro-American; (C) They have no evidence of damage to internal organs secondary to high blood pressure; (D) The blood pressure can be controlled by lifestyle modification and with use of no more than one anti-hypertensive drug; and (E) There is a reasonable guarantee they will undergo regular follow-up and treatment.

Any significant heart diseases, such as ischemic heart disease, heart failure, valvular valuation heart disease or significant arrhythmias is a contraindication to donation.[11]

Baseline evaluation should include electrocardiogram (ECG) and chest X-ray. Special tests include echocardiography (hypertensive patients, murmurs, dyspnea on exertion, elderly patients), Holter (suspected arrhythmias), cardiac stress tests (abnormal ECG, patient over 60 years old or a combination of risk factors: age >45 years old in men, >55 years old in women, tobacco smoking, dyslipidemia, high blood pressure, family history).

Renal Assessment

Though donors lose 50% of their GFR after nephrectomy it recovers almost entirely during the first postoperative week. One year post donor nephrectomy the remaining kidney can make up for approximately 20–40% the initial renal function.[12,13]

The Amsterdam Consensus has established that a creatinine clearance of <80 mL/min/1.73m^2 rules out the possibility of donation.[14] A creatinine clearance of >90 mL/min/173m^2 is desirable in patients less than 40 years old, while a lower clearance around 70 mL/min is acceptable in elderly donor >60 years old.[15, 16] If the difference between the kidney function of the two kidney is >5% then the kidney chosen to be extracted should be one with lower renal function.[17] Protein excretion should be measured from a 24-hour urine collection. Most transplant centers exclude patients with proteinuria >300 mg/day while others use a lower threshold >150 mg/day.[6]

Hematuria is defined as at least 10 red blood cells/high power field, while some centers use the criteria of 3 red blood cells/high power field. Donors with persistent hematuria should undergo complete urological evaluation and kidney biopsy if deemed necessary.[18] Structural abnormalities that rule out donation are, (A) Large differences in the size of the kidneys or significant unilateral atrophy; (B) Extensive cortical scarring; (C) More than 2–3 cysts in both kidneys or complex or multilocular cysts; (D) Angiomyolipoma, tumors; (E) Significant arteriosclerosis; (F) Fibromuscular dysplasia: (G) Multiple or large stones; (H) Dilatation or obstruction of ducts; and (I) Medullary sponge kidney.

Table 7.3: Clinical tests for donor evaluation

- Laboratory Tests
  - *Blood*
    - Complete blood count
    - General biochemical tests: Glucose, urea, creatinine, sodium, potassium, phosphorus, uric acid, blood gases
    - Liver function tests
    - Prothrombin time, partial thromboplastin time
    - Lipid profile
    - ABO blood typing
    - HLA assay
    - Serology—HIV, HTLV, cytomegalovirus, herpes simplex virus, epstein barr virus, varicella zoster and hepatitis B and C
    - Proteinogram: Immunoglobulin
    - Oral glucose overload test, if applicable
    - HbAIC
    - Prostate specific antigen (Men > 40 years)
    - Pregnancy test, where applicable.
  - *Urine*
    - Urinalysis with microscopy and urine culture
    - 24 hours urine test (creatinine clearance, proteinuria, calciuria, microalbuminuria)
    - Urine culture
  - Special Tests
    - Cardiology—electrocardiogram, echocardiography, holter, stress test
    - Respiratory-pulmonary function tests
    - Others—allergy, oncology and dermatology studies
  - Imaging studies
    - Chest X-ray
    - Abdominal ultrasound
    - CT angiogram/MR angiogram
    - Isotopic study of renal function , if applicable

Pulmonary Assessment

Pulmonary function tests are indicated in heavy smokers and when there are symptoms which would point to chronic lung disease. There is an increased risk for donors when FEV_1 or FVC is <70% or FEV_1/FVC is <65%.[5]

Cancer Detection

In men, a detailed physical examination should include testicular examination, and in those over 50 years, a measurement of prostate specific antigen (PSA) and digital rectal examination. Women should undergo breast examination, mammography (if age >40 years), pelvic examination and Papanicolaou smear. All potential donors >50 years of age should undergo colon cancer screening. Donation is ruled out if there is a previous diagnosis of hematological, gastrointestinal, testicular, melanoma, lung, breast, kidney or urinary cancer, choriocarcinoma or monoclonal gammopathy. [5,19]

Psychosocial Evaluation

Donors must be evaluated by a psychiatrist to rule out any mental disorder or intellectual deficiencies. It is important to assess donor knowledge about transplant, quality of life with one kidney and benefits for the recipient. It must also be assessed whether the donor is being pressurized to donote his/her organ. The donor must be correctly informed about the expected results before the living donor kidney transplant.[20,21]

The overall purpose of evaluation is to ensure that the potential donor is in good health, has normal kidney function and structure and is not a risk to the recipient with respect to transmission of infection.

Table 7.4: Contraindications for living kidney donation

- Absolute contraindications
  - Proteinuria and/or hematuria
  - Active infection
  - Impaired renal function (GFR < 80 mL/min/1.73m^2)
  - Markedly urologic and renal vascular abnormality
  - Active malignancy
  - Chronic active viral infection (HIV, HTLV, hepatitis B and C virus)
  - Clinically significant hypertension
  - Diabetes mellitus
  - Chronic illness, mainly pulmonary, liver, autoimmune, neurologic or cardiac disease
  - Nephrocalcinosis, bilateral kidney stones or recurrent nephrolithiasis
  - Pregnancy
  - Disorders requiring anticoagulation
  - Poorly controlled psychosis
  - Active substance abuse
- Relative contraindications
  - History of nephrolithiasis
  - Active peptic ulcer disease
  - Morbid obesity (BMI > 35 kg/m^2)
  - Age > 65 years or < 18 years
  - Strong family history of diabetes mellitus or hypertension
  - Family history of renal cell carcinoma

PREOPERATIVE ASSESSMENT AND MANAGEMENT OF KIDNEY RECIPIENT

The most common causes of end stage renal disease (ESRD) are diabetes, hypertensive nephrosclerosis, glomerulonephritis and autosomal dominant polycystic kidney disease. Because of the improvement in the quality of life and reduced mortality risk in patients with renal transplant when compared to those on maintenance dialysis several recipient groups previously considered as unsuitable candidates (e.g. patients with type II diabetes, advanced cardiomyopathy, various forms of vasculitis, sickle cell disease and morbid obesity) now may be considered suitable candidates for renal transplantation.[22,23,24]

Patients not yet requiring dialysis should not undergo renal transplantation until there has been an irreversible deterioration in renal function beyond a threshold level of clearance.

The 2005 Canadian Society of Transplantation Consensus guidelines suggest that transplantation should not be performed unless the GFR <20mL/min/1.73m^2 with evidence of progressive, irreversible deterioration in renal function over a period of 6 to 12 months.[25]

The Clinical Practice Guidelines 2010 for assessment of the potential kidney transplant recipient by the UK Renal Association recommends that kidney transplantation should be the renal replacement therapy of choice for the patient with chronic kidney disease stage 5 (predialysis, dialysis and transplant patients with GFR <15/mL/min/1.73m^2) who is considered fit for major surgery and for chronic immunosuppression.[26]

The kidney recipient should be carefully evaluated in order to detect and optimize any coexisting illness so as to minimize the risk of anesthesia and surgery.

Chronic renal disease affects multiple organ systems, therefore it is essential to optimize existing organ dysfunction.

The comorbid conditions which need to be assessed and optimized preoperatively are:

Cardiovascular Disease

Cardiovascular disease accounts for approximately 40% of deaths in patients undergoing dialysis and is the leading cause of death post kidney transplant.[27, 28]

Clinical evaluation beings with a history, physical examination and chest radiograph. The common cardiovascular disorders seen in patients with chronic renal disease are:

Coronary Artery Disease

The estimated incidence of coronary artery disease (CAD) in patients undergoing dialysis is 17 to 37%.[29] Non-invasive

Table 7.5: Contraindications for kidney transplantation

- Absolute Contraindications
  - Untreated current infection
  - Chronic illness with life expectancy of less than 1 year
  - Active malignancy with short life expectancy
  - Poorly controlled psychosis
  - Active substance abuse
- Relative Contraindications
  - Active infection
  - Coronary heart disease
  - Active hepatitis
  - Active peptic ulcer disease
  - Cereberovascular disease
  - Proven habitual medical noncompliance
  - HIV infection

testing is usually performed in patients with symptoms/signs of heart disease, previous history of coronary artery disease (such as myocardial infarction), symptoms/signs of heart failure, diabetes and/or multiple risk factors for heart disease.[30, 31]

Multiple risk factors include increased age (>45 years in male and >55 years in female), hypertension, dyslipidemia, diabetes, family history of heart disease, prolonged duration of chronic renal disease and history of smoking.[32]

Morbid obesity has been considered a contraindication to renal transplantation because of the increased perioperative mortality primarily caused by cardiac risk factors. Therefore careful screening for ischemic heart disease in obese patients is essential.

Non-invasive tests such as dipyridamole thallium stress test have limitations as a screening tool for coronary artery disease in diabetes, with a probability of having a negative image in presence of coronary artery disease being 38%. In patients with uremia the decreased sensitivity of dipyridamole thallium stress test is due to the altered microcirculatory response to dipyridamole.[33]

Dobutamine stress echocardiography has 52% sensitivity and 74% specificity to detect coronary artery disease and is a better tool than dipyridamole thallium stress test.[34] Patients with positive non-invasive test and those with symptomatic heart disease, should undergo coronary angiography and revascularization if indicated.[35] However, a prospective observational study done on 300 patients listed for kidney transplant showed that there was no significant survival difference between those patients referred for coronary angiography compared to those who were not.[36] Furthermore, trials in the non-renal population have shown that prophylactic coronary artery revascularization does not reduce the long term mortality or improve outcome in high-risk patients undergoing major non-cardiac surgery.[37]

Congestive Heart Failure

Congestive heart failure is present in over 50% of patients on chronic dialysis but when present before initiation of dialysis it is an independent prognostic indicator of mortality.[38] A major contributing cause of congestive heart failure in patients with chronic renal disease is uremic

Table 7.6: Pathophysiologic changes in chronic renal failure disease

Pathophysiological Changes	*Clinical Presentation*
Cardiovascular abnormalities	Congestive heart failure (CHF), coronary artery disease (CAD), uremic pericarditis, cardiac tamponade, dysrhythmias, systemic hypertension (left ventricular hypertrophy, cardiomyopathy)
Endocrine disturbances	Diabetes mellitus, secondary hyperparathyroidism, osteomalacia, renal osteodystrophy
Anemia	Decreased erythropoetin production, diminished erythrocyte production and survival (Normochromic normocytic anemia)
Hemostatic abnormality	Uremic coagulopathy—abnormal platelet function, decreased factor XIII and Von willebrand Factor production
Fluid, acid-base and electrolyte disturbances	Hypervolemia (congestive heart failure, pulmonary edema, pleural effusion), metabolic acidosis, hyperkalemia (dysrhythmia), hypocalcemia (osteoperosis), hypermagnesemia (hypotension, potentiation of muscle relaxants)
Neurologic dysfunction	Uremic encephalopathy (personality changes, drowsiness myoclonus, coma), peripheral neuropathy (peroneal nerve palsy with foot drop)
Gastrointestinal dysfunction	Uremic enteropathy (nausea and vomiting, peptic ulcer disease, gastrointestinal bleeding)
Dialysis related problems	Disequilibrium syndrome (cerebral edema), hypovolemia and electrolyte imbalance (hypokalemia, hypomagnesemia, hypophosphatemia), peritonitis (in patients on peritoneal dialysis), systemic anticoagulation (post dialysis)

cardiomyopathy. Echocardiography is the best screening test for cardiomyopathy.[35] Two distinct abnormalities of uremic cardiomyopathy are enlargement of the left ventricular end diastolic diameter and left ventricular hypertrophy.[39] Other contributing factors for congestive heart failure in patients on dialysis are hypoalbuminemia and anemia. The major independent risk factors associated with congestive heart failure are ischemic heart disease, old age, diabetes and systolic dysfunction.[38]

Improvement in uremic cardiomyopathy can be achieved by correcting anemia with erythropoietin. It is reversible and usually improves several months after successful transplant.[40]

The 2005 Canadian Society for Transplantation guideline suggests[25] that the following patients with coronary heart disease may be eligible for kidney transplant:

- Asymptomatic low-risk patients
- Asymptomatic patients in whom non-invasive testing is negative
- Patients on appropriate medical therapy with angiographic results showing non-critical disease
- Patients in whom successful interventions have been performed.

Hypertension

Hypertension is one of the commonest cause of end stage renal disease[41] and greater than 70% of patients with chronic renal disease are hypertensive before initiation of dialysis.[42] The commonly used antihypertensive medication in hypertensive patients are angiotensin-converting enzyme inhibitors, calcium antagonists, beta blockers and diuretics. Most antihypertensive medications should be continued throughout the perioperative period. Many centers discontinue the use of angiotensin converting enzyme inhibitors prior to surgery, as its use is associated with severe hypotension after induction of anesthesia. In patients awaiting kidney transplantation who are to be started on beta blocker therapy it should be started at least one month prior to transplantation so as to avoid perioperative bradycardia and hypotension.[43].

Aspirin therapy should be continued in the perioperative period as it reduces the severity of silent myocardial ischemia in patients with both stable and unstable angina. Aspirin use is not associated with an increased risk of bleeding or gastritis and its use in low dose perioperatively reduces the risk of renal vein thrombosis.[44, 45] Patients on clopidogrel are more likely to bleed perioperatively and require blood transfusions but should not be considered a contraindication to renal transplantation. Platelet infusion may be used to reduce the risk of bleeding. [46,47]

Peripheral Vascular Disease

Peripheral vascular disease is present or develops after surgery in a majority of renal transplant recipients. Although routine screening for peripheral vascular disease is not indicated, non-invasive doppler studies are useful in patients with diabetes mellitus and/or history of claudication. Decreased survival has been reported in renal transplant recipients with peripheral vascular disease.[48,49]

Diabetes Mellitus

In patients with type I diabetes mellitus and renal failure, renal transplant is widely acceptable, however patients with type II diabetes mellitus are not considered good candidates because of the high number of associated complications. A complete cardiac evaluation of transplant candidates with Type II diabetes is essential as myocardial infarction is the leading cause of death in these patients.[50,51]

There are several problems in patients with diabetes mellitus which are of concern to the anesthesiologist. Table 7.7 summarises the perioperative problems in patients with diabetes.

Anemia

Decreased erythropoietin production in patients with chronic renal failure results in normochromic normocytic anemia. The anemia of chronic renal failure can be severe with hemoglobin levels between 6 to 8 gm% and hematocrit value of 20% to 25%. The use of erythropoietin has resulted in a decreased need for blood transfusion and has improved the quality of life. The role of preoperative blood transfusion is questionable and has been abandoned in many transplant centers, as inappropriate blood transfusion increases the risk of transmission of infection, fluid overload and pulmonary edema. In patients with CAD associated with end stage renal disease, a hematocrit close to 30% results in a safer perioperative course. Hence, in patients in whom transfusion is indicated because of poorly tolerated harmotocrit values it should not be withheld.[52] Transfusion should be performed during dialysis so that the intravascular volume balance is maintained and hyperkalemia avoided.

Hemostatic Abnormality

Long standing uremia in patient with chronic renal disease leads to uremic coagulopathy, a complex syndrome that includes abnormal platelet function and ineffective production of both factor VIII and Von Willebrand factor. Prothrombin time and activated thromboplastin times are usually normal in patients with uremia.[53]

Table 7.7 Perioperative problems in patients with diabetes

Abnormality	*Clinical Relevance*
Stiff joint syndrome	Atlanto-occipital joint fixation may lead to difficult intubation of trachea
Autonomic neuropathy	Bradycardia, labile blood pressure, silent myocardial infarction, gastroparesis with delayed gastric emptying
Peripheral neuropathy	Glove-stocking distribution of sensory loss in lower extremities
Diffuse atherosclerosis	Systemic hypertension, myocardial infarction, stroke, peripheral vascular disease
Electrolyte imbalance	Cardiac arrhythmias
Ketoacidosis	Hyperglycemia, hyperkalemia, metabolic acidosis, coma
Hyperglycemia	Non ketotic hyperosmolar coma
Hypoglycemia	Sweating, tachycardia, hypertension, coma

Preoperative dialysis improves platelet function and prevents bleeding. Other therapies include the use of conjugated estrogen and desmopressin. Patients treated with conjugated estrogen 3 hours before surgery had fewer bleeding complications, this effect was long lasting and more effective than cryoprecipitate, fresh frozen plasma or desmopressin. Desmopression administration shortens the prolonged bleeding time, increases circulating levels of factors VIII and Von Willebrand antigen and reduces perioperative blood loss. Use of cryoprecipitate has the potential for transmission of infection.[54,55]

Fluid, Acid Base and Electrolyte Imbalance

In patients with chronic renal failure inadequate dialysis and dietary control may result in hypervolemia, pulmonary edema and hypertension, whereas overzealous dialysis and dietary restriction results in hypovalemia and dehydration but pulmonary edema may still be induced by positive fluid balance of as little as 500 mL.

These patients have chronic anion gap metabolic acidosis due to retention of sulfates and phosphates which are normally excreted by the kidney. The acidosis is usually mild and well compensated in patients on chronic dialysis.

Patients with chronic renal disease normally tolerate large variations of serum potassium concentrations, from 2.5 to 6.0 mEq/L. Serum potassium levels are frequently elevated due to decreased renal clearance, however patients may also develop hypokalemia post-dialysis.

Preoperative life threatening hyperkalemia is characterized by ECG manifestations such as prolonged PR interval, bradycardia, QRS widening, peaked T waves and AV block. Treatment includes calcium chloride or gluconate for cardiac membrane stabilization, infusion of insulin and dextrose to promote intracellular shift of serum potassium, correction of acidosis by sodium bicarbonate and methods to promote excretion of excess potassium which include diuretic therapy, cation exchange resins and hemodialysis.

Hypokalemia should be corrected using diluted intravenous potassium if it is associated with cardiac arrhythmias or presence of ECG changes such as flattened or inverted T waves, prominent U waves, ST depression, atrial and ventricular arrhythmias.[56]

Pulmonary Dysfunction

Hypoalbuminamia and low plasma oncotic pressure in patients with chronic renal disease makes them more prone to develop pulmonary edema in the presence of fluid overload. Decreased surfactant production along with a depleted lean body mass compromises the forced vital capacity (FVC) and increases the risk of postoperative pulmonary atelectasis. These patients have a impaired response to infection and are more likely to develop pneumonia as compared to patients with normal renal function.[56]

An increased risk of graft dysfunction and mortality has been seen in smokers.[25] One study reported a 30% higher risk of graft failure in patients with 25 pack years smoking history as compared to those who had never smoked or had smoked less.[57]

According to the 2005 Canadian Transplant Guidelines[25] patients with following clinical features should not be candidates for kidney transplant:

- Home oxygen therapy requirement
- Uncontrolled asthma
- Severe cor pulmonale
- Severe chronic obstructive pulmonary disease/pulmonary fibrosis/restrictive disease. This is defined by $FEV_1 < 25\%$ predictive value, PaO_2 on room air < 60 mm Hg, > 4 lower respiratory tract infection in last 12 months and/or moderate disease with progression.

Neurologic Dysfunction

Increased blood urea levels in patients with chronic renal disease leads to uremic encephalopathy. The signs and symptoms range from subtle personality changes to drowsiness, asterixis, myoclonus and seizures. The rapid increase in blood urea level rather than the absolute value is the determinant of progression of signs and symptoms of encephalopathy. Peripheral sensorimotor neuropathy with "glove and stocking" distribution is a common complication of chronic renal disease and an important indication for dialysis. The presence of peripheral neuropathy should alert the treating physician to the presence of co-existing autonomic neuropathy.[56]

Gastrointestinal Dysfunction

Urea is a potential mucosal irritant causing uremic enteropathy. In this condition the entire gastrointestinal tract becomes inflamed and irritable and is characterized by the presence of hiccups, nausea and vomiting. Protein restriction and dialysis helps in controlling the symptoms. Peptic ulcer disease occurs in upto 25% of patients with chronic renal disease. Uremic enteropathy along with autonomic dysfunction increases the risk of regurgitation and aspiration during induction of and emergence from anesthesia.[56, 58]

Patients on chronic hemodialysis have on increased risk of hepatitis B and C infection because of the frequent need of transfusion of blood and blood products. Many of the patients become asymptomatic carriers or have minimal abnormality of liver function tests. It is essential to treat all patients on dialysis as potentially infected and the medical personnel should take adequate precautions against exposure.[59, 60]

About 30 mL of sodium citrate given before induction of anesthesia increases the gastric pH and is excellent for preoperative acid aspiration prophylaxis. Metoclopramide 10 mg intravenously 30 minutes before anesthesia induction and any one of the H_{2-} receptor blockers (e.g. ranitidine, famotidine) improves gastric emptying, raises gastro-esophageal sphincter pressure and gastric pH. Dose reduction of the drugs is advisable as they undergo renal excretion.

Table 7.8: Investigation for a potential kidney recipient

- Complete blood count
- Renal function tests–blood urea nitrogen, creatinine, serum electrolytes–sodium, potassium, calcium, magnesium, phosphate
- Liver function tests
- Prothrombin time and partial thromboplastin time
- Urinalysis and urine or bladder wash culture
- HLA typing and blood grouping
- Serological testing for HIV, cytomegalovirus, varicella virus, Herpes simplex-virus, epstein barr virus, hepatitis A, B, and C virus
- Chest X-ray and ECG
- Ultrasonography-abdomen and pelvis
- Transthoracic echocardiography, thallium scintigraphy and/or dobutamine stress echocardiography
- In men: testicular examination and if the is age > 50 years, serum prostate specific antigen levels and a rectal examination
- In women: breast examination and if age > 40 years mammography

Preoperative Dialysis

Dialysis is essential to control acidosis, hyperkalemia and pulmonary edema. Excessive dialysis may result in hypovolemia and electrolyte imbalance (hypokalemia, hypomagnesemia, hypophosphatemia). This may precipitate a reduction in left ventricular ejection fraction and perfusion defects suggestive of myocardial ischemia without acute ECG changes and in the absence of a history of coronary artery disease. Acute neurological deterioration also known as disequilibrium syndrome occurs when an initial dialysis is done in the presence of severe uremia. This occurs as urea is rapidly removed from the intravascular compartment but not from the brain cells because of the blood brain barrier and the brain cells become relatively hypertonic. Fluid diffuses along the osmotic gradient and cerebral edema may occur.[56]

Patients presenting for kidney transplant are already on intermittent hemodialysis and ideal timing of dialysis is a day before surgery. The aim of the dialysis should be to optimize the fluid and electrolyte status and decrease the BUN to less than 100 mg/dL.

Surgery should not be performed on same day as hemodialysis because of the potential problems of anti-coagulation (due to heparinization during dialysis), rapid fluid shifts, hypokalemia, hypoxemia and neurological deterioration. On the other hand if the surgery is delayed for more than 48 hours post-dialysis, patients are more prone to develop fluid overload, hyperkalemia and acidosis.

CLINICAL PEARLS

- A detailed and comprehensive preoperative evaluation of potential kidney transplant recipient improves the outcome after transplant, thereby reducing morbidity and mortality.
- Donor protection is the most important criteria to be taken into account during the selection and assessment of a living donor.
- Any significant heart disease such as ischemic heart disease, heart failure, valvular heart disease or significant arrhythmias are a contraindication to surgery.

- Donors lose 50% of their GFR after nephrectomy which is recovered almost entirely during the first week following surgery.
- The UK renal association recommends kidney transplantation to be the renal replacement therapy of choice for patients with chronic kidney disease stage 5 with GFR <15 mL/min/1.73m^2.
- More than 70% patients with chronic renal disease are hypertensive before initiation of dialysis.
- The major cause of congestive heart failure in patients with chronic renal disease is uremic cardiomyopathy.
- Stiff joint syndrome in diabetic patients with chronic renal disease may lead to difficulty in intubation of the trachea.
- Long standing uremia causes abnormal platelet function and ineffective production of both factors VII and Von Willbrand factor leading to coagulopathy.
- Chronic anior gap metabolic acidosis and hyperkalemia are commonly seen in patients with chronic renal disease.
- Hypoalbuminemia and low plasma oncotic pressure in patients with chronic renal disease makes them more prone to develop pulmonary edema in the presence of fluid overload.
- Acute neurological deterioration, also know as disequilibrium syndrome, can occur if dialysis is done in the presence of severe uremia.

REFERENCES

1. Hou S. Expanding the kidney donor pool: ethical and medical considerations. Kidney Int, 2000;58:1820-36.
2. Ellison MD, McBride MA, Taranto SE, et al. Living kidney donors in need of kidney transplants: a report from the organ procurement and transplantation network. Transplantation, 2002;74:1349-51.
3. Davis CL. Evaluation of the living kidney donor: current perspectives. Am J Kidney Dis, 2004;43:508-30.
4. Port FK, Dykstra DM, Merion RM, Wolfe RA. Trends and results for organ donation and transplantation in the United States, 2004. Am J Transplant, 2005;5:843-9.
5. Govantes MAG, Palomo PP. Assessing and selecting a living kidney donor. Nefrologia, 2010;30:47-59.
6. Mandelbrot DA, Pavlakis M, Danovitch GM, et al. The medical evaluation of living kidney donors: a survey of US transplant centers. Am J Transplant, 2007;7:2333-43.
7. Textor S, Taler S. Expanding criteria for living kidney donors: what are the limits? Transplant Rev (Orlando), 2008;22:187-91.
8. Reese PP, Feldman HI, Asch DA, et al. Short-term outcomes for obese live kidney donors and their recipients. Transplantation, 2009;88:662-71.
9. Segev DL, Muzaale AD, Caffo BS, et al. Perioperative mortality and long-term survival following live kidney donation. JAMA, 2010;303:959-66.
10. Boudville N, Prasad GV, Knoll G, et al. Donor nephrectomy outcomes research (DONOR) Network. Meta-analysis: risk for hypertension in living kidney donors. Ann Intern Med, 2006; 145:185-96.
11. Garg AX, Prasad R, Thiessen-Philbrook HR, et al. For the donor nephrectomy outcomes research (DONOR) Network. Cardiovascular disease and hypertension risk in living kidney donors: an analysis of health administrative data in Ontario, Canada. Transplantation, 2008;86:399-406.
12. Stevens LA, Levey AS. Measured GFR as a confirmatory test for estimated GFR. J Am Soc Nephrol, 2009;20:2305-13.
13. Rule AD, Gussak HM, Pond GR, et al. Measured and estimated GFR in healthy potential kidney donors. Am J Kidney Dis, 2004;43:112-9.
14. Delmonico F. Council of the transplantation society. A report of the Amsterdam Forum on the care of the live kidney donor: data and medical guidelines. Transplantation, 2005;79:S53-66.
15. British Transplant Society and the British Renal Association: United Kingdom guidelines for living donor kidney transplantation, April 2005. www.bts.org.uk. Last accessed:17 October 2011.
16. Rook M, Bosma RJ, Van Son WJ, et al. Nephrectomy elicits impact of age and BMI on renal hemodynamics: lower postdonation reserve capacity in older or overweight kidney donors. Am J Transplant, 2008;8:2077-85.
17. Shokeir AA, Gad HM, El-Diasty T. Role of radioisotope renal scans in the choice of nephrectomy side in live kidney donors. J Urol, 2003;170:373-6.
18. Kido R, Shibagaki Y, Iwadoh K, et al. Persistent glomerular hematuria in living kidney donors confers a risk of progressive kidney disease in donors after heminephrectomy. Am J Transplant, 2010;10:1597-1604.
19. Kasiske BL, Ravenscraft M, Ramos EL, et al. The evaluation of living renal transplant donors: clinical practice guidelines. Ad Hoc Clinical Practice Guidelines Subcommittee of the Patient Care and Education Committee of the American Society of Transplant Physicians. J Am Soc Nephrol, 1996;7:2288-313.
20. Rowley AA, Hong BA, Martin S, et al. Psychiatric disorders: are they an absolute contraindication to living donation? Prog Transplant, 2009;19:128-31.
21. Rodrigue JR, Pavlakis M, Danovitch GM, et al. Evaluating living kidney donors: relationship types, psychosocial criteria, and consent processes at US transplant programs. Am J Transplant, 2007;7:2326-32.
22. Suthanthiran M, Strom TB. Renal transplantation. N Engl J Med, 1994;331:1719-20.
23. Xue JL, Ma JZ, Louis TA, Collins AJ. Forecast of the number of patients with end-stage renal disease in the United States to the year 2010. J Am Soc Nephrol, 2001;12:2753-8.
24. Kasiske BL, Cangro CB, Hariharan S, et al. American Society of Transplantation. The evaluation of renal transplantation candidates: clinical practice guidelines. Am J Transplant, 2001;1:3-95.
25. Knoll G, Cockfield S, Blydt-Hansen T, et al. Canadian Society of Transplantation consensus guidelines on eligibility for kidney transplantation. CMAJ, 2005;173:1181-4.
26. Dudley C, Harden P. UK Renal Association. Clinical Practice guideline assessment of the potential kidney transplant recipient. 5th edn. 2010. www.renal.org/guidelines. last accessed 17 October 2011.
27. Canadian Organ Replacement Register. 1991 Annual Report. Hospital Medical Records Institute. Ontario, Canada, Don Mills, 1993.
28. US Renal Data System. USRDS 1991 Annual Report. Bethesda, The National Institute of Diabetes and Digestive and Kidney Diseases, 1991.
29. Braun WE, Phillips D, Vidt DG, et al. Coronary arteriography and coronary artery disease in 99 diabetics and nondiabetic patients on chronic hemodialysis or renal transplantation programs. Transplant Proc, 1981;13:128-135.

30. Kasiske BL, Malik MA, Herzog CA. Risk-stratified screening for ischemic heart disease in kidney transplant candidates. Transplantation, 2005;80:815-20.
31. Rabbat CG, Treleaven DJ, Russell JD, et al. Prognostic value of myocardial perfusion studies in patients with end-stage renal disease assessed for kidney or kidney-pancreas transplantation: a meta-analysis. J Am Soc Nephrol, 2003;14:431-9.
32. Pilmore H. Cardiac assessment for renal transplantation. Am J Transplant, 2006;6:659-65.
33. Marwick TH, Steinmuller DR, Underwood DA, et al. Ineffectiveness of dipyridamole spect thallium imaging as a screening technique for coronary artery disease in patients with end-stage renal failure. Transplantation, 1990;1:100-103.
34. Herzog CA, Marwick TH, Pheley AM. Dobutamine stress echocardiography for the detection of significant coronary artery disease in renal transplant condidates. Am J Kidney Dis, 1999;33:1090.
35. Murphy SW, Parfey PS. Screening for cardiovascular disease in dialysis patients. Curr Opin Nephrol Hypertens, 1996;5: 532-540
36. Patel RK, Mark PB, Johnston N, et al. Prognostic value of cardiovascular screening in potential renal transplant recipients: a single-centre prospective observational study. Am J Transplant, 2008;8:1673-834.
37. McFalls EO, Ward HB, Moritz TE, et al. Coronary-artery revascularization before elective major vascular surgery. N Engl J Med, 2004;351:2795-804.
38. Harnett JD, Foley RN, Kent GM, et al. Congestive heart failure in dialysis patients: Prevalence, incidence, prognosis, and risk factors. Kidney Int, 1995;47:884-890.
39. London GM, Fabiani F, Marchais SG, et al. Uremic cardiomyopathy: An inadequate left ventricular hypertrophy. Kidney Int, 1987;31: 973-980.
40. Cho WH, Kim HT, Park CH, et al. Renal transplantation in advanced cardiac failure patients. Transplant Proc, 1997;29:236-8.
41. Rodicio JL. Does hypertensive therapy protect the kidney in essential hypertension? J Hypertens, 1996;14:569-576.
42. Zanchetti A, Stella A. Cardiovascular disease and the kidney: an epidemiologic overview. J Cardiovasc Pharmacol, 1999;33(1):S1-6; discussion S41-3.
43. Poldermans D, Boersma E, Bax JJ, et al. The effect of bisoprolol on perioperative mortality and myocardial infarction in high-risk patients undergoing vascular surgery. N Engl J Med, 1999;34:1789-95.
44. Mangano DT and the Multicenter Study of Peri-operative Ischemia Research Group. Aspirin and mortality from coronary bypass surgery. N Engl J Med, 2002;347:1309-17.
45. Robertson AJ, Nargund V, Gray DW, Morris PJ. Low dose aspirin as prophylaxis against renal-vein thrombosis in renal-transplant recipients. Nephrol Dial Transplant, 2000;15(11):1865-81.
46. Ozao-Choy J, Tammaro Y, Fradis M, et al. Clopidogrel and bleeding after general surgery procedures. Am Surg, 2008;74:721-5.
47. Bry W, Peddi V, Katznelson S, et al. Kidney transplantation on Plavix: Feasible or foolhardy? Am J Transplant, 2008;8:516.
48. Mäkisalo H, Lepäntalo M, Halme L, et al. Peripheral arterial disease as a predictor of outcome after renal transplantation. Transpl Int, 1998;11 Suppl 1:S140-3.
49. Sung RS, Althoen M, Howell TA, Merion RM. Peripheral vascular occlusive disease in renal transplant recipients: risk factors and impact on kidney allograft survival. Transplantation, 2000;70:1049-54.
50. Brynger H. Transplantation of the diabetic in 1994: A personal view. Nephrol Dial Transplant, 1995;10:56-57.
51. Hirschl MM. Renal transplantation in patients with type II diabetes mellitus. Nephrol Dial Transplant, 1995;10:58-60.
52. Opelz G. Blood transfusion. Current relevance of the transfusion effect in renal transplantation. Transplant Proc, 1985;27:1015-21.
53. Zachee P, Vermylen J, Boogaerts MA. Hematologic aspects of end-stage renal failure. Ann Hematol, 1994;69:33-40.
54. Greger B, Bockhom H, Reeb A, et al. Treatment of perioperative bleeding after kidney transplantation by conjugated estrogen. Transplant Proc, 1987;19:3704-3706.
55. Seth S, Geier TM. Use of conjugated estrogens to control gastrointestinal tract bleeding in two patients with chronic renal failure. Clinical Pharmacology, 1988;7:906-8.
56. Sladen RN. Anesthetic considerations for the patient with renal failure. Anesthesiol Clin North America, 2000;18:863-82.
57. Kasiske BL, Klinger D. Cigarette smoking in renal transplant recipients. J Am Soc Nephrol, 2000;11:753-9.
58. Reissell E, Taskinen MR, Orko R, et al. Increased volume of gastric contents in diabetic patients undergoing renal transplantation: Lack of effect with cisapride. Acta Anesthesiol Scand, 1992;36: 736-740.
59. Meyers CM, Seeff LB, Stehman-Breen CO, Hoofnagle JH. Hepatitis C and renal disease: an update. Am J Kidney Dis, 2003;42:631-57.
60. Fabrizi F, Martin P, Ponticelli C. Hepatitis C virus infection and renal transplantation. Am J Kidney Dis, 2001;38:919-34.

Perioperative Renal Replacement Therapy

Prabhat Kumar Choudhary

INTRODUCTION

Renal replacement therapy (RRT) has ushered a new era in the treatment of renal failure patients who, till now, have died of the complications of ureamia and fluid overload. Since, its documented use in treating symptoms of uremia in acute renal failure (ARF) it has come a long way and now RRT is used, in addition, to treat chronic renal failure (CRF), fluid overload, sepsis, drug overdose and poisoning.

As history goes, early research into *artificial kidney* (as it was popularly called) was conducted by **Abel** et al at John Hopkins University in 1913**. Hess** performed the first hemodialysis in 1924, Germany. **Ganter and Rosenak** performed first peritoneal dialysis in 1923 in guinea pigs and **Rhoads** on two nephritic patients in 1938. The first effective artificial kidney became available after outbreak of World War II when **Willem Koff** built it in 1943 in Holland, with cellophane, sausage casing, wooden slats, orange juice cans and a washing machine. Though it was labeled quackery by internists, later during the Korean War, the artificial kidney became the forefront of medicine in the advanced trauma centers.

The general goals of dialysis (RRT) are to avoid complications of advanced uremia which are debilitating and life threatening, maintain reasonable health and quality of life and prevent morbidity and mortality in the course of RRT.

Definite goals are to be discussed later in the chapter under goals of dialysis.

The RRT involves not only hemodialysis as commonly understood, but peritoneal dialysis, continuous renal replacement therapy and renal transplant too. Now researchers are also working on oral dialysis. So RRT though old, is still an evolving branch of medicine with newer modalities appearing on the horizon now and then. We here will present a brief and comprehensive account of RRT.

PHYSICS OF DIALYSIS

Dialysis is derived from a **Greek** word meaning '*to pass across*'. So all the mechanisms used in dialysis involves transport of solutes and water across a semipermeable membrane. The physical processes involved in dialysis are:

- **Osmosis**: Water moves from a solution of low solute concentration (plasma mainly) to a high solute concentration (dialysate mainly). It is the main mechanism involved during peritoneal dialysis.
- ***Diffusion***: Solutes move across a concentration gradient if the semipermeable membrane is permeable to them. Concentration gradient is the driving force for movement of the solute whereas the thickness and permeability of the membrane represents the resisting force for the particular molecule to move across.
- ***Convection***: It is the movement of solutes across a semipermeable membrane along with water. The force produced by water is called '*solvent drag*'. Many larger molecules can be moved across the membrane if the drag is stronger.
- ***Ultrafiltration***: If a transmembrane force is created across the semipermeable membrane, solvent moves from the high to low pressure area even against the concentration gradient. The necessary pressure gradient could be positive, as provided by the mean arterial pressure (MAP) or negative as created by the dialyzer for the movement of the fluid. The solvent thus obtained is called 'ultrafiltrate' and the process is called *ultrafiltration.*
- ***Adsorption***: It is the removal of solutes by clinging to the membrane. This is comparable with an air filter where impurities passing across it cling to its surface.

HEMODIALYSIS

It is based on a very simple mechanism where blood flows on one side of a semipermeable membrane and the dialysis fluid on the other side. The dialysis fluid is composed of osmotically balanced solution of electrolytes and a pH buffer (bicarbonate). Pores in the membrane allow small molecules to pass through but larger molecules—proteins and blood are upheld. This mechanism is called diffusion and is the main mechanism during hemodialysis.

When the physical mechanism of convection is applied, the process is called *"hemofiltration."*

Hemodialysis incorporates the following components.

1. Dialyzer, where blood comes in contact with the dialysate across the semipermeable membrane for purification
2. Extra-corporeal circuit to transport blood from the patient to the dialyzer and back to the patient
3. Vascular access for easy retrieval of blood in desired amounts for dialysis.

HEMODIALYSIS MACHINE (THE EXTRACORPOREAL CIRCUIT)

A typical hemodialysis machine consists of extracorporeal blood circuit and a dialysate circuit.

The part of the system through which blood traverses from the patient to the dialyzer and purified blood back to the patient constitute the *extra-corporeal circuit.* Blood is withdrawn from a vascular access (a needle or catheter) and carried to the dialyzer by an *arterial circuit* for purification. A *peristaltic roller pump* ensures adequate blood flow through the arterial blood circuit as it is a low pressure system. A compressible segment of the arterial tubing is inserted into the roller track in the pump. The rotation of the roller compresses the tubing, forcing blood out of the pump. After the passage of blood when the tubing regains its original shape, blood is drawn in. Blood forced out of the pump than reaches the *dialyzer.* Inside the dialyzer blood comes in contact with the purification fluid *(dialysate)* across a semipermeable membrane (the contact is never direct). Here the blood is filtered and the filtered blood is transfused back into the patient via a *venous circuit.* Typically the flow rates of blood and dialysate are kept around 200–300 mL/min and 500–800 mL/min respectively. Blood and dialysate move in opposite directions ensuring maximal exchange. Heparin is added into the system to prevent clotting in the blood circuit, either continuously (by a syringe pump or peristaltic pump) or by intermittent boluses. This is a simplified version of the actual functioning of the machine. Other integral parts include *air detectors and air traps. Clamps* are provided below the air traps to terminate the process and prevent air embolism if air enters the system. *Failure alarms* are provided if air enters the system (Fig. 7.1).

DIALYSATE

The fluid used for purification of blood across the semipermeable membrane is called dialysate. It consists of purified water along with desired concentration of *electrolytes* (Na^+, K^+, Ca^{++}, Mg^{++}, Ph^{++}) and a *buffer* (commonly bicarbonate). Dialysate is produced by adding sterile water to a dialysate concentrate. The sterile water can be obtained by treating tap water, in specialised water treatment plants, to remove particulate, chemical and biological contaminants.

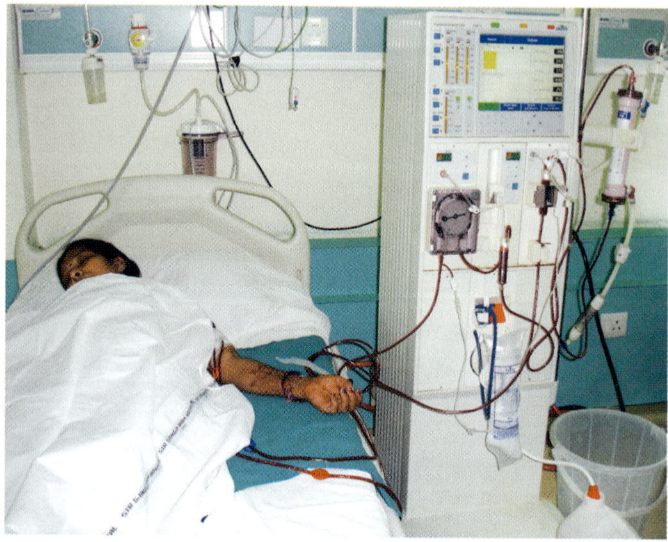

Fig. 7.1: Hemodialysis in progress

Composition of a Dialysate

Sodium

It is the **primary ion** to compensate for when urea is rapidly removed from extra-cellular space during dialysis. The decline in the osmolarity due to Na^+ movement creates an osmolar gradient causing fluid shift from extra- to intracellular space resulting in intracellular swelling and extracellular dehydration (and so intravascular hypovolemia). This can be ameliorated by adequate sodium concentration in the dialysate. A negative sodium balance may contribute to intra-dialysis hypotension and disequilibrium syndrome, fatigue, muscular cramps and headache. A positive sodium balance can cause hypertension, sometimes refractory to treatment. Hence the goal of dialysis is to remove the exact amount of sodium that has accumulated in the inter-dialysate period in order to obtain a zero balance. Since sodium concentration is strictly related to hemodynamic stability during dialysis, varying intradialytic sodium concentration is advocated. This is called sodium modelling.[1]

Potassium

It gets accumulated in the inter-dialysis period. So the goal of dialysis is to remove the excess potassium that has assimilated. Low potassium levels can cause ventricular ectopic activity (VEA), QT interval changes and changes in ventricular late potential. So potassium concentration of dialysate should be maintained at around 2.5–3.0 mmol/L (and potassium profiling should be introduced preferantially).[1]

Calcium

It plays an important role in the contractile process in both vascular and cardiac muscles and metabolic bone diseases. Changes in ionized serum calcium level may significantly affect hemodynamic stability. Therefore in patients with normal calcium level, the calcium concentration of dialysate should be kept at 1.50 mmol/L while for cardiac compromised patients calcium concentration should be 1.75 mmol/L, to improve hemodynamic stability.[2,3]

Acid Buffers

Metabolic acidosis [accumulation of H^+ ions] due to decreased kidney function is a major complication of CRF. H^+ accumulation is related to protein ingestion [approximately 0.77 mmol/gm of protein catabolized].[4] Since H^+ ions are buffered by serum bicarbonate it is used as a surrogate marker for acidemia (acid-base balance status is determined by plasma bicarbonate level). The usual bicarbonate concentration of a dialysate is 35 mmol/L.

At the end of 1980s, with development of convective dialysis techniques, *acetate free biofiltration (AFB)* was developed. It uses a dialysate without a buffer and concomitant post dialysis infusion of sterile sodium bicarbonate. So the net bicarbonate level in the patient is a result of loss from diffusion and gain from subsequent infusion.[5, 6]

Glucose

Earlier, in 1960s glucose concentrates was used to obtain osmotic ultrafiltration (to be discussed later). But with the development of hydraulic ultrafiltration its use has declined. Now glucose is used during dialysis to prevent hypoglycemia at a concentration of 100–200 mg/L. Other electrolytes that have been found useful during dialysis are magnesium and chloride.

DIALYZERS

They are also called artificial kidneys and constitute the center of dialysis system because the process of dialysis takes place in them. It consists of a blood compartment and a dialysate stream, separated by a semi-permeable membrane. The transfer of solutes and water occurs through this membrane. There are three basic designs of dialyzers.

Coil Dialyzers

It is an early and obsolete design. The blood compartment consists of two long membrane tubes wound around a plastic core *(coil)*. The membrane coil assembly was placed between two support screens. The dialysate flow around the membrane was erratic, limiting its performance. It was replaced by more efficiently working dialyzers.

Parallel Plate Dialyzers

It consists of multiple layers of membranes (2–20 or more) separated by flat supports. The dialyzer has a surface area of 1.1 m^2, the membrane has a surface area of 0.8–1.5 m^2 and the blood compartment size is of about 100 mL. The blood compartment volume can increase with increase in blood volume—a characteristic called *compliance of dialyzer*. It is advantageous over coil dialyzers as it has more uniform flow.

Hollow-Fiber Dialyzer

It consists of hollow fiber bundles of membranes encased in a plastic housing. It is then potted at both ends in a tight sealing material for support. Blood flows through an opening at one end of the dialyzer, in the fiber manifold, and comes out at the other end. Dialysate enters from the side of the dialyzer, flows around the fibers in a counter-current fashion and comes out of a hole at the other side. The surface area is about 1.2 m^2, the blood compartment is around 90 mL and it is non-compliant. Advantages of hollow fiber dialyzers are a small priming volume and the filter can be reused after proper cleansing.

DIALYSIS MEMBRANES

Dialysis membranes are semipermeable membranes and the most important constituent of a dialyzer. The membranes can be classified into three major types according to the material used for their manufacture–cellulosic, modified cellulosic and synthetic membranes.

Cellulosic Membranes

They are unmodified and produced from *celloboise*, a natural saccharides in the cell matrix. They are highly porous, have a low wall thickness *(6–15 mcm dry thickness)*, symmetric structure and a good diffusive transport for removal of small size uremic toxins. Some of the unmodified cellulosic membranes are cuprophan, cuproammonium rayon, saponified celluose ester. Though in use for a long time, they have a high hydroxyl group density that activates the complement pathway and neutrophils, a high hydrophilic character causing fouling (undesirable deposition on the surfaces) and ineffective removal of middle or larger size uremic toxins.[7]

Modified Cellulosic Membranes

They are produced by substitution of hydroxyl group and have larger pore sizes resulting in higher water permeability and greater middle molecule uremic toxins clearance. They are basically two types depending on the molecule replacement during modification:

Cellulose acetate membranes have their hydroxyl group replaced by acetate group to produce cellulose acetate membranes. About 75% substitution of hydroxyl group produces *diacetate* membranes and complete substitution *triacetate* membranes. Substitution results in decreased complement activation and decreased leukopenic response.

Hemophan membranes have low percentage of hydroxyl group replacement but tertiary amine replacement is significant. Complement activation and leukopenic response is same as the acetate group.

Synthetic Membranes

In order to solve the problems with cellulosic membranes and to achieve high filtration rate with low transmembrane pressure during hemodialysis, synthetic membranes were developed. The main difference is the chemical composition of the membrane as synthetic membranes are made of *thermoplastic* instead of natural polymers. Since 1970 when the first synthetic membrane was made, various polymers have been tried such as polysulfone, polyamide, poly-(methyl) methacrylate, polyethersulfone, polyarylethersulfone, polyamide, polyacrylonitrile and polycarbonate. Though they are referred by a single polymer name but actually they are made of more than one polymer.

An important characteristic of the membranes is pore sizes. Membranes with small pore sizes are called 'low-flux' and those with larger pore sizes are called 'high-flux' membranes. Since low-flux membranes cannot remove larger toxins, it is now a trend to use dialyzers with high-flux membranes.

It should be emphasized that dialysis membranes cannot be classified into two broad classes of (1) Cellulosic bio-incompatible, low efficiency, low-flux membranes and (2) Synthetic biocompatible, high-efficiency, high-flux membranes. There is substantial overlap between these categories so that the classification becomes meaningless.[8]

VASCULAR ACCESSES FOR HEMODIALYSIS

Vascular access can be divided into two types. Temporary and permanent.

Temporary Vascular Access

Temporary access is created when *immediate hemodialysis is necessary and rapid vascular access is required.* It is accomplished by inserting a catheter in the central veins—internal jugular, subclavian or femoral veins. These catheters are rigid double lumen, uncuffed or they are not tunneled. They can be inserted at bedside under ultrasound guidance as they do not require any fluoroscopy. They are made of *polyurethane, polyethylene and expandable-polytetrafluoroethylene (ePTFE).*

Indications

1. Prompt and immediate need for dialysis: as in a patient waiting for AV graft or AV fistula to mature or a patient with ESRD presenting in casualty with CHF
2. Non-compliance of patients for a permanent vascular access
3. Chronically ill patients unfit for permanent access
4. A patient with anatomical limitations such as superior vena caval syndrome.

Advantage is, when an early hemodialysis is required, it is a prompt, easy to conduct and less painful bed side procedure. In addition, the patients are more compliant.

Complications include infection, hemorrhage or hematoma, stenosis, clotting and other complications of central venous cannulation.

Permanent Vascular Access

It is done when long-term dialysis treatment is required. There are three ways to secure permanent access-central venous tunneled catheters, arterio-venous fistulae and arterio-venous grafts.

Central venous Tunneled Catheters

They differ from the temporary catheters in many ways. They are longer so they can be tunneled under the skin, thus called '*tunneled catheter*'. They have *Dacron cuffs* on their walls that initiate fibroblast ingrowth leading to scar tissue formation. This prevents infection to travel from the skin along the catheter into central blood pool and also serves as an anchor. They are softer, made of rubber like silicon (Sialistic), so require a rigid introducer for their placement. Flouroscopy is required to confirm the correct placement of the guide wire, dilator and finally the catheter. It also helps to reposition a misplaced catheter. Once the catheter has been placed, trans-catheter venography further confirms the intravenous placement of the catheter. The complications are same as discussed in the section of temporary catheter insertion.

Arteriovenous Fistula

It was first described by Brescia et al. (1966).[9] It is an *anastomosis between a high pressure artery and a low pressure vein* resulting in strengthening of the vein and increased blood flow. This will allow easier repeated needle insertions and the hemodialysis treatment more feasible. Its advantages are durability and ability to resist infection. An arterio-venous fistula takes 6–8 weeks to mature but it is recommended that it should be made 6–8 months in advance for proper functioning. Premature access of the fistula may result in hematoma formation or thrombosis of the fistula. *Maturation* refers to the progressive increase in diameter of the vein with thickening of the vein wall (arterialization).[10] The operation should preferably be done under local anesthesia or a regional block with intravenous sedation as it results in peripheral vasodilatation. General anesthesia is not recommended as it produces decreased cardiac output and reduced fistula flow.[11]

Four types of anastomoses are described: side-to-side, end of vein-to-side of artery, end-to end and end of artery-to-side of vein. Side-to side, end of artery-to-side of vein and end-to end anastomoses are not recommended in the wrist due to the risks of venous hypertension, arterial steal phenomena and insufficient fistula blood flow. The end of vein-to side of artery anastomosis avoids venous hypertension and allows maximum blood flow.[12] On completion of the procedure there is an evident thrill in the fistula and beyond. *Doppler examination* is used to confirm the adequacy of fistula flow. Flow rate increases rapidly in a successfully maturing fistula to >600 mL/min at the end of 6 weeks after creation.[14]

The preparations of the patient for arterio venous fistula formation should be initiated early. Withdrawal of blood from the extremity that has been selected to be used for an AV fistula should be stopped early, at stage 3 of CKD. The fistula should be made at stage 4 or within one year of anticipated start of dialysis.

Assessment of arteries and veins is done both by physical examination and doppler study for vascular mapping (both for arterial and venous system).

Arterio-venous Grafts

It is used to describe a bridge or conduit placed between a donor artery and a recipient vein. They could also be considered 'synthetic arteriovenous fistulae'. They could be of *biologic origin*- autologous saphenous vein, preserved cadaveric saphenous vein, denatured bovine grafts and human umbilical vein; or made of *synthetic materials* as Dacron and PTFE (expandable-polytetrafluoroethylene). The A-V grafts are then tunneled in the subcutaneous plane for needle access. The surgical procedure is, like any other bypass surgery, an anastomosis of an artery with the vein. The anastomoses are done in a side-to-end manner. It is preferably done under local or regional anesthesia while general anesthesia is avoided. Confirmation of a successful graft placement is done by a palpable thrill and then by doppler examination. Usual sites for putting AV grafts are forearm (brachial artery to antecubital vein), upper arm (brachial artery to axillary or proximal basilic vein) and in case of failing AV graft in the forearm, thigh (superior femoral artery to saphenous vein) or the chest wall.

The *principal benefit* of this procedure is that it can be put in patients in absence of adequate basilic or brachial veins and fistula formation is not feasible. A-V grafts take 10–14 days to mature before they can be used. Another use of an AV graft is putting it in a "*planned bridge*" manner. Here an AV graft is used to help mature the venous system by increasing the blood flow to the desired region.

Complications of vascular accesses are thrombosis, venous hypertension, infections, aneurysms and pseudoaneurysms, congestive heart failure and a rare complication called '*steal phenomenon.*' The ischemia of the limb distal to the fistula or graft is called vascular steal. Though some physiologic steal is common with high flow accesses at the time of creation but a symptomatic AV fistula and graft needs surgical attention. More common with upper arm grafts, the symptoms include pallor and coolness of the hand, neuropraxia and ischemic gangrene. If the symptoms are mild, they resolve within one or two months. If the patient has pain or paresthesias, urgent surgical revision is required.[13]

Biological grafts are more prone to develop aneurysms.

Subcutaneous Ports with Catheters

These devices consist of a subcutaneous port implanted beneath the clavicle and a catheter is attached to it. It is then tunnelled and put into the internal jugular vein. The port can be accessed with a dialysis needle through a trans-cutaneous approach. When used correctly, they provide higher blood flow and have lower infection rate thus increasing survival rate. Their future looks bleak as the manufacturers are not interested in continuing with the product in the market.

ANTICOAGULANTS DURING HEMODIALYSIS

During hemodialysis, thrombosis in the extracorporeal circuit is a known phenomenon hampering effective dialysis. Dialyzers, needle or catheters, tubings, venous and arterial bubble traps are components of thrombogenicity. Further risk factors are slow and turbulent blood flows with higher shear rates, increased hematocrit and blood transfusion into the extra-corporeal circuit. Clotting on an artificial surface occurs both by surface contact (intrinsic) and expression of tissue factors after endothelial damage (extrinsic) pathways.

Standard Anticoagulation During Hemodialysis

Routine anticoagulants interfere with the *plasmatic clotting cascade*. The anticoagulants are prescribed as per the clinical condition of the patient and tailored for specific hemodialysis sessions. Knowledge of the specific anticoagulant is important to monitor peri-operatve coagulation status and determine further course of action.

We will be discussing in short the specific anticoagulants with respect to their activity and side effects.

Unfractionated Hearin (UHF) consists of a mixture of anionic glucosamines of varying molecular sizes (5–40, mean 15 kDaltons). Its main action is indirect by binding with *antithrombin* (heparin binding factor 1). Anti-Th inactivates thrombin and factor Xa and to a lesser extent IXa, XIa, XIIa. It is ineffective against thrombin bound with fibrin or inside a thrombus. The dosing schedule is an initial loading dose or as an infusion into the arterial line of the dialysis machine. Alternatively, it can be given as intermittent boluses. Since UHF has a very narrow therapeutic window of adequate anticoagulation to bleeding, laboratory testing (aPTT, ACT) is required. Heparin causes many side effects but immune mediated thrombocytopenia is rare but life threatening complication. Two types of presentations of this complication have been described.[15]

Heparin induced thrombocytopenia type I (HIT I) occurs during first 2–3 days of heparin therapy when a modest drop in platelet count is seen due to de-granulation of platelets (and not due to any immunologic reaction). It is considered to be harmless. The platelet count improves even if heparin therapy is continued.

Heparin induced thrombocytopenia type II (HIT II) occurs from 4–10 days after initiating heparin therapy. It is an immune mediated disease caused by formation of antibodies —"HIT ANTIBODIES", against the platelet factor 4 and heparin complex. In HIT II, thrombocytopenia indicates platelet consumption, therefore low platelet count is not associated with bleeding but increased venous and arterial thrombosis. HIT is also called "*white clot syndrome*" because platelet rich white thrombi are formed in the arteries. The clinical picture is ischemia of one or more limbs and high rate of myocardial and cerebral infarction induced mortality. However, majority of thrombi are formed in the venous system including lungs which are frequently overlooked.

Management of HIT II is to stop all applications of heparin including heparin skin ointments, heparin coated catheters or even heparin rinsing of the circuits. In active HIT, if platelet count is low, systemic anticoagulation should always be considered by alternative anticoagulants. In this case regional anticoagulation in the extracorporeal system is done by citrate.

Low molecular weight heparin (LMWH) preparations consist of a mixture of anionic glucosamines with a smaller size (4–8 kDaltons). They bind to antithrombin but have lesser affinity as compared to UFH. Since anti-Xa activity is more pronounced, aPTT or ACT monitoring is unreliable and anti Factor Xa activity has to be measured.[16, 17] Though they are not interchangeable, their anticoagulant activity correlates with the body weight in normal renal function patients. But their dose has to be reduced during renal failure.

Danaparoid consists of *heparin sulfate (83%), dermatan sulfate and chondroitin sulfate*. The anticoagulant effect is by selectively binding to antithrombin, heparin cofactor 2 and to Factor X. Danaparoid has a low cross reactivity against HIT II antibodies. Monitoring of anticoagulant activity is done by anti Factor Xa. If applied appropriately, it has a favorable benefit/risk ratio, even for prolonged use.

Direct thrombin inhibitors directly bind to thrombin and block its activity and thus the conversion of soluble fibrinogen to insoluble fibrin. There are two thrombin inhibitors—*lepirudin* and *argatroban* approved for alternative anticoagulation in HIT.

Lepirudin is a recombinant hirudin preparation. It is mainly eliminated by the kidneys so its half life is markedly prolonged in renal failure, even after a single dose. With no antidote available only high volume hemofiltration is effective in reducing hirudin plasma level. Monitoring is performed by ecarin clotting time (ECT) or chromogenic substrate assays. Hirudin is a valid alternative anticoagulant in HIT patients if used with caution and monitoring.[18]

Argatroban is a arginine derived, synthetic, catalytic-site directed potent thrombin inhibitor. It is metabolised primarily in the liver. With periodic monitoring of anticoagulant activity the aPTT, ECT or ACT it is favored over lepirudin for alternate anticoagulation in chronic renal failure patients.[19]

Fondaparinux is synthetic pentasaccharide derived from the region of heparin that binds to antithrombin molecule. It exerts a high anti-Xa activity. The half life is prolonged in renal failure therefore its dose has to be reduced in patients with renal insuffiency and for hemodialysis procedures.

Citrate regional anticoagulation (described later) allows hemodialysis without systemic anticoagulants.

Anticoagulation in Patients with High Bleeding Risk

Dialysis is often required in patients with increased risk of bleeding as gastrointestinal or retinal bleeding or heparinization can be dangerous such as in pericarditis or following surgery. The risk can be reduced by following methods

1. *Minimal heparinization*—administration of 50% of the calculated dose
2. *Regional heparinization*—heparin is continuously neutralized by constant infusion of protamine before the blood returns to the patient. But in this case heparin rebound phenomenon can occur when reticuloendothelial cells breaks down the heparin-protamine complex and heparin reenters the circulation causing hemorrhage. This method is not recommended.
3. *Heparin free dialysis*—here both the dialyzer and blood lines are pretreated with 2500–5000 I U of heparin contained in one liter of saline and flushed every 10–15 minutes. Along with this, a high ultraflitration rate is required to remove a large amount of fluid given to the patient. It is the commonest method of heparin free dialysis.
4. *Regional citrate anticoagulation* is an effective alternative method of anticoagulation.[20] Citrate, in the form of *iso-smotic trisodium citrate solution*, is infused in the arterial line chelating calcium and magnesium. This inhibits the coagulation in extracorporeal circulation. The citrate-calcium complex is removed across the dialyzer. Calcium is substituted in the venous line to maintain calcium balance.

Problems of citrate coagulation are

a. Citrate is metabolized in the liver to form bicarbonate that may cause alkalosis

b. Trisodium citrate may induce hypernatremia. Therefore close monitoring is essential and necessary adjustments should be done.

COMPLICATIONS OF HEMODIALYSIS

Complications during hemodialysis could be

A. Mechanical complications due to malfunction of dialysis machine as dialyzer rupture or clotting, conductivity, high or low venous and arterial pressures, needle site bleeding, electric failures, etc.

B. Patient complications—procedural and related to the patients medical illnesses.

Intradialysis Hypotension

Symptomatic hypotension is a very common complication during hemodialysis. It is often accompanied by nausea, vomiting, muscle cramps and may lead to circulatory collapse. Causes include:

1. Decreased plasma volume due to rapid or high ultra-filtration rate, a low set or underestimation of dry weight
2. A low sodium or calcium content in dialysate
3. Increased blood and dialysate flow rate
4. Decreased compensatory vaso-constriction due to high dialysate temperature (37–38°C), acetate dialysate or anti-hypertensive medications
5. Decreased cardiac compliance: either failure to increase heart rate as with age or uremic autonomic neuropathy; or inability to increase cardiac output as with ageing, hypertension, atherosclerosis, amyloidosis or valvular heart diseases. Less frequent causes include pericardial tamponade, myocardial infarction, hemorrhage, septicemia, arrhythmias, anaphylaxis, hemolysis and air embolism.

Acute management include:

1. Trendelenburg position (if respiratory status allows)
2. Fluid resuscitation with boluses of 0.9% saline, 3% saline, 50% dextrose, 20% human albumin and mannitol
3. Pressor agents like dopamine
4. Other measures include reduction of ultrafiltration rate and discontinuation if the symptoms are severe.

For chronic and repeated cases foremost is the amelioration of the causative factors: maintain dry weight, antihypertensives only after the session, maintain sodium and calcium concentration of the dialysate, use cooler dialysate and check ultrafiltation rate. Oxygen supplementation, human albumin, and pressurized boots also help. If hypotension occurs during or after the procedure, follow as advised before.[21]

Disequilibrium Syndrome

Severely uremic patients, during dialysis, may develop neurological disturbances particularly due to fast removal of solutes (urea and osmolytes) from the blood.[24] Its occurrence is characterized by presence of cerebral edema because of increased brain osmolality, hence the term *'disequilibrium syndrome'*.[22,23] Rapid clearance of urea from the blood compared to the brain results in a higher concentration of urea in the brain. This results in severe osmotic fluid shift and cerebral edema.[22] Similar pathogenesis has been hypothesized due to accumulation of osmolytes-*sugars, aminoacids, polyols and methylamine and H^+ ions* in the brain tissue.

Symptoms include nausea, headache, blurred vision, disorientation and hypertension in mild cases. Severly affected patients can proceed to confusion, seizures, coma and even death. Predisposing factors are BUN >175mg%, older age, pediatric patients, severe metabolic acidosis and presence of other mental illnesses.[22]

Preventive measures include frequent (daily) and short (2–3 hours) dialysis session, sodium content of dialysate to be kept between 140–145 mmol/L and use of bicarbonate based dialysate.

Disequilibrium syndrome is usually self limiting, dissipating within hours but if severe symptoms persist, it can be reversed by raising the osmolality with hypertonic saline or mannitol.

Air Embolism

Air embolism is a serious and life threatening complication resulting in high mortality in spite of adequate and intensive therapy. It occurs due to air aspiration into the extracorporeal circuit that operates in the negative pressure range- between the arterial fistula needle and blood pump.
Causes include:

1. Air leaks around tubing joints and
2. Excessive (unattended or unmonitored) negative pressure due to inadequate fistula flow rate, for the demand of the pump or malposition of the arterial needle.

Manifestations depend on the *volume* of air entered into the vasculature, the *size* of the bubbles and *position* of the patient. In the upright position, cerebral symptoms predominate due to obstruction of cerebral veins leading to convulsions, coma and death.

In the recumbent position, air forms foam in the heart and cardiac symptoms predominate impairing cardiac performance and decreasing cardiac output. If the air passes into the pulmonary artery, pulmonary pressure will increase. Pulmonary symptoms include cough, dyspnea, cyanosis and chest tigtness. Subsequent passage into the left ventricle may cause arrhythmias and cerebral symptoms due to arterial embolism.

Management include clamping of venous line and stopping the blood pump. Place the patient in a left recumbent position, supplement oxygen and consider artificial ventilation, if required. In severe cases, air may be aspirated from the right ventricle by a transthoracic puncture. In some cases treatment in compressive chamber is of value. Air embolism is a life threatening that occurs almost always due to a human error and carries a mortality of 25%.

Dialysis Induced Hypoxemia

Hypoxemia is a complication of hemodialysis that becomes relevant in severely cardiac or pulmonary compromised patients. Hypoxemia is described with acetate dialysate due to

1. Hypoventilation caused by loss of CO_2 via the dialyzer (since PCO_2 in the dialysate is zero).
2. Complement activation by the hemodialysis membrane causing sequestration of white blood cells in the lungs and loss in the diffusion capacity.[26] Bicarbonate-based buffer also causes complement sequestration decreasing diffusion capacity and gain of bicarbonate from the dialysate, decreases respiratory drive as well.[27, 28]

Membrane Reactions

Reactions were commonly seen during first time use of dialyzers and so were called '*First-use Reactions*'**.** But later on they were also seen with subsequent reuses of the dialyzers and now they are called '*hypersensitivity reactions' or 'dialyzer reactions'* Thus the reactions were classified into two groups depending on their etiology.[29]

Anaphylactic Reactions (Type A) occur within 20–30 minutes but usually within 5 minutes of the start of the procedure. Clinical manifestations in milder forms include urticaria, pruritus, dyspnea, cough, coryza, abdominal pain, diarrhca, anxiety, angioedema and laryngeal edema. It can progress to severe hypotension and collapse and may lead to cardiac arrest and death.[30]

Etiology

1. Residual ethylene oxide (used for sterilization of dialyzers),
2. Complement activation,
3. Increased bradykinin level,
4. Bacterial endotoxins due to incomplete sterilization
5. Chemicals used for sterilization in reused dialyzers and
6. Acetate in dialysate (can act as a bonchoconstrictor).

Management is to *stop dialysis* and discard all the components including blood. Use *anti-histaminics, cortico-steroids, supplement oxygen and cardio-vascular support* if required. Switch to any non-acetate dialysate and a new non-complement activating membrane. All further dialysis should be done with disposable circuits after proper rinsing.

Non-specific Reactions (Type B) are non-specific, milder in symptoms and more common than anaphylactic reactions. Chest pain may be associated with these reactions. Etiology is complement activation due to contact. Thus, it is less common with reused dialyzers since they are coated with a protein layer. Management includes oxygen therapy and symptomatic treatment.

Arrhythmias

Arrhythmias during dialysis occur in the range of 30–45% and range from supraventricular to severe ventricular arrhythmias.[25] They occur frequently at the time of dialysis.

Predisposing factors include digitalis, increased LV mass, advanced age, preexisting IHD, hypokalemia, hypercalcaemia, hypomagnesaemia, and prolonged ESRD.

Management includes oxygen supplementation, sedation, ECG and further management depending on the type of arrhythmia. Anti arrhythmic drugs should be used sparingly; only for reccurrent severe or life-threatening manifestations.

Angina During Hemodialysis

Causes

1. Hemodynamic stress—hypotension, volume overload, air embolism, hemolysis
2. Hypoxemia
3. Predisposing factors for angina as coronary stenosis, hyperlipidemia, atherosclerosis or anemia.

Management include oxygen supplementation, sublingual NTG, sedation, ECG and further dialysis with acetate free (bicarbonate) dialysate, decrease blood flow and stop ultrafiltration. In severe cases, discontinue procedure.

Bleeding

Patients with uremia have an increased chances of bleeding due to platelet dysfunction.[31,32,33] This is increased during hemodialysis due to administration of heparin (heparin induced thrombocytopenia) and platelet membrane interactions. Petechial hemorrhage and bruising around fistula puncture or skin blood blisters are common. Serious bleeding can occur during hemodialysis like intracerebral bleed, subdural hematoma, subarachnoid hemorrhage (in patients with polycystic disease), subcapsular liver hematoma, retroperitoneal bleed and gastro-intestinal bleed.[34] In presence of pericarditis (a frequent occurence in renal failure) heparin used during dialysis can cause hemopericardium and subsequent cardiac tamponade (so heparin is preferably avoided). It is a life threatening situation and should be immediately managed.[35]

Muscle Cramps

It is not a critical complication but the incidence is 5–20%. Common causes are hypotension, excessive ultrafiltration causing intracellular dehydration or electrolyte disturbances (mainly decrease in sodim and potassium). Correction of the causes may take care of this symptom.

Treatment include quinine, diazepam/oxazepam given 2 hours before dialysis and stretching exerercises.

CONTINUOUS RENAL REPLACEMENT THERAPY (CRRT)

Intermittent (or traditional) hemodialysis (IHD) therapy needs to be done every 2–3 days and it causes hemodynamic instability. Critically ill patients are unable to tolerate these sudden fluid and electrolyte changes and the ensuing hypotension can further damage the kidneys.[37,38] These patient also require a large amount of fluid and proteins. So in 1980s, CRRT was developed to overcome these limitations, for those who could not tolerate IHD.[36]

The CRRT provides a slow continuous removal of water, toxins and solutes mimicking a normal kidney so there is no sudden hypotension, proteins could be administered with ease and toxins and solutes can be removed at will prior to build up, thus avoiding metabolic disturbances after dialysis.[39,40] The chances of renal recovery are better with continuous than intermittent therapies,[40,41] although it is similar to hemodialysis and involves all the mechanisms of transport—diffusion, convection, adsorption and ultrafiltration.

Vascular access can be achieved both by *arterio-venous route* (artery for drawing blood and vein for infusing purified blood) and *veno-venous route* (a double lumen single catheter). The inability of critically ill patients to produce enough pressure for forward flow in the circuit and with the introduction of blood pumps, veno-venous route is preferred. Vascular access for CRRT are femoral, subclavian or internal jugular veins. It should preferentially be put away from any other vascular site used for routine infusion of drugs or parenteral nutrition because then these substances will also be filtered.

Indications of CRRT: The most common indications for CRRT is acute renal failure (ARF) complicated with heart failure, volume overload, hypercatabolism, acute or chronic liver failure, and/or brain swelling. Less common indications include systemic inflammatory response (SIRS), sepsis, multi-organ failure (MOF), ARDS, and chronic heart failure. CRRT could be used during or after open heart operations, heart, lung or/and liver transplantation in adults and children.[42]

Contraindications include refusal for dialysis or life sustaining therapy by the patient or family and inability to establish vascular access.

REPLACEMENT FLUIDS

The replacement fluids are crystalloids administered to replace the ultrafiltrate removed during hemofiltration or hemodiafiltration. The fluid is infused either before the blood enters the filter (*pre-dilution*) or after the blood leaves the filter (*post-dilution*). Additives can be added to replace certain solutes and nutrients. The increased fluid flow, through the filter, allows more molecules to be carried away across the filter.

Types of CRRT

Four of types CRRT have been described.

1. Slow continuous ultrafiltration (SCUF)
2. Continuous veno-venous hemofiltration (CVVH)
3. Continuous veno-venous hemodialysis (CVVHD)
4. Continuous veno-venous hemodiafiltration (CVVHDF).

Slow continuous ultrafiltration (SCUF) primarily removes water with solutes being carried in small amounts with it (not significant clinically). The blood is run through a filter with no dialysate or replacement fluid. The primary indication is fluid overload without uremia or any significant electrolyte imbalances. Fluid removal rate is typically around 100 mL/hr and a net of 2 liters/day.

Continuous veno-venous hemofiltration (CVVHF) is an extremely useful method of solute removal and indicated in severe electrolyte or pH imbalances with or without fluid overload. In this method, replacement fluid is added but no dialysate is used.

Continuous veno-venous hemodialysis (CVVHD) is similar to the classical dialysis technique (but continuous) and good for removing small and medium sized molecules. The patient is put on CRRT and dialysate is run but no replacement is added. Fluid removal also takes place along with the solutes.

Continuous veno-venous hemodiafiltration (CVVHDF) combines benefits of both diffusion and convection and adds more flexibility to dialysis treatment. The patient is put on CRRT with dialysate and replacement fluids added to it. The replacement fluids allow better solute removal with a net positive or zero fluid balance.

COMPLICATIONS OF CONTINUOUS RENAL REPLACEMENT THERAPY

1. *Bleeding:* Bleeding could be *local or systemic. Local bleeding* occurs from the site of the vascular catheter—ecchymoses, hematoma or external bleeding. Invisible bleeding can occurs from subclavian or femoral site. Hemoglobin and hematocrit should be monitored to find any internal bleeding. Inadvertent disconnection of the tubings also cause bleeding. *Systemic bleeding* can occur due to anticoagulation or systemic manifestation of the disease in critically ill patients. So additional lab test for thrombocytopenia or DIC—PT, aPTT, platelet count, FDP, fibrinogen a bleeding time should be monitored regularly.
2. *Hypothermia:* These patients are always at risk because blood is circulated outside the body. It is important to keep body temperature above 36°C by warming blankets and increased ambient temperature of the room. Warming of IV fluids prior to administration should be done. *[Bicarbonate containing solutions should not be warmed as CO_2 diffuses out as bubbles].*
3. *Electrolyte Imbalances:* CRRT is employed in critically ill patients for correction of electrolyte abnormalities. But over-correction can happen as non-physiological fluids (dialysate or replacement fluids) are used or electrolytes are added to these fluids to correct certain imbalances.
4. *Acid-base Imbalances:* Though a complication of the critically ill, CRRT can also cause these abnormalities from over-correction. Correction of pH is done along with electrolytes. But CRRT only corrects metabolic acidosis of renal origin and not the one arising from tissue hypoperfusion or respiratory causes.
5. *Dose Adjustments of Medications:* Renally cleared drugs are efficiently cleared by all types of CRRT so their doses need not be adjusted. But if CRRT is planned to be discontinued then their level can build upto toxic levels and adjustments are required.

SLOWER METHODS OF RENAL REPLACEMENT THERAPY

Sustained low efficiency dialysis (SLED) and extended daily dialysis (EDD) are slower modalities of RRT. They were introduced as a *hybrid technique* between IHD and CRRT for patients in ICU as they incorporate both their advantages and overcome the disadvantages.[43]

They run on conventional IHD machines for prolonged periods using low pump speeds *(around 50–200 mL/min)* and low dialysate flow *(around 200–400 mL/min)* for 6–12 hours daily, providing better hemodynamics stability (as in CRRT) and avoid the need for expensive CRRT machines. SLED can be done in the daytime or in the night. EDD is done in the day with the above settings for a longer period. Since SLED and EDD can be done intermittently based on the need of the patient, interruption of the various diagnostic and therapeutic procedures required in the patient may be avoided. Also a single machine can be used in all types of clinical situations either in ICU or in outside-day-care patients. This adaptability for flexible regimen makes it useful in all types of ICU patients. Prospective studies have found no difference in mean arterial pressure or inotrope support and overall mortality in patients treated with EDD and CVVH.[43,44]

PERITONEAL DIALYSIS

Peritoneal dialysis is a common modality of renal replacement therapy though poorly understood by physicians and anesthesiologists. The origin of peritoneal dialysis can be traced back to Ganter et al in 1923, when they first tried it on guinea pigs and rabbits.[45] Rhoads, in 1938, used it to treat two nephrotic patients, with some success.[46] But it was in 1968 when Tenckhoff and Schecter modified the silicone indwelling peritoneal catheter for long-term peritoneal dialysis (attached 'the cuffs') that the modality gained popularity and usefulness.[47] Peritoneal dialysis was developed along with hemodialysis to teat uremia but, by 1960s it use was limited to treat ARF only. In 1976 Popovich et al introduced CAPD as an alternative treatment of ESRD and since then it has come to the forefront in treatment of renal failure.

Anatomy and Physiology in Peritoneal Dialysis

Peritoneal dialysis is similar to hemodialysis. Here the peritoneum (visceral peritoneum) acts as a semi-permeable membrane between the blood and dialysate. The peritoneal dialysate is instilled in peritoneal cavity by a peritoneal catheter. The dialysate, thus instilled allows exchange of solutes and water between capillary blood and dialysate fluid. The rate of exchange diminishes with time and eventually stops after attaining equilibrium between plasma and dialysate. The used dialysate is later drained from the body by the catheter. Every cycle of refilling and drainage is called an *'exchange'* and the time spent by the dialysate inside the peritoneum is *'dwell time.'*

Histologically, the visceral peritoneum which lines the abdominal organs and also overlays the blood vessels, lymphatics and connective tissues is composed of a single layer of mesothelial cells. Mesothelial cells also extend microvilli on their free surface thus increasing the areas of solute and water transport.

Physics of Peritoneal Dialysis

Physical forces active in peritoneal dialysis are similar to that in hemodialysis as:

- *Diffusion:* It is the primary mechanism through which solutes move between the peritoneal capillaries and dialysate along a concentration gradient across the peritoneum.
- *Osmosis:* It is the movement of water (solvent) across the peritoneum along the concentration gradient. This process produces ultrafiltrate and so it is called 'osmotic ultrafiltration.' Osmosis during peritoneal dialysis is achieved by using a hyperosmolar dialysate. It differs from the hemodialytic ultrafiltration as that is driven along a hydrostatic pressure gradient. *[Hydrostatic ultrafiltration is difficult to achieve in peritoneal dialysis]*

  Plasma proteins removed during peritoneal dialysis serve as a means for excreting uremic toxins that are tightly bound to proteins.

Peritoneal Dialysate

Peritoneal dialysate, like the hemodialysate, is a balanced salt solution designed to create a concentration gradient across the peritoneal membrane and remove endogenous waste products and maintain electrolytes, pH and fluid volume to near normal. But peritoneal dialysis uses osmotic rather than convective ultrafiltration. So, peritoneal dialysate is deliberately rendered hyperosmolar relative to plasma (by adding an osmotic agent to create an osmotic gradient) to favor net movement of water across the peritoneal cavity. They are available in prefilled bags of 0.5–3.0 liter capacity depending on the size of the patient from pediatric to big adults.

The various components of peritoneal dialysate are:

- *Osmotic agent (Glucose)*: In commercially available peritoneal dialysates, glucose serves as the osmotic agent to enhance ultrafiltration. The glucose concentration ranges from 1.36% (1.5% dextrose) to 3.86% (4.5% dextrose). Over a period, the osmolality of the dialysate declines as a result of water moving into the peritoneal cavity and absorption of dialysate glucose.
- *Sodium:* The role of sodium in maintaining hemodynamics during dialysis has been discussed earlier. Since peritoneal dialysates are hyperosmolar they can cause dehydration and hypernatremia due to increased water loss. Frequent cycling can further result in significant dehydration and hypernatremia. Still, low sodium dialysates have not shown much clinical benefit in these situations. Commercially available peritoneal dialysates have a sodium concentration of 132 mEq/L.[48]
- *Potassium:* Potassium intake is greater than the clearance affected with peritoneal dialysis. But significant hyper-

kalemia is rare because colonic secretion and residual renal functions take care of it. So potassium is not routinely added in peritoneal fluid. However hypokalemia can occur in patients undergoing frequent exchanges, so potassium is added to a concentration of 2–3 mEq/L.[48]

- *Calcium:* Calcium concentration of commercially available peritoneal dialysates is either 1.25% or 1.75%. The decision to use one concentration or the other is to be made on an individual basis. Most patients are dialyzed with 1.75% solutions but a lower concentration is used in a patient treated with calcium containing phosphate binders and calcitriol to avoid hypercalcemia.
- *Magnesium:* Commercially available peritoneal dialysates have a magnesium concentration of 0.5 mEq/L.
- *Dialysate Buffer:* The pH of the peritoneal buffer is rendered acidic (by adding HCl) to prevent caramelization of glucose and prevent precipitation of calcium and magnesium during sterilization of the solution. The buffer commercially used is lactate, as it is converted to bicarbonate, after instillation, on a molar basis in patients with intact liver function (1 mmol of lactate generates 1 mmol of bicarbonate).

The conventional PD fluids have some drawbacks related to the glucose content and low pH.[48,49] The absorption of glucose contributes substantially to the calorie intake of patients on peritoneal dialysis. This carbohydrate load contributes to decreased nutrition as a result of loss of appetite and decreased protein intake. It also causes progressive obesity, hyperinsulinemia, hyperlipidemia and decreased peripheral sensitivity to insulin. The high glucose content and toxicity of advanced glycosylated end products and glucose degradation products have an inhibitory effect on the function of leukocytes, peritoneal macrophages, and mesothelial cells resulting in peritoneal sclerosis and ultrafiltration failure and patients being transferred to hemodialysis.[48] So, in an attempt to develop a more physiologic (biocompatible) solution, various new osmotic agents were under investigation namely icodextran, fructose, sorbitol, xylitol, dextran, gelatin, glycerol, and aminoacids. Some of these have proved useful as alternatives to the standard glucose, i.e icodextrin (a glucose polymer that is not absorbed) and aminoacids. Dialysates with amino acids have received the most attention. This may be used to provide additional nutrition but its use is limited by uremic byproducts, an additional load that has to be taken care of during dialysis.[48]

The second modification in making the peritoneal fluid more biocompatible, is replacing lactate with bicarbonate as a buffer.[48] Use of bicarbonate increases the pH that decreases the pain during instillation, has no adverse effect on peritoneal transport, lessens the incidence of peritonitis, renal functions are better preserved and a better survival benefit compared to conventional solutions. The advancements in sterilization process and delivery systems (separate bags or two-chamber single bags to separate the precipitating components) have made it possible to use a bicarbonate buffer. Bicarbonate alone or a combination of lactate and bicarbonate is being advocated for future dialysates.

Peritoneal Catheter

Peritoneal catheters are accesses for peritoneal dialysis. They have a similar basic design despite the presence of a bewildering variety.[51] The catheter consists of three parts—peritoneal part that indwells inside the peritoneum with the tip placed into the pelvis, the middle or subcutaneous portion is from the peritoneum to the skin exit site and the external part that is present outside the skin. The external part is used to fill and empty the peritoneum during dialysis. They have radio-opaque stripe for X-ray visualization. An ideal peritoneal catheter should allow adequate amount of flow of dialysate, drain the abdomen to less than few hundred milliliters of residual dialysate, minimize infection and a successful resolution if it occurs, avoid pericatheter leaks and hernias and should easily be implantable without any major surgery.

Catheters can be classified depending on the duration of peritoneal dialysis as acute and chronic catheters.

Acute PD catheters are a length of straight or slightly curved relatively rigid tubings with numerous side holes at the distal end. A metal stylet or flexible guide wire is used to slide the catheter during insertion. They are designed to be placed 'medically' at bedside because even a short delay for surgical consultation and implantation is not acceptable for the patients with ARF. They should not be used beyond three days, as risk of peritonitis increases due to lack of cuffs and chances of bowel perforation is high. Nowadays single cuff silicone Tenckhoff catheters are also used for acute peritoneal dialysis.

Chronic PD catheters are the most successful transcutaneous access devices with success measured in years and not in days or months.[51] They are made of silicone or soft rubber as polyurethane. They have one or two Dacron cuffs that provide tissue ingrowth (fibroblast growth) thus acting as an anchor, prevent fluid leaks and prevent infection from travelling into the peritoneum. The most commonly used peritoneal catheter is the Tenckhoff cuffed catheter first introduced in 1968 and modified thereof to the present shape.[50]

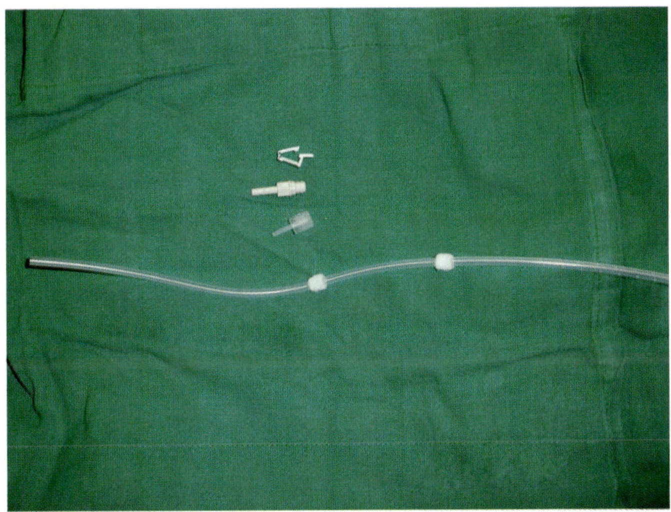

Fig. 7.2: Double Dacron cuff Tenckhoff peritoneal catheter with connections (note the two cuffs)

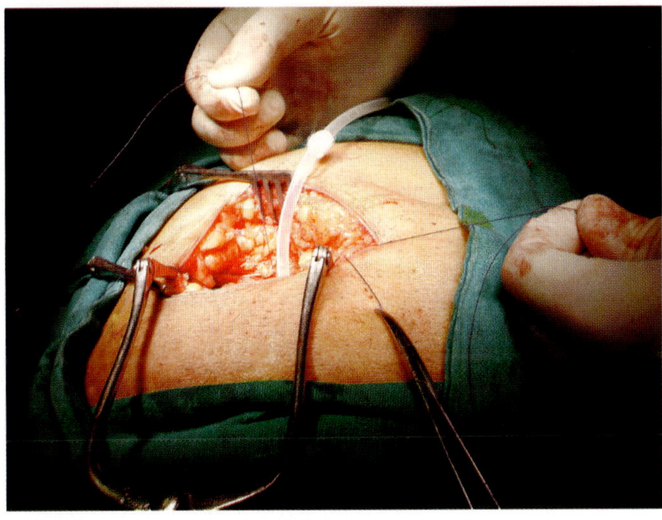

Fig. 7.3: Operative placement of Tenckhoff peritoneal catheter in progress

The Tenckhoff catheters commonly used have two Dacron cuffs approximately 5 cms apart. The inner cuff is placed in the rectus muscle and the external cuff is placed in the subcutaneous tissue about 2 cms away from exit site. The peritoneal part of the catheter has multiple holes and an open pelvic end. The side holes are helpful in better evacuation of the dialysate at the end of the procedure (Fig. 7.2). Peritoneal catheters come in various sizes to accomodate different age groups-from pediatric to obese adults. There are various modifications in the peritoneal catheters to diminish outflow obstruction in the intraperitoneal portion (curved or coiled) and prevent catheter migration in the subcutaneous portion (150 degree curve in Swan Neck and double 90 degree curves in Pail Handle catheter).

The catheter can be placed in the following ways:

- Open dissection surgical placement
- Laparoscopic surgical placement
- Percutaneous blind puncture after filling the abdomen with fluid and
- Peritoneoscopy: a device used to first visualize the peritoneum, then create pneumoperitoneum with one liter of air and choose a proper location for implantation of the catheter.

Percutaneous technique is reserved mainly for the temporary catheters. It is less expensive and efficient procedure. It is done under local infiltration with inrtravenous sedation and anti *Staphylococcus* prophylaxis. A guide wire is first introduced followed by the catheter into the peritoneal cavity and placed in the pelvis.

Open technique is preferred for longer indwelling (long-term) peritoneal catheters.[52] It should be inserted in the operation room (theater) for patient comfort and a strict sterile environment. Local or regional anesthesia is preferred. General anesthesia is reserved for children or certain group of uncooperative patients where muscle relaxation of abdominal muscles is required. The preferred incision is infraumbilical so that the catheter exit site is positioned below the belt-line. Any handling of the catheter should always be done under strict sepsis (Fig. 7.3). The catheter should be flushed daily. Dialysis, if required to be started early, should be done with small amount of fluid.

Laparoscopic placement of peritoneal catheters was introduced by Ash and colleagues in 1981.[53] It requires general anesthesia. This technique also allows documentation of correct placement of peritoneal catheter and lowers the incidences of surgical complications such as wound infection.

Types of Peritoneal Dialysis

Depending on the duration of peritoneal dialysis it could be classified into two categories:

1. Short term peritonel dialysis
2. Long term peritoneal dialysis.

Short term or acute peritoneal dialysis is reserved for patients with ARF. The indications for short term PD include electrolytes disburbances (e.g. hyperkalemia), hypercatabolic ARF, metabolic acidosis or other metabolic disturbances (e.g. hyperuricemia), congestive heart failure, drug intoxication or poisoning.[54-59] Short term PD should not last for more than

3–4 days. Acute PD was once the mainstay of ARF due the potential drawbacks of intermittent hemodialysis viz. highly trained personnel, systemic anticoagulation, complex and expensive procedure and hemodynamic instability. But due to its inadequate small solutes clearance, inability during severe illnesses and the growth of CRRT, it fell into disregard. Acute PD still holds its place as a safe and economic modality for severely ill patients with hemodynamic instability, with increased risk of bleeding, severe coagulation disorders, in infants and children and where facilities for CRRT or SLED are not available.

Long term peritoneal dialysis may last for months to years. The indications for long term PD include patients with end stage renal disease who do not prefer IHD or do not have facilities for the same. Patients with congestive heart failure, diabetes, contraindication to heparinization and children and adults who have smaller arteries where fistulas are not possible, can also be considered for peritoneal dialysis.

Modalities of Peritoneal Dialysis

1. Intermittent peritoneal dialysis (IPD) is the oldest modality of PD where peritoneal dialysis is done intermittently, i.e. thrice a week with a dwell time of 20–30 minutes or as overnight dwells on alternate nights. Once a common modality, it is seldom practiced now except for a few indications viz refusal by the patient for whatever reason, immediately following catheter insertion, during severe peritonitis and patients with high peritoneal permeability resulting in loss of ultrafiltration. Its efficiency is low so it has been replaced by more efficient continuous techniques.
2. Continuous ambulatory peritoneal dialysis (CAPD) is a home based therapy that does not require any hospital admission. First proposed by Popovich in 1976, as *continuous equilibrium peritoneal dialysis (CEPD)*[60], it is a closed system where dialysate is instilled into the peritoneal cavity by gravity and drained after a dwell time of several hours. The basic equipment consists of a plastic bag containing PD fluid, a transfer set (rubber tubings to deliver and drain the fluids) and a permanent indwelling catheter. The procedure is done 4–5 times a day under strict sterile, non-touch technique. Since, the connection is broken several times a day the chances of contamination is still high. A modification, night exchange device (NXD), has been designed to provide an extra exchange overnight. It uses a 'cycler' to deliver the required dose during sleep.
3. Automated peritoneal dialysis (APD): This refers to all forms of PD where a mechanical device, a cycler, is used to automatically deliver and drain multiple exchanges of a prescribed volume of the peritoneal dialysate . It reduces the patient involvement in performing the procedure. The various regimens are:
   a. Continuous cyclic peritoneal dialysis: It is performed as 3–5 exchanges during the night with one long day time dwell for exchange (a reverse of CAPD). It was developed for patients who preferred their daytime free. It has an added advantage of reduced risk of peritonitis, hernias and pericatheter fluid leaks. It is preferred for children and those with high peritoneal permeability (called high transporters).
   b. Nightly IPD: It is done every night without any daytime dwell. Though a low efficiency technique, it is preferred in patients with recurrent abdominal hernias, bladder prolapse, poor ultrafiltration and during fluid leaks.
   c. Tidal PD: It is a technique where a portion of dialysate (usually one half) is drained and replaced with fresh dialysate so a majority of dialysate is in constant contact with the peritoneum. Though a costly technique, it results in 10–40% increase in clearance.

   Cyclers were initially developed to provide short and frequent IPD exchanges.

Benefits of Peritoneal Dialysis

The benefits of peritoneal dialysis are cost effectiveness, better preservation of hemodynamic profile, better preservation of residual renal function, better lipoprotein profiles, higher hemoglobin levels and easy to perform home procedure. The survival rate of peritoneal dialysis is similar to hemodialysis in absence of serious complications as peritonitis, diabetes mellitus or in elderly subjects.

Complications of Peritoneal Dialysis

1. Catheter related complications:
   a. Outflow problems due to catheter malposition, kink or clot, or side hole obstruction by omentum
   b. Inflow pain due to catheter malposition or low pH of the dialysate
   c. Visceral perforation, peritonitis and significant intra-peritoneal bleeding immediately or late after catheter placement, (Late bleeding noted after a month needs further evaluation)
   d. Pericatheter leakage of dialysate, pericatheter hernias or worsening of previous hernias
   e. Local infections due to poor hygienic conditions.
2. Metabolic complications
   a. Dehydration or overhydration depending on the osmolality of the dialysate

b. Increased calorie load (glucose). In diabetics this could lead to hyperglycemia and hyperosmolar coma
c. Electrolytes disturbances: hypo-or hypernatremia and hypo-or hyperkalemia
d. Disequilibrium syndrome (as discussed earlier)

3. Peritoneal membrane dysfunction
4. *Complication due to increased intraabdominal pressure,* i.e. increased gastric emptying time and gastroesophageal reflux, worsening of pulmonary status in already compromised patients, decreased cardiac output and stroke volume due to reduced preload and worsening of CHF symptoms.

Goals of Dialysis

The goal of dialysis treatment is (1) To control all the symptoms of uremia; (2) Ensure adequate nutrition, hemoglobin >11.5/dL and albumin of >40 gm/L; (3) A pre-dialysis plasma potassium concentration of <5.5 mmol/L, plasma phosphate of <1.6 mmol/L and bicarbonate of >24 mmol/L; (4) Control hypertension (pre-dialysis BP of <140/90 mm Hg) and avoid pulmonary edema.

Dialysis Dose: Adequacy of Dialysis

Dialysis dose was coined as a concept for the prescription of dialysis for a uremic patient equating to any other pharmacological treatment. RRT, like any other therapy, is a therapeutic intervention so its adequacy should be measured to deliver the correct dose and modify if neccessary. *Adequate dose* is defined as the dose of dialysis below which a significant worsening of mortality and morbidity is observed. *Optimal dose* is the one above which no further improvement in the outcome is seen. Adequacy of dialysis is now calculated in terms of long-term survival of the subject on dialysis. The survival of the patient on dialysis is directly related to the clearance of small solutes. Urea is the most abundant small solute with favorable kinetics during dialysis. It is a non-toxic surrogate for other similar molecules which are toxic and hypothesized to accumulate in ureamia. So urea clearance became the *'gold standard'* for calculating dose and adequacy of dialysis.

The dose of dialysis is measured by the following parameters:

1. Urea reduction ratio (URR): It is the simplest method of calculating urea removal. It is calculated as the ratio of post-dialysis urea concentration to pre-dialysis urea concentration, urea reduction ratio (URR) is calculated as 1-R multiplied by 100%. Data has shown exponential decline in mortality as URR approaches 65%. In hemodialysis URR is calculated per session and during PD it is calculated on a weekly basis (calculated by multiplying by 7). So the recommended URR for hemodialysis is >65% per session and for CAPD > 70% per week.
2. Fractional clearance of urea (Kt/V): Despite the simplicity of URR the centers now use a more complex measure of urea removal, the 'fractional clearance of urea–'Kt/V'. *K* is clearance of urea by the dialyzer, *t* is the duration of dialysis, *V* is volume of distribution of urea. In hemodialysis Kt/V is calculated per session and during PD it is calculated on a weekly basis (multiplied by 7). Minimum Kt/V for hemodialysis should be >1.2 (ideal >1.7), for CCPD >2.1 and for CAPD >2.0 on a weekly basis.
3. Creatinine clearance: Due to the problems in urea kinetics during PD, **total creatinine clearance (TCC)** have also been used to measure dialytic dose. As a consensus, the target dose of TCC should be around >60 liters/wk normalized to 1.73 sqm surface area for CAPD and a slightly higher for IPD patients due to its intermittent nature.

LIMITATION OF RENAL REPLACEMENT THERAPY

The RRT, despite being a century old modality, only replaces the excretory functions of the kidney but not the metabolic or hormonal functions. Dialysis is generally effective in removing small uremic solutes but larger molecules like b-amyloid, homocysteine, leptin and a host of other molecules are difficult to remove and require expensive advanced machines and expert personnel. The success of RRT still depends on expertise of the caregiver and this subjectivity of the therapy makes it difficult to succeed in all centers and situations. Some dialysis modalities like CAPD and CCPD are ambulatory household procedures but sometimes they also need handlers (as for debilitated, elderly and children) and bulky sophisticated machines (e.g. cyclers).

The quality of dialysis fails with dwindling residual functions of the kidney increasing incidences of complication especially with PD. In addition, the frustrating schedule of the therapy leads to non-compliance by the subjects. So, the researches are developing ways to make the procedure more physiological and compliant; even they are working on an oral dialysate. Still, RRT is not a complete cure for the excretory function of the kidney till now but a time bying procedure for a future successful kidney transplant. Though this may sound disheartening, RRT will always be a ray of hope for all the subjects suffering from renal failure to have a decent productive life if not a complete cure for their disease till some new effective treatment springs on the horizon.

CLINICAL PEARLS

- The RRT replaces only the excretory functions of the kidney but not the endocrine or metabolic functions
- Dialysis involves transport of solutes and water across a semi-permeable membrane
- All dialysis procedures involves diffusion/osmosis
- Most preferred vascular access is A-V fistula made in the wrist
- CRRT and made it possible to deliver RRT in hemodynamically unstable patients
- Other slower modalities as SLED and EDD achieved the goals of CRRT at reduced costs
- CAPD made peritoneal dialysis a household affair by bringing RRT from the clutches of hospital into individual hands.

REFERENCES

1. Locatelli Francesco, Covic Adrian, Charles Chazot, Leunissen Karot, Yaqoob Mohammed. Optimal composition of the dialysate, with emphasis on its influence on blood pressure. Nephrol Dial Transplant, 2004;19(4):785-96.
2. Van Kuijk WH, Mulder AW, Peels CH, Harff GA, Leunissen KM. Influence of changes in ionised calcium on cardiovascular reactivity during hemodialysis. Clinical Nephrology, 1997;47(3):190-6.
3. Van Der Sande FM, Cheriex EC, Van Kuijk WH, Leunissen KM. Effect of dialysate calcium concentration on intradialytic blood pressure course in cardiac-compromised patients. American Journal of Kidney Diseases, 1998;32:125-31.
4. Weiner IM, Blanchard KC, Mudge GH. Factors influencing renal excretion of foreign organic acids. American Journal of Physiology, 1964;207:953-963.
5. Oettinger CW, Oliver JC. Normalisation of uremic acidosis in hemodialysis patients with a high bicarbonate dialysate. Journal of American Society of Neprology, 1993;3:1804-7.
6. Albertazzi A, Palmeri PF, Mastrangelo E. Efficacy and tolerance of acetate free biofiltration: a central Italian multicenter trial. Kidney International. Suppl, 1993;41:S188-94.
7. A thesis by Filiz Yasar Machlichi for Master of Science in Chemical Engineering—Preparation and characterization of hemodialysis membranes. IZMiR; January 2007.
8. Foret Leslie L, Ward Richard A, Cheung Alfred K. Choice of Hemodialysis Membranes; Principle and Practice of Dialysis.
9. Brescia M, Cimino J, Appel K, et al. Chronic hemodialysis using venipuncture and surgically created arteriovenous fistula. New England Journal of Medicine. 1966;275:1089-92.
10. Bennion R, William R. The Radiocephalic Fistula. Contemporary Dialysis, 1982;3:12-6.
11. Monquet C, Bitker M, Bailliant O, et al. Anaethesia for creation of forearm fistula in patients with end stage renal failure. Anaesthesiology, 1980;70:909-14.
12. Wedgwood KR, Wiggins PA, Guillou PJ. A prospective study of end-to-side vs. side-to-side arteriovenous fistulas for haemodialysis. Brit J Surg, 1984;71:640-2.
13. Schanzer H, Schwartz M, Harrington E, Haimov M. Treatment of ischemia due to "steal" by arteriovenous fistula with distal artery ligation and revascularization. Journal of Vascular Surgery. 1988;7:770-3.
14. National Kidney Foundation. NFK/DOQI, Clinical Practice Guidelines for Vascular Access. Am J of Kidney Diseases. 2006;48(1):S176-307.
15. Fischer KG. Mechanism and clinical presentation of heparin induced thrombocytopenia. Hemodialysis Ineternational, 2000;5: 74-80.
16. Greiber S, Weber U, Galle J, Bramer P, Schollmeyer P. Activated clotting time is not a sensitive parameter to monitor anticoagulation with low molecular weight heparin in hemodialysis. Nephron, 1997;76:15-19.
17. Frank RD, Brandenberg VM, Lanzmich R, Floege J. Factor Xa-activated whole blood clotting time (Xa-ACT) for bedside monitoring of deltaparin anticoagulation during hemodialysis. Nephrology Dialysis Transplant, 2004;19:1552-8.
18. Vanholer RC, Camez A, Vyes N, et al. Pharmacokinetics of recombinant hirudin in hemodialysed end stage renal failure patients. Thromb Haemost, 1997;77:650-5.
19. Swan SK, Hurstring MJ. The pharmacokinetics of argatroban: Effects of age, gender and hepatic or renal dysfunction. Pharmacotherapy, 2000;20:318-9.
20. Asper R, Buchameyer H, Lang T, et al. Simplified citrate anticooagulation for high-flux hemodialysis. American Journal of Kidney Diseases, 2001;38:979-87.
21. Emili S, Black NA, Paul RV, et al. A protocol-based treatment for intradialytic hypotension in hospitalized hemodialysis patients. Am J Kidney Dis, 1999;33:1107-14.
22. Aireff AJ. Dialysis disequilibrium syndrome: Current concepts on pathogenesis and prevention. Kidney International(italics), 1994; 45:629-35.
23. Kennedy AC, Linton AC, Eatons JC. Urea level in cerebrospinal fluid after hemodialysis. Lancet, 1.1962;410-11.
24. Petersons HD. Acute encephalopathy occurring during hemodialysis. Archives of Internal Medicine, 1964;113:8777-800.
25. Copplino G, Luscisano G, Bolignano, Buemi M. Acute cardiovascular complications of hemodialysis. Minerva Urol Nefrol, 2010; 62(1):67-80.
26. Dolan MG, Whipp BJ, Davidson WD, Weizman RE, Wasserman K. Hypoapnoes associated with acetate hemodialysis: carbon dioxide – flow-dependent ventilation. New England J of Medicine, 1981;305:72-5.
27. DeBacker WA, Verpooten GA, Borgonjen DJ, Vermiere PA, Lins RL, Broc ME. Hypoxaemia during hemodialysis: effects of different membranes and dialysatecomposition. Kidney International, 1983; 23:738-43.
28. Hunt JM, Chappel TR, Henrich WL, Rubins LJ. Gas exchange during dialysis. Contrasting mechanisms contributing to comparable alterations with acetate and bicarbonate buffers. Am J Med, 1984;77:255-60.
29. Daugirdas JT, Ing TS. First use reactions during hemodialysis- a definition of subtypes. Kidney International, 1988;24:537-43.
30. Ing TS, Daugirdas JT, Popli S, Gandhi VC. First use syndrome with cuprammonium cellulose dialysers. International Journal of Artificial Internal Organs, 1983;6:235-9.
31. DeMunnio C, Martinez J, McKean M, DeLaRosa J, Burke JE, Murphy S. Platelet dysfunction in ureamia. Multifaceted defect partially corrected by dialysis. Am J Med, 1985;79:552-7.

32. Noris MRG. Uremic bleeding: closing the circle after 30 years of controversies? Blood, 1999;94:2569-74.
33. Escolar G, Cases A, Bastida E, Garrido M, Lopez J, Revert L, et al. Uremic platelets have a functional defect affecting the interaction of von Willebrand factor with glycoprotein IIb-IIIa. Blood, 1990;76:1336-40.
34. Zuckerman GR, Cornette GL, Clouse RE, Harter HR. Upper gastrointestinal bleeding in patients with chronic renal failure. Ann Intern Med, 1985;102:588-92.
35. Lindsay Jr J, Crawley IS, Callaway Jr GM. Chronic constrictive pericarditis following uremic hemopericardium. Am Heart J, 1970;79:390-5.
36. Bucchardi H. History and development of continuous renal replacement techniques. Kidney International, 1998;vol. 53, suppl 66:120-4.
37. Manns M, Sigler M, Teehan BP. Continuous renal replacement therapy: an update. Am J Kidney Dis, 1998;32:185-207.
38. Conger J. Dialysis and related therapies. Semin Nephrol, 1998; 18:S33-40.
39. Briglia A, Paganini E. Acute renal failure in the intensive care unit. Clin Chest Med, 1999;20:347-66.
40. Mehta R, McDonald B, Gabbai F, et al. A randomized, clinical trial of continuous versus intermittent dialysis for acute renal failure. Kidney Int, 2001;60:1154-63.
41. Ronco C, Bellomo R, Homel P, et al. Effects of different doses in continuous veno-venous hemofiltration on outcomes of acute renal failure: a prospective, randomized trial. Lancet, 2000; 356:26-30.
42. Kes P, Liutic-Jukic N, Brunetta B. Indications of continuus reanal replacement therapy. Acta Med Croatian, 2003;57(1):71-5.
43. Kumar VCM, Depner T, Yeun J. Extended daily dialysis: a new approach to renal replacement for acute renal failure in the intensive care unit. Am J Kidney Dis, 2000;36:294-300.
44. LornoyW, De Meester J, Demeyer I,Waterschoot M, De Cooman S, Billiouw JM, et al. Outcome of critically ill patients with acute renal failure treated with slow, extended daily, on-line hemodiafiltration [abstract 21]. Abstracts of the Sixth International Conference on Continuous Renal Replacement Therapies (CRRT): Blood Purification, 2001;19:338.
45. Michael M Farooq, Julie A Freischlag. Peritoneal dialysis. Ruthereford Vascular surgery, 5th edn. (2000), WB Saunders Company.
46. Rhoads JE. Peritoneal lavage in the treatment of renal insufficiency. Am J Med Science, 1938;192:642.
47. Twardowski, ZJ. History of peritoneal access development. Int J Artif Organs, 2006;29(1):2-40.
48. Biff F Palmer. Dialysate Composition in Hemodialysis and Peritoneal Dialysis. Chapter 2 Principle and Practice of Dialysis.
49. W L EE, L C HAN. New perspectives in peritoneal dialysis fluids. Hong Kong Journal of Nephrology, Volume 1, Issue 1, Pages 4-10; 1999.
50. Tenckhoff H, Schecter H. A bacteriologically safe peritoneal access device. Trans Am Soc Artif Intern Organs, 1968;14:181.
51. Ash Stephen R. Chronic peritoneal Dialysis Catheters: Overview of Design, Placement, and Removal Procedures. Seminars in Dialysis- vol. 16: pp 323-334; No 4 (July- August) 2003.
52. Olcott C, Feldman CA, Coplon NS, et al. Continouous ambulatory peritoneal dialysis: Technique of catheter insertion and management of associated surgical complications. Am J Surg, 1983;146:98.
53. Ash SR, Wolf GC, Bloch R. Placement of the Tenckhoff peritoneal dialysis catheter under peritoneoscopic visuliasation. Dial Transplant, 1981;10:383.
54. Rubin J, Ball R. Continuous ambulatory Peritoneal Dialysis for treatment of severe CHF in face of CRF. Arch Intern Med, 1986;146:1533.
55. Wincester JF, Gelfar MC, Knepsshield JH, Schreiner GE. Dialysis and hemoperfusion of poisons and drugs- Update. Trans Am Soc Artif Intern Organs, 1977;23:762.
56. Maher JF. Principles of dialysis and dialysis of drugs. Am J of Med, 1977;62:475.
57. Maher JF, Rath CE, Schreiner GE. Hyperuricaemia complicating leukemia: treatment with allopurinol and dialysis. Arch Intern Med, 1987;123:198.
58. Aamir P, Khanna R, Libel B, et al. CAPD in diabetes with ESRD. N Eng J of Med, 1983;306:625.
59. Fine RN, Salusky JB. CAPD/CCPD in children: Four years experience. Kidney Intern, 1986;30:571.
60. Popovich RP, Moncrief JW, Nolph KD, et al. Continuous ambulatory Peritoneal Dialysis. Ann Intern Med, 1978;88:449.

Surgical Technique in Renal Transplantation

Harsha Jauhari, Sudhir Chadha, Vipin Tyagi

INTRODUCTION

Renal transplant is a major surgical procedure that has enjoyed remarkable progress in the last century. Carrel and Guthrie[1] pioneered the method of vascular anastomosis in an animal model. Using this, the first clinical deceased renal transplant was performed in 1933 by Ukrainian surgeon, Voronoy, with an unsuccessful result secondary to immunologic barriers.[2] In 1951, Kuss used the retroperitoneal technique to place the graft kidney and then this technique was used by Murray et al[3,4] in 1955 to perform a transplant between monozygotic twins that resulted in excellent long-term graft survival rates. The era of modern renal transplantation began with the introduction of immunosuppressive agents and now renal transplantation is established as the most appropriate available option for treatment of end stage renal disease (ESRD).

Transplantation results in superior survival, improved quality of life and lower cost as compared with dialysis for majority of individuals with ESRD. There are very few absolute contraindications, so most of the patients with ESRD should be considered as potential candidates for transplant.

Renal transplantation surgery includes:

A. Retrieval of kidney from live/deceased donor—Donor nephrectomy—Live/Cadaveric

B. Placement of donor kidney into the recipient's body—renal transplantation is a major surgical procedure which involves vascular and urological components.

A uremic recipient, who also receives immunosuppressive drugs and is anemic or malnourished, merits meticulous surgical technique, strict aseptic environment and perfect hemostasis during the surgery. The need for a perfect surgical procedure cannot be stressed enough, bearing in mind that renal transplantation could be the only opportunity that the recipient has which can make a dramatic change in his/her quality of life.

DONOR NEPHRECTOMY

The appropriate identification and preparation of donors for retrieval of the kidney is critical for the success of the transplant. The donor may be live or deceased. There are wide variations in use of living and deceased kidney donations around the world, due to varying medical and social cultural values. The proportion of living donors is currently variable —approximately 12% in Europe, 35% in USA, 50% in Latin America and 90% in Asia. In India, cadaveric kidney donation makes an insignificant contribution in kidney transplant program. Surgical techniques are different for retrieval of kidney from a deceased and live donor.

Living Donor Nephrectomy

The presence of 2 kidneys in most individuals, each with physiological reserve capable of providing 4 to 5 times the minimal required function has led to acceptance of renal transplantation using living related resources as the source of kidney.

Living kidney donation is accepted by law, religion and bioethics, provided that the donor is aware of the consequences of his/her act and makes the decision without outside prenure or commercialism.

Once the prospective donor is medically fit for donation, the last step is surgical evaluation. The term 'surgical evaluation' is the assessment of the anatomic features of the donor kidney to determine if nephrectomy can safely be performed, which kidney should be removed and to determine which nephrectomy technique is to be employed.

Preoperative spiral CT angiography is the preferred tool for surgical assessment of kidney donors because it not only provides the status of vasculature of both the kidneys but also provides other anatomic details like cyst, calculus and even function. Usually the left kidney is selected for donation because of the long left renal vein . The right kidney is selected for donation if:

- The left kidney has more complex vascular anatomy as compared to right.
- The right kidney has minor renal abnormalities like cyst, UPJ obstruction and left kidney is normal.
- In women who may become pregnant.

The kidney removal from a prospective live kidney donor is either by an open approach or by a laparoscopic approach. Whatever approach is used, following principles merit emphasis:

- Adequate exposure
- Careful handling of the kidney, especially during periarterial dissection
- Preservation of adequate perihilar and periureteral fat to ensure vascularity to ureter
- Maintenance of active diuresis, which makes prompt post transplantation function more likely.

Open Nephrectomy

This is the traditional method for removal of kidney and can be performed via following approach:
- Flank approach
- Anterior extraperitoneal approach—not usually preferred.

Flank Approach

This is an extra pleural and extra peritoneal approach to the kidney. It involves minimal disturbances to other viscera and also avoids contamination of the peritoneal cavity. This approach can also easily be used in obese donors as most of the panniculus falls forward, making this incision relatively straight forward.

It has two variations: Intercostal approach or through the bed of 11th and12th rib after resection of the rib.

The choice of either *intercostal* or *transcostal* depends on the surgeon's preference. We are comfortable using the intercostal approach because it avoids resection of the rib and provides stable retraction.

Position of the Donor

The donor is placed in the lateral position . The back is placed close to the edge of the operating table with the tip of 12th rib over the kidney rest. The lower leg is flexed to 90 degrees with the top leg straight to maintain stability. A pillow is placed between the knees and a sponge pad is placed under the axilla to prevent compression of the brachial plexus. Flexion of the table and elevation of the kidney rest should be performed slowly. Flexion increases the space between the costal margin and iliac rest and puts the flank muscles and skin on tension. In patients who have a stiff spine, care must be taken to ensure that their extremities remain in contact with the table because their range of lateral flexion is limited.

After flexion and elevation of the kidney rest, the patient is secured in this position with a wide adhesive tape over the greater trochanter and attached to the moveable portion (Fig. 7.4).

The extended upper arm can be supported on a padded Mayo stand, which is adjusted to an appropriate height to maintain the arm in a horizontal position with shoulder rotated slightly forward (Fig. 7.5).

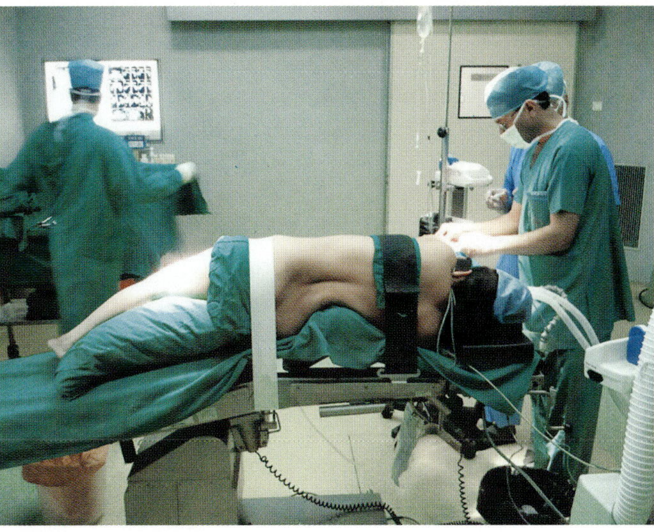

Fig. 7.4: Right lateral position for left nephrectomy

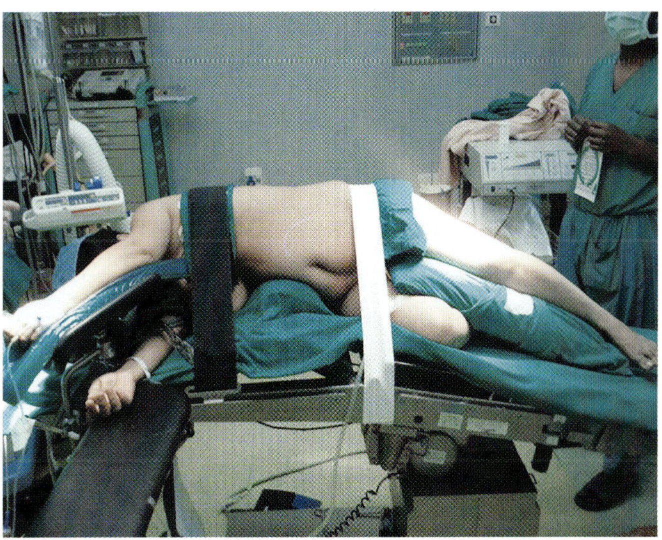

Fig. 7.5: Right lateral position with upper arm extended

It is important to check the blood pressure of the donor after flexion of table and elevation of the kidney rest because this position may cause hypotension. This may not be tolerated by elderly patients and by those with impaired cardiopulmonary function.

Intercostal Approach

After induction of general anesthesia, the donor is placed in the lateral position as described earlier.

Incision

In the *intercostal approach* the incision can be above the 11th or 12th rib, determined by examining the position of the kidney in relation to 11 and 12th rib on the X-ray KUB.

Intercostal incisions above the 11th rib offer an advantage of providing good direct access to hilum and upper pole and is also shorter as compared to that above the 12th rib.

We usually prefer supra 11th incision on the left side and supra 12th on the right owing to inferior position of right kidney as compared to left.

The *transcostal approach* merits resection of rib which not only increases the operative time but also results in more post operative pain. The transcostal incision is either through the bed of 11th or 12th rib. Again the choice is 11th rib on left side and 12th on right, making the decision only after evaluation of X-ray KUB.

Operative steps: In both intercostal or transcostal approach, the operative steps are essentially same except that rib resection is done in the transcostal approach.

- Skin incision is made extending from 3–4 cm anterior to the rib to either over the rib or in between the ribs posteriorly.
- The anterior external oblique and posteriorly the latissimus dorsi and slips of serratus posterior inferior muscles are divided.
- The lumbodorsal fascia is cut and after sweeping the peritoneum forward, the internal oblique and transversus abdominis muscles are cut.
- Posteriorly, in the intercostal approach the intercostal muscles are cut, while in the transcostal approach the rib is resected after reflecting the periosteum off the rib. In both the approaches, extra care is to be taken to avoid injury to pleura.
- For better retroperitoneal space, the pleura may be reflected upward by sharply dividing the fascial attachments to the diaphragm. This step makes an easy access to the upper pole.
- A Finochietto retractor is used to maintain exposure.
- The paranephric fat and Gerota's fascia, lying in the central part of wound are entered.
- Now the kidney is examined to exclude occult polycystic disease, scarring or any other malformation which either demands another maneuver or precludes donor nephrectomy.
- The kidney surface is then dissected free of the underlying perinephric fat all around except in the renal hilum and in the area between the lower pole and the ureter.
- Hilum dissection is then started. Anteriorly, the renal vein is dissected to its junction with the vena cava on the left side, the adrenal, gonadal and lumbar tributaries being ligated and divided. On right along with renal vein, anterior and posterior surface of IVC at level of its junction with renal vein is also cleared, making it easy to take of patch of IVC along with renal vein.
- At the hilum, posteriorly the renal artery is skeletonized till its origin from aorta taking care to avoid injury to branches of renal artery.
- It is essential to be gentle while manipulating the kidney for anterior or posterior dissections, especially adjacent to the renal artery so as to avoid renal artery spasm.
- The ureter is then freed with its investing vessels and fat, down to or below the pelvic brim and then transected.
- Brisk diuresis should be evident from the cut ureter, mannitol, furosemide and adequate crystalloid solution having been infused during dissection of the kidney.
- Once the recipient is ready, the kidney is retrieved by clamping the renal artery first followed by the renal vein.
- The stumps of the renal artery and the renal vein are then secured properly.
- The wound is then closed after lowering the bridge.

Laparoscopic Donor Nephrectomy[5]

Laparoscopic donor nephrectomy (LDN) was developed with intent to limit the morbidity of open donor nephrectomy (ODN). In 1995, since the first laparoscopic retrieval of live kidney was done by Ratner and Kavoussi, laparoscopic procurement of donor kidney has become widely adopted and is now becoming the standard technique for live donor procurement in most of the centers. LDN has been shown to reduce the disincentive to living renal donation and thus potentially increasing the supply of willing donors.

Troppmann and colleagues analyzed the outcomes of kidney transplants following ODN and LDN. They concluded that although LDN recipient experienced slower early post transplant graft function, there was no significant difference in graft survival at 1 year.[4] In addition, there was no difference in the incidence of acute rejection between the two groups. Thus LDN offers the advantage of less morbidity as compared to ODN without compromising the functional outcome. The preoperative preparation is identical to those for ODN.

Intraoperative Management

Good communication between the surgeon and anesthesiologist is of paramount importance during LDN. The anesthesiologist and surgeon should understand the pathophysiological changes of pneumoperitoneum and increased intra-abdominal pressure on major organs especially renal blood flow which dramatically alters the intraoperative fluid requirement as compared to ODN. Adequate muscle relaxation is essential in order to obtain sufficient working space. Nitrous oxide should be avoided since its use is associated with bowel distension and obscuring of surgeon's view and it has also been implicated in postoperative nausea and vomiting.

Position

Modified lateral decubitus position with hips rotated back and arm extended above the head. The table is flexed to expand the area between the costal margin and pelvic brim.

Pneumoperitoneum is established either by the blind method using Veress needle or by open method using Hasson's cannula. Veress needle is mostly used for this purpose, except when there is possibility of intraperitoneal adhesions as in previous abdominal surgery, when Hasson's cannula is introduced by the open technique.

The Veress needle is introduced lateral to the rectus muscle at the level of umbilicus and introduced across the anterior abdominal wall. Often two pops are felt, one at the anterior rectus sheath and second at the level of peritoneum. Once the needle is in the peritoneal cavity, following tests should always be performed to confirm its placement:

1. Aspirate the needle to ensure that it is not in any viscus or vessel.
2. Water drop test: Put a few drops of saline on the hub of the needle, it should fall freely into the peritoneal cavity.
3. Inject a little saline into the needle and aspirate it. If the needle is in the peritoneal cavity aspiration of saline is not possible, while aspiration of saline suggests that needle is in the preperitoneal space.

Insufflation with CO_2 is now done. Once adequate pneumoperitoneum is established (15 mm Hg), ports are placed as follows:

- 12 mm port in midline just above umbilicus.
- 12 mm port at the level of the umbilicus or slightly below along lateral border of the rectus sheath.
- 5 mm port in midline two or three fingers breadth below xiphoid process.

After proper inspection of the peritoneal cavity, the lateral colonic attachments are incised using a laparoscopic Debakey forceps and scissors or endoshears and the descending colon and sigmoid are fully mobilized medially after incising the phrenocolic ligaments.

The colon is mobilized to expose the psoas muscle and identify the gonadal vein and ureter along the medial border of the muscle. The ureter is dissected caudally till the level of iliac vessels. The ureter should be dissected enbloc with the gonadal vein in order to preserve the periureteral tissue.

The gonadal vein is traced till it empties to its insertion into the main renal vein. This dissection should be medial to the gonadal vein to avoid devascularization of ureter in the hilum region. Renal vein is cleared completely off the investing tissue and the gonadal, lumbar and adrenal branches are clipped and cut. It is not uncommon to find few abnormal tributaries of the renal vein, which should be clipped as well.

The lower pole of the kidney is elevated with the Debakey grasper, and the renal artery is identified posterior and cranial to the renal vein. The artery is dissected off the nervous plexus and lymphatics till its origin from the aorta. Use of excessive cautery and undue stretch of renal artery should be avoided so as to prevent arterial spasm and thus decreasing the incidence of delayed graft function. The kidney is now dissected away from the adrenal gland by clipping the vascularized tissue in this region. The upper pole is shelled out of the envelope of Gerota's fascia, the posterior attachments are lysed by elevating the upper pole and teasing the adherent tissue away. Mannitol and furosemide are administered during dissection to ensure good diuresis.

At this point, an incision is made for retrieval of kidney. Usually a Pfannenstiel incision is preferred, but a low transverse or oblique skin incision may also be used, to accommodate just one hand, but the peritoneum is not incised.

The ureter which has already been dissected till the iliac vessels is clipped as distally as possible and cut above the clip.

The kidney is now left only with renal artery and vein. Using a multifire endo GIA 30 stapling device with 2.0 sized staple loads, the renal artery is divided flush to aorta followed by division of renal vein below the adrenal vein, using the same.

The peritoneum is now opened and kidney is held by introducing the hand. The endo catch bag may also be used for kidney removal. The kidney is placed in ice slush and immediately transferred to the recipient operative suite (Fig. 7.6).

The peritoneal cavity is inspected under low pressure to check for hemostasis with particular attention to staples line. All the trocars are removed under direct vision and all trocar sites and retrieval incision are closed.

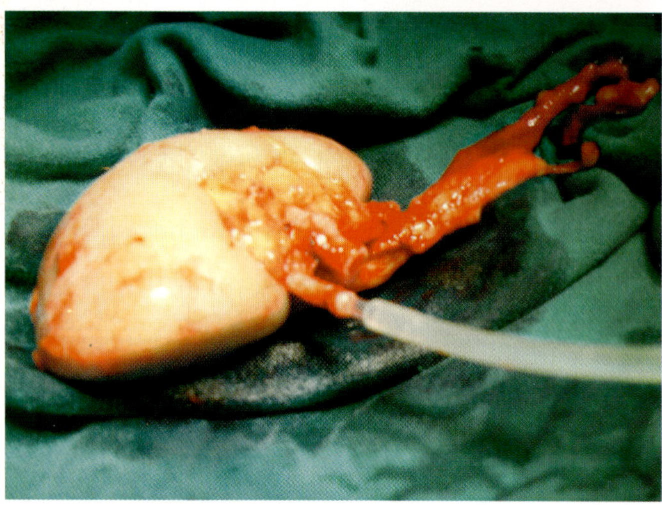

Fig. 7.6: Perfusion of kidney

Right Donor Nephrectomy

The right kidney is generally not favorable for donation because of the short length of the renal vein. In case of LDN, this limitation becomes more relevant. There are few modifications which can be made to achieve maximal length of renal vessel.

Port placement is mirror image of that used for left side procedure, although an additional port may be required for retraction of the liver.

Following modifications can be made to achieve maximal length of the renal vessels:

1. Division of the renal vessels in a plane parallel to the inferior vena cava by the endoscopic GIA device.
2. Make a 5–6 cm transverse incision in right upper quadrant at a point overlying the confluence of right renal vein and inferior vena cava.
3. Introducing a hand port at the level of the 11th rib in order to lift up the kidney on its pedicle.

Deceased Donor Nephrectomy

The process of deceased donor transplantation from identification of a potential donor to the operation is complex. Organ donor management fundamentally occurs in the following sequence:

- Surveillance to identify patients with severe neurological injury likely to progress to brain death.
- Declaration of brain death using standard methodology and a standard protocol for withdrawal and deceleration in case of donation after cardiac death.
- A uniform request for consent.
- Optimal medical management of potential donor.

The above process represents the epitome of coordinated team work and institutional co-operation.

Once the declaration of brain death is done using standard protocol, the medical stabilization of the donor is commenced.

It includes:

- BP should be maintained at a greater than 100 mm Hg by aggressive administration of crystalloids, colloids or blood products.
- Central venous pressure should be maintained greater than 10 mm Hg.
- If urine output decreased to less than 40 mL/hr in a well hydrated donor, furosemide or mannitol may be given.
- Low dose inotropic support is sometimes required if BP remains low inspite of proper hydration.
- Insulin administration may be necessary to minimize hyperglycemia and glycosuria.
- Hormonal resuscitation with methylprednisolone, triiodo thyronine and arginine vasopressin may improve quality of retrieved organ.

Surgical Technique for Cadaveric Organ Retrieval

Kidneys are usually retrieved together as a part of multiorgan harvesting. We will be here describing only the retrieval of kidneys.

- A midline incision extending from sternal notch to symphysis pubis is usually given but occasionally, a combined midline and transverse abdominal incision is used for obese donor.
- The abdominal flaps can be folded back and held in place with sharp towel clips.
- After proper retraction of sternum and abdominal flap, a thorough abdominal exploration is quickly performed in order to rule out contraindication to procurement such as malignancy or intra-abdominal sepsis.
- For kidney retrieval, a cattle-Braasch maneuver is done with incision of the posterior peritoneum lateral to ascending colon and extending medially around the cecum and upward to the ligament of Treitz completely mobilizing the distal small bowel, right colon and duodenum. Similarly, the white line of Toldt is also incised lateral to descending and sigmoid portion of colon.
- The right colon, small bowel and left colon are reflected superiorly by developing a plane superficial to the gonadal vein to explore the distal part of abdominal aorta and IVC just proximal to the iliac bifurcation. Both IVC and aorta are individually encircled with umbilical tapes.

- The inferior mesenteric artery is divided at its aortic origin between ligatures in order to facilitate the dissection of aorta. During the dissection, care is taken to avoid injury to polar renal arteries.
- During cephalad reflection of bowel and its mesentery, the left renal vein is identified as it crosses anterior to the aorta, it serves as a landmark for the origin of superior mesenteric artery (SMA).
- The superior mesenteric artery is dissected free from its surrounding of thick cover of lymphatic, neural and connective tissue. This allows free encircling of the SMA in order to occlude it, at the time of flushing.
- In preparation to obtain control of the supraceliac aorta, the left triangular ligament of the liver is divided and gastro hepatic ligament is examined and divided if no aberrant left hepatic artery is noted. The right diaphragmatic crus is divided and the supraceliac aorta is identified and mobilized.
- The supraceliac aorta is encircled with an umbilical tape. In an unstable donor, cold perfusion may be done at this point.
- Proximal control of the vena cava is usually provided by the liver retrieval team, but in instances in which hepatic recovery does not occur an umbilical tape is placed just below the liver.
- Systemic heparinization (100–300 units/kg) is now performed.
- A cannula is placed into the distal aorta and passed retrograde from above the iliac bifurcation to the origin of the renal arteries. The distal vena cava is ligated with an umbilical tape after a larger bore cannula has been placed for drainage by gravity.
- The supradiaphragmatic portion of IVC is then incised to allow venous blood to vent into the chest cavity.
- A clamp is applied just below the diaphragm to occlude its proximal segment, the abdominal aorta is perfused in a retrograde fashion with University of Wisconsin preservation solution to an achieve in situ flushing of kidney, taking care to avoid introducing air into the aorta which may embolize subsequently.
- Slushed ice of sterile saline solution is then applied to the kidneys to achieve surface cooling.
- Kidney retrieval then begins by mobilizing and dividing the ureters deep in the pelvis near their entrance into the urinary bladder.
- The kidneys are mobilized by sharply dissecting Gerota fascia off the iliopsoas muscle and dividing the peritoneal reflections.
- The left kidney is freed from the spleno-renal ligament and brought out through a mesenteric window created in the mesocolon.
- The aorta and vena cava are transected above the level of celiac axis and the flushing procedure is terminated.
- Both the kidneys with their ureters attached are gently lifted from the field by dividing restraining bands of paraverterbral muscles and establishing a plane above the bodies of last thoracic vertebra and lumbar vertebrae to the sacral promontory. Injury to posterior wall of aorta and vena cava during dissection has to be prevented.
- The distal aorta and vena cava are divided above iliac ligament to release the en-bloc organ.
- The en-bloc specimen of kidneys is placed in cold preservation solution and are separated on back table.

Via an anterior approach the left renal vein is identified and divided flush with vena cava to preserve adequate length. Then the posterior wall of aorta is exposed by turning the specimen, which is then divided longitudinally down its center aspect which allows for inspection of renal artery orifices from within the aortic lumen. After incision of anterior wall of aorta, the two kidneys are separated leaving the right renal vein attached to IVC to permit extension of short renal vein if necessary. Excess adherent fat is dissected from the kidney surface taking care to preserve the triangular wedge of tissue between the lower pole and the ureters. The kidneys are then placed in a sterile plastic jar barrier and packed in ice for storage and transportation. In addition 15–20 lymph nodes and 15 gm of splenic tissue is removed for histocompatibility testing. Incision is closed with continuous nylon 1.0 sutures.

RECIPIENT SURGERY

The general preparation and selection of recipient for kidney transplantation commences with the nephrological evaluation and ends with evaluation by the transplant surgeon.

In absence of any possible contraindication for transplantation, the recipient is ready to receive a new kidney. The preoperative and anesthetic considerations have already been discussed. After induction of anesthesia and placement of central and arterial lines, the recipient is prepared and draped from nipple to mid thigh. A third generation cephalosporin is given at time of induction. A three way urinary catheter is placed with full aseptic precautions and unobstructed drainage is ensured.

Since, its early description, the right iliac fossa has been used for implantation of the kidney[4,6,7] (Fig. 7.7).

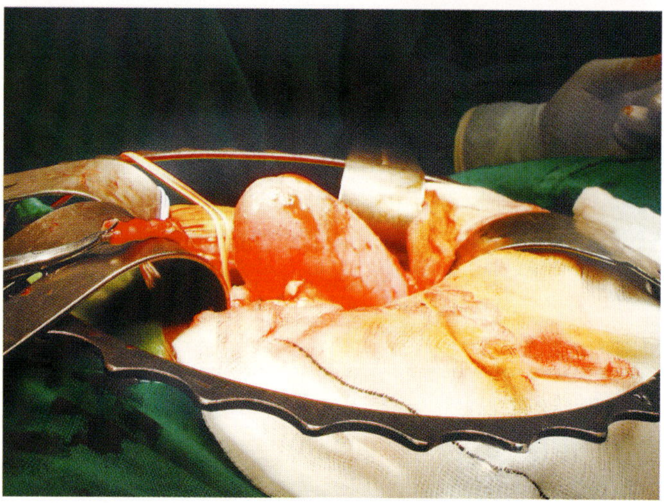

Fig. 7.7: Kidney in right iliac forssa

The advantage of placing the kidney in the right iliac fossa is that external iliac vein is more superficial as compared to left iliac fossa, making venous anastomosis an easy procedure.

The right iliac fossa is used for implantation of either kidney in most of the centers, however in some centers, while the left kidney is placed it in the right iliac fossa, the right kidney is placed in the left iliac fossa. The advantage of placing in the contralateral fossa, is that the pelvis and ureter face anteriorly which will make subsequent urological intervention easy, if required. It is also not uncommon to place the kidney in the ipsilateral fossa which will simulate the anatomy of normal kidney.

In children, who weigh more than 20kg, the extraperitoneal placement of kidney is preferred, but in pediatric patients who are less than 20 kg, the kidney can be placed either in the extraperitoneal space which is created by extending the incision to right costal margin, or may be placed intraperitoneally by a transperitoneal approach.

In both approaches, partial occluding side clamps are used to isolate a part of IVC and aorta to which the renal vessels are anastomosed.

Incision

An oblique Rutherford Morison or curvilinear incision in right or left quadrant of the abdomen is used for renal transplantation. This incision begins almost in the midline and curving upward parallel to the inguinal ligament and approximately 2 cm above it and ending just above the anterior superior iliac spine. The external oblique muscle and fascia are divided in line of incision till lateral extent of the wound.

Medially the anterior rectus sheath is cut, but the rectus muscle is preserved. The inferior flap of anterior rectus sheath is reflected away from rectus sheath for exposure of the urinary bladder.

The internal oblique and transverse muscles are either divided with cautery in the line of incision or may be divided at confluence of the oblique muscles and rectus sheath, which avoids the cutting of muscles.

The inferior epigastric vessels are found in the medial half of the incision. They are ligated and divided unless there are multiple renal arteries, in which case inferior epigastric artery may be used for anastomosis to one of the renal arteries. The spermatic cord is dissected and preserved unless the patient is elderly. In females, the round ligament can be divided. The peritoneum is now swept superiorly and medially after division of transversalis fascia. Small vessels overlying the peritoneum are coagulated well. The self retaining ring retractor should be applied so that both the hands of the assistant are free to assist during anastomosis.

The target vessels are now dissected. For revascularization, the renal artery can be anastomosed to the internal iliac artery or to the external iliac artery but the vein is anastomosed to the external iliac vein. The lymphatics which course along and over the vessels must be ligated and cut. The external iliac artery and vein are dissected from bifurcation of common iliac artery to the inguinal ligament. All the tributaries of vein and branches of artery are ligated and cut.

If the internal iliac artery is to be used, it is important to mobilize a length of common and external iliac arteries so that the internal iliac artery can be rotated laterally without kinking for easy anastomosis.

Once the vessels are prepared, the kidney is ready to be implanted. Kidney transplantation includes revascularization by vascular anastomosis followed by urinary tract reconstruction.

REVASCULARIZATION

Arterial Anastomosis

The graft kidney from cadaveric/live donor after adequate perfusion is anastomosed to either the internal or external iliac artery depending on the choice of the surgeon.

We prefer to do an end to side anastomosis of renal artery to external iliac artery.

The advantages of using external iliac artery are the following:

- A kidney with multiple arteries can easily be anastomosed to external iliac artery.
- There is no disparity of size of lumen of graft and recipient vessels as will occur while using internal iliac artery.

- The renal artery can be placed according to the acceptable position of the kidney.

Venous Anastomosis

Renal vein to external iliac vein: End to side.

All anastomosis are done by 6.0 monofilament vascular suture.

The question of whether the arterial anastomosis or venous anastomosis should be done first depends on final position of kidney and the ease with which the second anastomosis may/may not be done. It also depends on surgeon's choice. Usually if renal artery is to be anastomosed to external iliac artery, then the venous anastomosis should be the first anastomosis and in case where internal iliac artery has to be used it is usual to do arterial anastomosis first.

Once the vascular anastomosis is complete, the clamps are opened. The venous clamp is open first followed by opening of arterial clamp. The rational of opening the venous clamp first is to avoid congestion of renal vasculature which would happen if arterial clamp is opened first.

The following parameters have to be observed after the opening of renal clamp:

- Color and consistency of kidney
- Hemostasis at the anastomotic site and in renal hilum
- Urine output (Fig 7.8).

A pink and firm kidney with immediate, brisk and profuse diuresis is an ideal outcome.

In case of soft kidney with no or little urine output, watch both the anastomosis for possible kink or obstruction, apart from anesthetic and immunological factors.

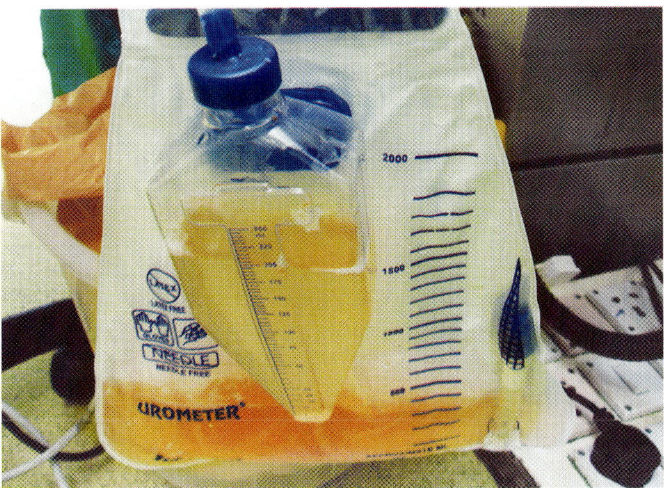

Fig. 7.8: Urine after renal anastomosis and release of clamps

Proper and adequate hemostasis has to be achieved following which urinary tract reconstruction is done.

RECONSTRUCTION OF URINARY TRACT

After renal revascularization, the kidney is placed in its final acceptable position and re-establishment of urinary tract begins. The factors that determine the type of urinary tract reconstruction are the length and condition of the donor ureter, the condition of the recipient's bladder or bladder substitute, the condition of the recipient's ureter and familiarity of the surgeon with the technique.

The options available are ureteroneocystostomy, pyelo-ureterostomy, uretero-ureterostomy and pyelovesicostomy. Ureteroneocystostomy is the usual form of urinary tract reconstruction while other options are used, if required. Ureteroneocystostomy offers following advantages-

- It can be performed regardless of the quality or presence of the recipient ureter
- It is several centimeters away from vascular anastomosis
- The native ureter remains available for the treatment of ureteric complications
- Native nephrectomy is unnecessary

The goal of ureteroneocystostomy is to create a 2–3 cm submucosal tunnel with muscle backing of the ureter so that when the bladder contracts, there is valve mechanism to prevent reflux of urine.

We use the extravesical technique of ureteroneo-cystostomy based on the procedure described by Lich and associates and was adapted for renal transplantation by Woodruff in 1962.[8-10]

The bladder is distended with an antibiotic solution through the urethral catheter. The lateral surface of bladder is cleared of fat and peritoneal reflection. A 3 cm longitudinal oblique incision is made over the lateral surface of bladder, until bladder mucosa bulges into the incision.

The mucosa is dissected away from the detrussor muscle to make a submucosal tunnel for the ureter. At the upper most end of mucosa, a stay suture is taken which will later be used to invaginate the mucosa with ureter below the dissected detrussor muscle. Mucosa is then incised. The ureter is laid in the trough, spatulated and anastomosed to the bladder mucosa with running or interrupted fine absorbable sutures, over a Double J stent. The mobilized detrusor muscles are then closed over the ureter without giving pressure over the ureter, in order to make a submucosal tunnel.

After ensuring proper hemostasis, the wound is then closed after placing a drain.

Postoperative Care

The recipient is managed in dedicated kidney transplant unit, after the surgery.

The Foley's catheter is removed after 7 days of surgery. The drain is removed if the drain output is less than 50 mL for 3 consecutive days or after 3 weeks. The stitches are removed after 3 weeks of surgery. After one month of transplant the DJ stent is removed.

CLINICAL PEARLS

- Renal transplant in now one of the most common transplant procedures.
- Anesthesiologists working in non-transplant centers should be able to manage them.
- Transplanted patients may require surgery for procedures unrelated to the transplant.

REFERENCES

1. Carrel A. Le technique operatoire des anastomoses vasculaire et al transplantation des visceres. Lyon Med. 1902;98:859.
2. Voronoy Yu Yu. Sobre el bloqueo delaparato reticulo-endothelial. Singlo Med. 1936;97:296.
3. Kuss R, Tsenturier J, Milliez P. Quelgues ess ais de greffos du rein chez l'homme. Med Acad Chir. 1951;77:755.
4. Merrill JP, Murray JE, Harrison JH, Guild WR. Successful homotransplantations of the human kidney between two identical twins. J Am Med Assoc. 1956;28:160(4):277.
5. Ratner LE, Ciseck LJ, Moore RG, et al. Laparoscopic live donor nephrectomy. Transplantation. 1995;60:1047-49.
6. Michon L, Hamburger J, Oeconomos N, et al. Une tentative de transplantation renale chez l'homme aspects medicaux et abiologiques. Presse Med. 1953;61:1419.
7. Starzl TE, Marchioro TL. Technique of renal homotransplantations: experience with 42 cases. Arch Surg. 1964;89:87.
8. Lich R, Howerton LW, David LA. Recurrent urosepsis in children. J Urol. 1961;86:554.
9. Paquin AJ Jr. Ureterovesical anastomosis: the description and evaluation of a technique. J Urol. 1959;82:573.
10. Politano VA, Leadbetter WF. An operative technique for the correction of vesicoureteral reflux. J Urol. 1958;79:932.

Anesthetic Considerations for Kidney Transplant in an Adults

Rashmi Jain

INTRODUCTION

The incidence of end stage renal disease (ESRD) has increased over the past several decades due to an increased incidence of diabetes, obesity and hypertension and in part due to improved care of concurrent diseases like ischemic heart disease and stroke. Patients with ESRD may receive replacement therapy by dialysis or by renal transplant from a living, related donor or a cadaver donor. The number of patients with ESRD who receive treatment has increased because of more liberal acceptance of candidates for dialysis therapy. Kidney transplantation is the preferred therapy for end-stage kidney disease but requires life long immunosuppression. The relative risk of death is increased at the time of surgery approximately three fold, but by postoperative day 180 the relative risk is the same as the patients remaining on dialysis and by one year patients, who received a transplant were close to one third less likely to die than those who stayed on dialysis.[1]

Survival and health related quality of life is better after kidney transplantation than after dialysis therapy. Dialysis therapy is associated with high mortality rate along with impairment in physical and cognitive function.

Despite improvement in immunosuppression regimens which have reduced rates of acute transplant rejection, long-term allograft survival remains sub-optimal. To improve long-term outcomes, physicians need to understand the mechanisms underlying transplant rejection and tolerance in humans.

Patients with renal failure undergoing surgery are at a substantial risk for increased morbidity and mortality due to multisystem dysfunction including:

1. Cardiovascular
   Hypertension, ischemic heart disease, cardiac failure, pericarditis
2. Respiratory
   Pulmonary edema, pleural effusion, respiratory infection
3. Gastrointestinal
   Stress ulceration, delayed gastric emptying, malnutrition
4. Central nervous
   Peripheral neuropathy, autonomic neuropathy, mental slowing, convulsions, coma
5. Renal
   Fluid and electrolyte imbalance, altered pharmacokinetics and pharmacodynamics
6. Hematological
   Anemia, coagulopathies
7. Immunological
   Immunosuppression
8. Dialysis related problems
   a. Peritonitis (peritoneal dialysis)
   b. Systemic anticoagulation
   c. Vascular access
   d. Dementia.

Cardiovascular System (Fig. 7.9)

The main cardiovascular problems of chronic renal failure are arterial hypertension, atherosclerosis and hyperlipidemia leading to ischemic heart disease. Hypertension may be controlled with dialysis and appropriate antihypertensive therapy. Sometimes an abnormal relationship exists among plasma renin activity, intravascular fluid volume and blood pressure, and there may be an inappropriate level

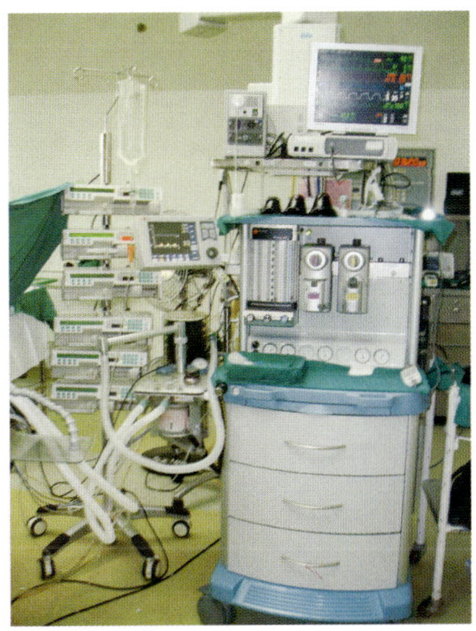

Fig. 7.9: Anesthesia machine

of sympathetic activity requiring large doses of combination of antihypertensive agents. This may cause drug interaction with volatile and intravenous anesthetic agents. Immunosuppression including cyclosporine therapy may also produce hypertension and increase tendency to CVS disease.

Inspite of adequate therapy, 50–70% patients experience marked swings in blood pressure during surgery. Exaggerated vascular response to induction of anesthesia, laryngoscopy, intubation and extubation can take place. Induction of anesthesia should include hypnotic agent along with an opioid. Left ventricular function may be compromised by uremic cardiomyopathy and pericarditis.

Proteinuria indicates graft dysfunction and cardiovascular risk. ACE inhibitors reduce proteinuria and improve survival in kidney recipients.

Left ventricular hypertrophy (LVH) begins early in chronic renal failure patients often by the time the creatinine clearance has fallen below 25 mL/min and 70% at the start of dialysis. LVH increases with increasing time on dialysis. The LVH regresses following transplantation as the mechanisms of anemia and fluid overload cease to operate.

Effective blood pressure control following transplantation is beneficial to graft and patient survival. It also reduces the degree of LVH.

Cardiovascular disease including coronary artery disease, acute myocardial infarction, arrhythmia, cardiomyopathy, heart failure and stroke are the leading causes of death in renal transplant recipients.[2]

Parathyroid hormone adversely affects lipid metabolism and causes hyperlipidemia in CRF, has a permissive role in arteriolar wall thickening and myocardial interstitial fibrosis. It also contributes to hypertension. This effect can be blocked by calcium channel blocker, verapamil[2] (Flow chart 7.2).

Respiratory System

Pulmonary congestion and edema can occur between dialysis sessions, causing hypoxemia and hypocapnia. Peritoneal dialysis can cause problems because the intraperitoneal fluid causes diaphragmatic splinting with basal pulmonary atelectasis and shunting. Uremic lung is characterized by perihilar pulmonary venous congestion secondary to fluid retention and can also cause pleuritis. Immunosuppressed transplant patients are susceptible to pulmonary infections.

Flow chart 7.2: Risk stratification of cardiovascular disease in ESRD patient

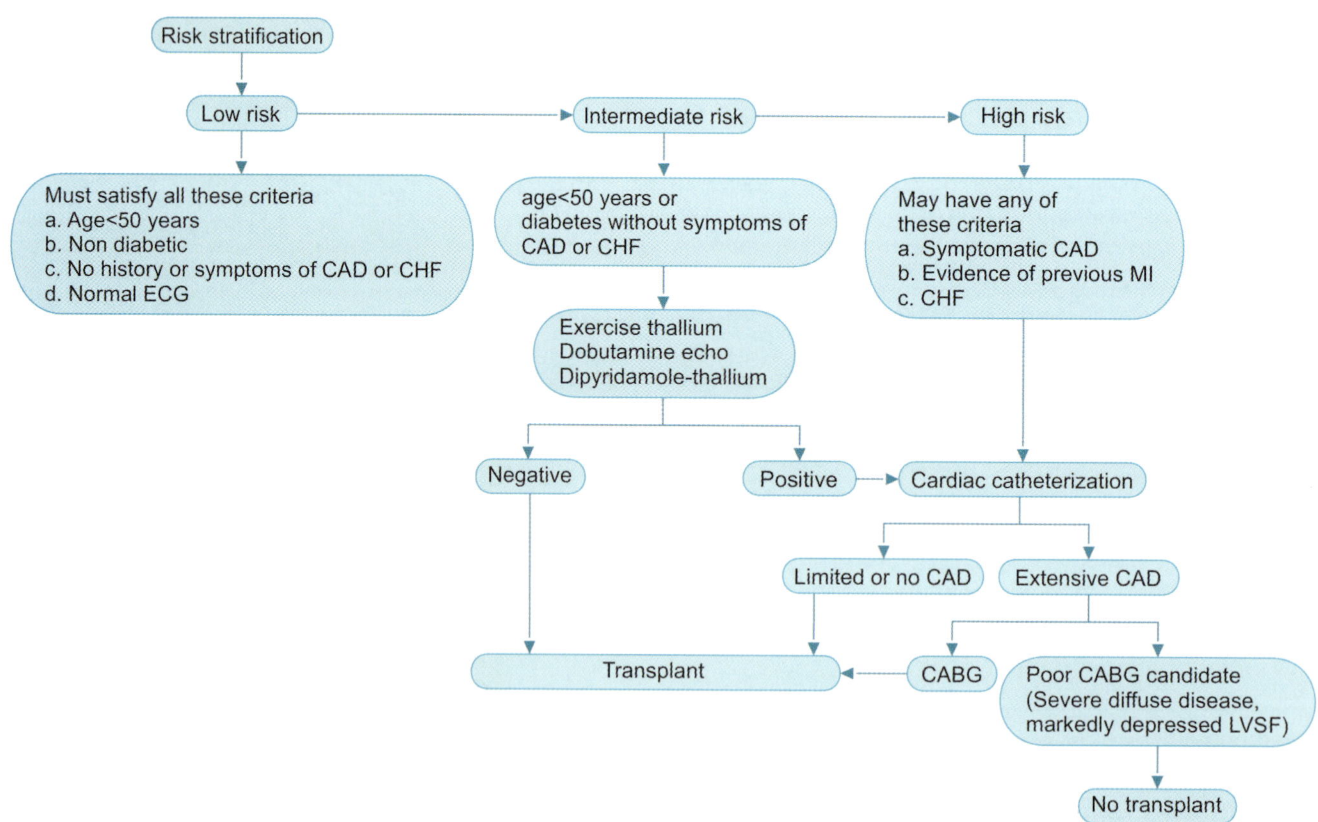

Gastrointestinal Tract System

Patients in renal failure have delayed gastric emptying in addition to increase in acidity and gastric volume. H_2 receptor antagonists should be administered as part of premedication. An important complication is ascites (along with hypoalbuminemia) which may lead to splinting of the diaphragm and basal pulmonary atelectasis resulting in hypoxemia.

Central Nervous System

Uremia may result in reduced mental ability, myoclonus, seizures, coma and even death. Sudden change in extracellular volume and electrolytes can cause cerebral edema. The disequilibrium syndrome is characterized by dehydration, weakness, nausea, vomiting, hypotension and sometimes convulsions and coma. Treatment is symptomatic.

Anemia

Anemia (normochromic, normocytic) is a major problem in the anesthetic management of patients with renal failure. It is due to impaired erythropoiesis, secondary to decreased erythropoietin synthesis and release. The other factors are reduced red blood cell life span, increased hemolysis and bleeding, repeated blood loss during hemodialysis, aluminium toxicity, uremia induced bone marrow suppression, iron, folate, vitamin B_6, B_{12} deficiency, and the presence of uremic inhibitors like parathyroid hormone.

Various compensatory mechanisms exist to overcome the decrease in oxygen carrying capacity.

a. Increase in cardiac output which results in LVH and cardiovascular mortality.
b. Increase in the red blood cell 2,3 diphosphoglycerate, which shifts the oxygen dissociation curve to the right improving tissue oxygenation. The shift is greater in uremic patients who are well controlled with hemodialysis. Severe anemia affects the blood gas partition coefficient for the volatile anesthetic agents with an increase in the role of onset and recovery from anesthesia.

Coagulation

Platelet dysfunction and decreased levels of platelet factor III result in poor adhesiveness and thrombocytopenia. Laboratory investigations show normal prothrombin or partial thromboplastin time, but the bleeding time is prolonged. Platelet function may be corrected by dialysis. Thromboelastography (TEG) may be done preoperatively to know any abnormality in platelet adhesion and aggregation. Heparin is used during dialysis which can also cause abnormality in the coagulation parameters. Basta and Sloan reported a case of epidural hematoma in a patient with chronic renal failure about 60 hours after catheter placement.[3]

Despite these problems, blood loss during transplantation is less than 500 mL but if it occurs then it is rapid and should be replaced through large venous catheters.

Acid Base Status

Patients with renal failure have an impaired ability to excrete water, electrolytes and free acids. Preoperative electrolyte disturbances have largely disappeared due to routine dialysis before transplantation. Methods for the correction of hyperkalemia include glucose insulin therapy and administration of sodium bicarbonate, or continuous hemodialysis leading to increased potassium elimination. Infusion of stored blood and hypoventilation causes respiratory acidosis which can further increase plasma potassium concentration and are best avoided.

Endocrine System

Diabetic nephropathy is a common cause of end stage renal disease. Diabetic autonomic neuropathy can cause gastroparesis and homodynamic instability. Long-term problems include stiffening of the temporomandibular joints and difficulty with laryngoscopy and intubation.

Uremic osteodystrophy includes osteomalacia, osteosclerosis and osteitis fibrosa cystica. Failure to convert 1-hydroxyvitamin D to 1,25-dihydroxyvitamin D leads to reduced absorption of calcium, which results in hyperparathyroidism. It causes bone demineralization and spontaneous fractures. Phosphate excretion declines resulting in hyperphosphatemia.

Depression

Depression can cause increased morbidity and mortality and poor quality of life in patients with ESRD. Prevalence of depression has been found to be lower in transplant recipients than in wait listed patients. One fifth of transplant patients are still at high-risk of depression depending upon socioeconomic status, comorbid conditions and treatment modalities.[4]

Absolute Contraindications

i. Patients with chronic, irreversible and terminal illness in other organ systems may not survive the challenge of anesthesia and surgery. The predicted patient survival is less than 5 years after transplant in such patients

ii. Patients with severe, refractory cardiac disease or severe respiratory failure are poor surgical patients
iii. Disseminated metastatic carcinoma
iv. Persistent chronic infection
v. Predicted risk of graft loss greater than 50% at 1 year
vi. Patients unable to comply with immunosuppressant therapy
vii. Immunosuppression predicted to cause life threatening complication.

PATIENT SELECTION

Advanced age is not a contraindication to renal transplant, although older recipients are at greater risk of perioperative complications including death. Infants less than 1-year of age and geriatric patients aged 70 years and older are considered eligible for renal transplant.

Sickle Cell Disease

Patients with sickle cell disease have several renal pathologies like glomerulonephritis, pyelonephritis and nephrotic syndrome.

Obesity

Patients who are obese gain a significant advantage after transplantation rather than staying on the waiting list. Many centers use a body mass index (BMI) of 30–35 kg/m^2 as a limit for transplant eligibility. This is due to the belief that obese patients have more complications and shorter patient survival than ideal weight patients. In the study by Kavitha Potluri these patients should not be excluded from the list of transplant although they observed increased risk of postoperative wound complications.[5] Nutritional counseling should be available immediately after transplantation for all patients. Weight gain after transplantation is associated with higher dose steroid and renewed sense of well being.

SPECIAL SITUATIONS

Mental Retardation

Transplantation is cost effective and it is easier to manage these patients after transplant since dialysis can be discontinued. Improvement in quality of life can justify renal transplant in these patients.

Retransplantation

Patients with three or more transplants may have surgical difficulty. They are sensitized by previous transplants and blood transfusions and therefore cross-matching and immunosuppression may become difficult.

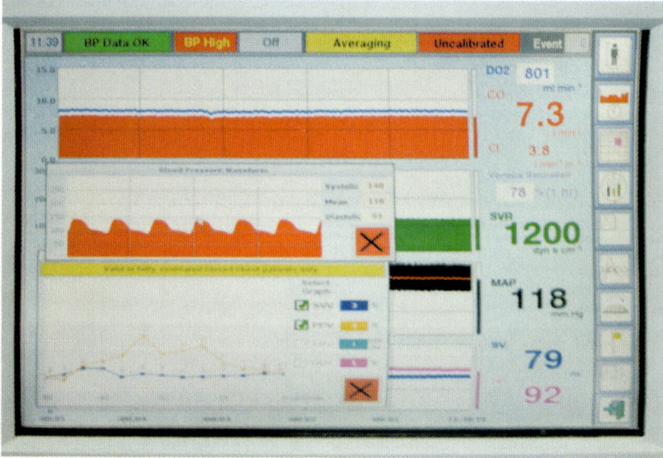

Fig. 7.10: Cardiac output monitor[1]

Female renal transplant candidates are prone to be sensitized by prior pregnancies.

The HIV positive status, Renal transplantation is not a contraindication in carefully selected HIV infected patients.[6] Historically HIV positive patients were considered a contraindication for renal transplant. After 1996, with the introduction of highly active antiretroviral therapy (HAART) the retropositive patients live longer and therefore end stage organ disease is now an increasingly important cause of mortality and morbidity in these patients. Guidelines regarding use of immunosuppressives in HIV positive patients who are on HAART and drug interaction is critical to patient management. In most cases patients continue their pretransplantation autiretroviral regimen. Doses of drugs depend on the level of kidney function with frequent adjustments in the early post-transplant period and during periods of graft dysfunction. Potential nephrotoxicity of antiretroviral agents used to prevent opportunistic infections can occur and medication is changed accordingly.[7] If the patient had hepatitis B virus coinfection then a liver biopsy is done to rule out cirrhosis (less than stage 2 fibrosis). They should have undetectable hepatitis B virus surface antigen while on anti-viral therapy.

Transplantation is a reasonable option for selected HIV-infected patients. One and 3-year kidney patient and graft survival are comparable to the general kidney recipient population. HIV specific outcomes are excellent.[8]

Patients with HCV coinfection are advised about the potential immunostimulatory effects of posttransplant interferon therapy. They could elect to have pretransplant interferon treatment.

Diabetes Mellitus Type II

Conventionally they were not considered suitable for transplantation and were maintained on dialysis. However recently its been seen that in the absence of vascular complications these patients have an improved survival rate with transplantation versus dialysis.

PREOPERATIVE PREPARATION

Appropriate anesthesia for renal transplantation requires minimal toxicity for the patient and transplanted kidney in addition to maintenance of vital functions and sufficient pain relief.

Hemodialysis (Fig. 7.11)

Hemodialysis optimizes the acid base and overall volemic status. Preoperative dialysis reduces perioperative mortality and delayed graft function, which has been reduced to almost 0%.[9] It should be scheduled about 12–24 hours prior to surgery. The ionic content of the dialysate may be altered to influence the amount and composition of the fluid to be removed. A post dialysis measurement of serum electrolytes is required before surgery as dialysis induced electrolyte disturbances can predispose to intraoperative cardiac dysrhythmias. When the patient is on chronic hemodialysis the need for acute pre-surgery hemodialysis is very rare. In many units a serum potassium level of 5.5 mmol/L or greater will trigger an acute hemodialysis treatment. If it is decided to use acute hemodialysis prior to surgery, then a short treatment of about two hours is usually all that is necessary as that will reduce the potassium by approximately 2 mmol/L. Patients undergoing hemodialysis have a target "dry weight" that is achieved at the end of each treatment session. In fact on an average at that weight most patients are intravascular depleted. Coagulation defects caused by reduced platelet adhesion and aggregation are also reversed by dialysis. Residual anticoagulation after recent hemodialysis may cause problems. Acute hemodialysis treatment requires some degree of anti-coagulation. Therapeutic anticoagulation can be minimized but platelet consumption in the dialyzer increases the risk of bleeding.

For patients treated with peritoneal dialysis, which is a "continuous" treatment, wide fluctuations in serum electrolytes are rare but they are usually fluid overloaded. However, there is no need to make changes to peritoneal dialysis prescription prior to surgery (Fig. 7.12).

Vascular Access

Patients for renal transplant may have difficult intravenous access. Current or potential future fistula sites should be avoided, including all forearm and anticubital veins, if possible. Central venous cannulation may also be difficult if hemodialysis catheters have previously been sited in the central veins. Use of ultrasound guidance may be required. Central venous access to enable monitoring of central venous pressure is important to guide fluid management in these patients who are oliguric or anuric.

Antihypertensive Medication

Most patients are on antihypertensive medication. Angiotensin converting enzyme (ACE) inhibitors decrease mortality in congestive heart failure and hypertension, slow progression of established diabetic nephropathy, and other

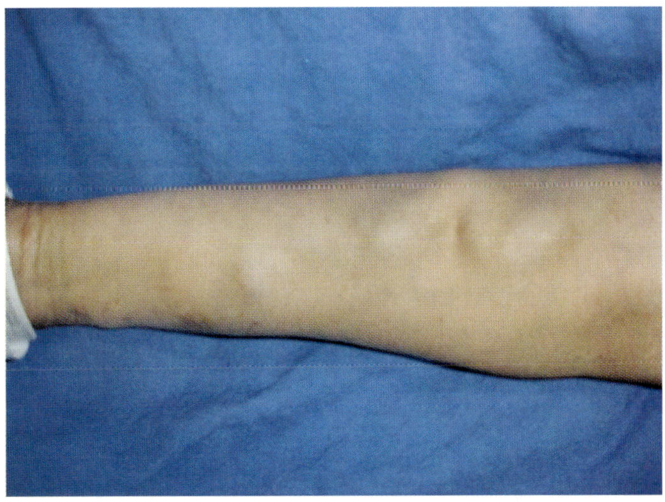

Fig. 7.11: Arteriovenous fistula for hemodialysis

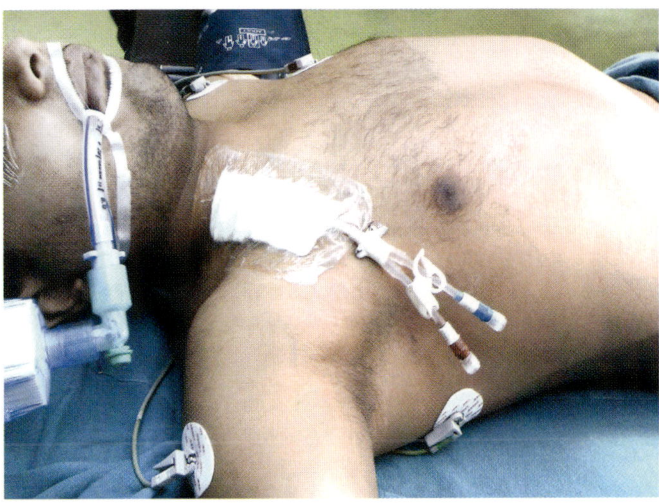

Fig. 7.12: Percutaneous tunnelling of hemodialysis catheter inserted in the right internal jugular vein

proteinuria associated glomerulonephritides. Both ACE inhibitors and angiotensin receptor blockers can reverse left ventricular hypertrophy and improve left ventricular diastolic dysfunction in renal transplant recipients, independent of blood pressure reduction. Antihypertensive agents with significant renal elimination need to be administered at lower dosages and sometimes, less frequently.

Most of the antihypertensives like clonidine and β-blockers, if stopped, can cause perioperative rebound hypertension, tachycardia or myocardial infarction, and therefore these agents should be continued throughout the perioperative period. Chronic use of ACE inhibitors for control of hypertension or maintaining therapy till the day of surgery may increase the probability of hypotension after anesthetic induction. It is advisable to withhold ACE inhibitors in the immediate perioperative period, especially in those who are hypovolemic and if large fluid shifts are anticipated.[10]

If blood pressure remains high despite treatment but the patient is fit for surgery in other respects, the procedure should not be deferred simply on account of an elevated arterial pressure. If the arterial pressure is consistently elevated to levels of ≥180 mm Hg systolic or ≥110 mm Hg diastolic, surgery may proceed, but care should be taken to ensure perioperative cardiovascular stability.[9,11]

Blood Transfusion

Nowadays perioperative blood loss is minimal. Although blood should be available for intraoperative transfusion, it is rarely administered. Blood transfusion does not improve transplantation outcome.[12]

Preoperative Assessment

Patients with renal failure have other comorbidities including hypertension, diabetes, peripheral vascular disease and cardiac disease. Renal failure not only causes water and electrolyte abnormalities but affects other organ systems also thus making the intraoperative management especially challenging.

History and physical examination along with review of the laboratory investigations is essential.

These patients are hemodynamically labile during anesthesia and surgery.

a. ***Ischemic heart disease:*** It should be optimized to reduce perioperative morbidity and mortality. Baseline electrocardiogram, echocardiography and dobutamine stress testing is able to predict patients at high risk of perioperative cardiovascular mortality and morbidity. Pericardial effusion, uncontrolled hypertension, unstable angina and diabetes mellitus should be addressed when patient is selected for transplantation.
b. ***Consideration of the renal history***
   - Usual fluid intake may be restricted
   - Daily urine output
   - Regime of renal replacement therapy (frequency of dialysis)
   - Renal function
     - Glomerular filtration rate
     - Serum electrolytes, sodium and potassium
     - Serum urea and creatinine concentration
c. ***Serum potassium abnormalities:*** These patients may present with hyper or hypokalemia. Hyperkalemia is due to impaired renal potassium elimination while hypokalemia is due to excessive removal by dialysis. These patients are normally tolerant of large variations of serum potassium concentration. Emergency treatment of hyperkalemia is indicated if there are ECG manifestations such as bradycardia, PR prolongation, QRS widening, peaked T waves and AV block.

Treatment

a. Continuous cardiac monitoring
b. Large bore IV access
c. Cardiac membrane stabilization using calcium chloride or calcium gluconate
d. Intracellular shift of serum potassium using an infusion of insulin and dextrose while monitoring plasma glucose concentration
e. Cation exchange resins and renal replacement therapy using dialysis or hemofiltration
f. Basic and advanced life support measure

Hypokalemia can cause flattened or inverted T waves, prominent U waves that appear as QT prolongation, ST depression, atrial and ventricular tachyarrhythmias.

Potassium replacement should be done under the supervision of the nephrologist/anesthesiologist and with ECG monitoring.

Gastrointestinal system: They are prone to reflux and delayed gastric emptying. Antacid prophylaxis should be given. Anesthesia technique that will protect the airway should be the method of choice.

Neurology these patients are prone to peripheral neuropathy. Positioning on the operating table should be done with care. Pressure areas should be adequately padded.

Autonomic neuropathy causes intraoperative hemodynamic instability hence invasive blood pressure monitoring is done. Anesthetic drug dose alteration may be required frequently.

Anemia: Despite anemia (sometimes hemoglobin as low as 5g%) blood transfusion is not recommended since, it can cause primary sensitization.[12]

These patients are immunosuppressed hence steroid supplementation and antibiotic prophylaxis is given. Immunosuppression is induced before anesthesia and maintained postoperatively.

A patient requiring renal transplant receives a range of medications, including beta blockers, calcium channel antagonists, furosemide, angiotensin converting enzyme inhibitors, antacids, iron, vitamin supplements, erythropoietin and immunosuppressants.

Neurological sequelae, including confusion, sedation or obtundation can result from uremic encephalopathy. Intubation for airway protection may be necessary. Volume overload can lead to pulmonary edema and hypoxia. Ventilatory support is necessary until adequate fluid removal has been achieved with dialysis or diuresis. Renal failure causes metabolic acidosis and mechanical ventilation may be required until the acidosis is corrected. Blood gas analysis at the point of care helps the anesthesiologist to treat metabolic derangements and hypoxemia.

Premedication

Benzodiazepine like diazepam or alprazolam take care of anxiety of the patient. H_2-receptor blocker like pantocid are prescribed. Morning dose of immunosuppressants and antihypertensives should be taken.

CHOICE OF ANESTHESIA (FIG. 7.13)

General anesthesia with controlled ventilation is the technique of choice for renal transplant patients. Regional anesthesia is also practiced in some centers. Surgery may last four hours or more and large volume of fluid may be infused.

The patient is placed supine on the operating table. Care is taken to protect the arterio-venous fistula. Intravenous or arterial lines or the blood pressure cuff should not be placed on the same extremity as the fistula. An intravenous drip is usually in situ which had been used for giving immunosuppressive therapy the previous day. The same venous access is used for induction of anesthesia. The regime used for immunosuppressive therapy is discussed in another chapter. The monitors are attached to the patient and baseline recording is done. Intraoperative monitors include the following:

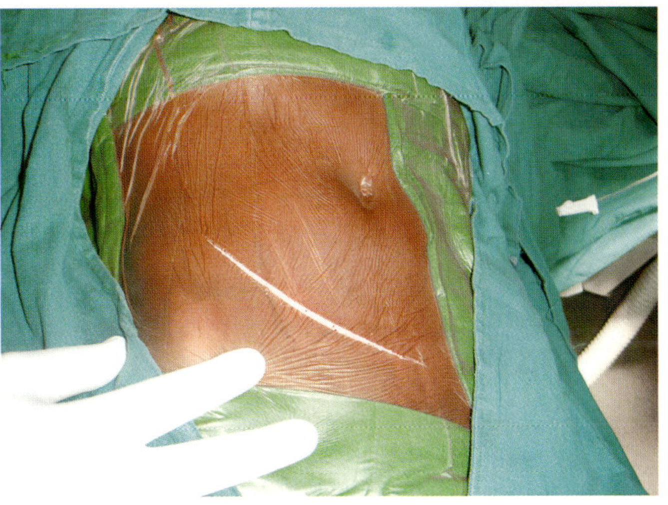

Fig. 7.13: Incision at the right illiac fossa

- Electrocardiogram
- Noninvasive blood pressure
- Pulse oximeter
- Temperature maintenance (Fluid warmer, Warming blanket (upper body)) (Fig. 7.14A and B).

After induction of anesthesia and endotracheal intubation invasive monitoring is started, which includes end tidal carbon dioxide (capnography), central venous pressure, temperature probe, intra-arterial monitoring and urine output monitor (to assess output once the kidney function starts) (Figs 7.15A and B).

Lower body warming blankets are not applied because they can cause burns during the time of arterial clamping (Fig. 7.16). Routine use of pulmonary artery catheters is not required. Strict asepsis has to be maintained because these patients are on immunosuppressants and hence prone to infection.

Intraoperative arterial blood gas analysis along with serum electrolytes is done, after induction, before and after reperfusion. Metabolic acidosis after reperfusion can be corrected by bicarbonate therapy. Acid base balance and ventilation should be maintained because hyperventilation may shift the oxyhemoglobin dissociation curve to the left, decreasing the ability of hemoglobin to release oxygen to the peripheral tissues. This is specially important in these patients who are severely anemic.

Hypovolemia and hypotension should be avoided at all cost because it is detrimental to the newly transplanted kidney. Usually chronic renal failure patients are kept dry to prevent fluid overload and to avoid the need for postoperative dialysis.

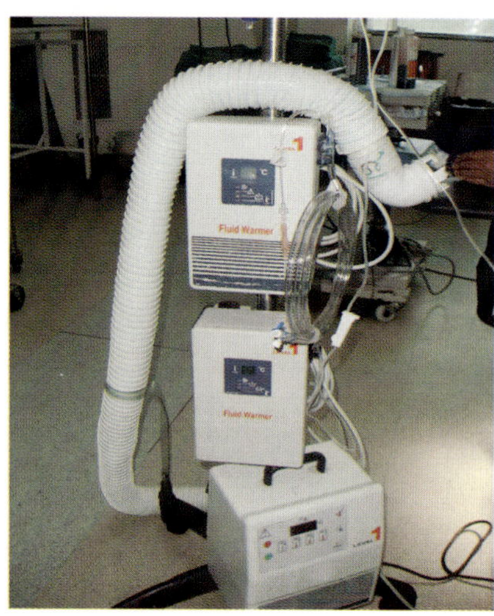

Fig. 7.14A: Fluid and patient warmer

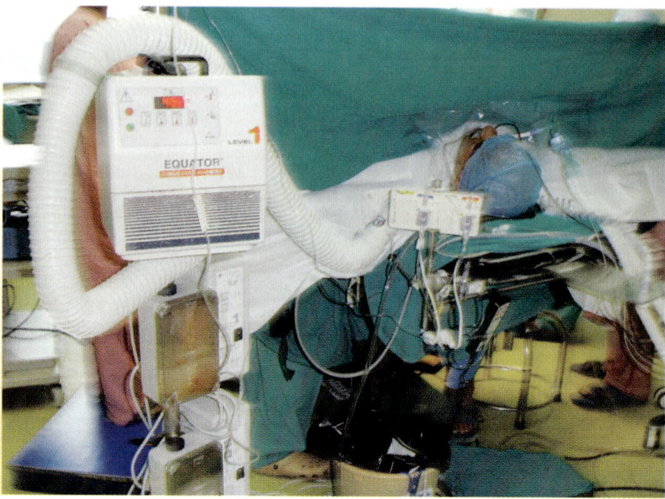

Fig. 7.14B: Warming blanket to maintain the temperature

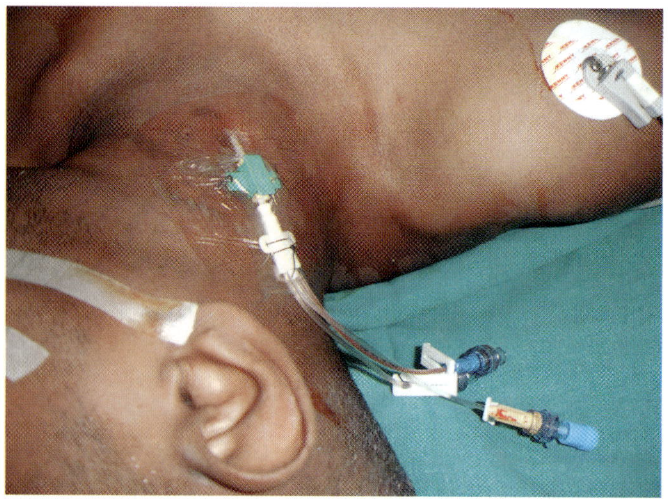

Fig. 7.15A: Internal jugular vein cannulation

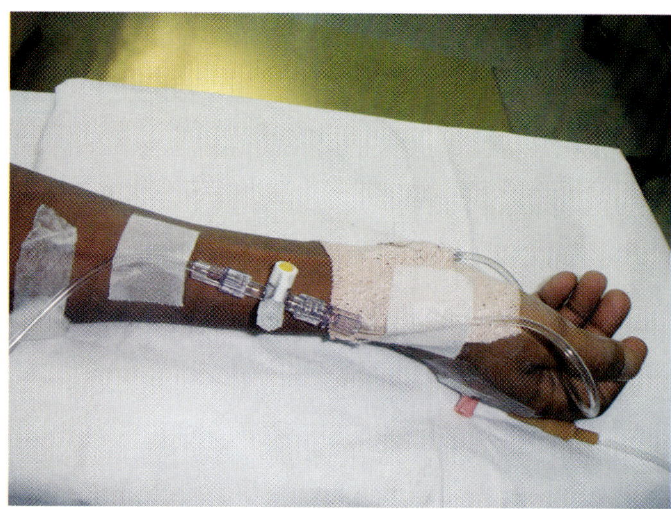

Fig. 7.15B: Radial artery cannulation

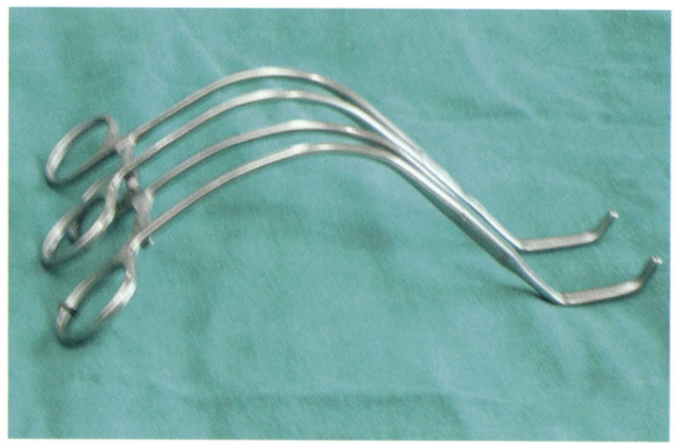

Fig. 7.16: Vascular clamps

The transplanted patient should be "wet" with a "supernormal intravascular volume" to ensure adequate flow to the new renal graft after opening the clamps. Central venous pressure of 15–20 mm Hg at the time the arterial clamps are released is recommended. Administration of albumin (1.2 g/kg) was associated with a reduced incidence of delayed graft function.

Inotropes like dopamine should not be used routinely. Inhalational anesthetic agents and opioids are tailored in such a manner to maintain systolic blood pressure at or above 140 mm Hg to ensure adequate flow to the new graft.

The new kidney requires adequate perfusion to ensure optimal function. Appropriate hydration during renal transplant is of utmost importance. Central venous pressure reflects the pulmonary artery diastolic pressure. Intra-arterial pressure monitoring is useful especially in patients with significant cardiovascular or lung disease or poorly controlled hypertension. Arterial cannulae should not be inserted on the same side as an AV fistula is located.

Drawbacks like prolonged paralysis requiring post-operative mechanical ventilation, iatrogenic pulmonary infection and adverse effects of inhalation agents may be seen.

Avoiding intraoperative renal insults and maintaining isovolemia, adequate cardiac output and renal perfusion pressure are more important than the choice of a specific anesthetic technique (Figs 7.17 and 7.18).

Many drugs used during anesthesia are dependent on renal excretion for elimination. Patients with renal disease are sensitive to barbiturates and benzodiazepines secondary to decreased protein binding. Narcotics including morphine and pethidine should be used judiciously as they have active metabolites and may have prolonged activity. Fentanyl or remifentanyl are better choices.

Succinylcholine may be used if the patient's serum potassium level is normal. Atracurium does not rely on renal function for its elimination and therefore is the nondepolarizing muscle relaxant of choice. However vecuronium can also be used but its effect may be prolonged. Vecuronium may be clinically useful and even beneficial with proper neuromuscular monitoring due to its marked absence of systemic and cardiovascular side effects. Neuromuscular reversal agents rely on renal excretion. Nonsteroidal anti-inflammatory agents (NSAIDs) should be avoided.

Intraoperative Fluid Therapy

Crystalloids are distributed mostly to the interstitial space whereas colloids remain in the intravascular space. 0.9% saline is most frequently administered crystalloid during renal transplant because it is devoid of potassium thus minimizing the risk of electrolyte induced cardiac dysrhythmias. Thirty minutes after infusion of 1000 mL normal saline, plasma volume is typically expanded by just 180 mL with the balance extravasated to the interstitial space. In a recent study no difference was found when 0.9% sodium chloride, Ringer's lactate or plasmalyte were given during renal transplant. Plasmalyte showed the best metabolic profile. Some protocols recommend normal saline containing sodium bicarbonate (20 mmol/L) for volume expansion.[13]

Patients with chronic renal failure have a narrow margin of safety for intravenous hydration. The anesthesiologist must carefully adjust intravascular volume and arterial blood pressure to effectively perfuse the graft after vascular anastomosis.

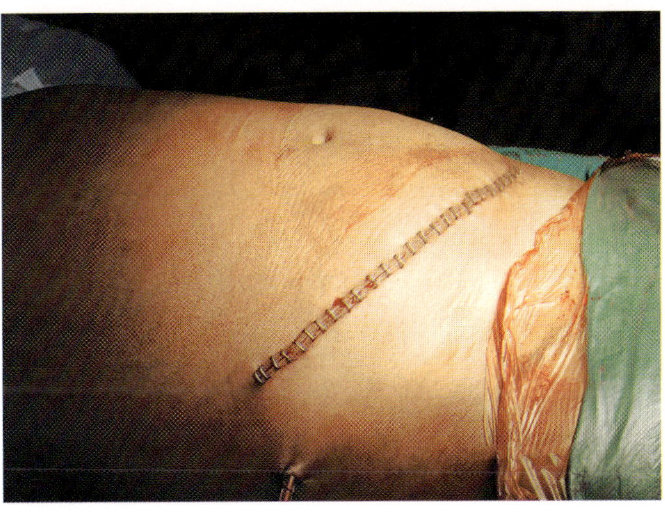

Fig. 7.17: Site of incision

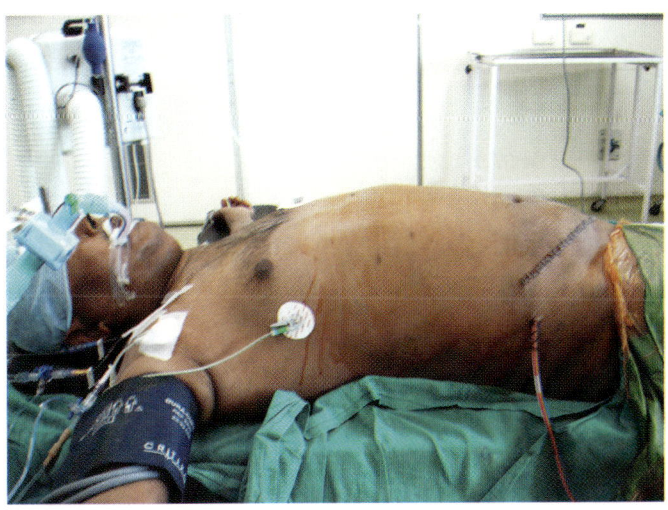

Fig. 7.18: Extraperitoneal placement of the transplanted kidney in the right flank kidney

Delayed return of renal function is usually associated with 20% to 40 % decrease in graft survival.

One year graft survival decreased from 75% with immediate urine output to only 49% when onset of diuresis was delayed >12 hours. Hence the anesthesiologist should aggressively expand the vascular volume to promote early diuresis during anesthesia for kidney transplant.[14]

Post recovery graft function was evaluated by estimation of fraction extraction sodium ratio (FENa^{+}%) at 0, 2, 4, 6 hours after surgery to assess renal concentrating power. High CVP at the time of unclamping the renal artery after anastomosis provides a more favorable outcome. Carlier et al showed that maximum hydration during anesthesia (100 mL/kg normal saline) and elevated right heart pressure is associated with early graft function.[15]

According to the study done by Othman MM et al, two groups of patients were studied. This clinical trial showed that a regimen targeting low CVP before cross-clamp of the donor kidney, and then a high CVP until unclamping the renal artery after anastomosis (CVPT group), provides a more favorable outcome than the continuous infusion rate (CIR) regimen used in this study. Recipients in the CVPT group had better intraoperative graft turgidity, arterial blood pressure stability, earlier diuresis, and rapid improvement of postoperative graft function. This was achieved in the CVPT group without an overall increase in infused saline volume, vasopressor use, and diuretic doses compared with the CIR group. Patients in the CVPT group also had less tissue edema than patients in the CIR group.[16]

However patients with preexistent cardiac disease or poor myocardial function are at overt risk of fluid overload, acute pulmonary edema, acute respiratory failure and prolonged intubation. If there is no urine output, then slow the IV infusion.

Measures used to Enhance Urine Output During Kidney Transplant (Figs 7.19 to 7.21)

1. Mannitol: It confers protection against renal ischemia by increasing tubular urine formation and by scavenging free radicals. It is given in the dose of 0.7–1 g/kg. Mannitol infusion is started when renal anastomosis is commenced. However large doses of mannitol can induce renal vasoconstriction and pulmonary edema.
2. Loop diuretics: Inhibit Na^+ K^+ ATPase decreasing tubular oxygen consumption which may offer some protection against ischemic injury.

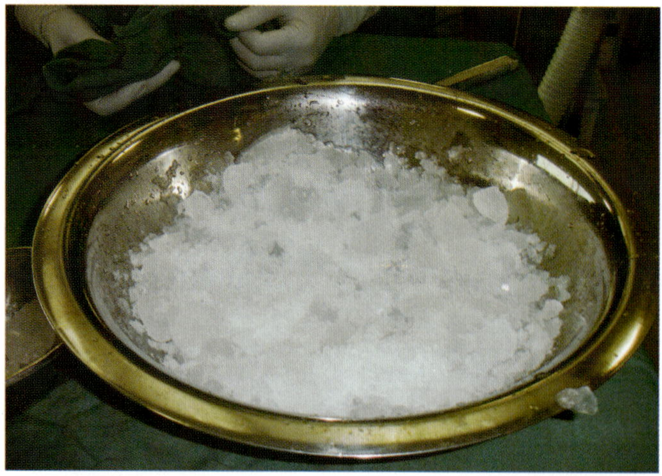

Fig. 7.19: Ice for keeping the graft cold

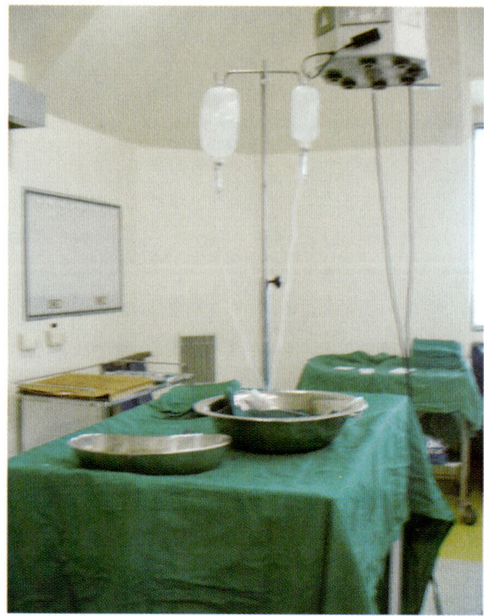

Fig. 7.20: Ice cold Ringer Lactate used for cold perfusion of graft kidney

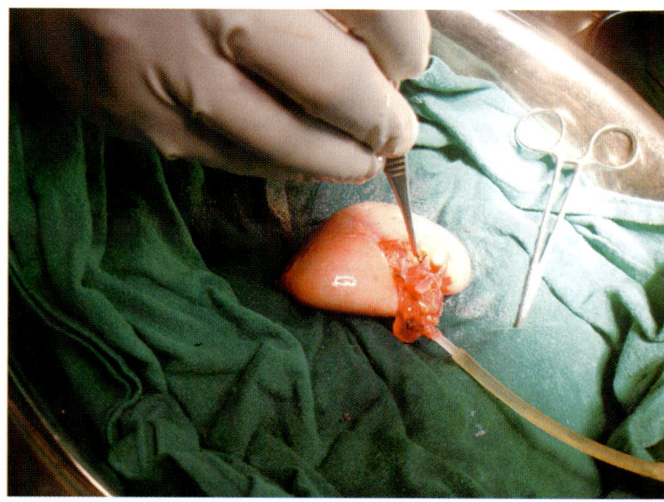

Fig. 7.21: Perfusion of donor kidney on the side table

3. An aggressive intraoperative volume expansion by keeping CVP between 10–15 mm Hg is recommended to avoid acute tubular necrosis secondary to inadequate intraoperative hydration. 20% albumin, 0.8–1.6 mL/kg may improve the graft survival, urine volume and early graft function.

Whether mannitol, loop diuretic or dopamine influence the rate of delayed graft function (DGF) is difficult to decide. These strategies are based on observational studies only.

Influence of Renal Disease on Pharmacokinetics and Pharmacodynamics of Drugs used During Anesthesia

Many changes occur in the uptake, metabolism and excretion of drugs in the patients with chronic renal failure.

Midazolam

Total drug clearance and apparent volume of distribution was greater in patients with chronic renal failure than in healthy controls. There is no difference in drug kinetics and elimination half-life. The unbound drug is rapidly distributed to the vascularized tissues hence it should be administered slowly, titrating dose to effect.[17]

Thiopental Sodium

There is no difference in the dose of thiopental required to induce anesthesia in healthy patients and in patients with renal failure.

There is no alteration in brain sensitivity to the thiobarbiturate. The kinetics and total drug elimination half life is unaltered.[18]

Propofol

There is no major alteration in elimination half life or clearance in patients with renal failure. There is no significant effect on the plasma protein binding of propofol. There is a greater dose requirement of propofol for attaining hypnosis and a bispectral index monitor level of 50 in patients with renal failure. This may be due to increased cardiac output accompanying the anemia seen in renal failure.[19]

Infusion of propofol is also used for maintenance of anesthesia for renal transplantation.

Morphine

Most studies show that renal failure has little effect on morphine clearance but accumulation of its various metabolites takes place. The longer half lives of morphine 3 glucuronide and morphine 6 glucuronide in patients with renal failure can cause prolonged effect of the parent drug.

Fentanyl, Alfentanil and Sufentanil

Many anesthesiologists prefer fentanyl, alfentanil and sufentanil to provide intraoperative analgesia. A small fraction of these three drugs is excreted by the kidney unchanged and their metabolites are inactive. There is no alteration in fentanyl binding in patients with uremia. There is no relationship between preoperative creatinine and the disposition parameters of fentanyl.[20]

Remifentanil

Remifentanil is a piperidine derivative. Its elimination does not depend on either hepatic metabolism or renal elimination, but on plasma and tissue esterase hydrolysis. The kinetics of remifentanil is unaltered in awake, end stage renal disease patient.[21]

Neuromuscular Relaxant Drugs

Rapid sequence intubation in renal transplant recipients in the absence of hyperkalemia, may be done with suxamethonium. Large doses of nondepolarizing drugs like atracurium, cisatracurium, mivacurium and rocuronium are the other alternatives in patients with hyperkalemia. There is a decreased activity of the enzyme pseudocholinesterase in patients being treated for renal failure by hemodialysis; however this is not a significant problem with current hemodialysis technique.

In order to minimize the increase in plasma potassium levels after suxamethonium, some pretreatment is advised like nondepolarizing neuromuscular blocking agent, benzodiazepines or magnesium sulfate.

Nondepolarizing Neuromuscular Blocking Agents

Atracurium

Many clinical studies found no difference in the duration of neuromuscular blockade from an initial dose of atracurium or from repeated doses when the drug was administered to patients with normal function compared with patients who were anephric.[22]

After continuous infusion of atracurium or by bolus dosing, rapid recovery has been reported in patients with renal failure. Peak laudanosine concentration was not significantly different in healthy patients and in patients with renal failure. Although elimination of laudanosine is principally via the kidneys, there are evidence that in humans other organs may be involved in its elimination (e.g. liver).

Vecuronium

The kinetics of vecuronium was studied in renal failure and in control group of healthy patients.[23] There was no significant effect on the elimination half life or the systemic clearance of vecuronium but the duration of neuromuscular blockade and recovery from blockade was significantly prolonged in the renal failure group. Sakamoto and colleagues confirmed that the duration of action of vecuronium is prolonged in patients with end stage disease as a result of a higher sensitivity to the drug and not because of altered kinetics.[24]

In the uremic patient undergoing transplant surgery, potentiation of the block may occur secondary to hypokalemia, hypocalcemia, hypermagnesemia, use of aminoglycoside antibiotics, furosemide, mannitol and methylprednisolone. We have to be absolutely sure that complete return of neuromuscular function occurs if multiple increments or infusion of the drug is used during prolonged surgery in anephric patients.

Rocuronium

Rocuronium has a rapid onset of effect and intermediate duration of action and may be an alternative to suxamethonium for rapid sequence intubation. It is rapidly metabolized in the liver, with only 9% of the injected dose being recovered unchanged in the urine.

In a single dose comparison of vecuronium, atracurium, cisatracurium and rocuronium in healthy controls and in patients undergoing renal transplantation there were no significant differences within patient groups of onset time or duration of action. Recovery index was slower in the renal patients for all neuromuscular blocking drugs. There is a prolonged duration of effect after repeat doses of rocuronium and veuronium in these patients.[25]

Although most anesthesiologists favor atracurium as the drug of choice, rocuronium can be used for neuromuscular blockade in patients with renal impairment using neuromuscular monitor.

Anticholinesterases

All anticholinesterases are excreted through the kidney by glomerular filteration and tubular secretion. Significant decrease in the clearance of anticholinesterases is seen in anephric patients. Pharmacokinetic parameters similar to those in patients with normal renal function can be shown in patients to whom the drugs are given approximately 1 hour after receiving a living related renal transplant and the graft function is normal.[26]

Inhalational Anesthetic Agents (Fig. 7.22)

All volatile anesthetic agents are myocardial depressants and reduce the cardiac output and blood flow to the transplanted kidney. Enflurane and sevoflurane are biotransformed in the liver, causing increased serum levels of inorganic fluoride. This ion can lead to high output renal failure. Enflurane should not be used to supplement anesthesia for renal transplantation.[27]

Isoflurane undergoes only limited biotransformation to inorganic fluoride and is the agent of choice for a balanced anesthetic technique.[28]

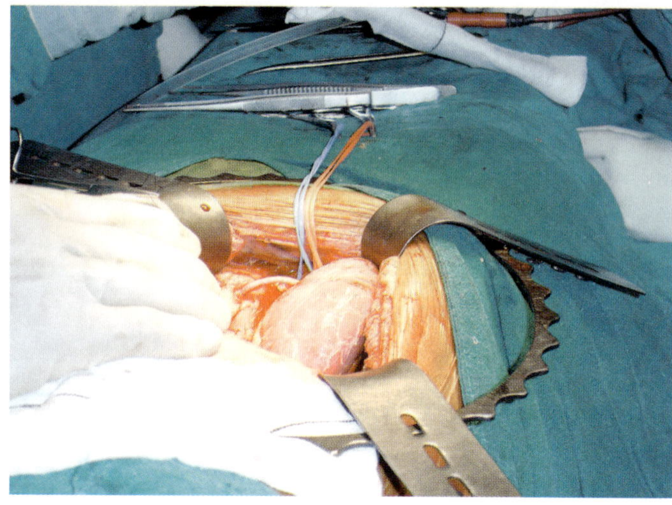

Fig. 7.22: Kidney graft in the recipient after reperfusion

Desflurane does not undergo breakdown either by the liver or by contact with sodalime. Desflurane also has no deleterious effects on routine laboratory tests of renal function when given to patients with chronic renal disease.[29]

Sevoflurane is less stable. 3% of the absorbed dose undergoes hepatic biotransformation. Kharasch et al[30] have shown that increased systemic fluoride concentration causes nephrotoxicity. To predict the occurrence of renal damage neither the peak concentration nor the duration of the fluoride concentration increase alone is sufficient. It is the site of the fluoride production that is important. For sevoflurane, this site is extra renal. In a study by Conzen et al[31] 38 patients with chronically impaired renal function, peak fluoride concentrations were significantly higher after sevoflurane administration compared with enflurane but no permanent deterioration of preexisting renal insufficiency was observed. Sevoflurane is degraded to a vinyl metabolite (compound A) when administered by low flow with a carbondioxide absorber containing either baralyme or to a lesser extent, sodalime. Reductions in anesthetic fresh gas flow and an increase in temperature would result in increased compound A concentration. There is no evidence of nephrotoxicity of this metabolite in humans.[32]

The safety of sevoflurane in patients with renal impairment is unclear.

Desflurane

No renal toxicity has been reported after inhalation of desflurane.[33]

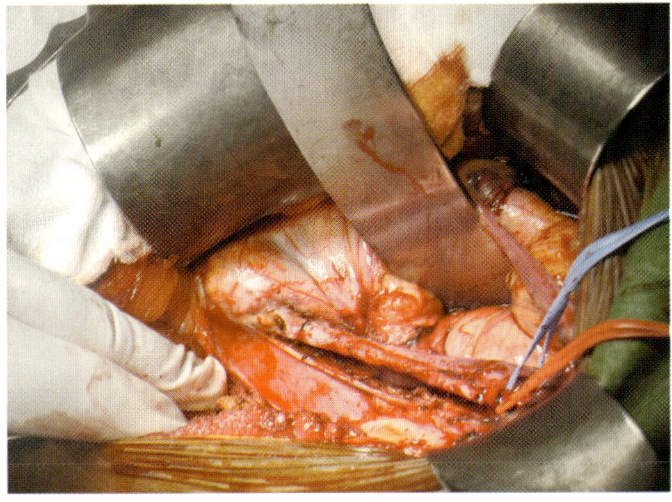

Fig. 7.23: Surgical site showing the anastomosis

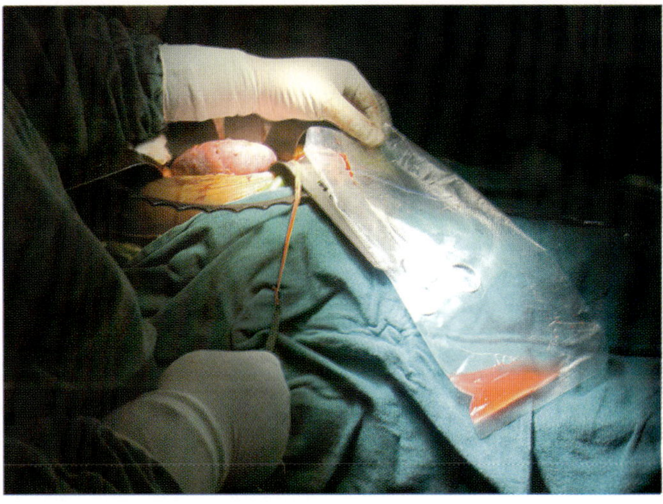

Fig. 7.24: Immediate graft function seen from the cut end of the ureter

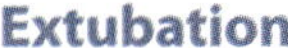

Extubation

Patients with ESRD can experience prolonged effects from intraoperative analgesia and neuromuscular agents but in clinical practice it is not a big issue. Most patients are awake and can be extubated at the end of the procedure provided the transplanted kidney has started functioning. Maintaining fluid balance and adequate perfusion of the transplanted kidney is the main task. Arterial blood gas analysis is important to ascertain the hemodynamic status of the patient and corrective measures should be taken accordingly. Oral hydration can be allowed a couple of hours post transplant.

Postoperative Management (Figs 7.23 and 7.24)

A vast majority of patients will be awake and trachea can be extubated after completion of surgery. After leaving the recovery room they are nursed in a high dependency unit; In our center there is a kidney transplant unit where skilled staff looks after these patients. The aim of a warm, well perfused, patient continues postoperatively. Fluid regimes are variable, depending upon CVP and urine output of the previous hour. In a stable patient, oliguria should trigger a surgical review and urgent doppler imaging of the graft blood supply.

Acidosis is common and is due to impaired renal excretion and an overproduction of acid. Hyperventilation of the mechanically ventilated patient helps to normalize pH but the spontaneously breathing patient is unable to maintain an adequate minute ventilation to restore a normal pH. It is essential to recognize impending respiratory failure early and to intubate and mechanically ventilate the patient before cardiorespiratory collapse ensues. The patient with severe metabolic acidosis at the end of surgery should not be extubated until the metabolic derangements are corrected sufficiently to support spontaneous ventilation.

Sodium bicarbonate should be given intravenously in the mechanically ventilated patient when the pH is below normal as indicated by arterial blood gas analysis, 100% correction can be done. There is catecholamine based vasoconstriction. Sodium bicarbonate restores the effectiveness of exogenous catecholamines and vascular tone. Sodium bicarbonate should be given slowly to avoid overproduction of carbon dioxide since it can easily traverse intracellularly converting to carbonic acid and causing intracellular acidosis (Fig. 7.25).

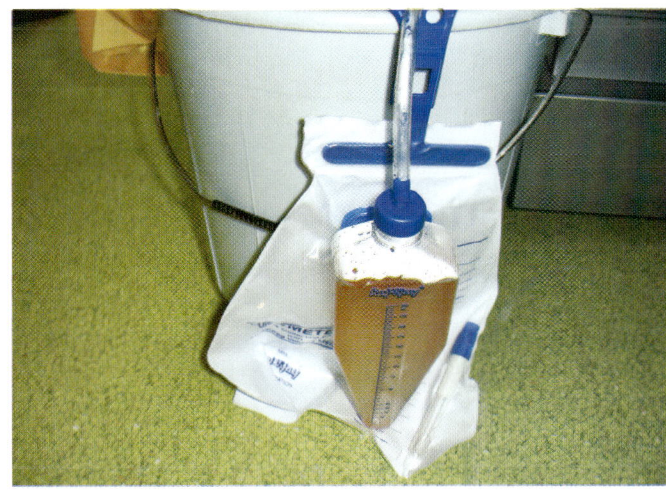

Fig. 7.25: Graft function is assessed by counting the urine drops in the urometer

Postoperative Analgesia

Effective postoperative pain management contributes to successful outcome after renal transplant. Inadequately controlled pain may lead to agitation, tachycardia, hypertension and increased risk of respiratory complications. Intravenous opioids are the mainstay of analgesia. Morphine and fentanyl are both used with equal frequency. There is no evidence to support the use of one opioid over another in patients with renal transplant.[34] A functioning graft contributes to effective analgesia.[35]

Patient controlled analgesia (PCA) can be used in post transplant patient. Analgesia is titrated by the patient according to his pain. The drugs should be carefully selected because accumulation of active metabolites of pethidine and morphine can occur in a patient with nonfunctioning allograft. The patients may suffer from delayed respiratory depression, sedation and convulsions. Patient controlled analgesia may aid in safe titration of dosage to desired effect in the uremic patient. This allows fast onset pain relief and patient is in control of his pain. However it requires intravenous access and the availability of experienced staff. In several centres a background infusion of opioid as part of the PCA is not used.

Nurse administered oral or intramuscular analgesia is frequently employed. Regional blocks like paravertebral block or transversus abdominal plane block also give good results and decrease opioid consumption.

Epidural analgesia with narcotics is superior to parenteral analgesia for postoperative pain relief. It blocks afferent nociceptive stimuli with fewer side effects.[36]

Nonsteroidal anti inflammatory drugs (NSAIDs) can cause reversible kidney damage with reduction of renal blood flow and glomerular filtration rate. They can cause edema, interstitial nephritis and papillary necrosis in the kidneys. These effects are due to action of NSAIDs on prostaglandin synthesis which is integral for renal blood flow and glomerular filtration rate autoregulation. Few NSAIDs are eliminated unchanged via the kidneys however there is evidence of reduced clearance of ketoprofen, fenoprofen and paproxen in renal failure as a result of deconjugation of acylglucuronide metabolites.

These drugs should be avoided in the post transplant patient and in all patients with renal impairment.

POSTOPERATIVE COMPLICATIONS

Delayed graft function (DGF) implies delayed decrease of serum creatinine. In DGF there is a 40% increased risk of acute rejection as well as increased graft loss within three years post procedure. The most common cause of DGF is acute tubular necrosis resulting from ischemic damage to kidney before engraftment or renal hypoperfusion during and after the procedure. Hypoperfusion can be induced by vasoactive agents (cyclosporin, NSAIDs) or unrecognized hypovolemia.[37] Hemodialysis in the immediate period before transplantation is associated with a poorer outcome. The causes implicated are complement activation by the dialysis membrane or intravascular hypovolemia due to haemodialysis.[38]

Opportunist Infections

These patients are on immunosuppressive therapy and opportunist infections post renal transplant can become problematic. The patients can deteriorate rapidly and empirical broad spectrum treatment should be started while awaiting the results of various cultures.

Transplanted kidneys are supplied by single artery with no collateral supply, unlike native kidneys. Immunosuppressive drugs cause nephrotoxicity. Precautions to minimize the effects include hemodynamic stability and prevention of hypovolemia. Treatment with intravenous fluids, inotropes and vasoconstrictors should be guided by invasive monitoring.

If the patient has a functioning peripheral arterio-venous fistula (AVF), placement of an ipsilateral central line can narrow the lumen to a critical level and cause limb or facial edema.

The risk of acute rejection is low one-month post-transplant. Renal transplant recipients have to return to dialysis therapy if acute rejection takes place.

Sleep Disorders

The prevalence of insomnia and restless legs syndrome is reduced in kidney transplant patients compared to dialysis patients, and it is similar to the prevalence observed in the general population. The prevalence of sleep apnea is very high, around 30%. These factors are responsible for the impaired quality of life in the kidney transplant population.[39]

Weight Gain

After transplantation it is considered undesirable by the physicians as it complicates the management of hypertension and hyperlipedimia. Many centers deny transplant to patients who are obese unless they reach a specified body mass index before transplantation, although there are no studies which demonstrate the benefit of this practice.

Regional Anesthesia

Renal transplant can be done under regional anesthesia–spinal, epidural and CSE. Intravenous agents that require renal excretion such as muscle relaxants and opiates can be avoided. The other advantages include avoidance of tracheal intubation in the immunosuppressed patient.

In chronic renal failure, the onset of sensory analgesia occurs faster after subarachnoid blockade because of the combined effects of the metabolic acidosis which causes greater degree of ionization, reduction in the volume of the epidural space secondary to distension of the epidural and spinal veins by a hyperdynamic circulation and shorter duration of sensory and motor blockade (20%) in patients with renal failure because the increased cardiac output in these patients results in a faster washout of the local anesthetic from its site of action.[40]

Disadvantages

- The central venous pressure lines and arterial lines have to be inserted while the patient is awake.
- There is a concern over the possibility of extradural hematoma formation in patients with coagulopathies.
- There is difficulty in handling major blood loss in a vasodilated patient.
- An unpredictable response of a hypertensive renal patient on drug therapies to vasopressors.
- Maintenance of an awake patient's well being during a long procedure.
- Medicolegal implications of a postoperative peripheral neuropathy.
- Postdural puncture headache.[41]

PEDIATRIC RENAL TRANSPLANTATION

Introduction

The major causes of ESRD in the pediatric age group include:

- Glomerulonephritis
- Congenital and hereditary diseases
- Collagen vascular diseases
- Obstructive nephropathy, secondary to posterior urethral valves

Young patients undergo transplantation as the 1st line of treatment as compared to hemodialysis or peritoneal dialysis in the adult population.

Several factors influence the selection of transplantation over dialysis in children:

- Transplantation is associated with a longer survival and improved quality of life[42]
- Transplant improves neurologic development and cognitive performance, especially learning and problem solving skills.[43]
- Children less than 7 years of age have normalization of growth after transplantation, whereas children older than 7 years usually do not.[44]

Risk Factors for Pediatric Kidney Transplants[45]

Recipient age—Poor outcomes are seen in teenagers due to non compliance.

1. Donor type—Living donor kidneys are associated with longer half-lives than deceased donor kidneys.[46]
2. Delayed graft function—is associated with inferior graft survival. It is also associated with acute rejection.
3. Rejection—Acute rejection is not associated with worse long-term outcomes, if it is completely reversed.
4. Recipient race—African, American race is associated with more rejection and worse long-term outcomes.
5. Recurrent disease:
   - Focal segmental glomerulosclerosis (FSGS)
   - Membrano proliferative glomerulonephritis (MPGN) type II
   - Hemolytic uremic syndrome (HUS)

   have the potential to recur in the transplanted kidney.
6. Sensitization: Sensitized patients have inferior outcomes after kidney transplantation.
7. In the population of small recipients of adult sized donor kidneys the renal perfusion pressure is lower in the recipient (50–70 mm Hg MAP) as compared with adults (80–100 mm Hg MAP). Vascular anastomoses to the aorta or proximal common iliac artery and inferior vena cava can optimize the renal perfusion. To avoid kinking of renal vessels the vascular pedicle is shortened to assure a direct route to the aorta and IVC.[47]
8. There is a technical challenge of finding proper placement for the adult size kidney and the anastomosis of the adult size renal artery and renal vein to an infant or small child's aorta and vena cava and demands absolute preciseness.

Contraindications for Kidney Transplantation

1. Active infection
2. Human immunodeficiency virus infection
3. Malignancy.

Isolated mild mental retardation is not per se a contraindication and intellectual catch-up growth can be seen routinely in pediatric patients.

Donor evaluation

It has been dealt with in another chapter. Donor selection in living donation is superior for pediatric recipients as it allows preemptive transplantation and limits waiting time.

Patients receiving living related donor allograft have improved graft survival compared with cadaver graft. For patients with live related donor grafts, the most important factors associated with poor graft survival are

- Recipient age < 2 years
- Black race
- More than five prior blood transfusions
- Failure to provide induction therapy with a monoclonal antibody preparation within 1 day of transplantation
- Delayed graft function (DGF).

In the absence of live related donor, it is best to consider dialysis before cadaver transplantation and to optimize the controllable risk factors, such as donor age, HLA mismatching and cold ischemia time.[46]

Recipient Evaluation

Pediatric patient evaluation is not different from that used in adults. A history, physical with routine comprehensive laboratory studies, chest radiograph and electrocardiogram are done. Urinalysis and urine culture, 24 hour urine collection and renal biopsies are routinely obtained. Urological evaluation is performed in patients with history of reflux due to posterior urethral valves or other congenital anomaly. Psychosocial evaluation is an important part of preoperative assessment.

Effect of ESRD on New Muscle Relaxants, Opioids and Inhaled Anesthetic Agents

Mivacurium

The effect of mivacurium in a dose of 0.15 mg/kg is prolonged with renal disease.[48] This increased duration of action is due to decrease in plasma cholinesterase activity.[49]

Mivacurium is composed of cis-cis, cis trans and trans – trans isomers. The clearance of cis-cis isomer is prolonged in patients with ESRD and chronic renal insufficiency and it may accumulate in patients with renal failure who are receiving prolonged infusions.

Cisatracurium

The pharmacodynamics of an intubating dose of 0.1 mg/kg (2X ED_{95}) of cisatracurium has been studied in both healthy patients and those with chronic renal failure. Renal failure slightly delays the time to 90% twitch depression, but there was no difference in time to maximum block. The time to 75% and 90% recovery of T_1:T_0, the recovery index and the train of four (TOF) to 0.7 were not significantly different.[50] Its half life was slightly prolonged and the clearance was reduced by 13% in patients with renal failure.[51]

Rocuronium

Renal failure patients given a dose of 0.6 mg/kg of rocuronium had prolonged time to 25% recovery of T1 but it was not statistically significant. Prolonged recovery time to 0.7 and greater variability among patients was seen.[52]

Opioids

Patients with renal failure are sensitive to morphine and pethidine because of accumulation of metabolites. The pharmacokinetics of the opioids alfentanil, sufentanil and remifentanil change little in patients with renal failure. Remifentanil is an ultra short acting mu receptor agonist and is unaffected by renal insufficiency. It is metabolized by plasma and tissue esterases, hence end organ failure does not affect its pharmacokinetic profile.[53]

Isoflurane

It is the agent of choice for maintenance of anesthesia in patients with renal insufficiency. It has minimal toxicity and minimal biotransformation and provides patients with hemodynamic stability. The vasodilating properties of isoflurane increase vascular capacitance which allows volume expansion.

Desflurane

It is the least metabolized inhaled anesthetic agent. In studies comparing desflurane with isoflurane in patients with or without renal disease or with sevoflurane in healthy volunteers, desflurane produced no renal injury.[33,54]

Sevoflurane

It is the newest inhaled anesthetic which undergoes biodegradation into inorganic fluoride and degradation by the CO_2 absorbents to a vinyl ether—compound A. Sevoflurane does not produce renal injury in either patients or volunteers.[55]

Anesthetic Management

Preanesthetic evaluation and preparation is similar to as in adults.

Monitoring

Routine monitors include noninvasive SpO_2, $EtCO_2$, BP, ECG, core temperature are used.

Invasive monitors include

1. Intra-arterial monitoring is required for small children undergoing anastomosis of the allograft to the great vessels. Older children, where iliac vessels are used for anastomosis, do not require arterial monitoring. This is to preserve sites for future arteriovenous fistula.
2. CVP monitoring is required for all patients in order to guide volume management and for postoperative vascular access. Triple lumen CVP line is placed in a jugular or subclavian vein.
3. Swan-Ganz monitoring of PA pressure is required in patients with hypertensive cardiomyopathy or other cardiac dysfunctions.
4. Bladder catheterization is done in all patients.
5. Acid base status, electrolytes and hematocrit is monitored every 1–2 hours.

General anesthesia is recommended. Induction of anesthesia with thiopentone sodium, benzodiazepine and opioids is done. Atracurium is the muscle relaxant of choice.

Lumbar epidural catheters may be inserted in lumbar or caudal space before or after induction of anesthesia for perioperative analgesia. Local anesthetic (bupivacaine) ± opiates (fentanyl) are used in the epidural space.

During the time of vascular anastomosis, volume load with crystalloid is given to maintain CVP between 15–20 mm Hg and prevent hypotension. Before unclamping of the vessels (first vein, then artery) mannitol 0.25 mg/kg and furosemide 2 mg/kg is administered. Watch for urine output during ureteral anastomosis or implantation of graft ureter into the bladder. Appropriate fluids are Ringer lactate or normal saline taking care not to aggravate metabolic acidosis.

Adult kidneys in small infants can take up a large percentage of the cardiac output and appropriate volume loading is necessary to ensure good perfusion of the new kidney (systolic blood pressure of 130 mm Hg should be the aim). After unclamping of the vessels there is a large drop in systemic vascular resistance (SVR) and vascular volume. There is potential for blood loss if there is anastomotic leak. Post unclamping renal graft functions are best with high CVP which is evidenced by brisk diuresis. Replace the diuresis volume by volume with crystalloid to prevent dehydration from the mannitol induced osmotic diuresis. Urine volumes are generally large during this phase of surgery requiring very large volume infusions.

Recovery

1. Tracheal extubation is usually done in the older children with blood pressure in the range of donor's normal blood pressure (80–90 mm Hg) and slightly hypervolemic.
2. Patients < 10–15 kg require postoperative mechanical ventilation because
   - Smaller kidney recipients require more intraoperative fluid on a mL/kg basis to diminish the incidence of acute tubular necrosis (ATN)
   - The crystalloid/colloid infusions result in pulmonary edema, which is less well tolerated by infants and children in this weight group.
   - The implantation of a large adult kidney into the abdomen of a small child further diminishes pulmonary compliance and limits diaphragmatic mobility, leading to transient respiratory insufficiency.
   - Efforts to maintain an adult blood pressure will cause further hypervolemia and pulmonary edema for 24–48 hours.

Postoperative Analgesia

- If an epidural catheter is placed it should be used to provide postoperative analgesia. A local anesthetic infusion with 0.0625% bupivacaine + 0.05 mg/mL morphine at an infusion rate (0.3 mL/kg/hr) is used. If the blood pressure is below the target range then use opioid without local anesthetic to eliminate sympathectomy.
- Morphine PCA should be limited to prevent accumulation of the 6-glucuronide metabolite which is poorly cleared with renal insufficiency. Fentanyl can be used alternatively.
- Pethidine should not be used because of poor clearance of norpethidine with renal insufficiency.
- Nonsteroidal anti-inflammatory drugs (NSAIDs), ketorolac should not be used because of the resultant diminished renal blood flow.

Risk Factors and Complications

1. **Graft dysfunction**: Delayed graft function (DGF) is defined as the need for dialysis in the first week after transplantation. It is related to ischemia—reperfusion injury. Deceased donor kidneys with long cold ischemia time are at higher risk for DGF.
2. **Rejection**: This is another important source of graft dysfunction. Rejection is a function of the immune system recognizing the transplanted organ as a foreign body and attempting to destroy it. It can occur early after transplantation and is called acute rejection, or it can occur late after transplantation. Late rejection is called chronic rejection or chronic allograft nephropathy or tubular atrophy/interstitial fibrosis.

3. **Technical complications include:**
   - Arterial thrombosis or stenosis
   - Venous thrombosis
   - Ureteral leak
   - Stenosis or reflux
   - Development of fluid collections like hematoma, seromas, lymphoceles, etc.
   - Post-transplantation adjustment of immunosuppressant therapy and initiation of growth hormone therapy may improve growth but its use is controversial. Growth hormone may have detrimental effect on renal function and the immune system.[56]

While short and medium term outcomes have improved, the 10 year graft survival has not improved. Chronic calcineurin inhibitors (CNI), e.g. cyclosporine, tacrolimus, toxicity has a negative effect on graft and patient survival. Chronic corticosteroids cause growth retardation in children.

CONCLUSION

Kidney transplant under general anesthesia is the preferred therapy for chronic kidney disease patients. Regional anesthesia for kidney transplant is safe, if there is no coagulopathy in the adult patient.

CLINICAL PEARLS

- Patient with renal failure have multisystem dysfunction; hence patients undergoing surgery have increased morbidity and mortality.
- Chronic renal failure leads to chronic anemia due to impaired erythropoiesis. Low hemoglobin is tolerated well by the patient due to compensatory mechanisms; hence blood transfusion is not required to raise hemoglobin unless there is acute blood loss.
- Hemodialysis a day before surgery is important to optimize the fluid and electrolyte status of the patient.
- Intraoperative fluid therapy is important. Rapid rise in CVP causes less tissue edema than continuous infusion.
- In majority of patients trachea can be extubated at the end of procedure. In cases of delayed graft function postoperative ventilation will be required till the time graft function is satisfactory.

REFERENCES

1. Wolfe RA, Ashby VB, Milford EL, Ojo AO, Ettenger RE, Agodoa LY, et al. Comparison of mortality in all patients on dialysis, patients on dialysis awaiting transplantation, and recipients of a first cadaveric transplant. N Engl J Med, 1999;341(23):1725-30.
2. Ostovan MA, Fazelzadeh A, Mehdizadeh AR, Razmkon A, Malek-Hosseini SA. How to decrease cardiovascular mortality in renal transplant recipients. Transplant Proc, 2006;38(9):2887-92.
3. Basta M, Sloan P. Epidural hematoma following epidural catheter placement in a patient with chronic renal failure. Can J Anaesth, 1999;46(3):271-4.
4. Szeifert L, Molnar MZ, Ambrus C, Koczy AB, Kovacs AZ, Vamos EP, et al. Symptoms of depression in kidney transplant recipients: a cross-sectional study. Am J Kindey Dis, 2010;55(1):132-40.
5. Potluri K, Hou S. Obesity in kidney transplant recipients and candidates. Am J Kidney Dis, 2010;56(1):143-56.
6. Szczech LA. Tackling the unknowns in the HIV-related Kidney diseases. The New England Journal of Medicine, 2010;363(21): 2058-59.
7. Frassetto LA, Browne M, Cheng A, Wolfe AR, Roland ME, Stock PG, et al. Immunosuppressant pharmacokinetics and dosing modifications in HIV-1 infected liver and kidney transplant recipients. Am J Transplant, 2007;7(12):2816-20.
8. Rolanda ME, Barinb B, Carlsona L, Frassettoa LA, Terraulta NA, Hirosea R, et al. HIV-Infected Liver and Kidney Transplant Recipients: 1- and 3-Year Outcomes. American Journal of Transplantation, 2008;8(2):355-65.
9. Jankovic Z, Sri-Chandana C. Anaesthesia for renal transplant: Recent developments and recommendations. Current Anaesthesia & Critical Care, 2008;19(4):247-253.
10. Coriat P, Richer C, Douraki T, Gomez C, Hendricks K, Giudicelli JF, et al. Influence of chronic angiotensin-converting enzyme inhibition on anesthetic induction. Anesthesiology, 1994; 81(2):299-307.
11. Howell SJ, Sear JW, Foex P. Hypertension, hypertensive heart disease and perioperative cardiac risk. Br J Anaesth, 2004;92(4): 570-83.
12. Jeroen Aalten, Frederike J Bemelman, Ella M van den Berg-Loonen, Frans H Claas, Maarten H Christiaans, Johan W de Fijter, et al. Pre-kidney-transplant blood transfusions do not improve transplantation outcome: a dutch national study. Nephrology, dialysis, transplantation: official publication of the European Dialysis and Transplant Association-European Renal Association, 2009;24(8):2559-66.
13. Hadimioglu N, Saadawy I, Saglam T, Ertug Z, Dinckan A. The effect of different crystalloid solutions on acid-base balance and early kidney function after kidney transplantation. Anesth Analg, 2008;107(1):264-9.
14. Sprung J, Kapural L, Bourke DL, O'Hara JF Jr. Anesthesia for kidney transplant surgery. Anesthesiol Clin North America, 2000;18(4):919-51.
15. Carlier M, Squifflet JP, Pirson Y, Gribomont B, Alexandre GP. Maximal hydration during anesthesia increases pulmonary arterial pressures and improves early function of human renal transplants. Tranplantation, 1982;34(4):201-4.
16. Othman MM, Ismael AZ, Hammouda GE. The impact of timing of maximal crystalloid hydration on early graft function during kidney transplantation. Anesth Analg, 2010;110(5):1440-46.
17. Vinik HR, Reves JG, Greenblatt DJ, Abernethy DR, Smith LR. The Pharmacokinetics of Midazolam in Chronic Renal Failure Patients. Anesthesiology, 1983;59(5):390-94.
18. Christensen JH, Andreasen F, Jansen J. Pharmacokinetics and pharmacodynamics of thiopental in patients undergoing renal transplantation. Acta Anaesthesiol Scand, 1983;27:513.
19. Goyal P, Puri GD, Pandey CK, et al. Evaluation of induction doses of propofol, comparison between endstage renal disease and normal renal function patients. Anaesth Intensive Care, 2002;30: 584.

20. Sear JW, Hand CW. Fentanyl disposition in anaesthetized patient with renal failure using an iodine- labeled RIA. Br J Anaesth, 2000; 84:285.
21. Hoke FI, Shlugman D, Dershwitz M, et al. Pharamcokinetics and pharmacodynamics of remifentanil in persons with renal failure compared with healthy volunteers. Anesthesiology, 1997;87:533.
22. Hunter JM, Jones RS, Utting JE. Use of atracurium in patients with no renal function. Br J Anaesth, 1982;54:1251.
23. Lynam Dp, cronnelly R, Castagnoli KP, et al. The pharmacodynamics and pharmacokinetics of vecuronium in patients anesthetized with isoflurane with normal renal function or with renal failure. Anesthesiology, 1988;69:227.
24. Sakamoto H, Takita K, Kemmotsu O, et al. Increased sensitivity to vecuronium and prolonged duration of its action in patients with end-stage renal failure. J Clin Anesth, 2001;13:193.
25. Della Rocca G, Pompei L, Coccia C, et al. Atracurium, cisatracurium, vecuronium and rocuronium in patients with renal failure. Minerva Anesthesiol, 2003;67:605.
26. Cronnelly R, Morris RB. Autogonism of neuromuscular blockade. Br J Anaesth, 1982;54:183.
27. Loehning RW, Mazze RI. Possible nephrotoxicity from enflurane in a patient with severe renal disease. Anesthesiology, 1974;40:203.
28. Goldberg ME, Cantillo I, Larijani GE, et al. Sevoflurane versus isoflurane for maintenance of anesthesia: are serum inorganic fluoride ion concentrations of concern? Anesth Analg, 1996;82:1268.
29. Litz RJ, Hublea M, Lorenz W, et al. Renal response to desflurane and isoflurane in patients with renal insufficiency. Anesthesiology, 2002;97:1133.
30. Kharasch E, Hankins DC, Thummel KE. Human kidney methoxyflurane and sevoflurane metabolism: intrarenal fluoride production as a possible mechanism of methoxyflurane toxicity. Anesthesiology, 1995;82:689.
31. Conzen PF, Nuscheler M, Melotte A, Verhaegen M, Leupolt T, Van Aken H, et al. Renal function and serum fluoride concentrations in patients with stable renal insufficiency after anesthesia with sevoflurane or enflurane. Anesth Analg, 1995;81(3):569-75.
32. Mazze RI, Callan CM, Galvez ST, et al. The effect of sevoflurane on serum creatinine and blood urea nitrogen concentration: a retrospective, twenty two centre, comparative evaluation of renal function in adult surgical patients. Anesth Analg, 2000;90:683.
33. Eger EI 2nd, Koblin DD, Bowland T, Ionescu P, Laster MJ, Fang Z, et al. Nephrotoxicity of sevoflurane versus desflurane anesthesia in volunteers. Anesth Analg, 1997;84(1):160-8.
34. Perico N, Cattaneo D, Sayegh MH, Remuzzi G. Delayed graft function in kidney transplantation. Lancet, 2004;364(9447):1814-27.
35. Chas Newstead. Management of the peri-operative and critically ill renal transplant patient. Current Anaesthesia and Critical Care, 2010;21(2):75-77.
36. Molnar MZ, Novak M, Mucsi I. Sleep disorders and quality of life in renal transplant recipients. Int Urol Nephrol, 2009;41(2):373-82.
37. Jankovic Z, Sri-Chandana C. Anaesthesia for renal transplant: Recent developments and recommendations. Current Anaesthesia and Critical Care, 2008;19(4):247-53.
38. Williams M, Milner QJ. Postoperative analgesia following renal transplantation-current practice in the UK. Anaesthesia, 2003;58(7):712-13.
39. Davies MJ. Perioperative epidural anaesthesia and analgesia--an appraisal of its role. Anaesth Intensive Care, 2007;35(4):593-600.
40. Orko R, Pitkanen M, Rosenberg PH. Subarachnoid anaesthesia with 0.75% bupivacaine in patients with chronic renal failure. Br J Anaesth, 1986;58:605-09.
41. Bhosale G, Shah V. Combined spinal-epidural anesthesia for renal transplantation. Transplant Proc, 2008;40(4):1122-4.
42. Almond PS, Morell P, Matas AJ, Gillingham KJ, Chau KS, Brown A, et al. Transplanted children with long-term graft function have an excellent quality of life. Transplant Proc, 1991;23:1380-81.
43. Davis ID, Chang PN, Nevins TE. Successful renal transplantation accelerates development in young uremic children. Pediatrics, 1990;86(4):594-600.
44. Ingelfinger JR, Grupe WE, Harmon WE, Fernbach SK, Levey RH, et al. Growth acceleration following renal transplantation in children less than 7 years of age. Pediatrics, 1981;68(2):255-59.
45. Montenegro LM, Ward A, McGowan FX, Davis PJ. New directions in perioperative management for pediatric solid organ transplantation. J Cardiothorac Vasc Anesth, 1998;12(4):457-72.
46. Shapiro R, Sarwal MM. Pediatric kidney transplantation. Pediatr Clin North Am, 2010;57(2):393-400.
47. Healey PJ, McDonald R, Waldhausen JHT, Sawin R, Tapper D. Transplantation of Adult Living Donor Kidneys Into Infants and Small Children. Arch Surg, 2000;135(9):1035-41.
48. Cook DR, Freeman JA, Lai AA, Kang Y, Stiller RL, Aggarwal S, et al. Pharmacokinetics of mivacurium in normal patients and in those with hepatic or renal failure. Br J Anaesth, 1992;69(6):580-85.
49. Phillips BJ, Hunter JM. Use of mivacurium chloride by constant infusion in the anephric patient. Br J Anaesth, 1992;68(5):492-98.
50. Boyd AH, Eastwood NB, Parker CJ, Hunter JM. Pharmacodynamics of the 1R cis-1'R cis isomer of atracurium (51W89) in health and chronic renal failure. Br J Anaesth, 1995;74(4):400-04.
51. Eastwood NB, Boyd AH, Parker CJ, Hunter JM. Pharmacokinetics of 1R-cis 1'R-cis atracurium besylate (51W89) and plasma laudanosine concentrations in health and chronic renal failure. Br J Anaesth, 1995;75(4):431-35.
52. Cooper RA, Maddineni VR, Mirakhur RK, Wierda JM, Brady M, Fitzpatrick KT. Time course of neuromuscular effects and pharmacokinetics of rocuronium bromide (Org 9426) during isoflurane anaesthesia in patients with and without renal failure. Br J Anaesth, 1993;71(2):222-26.
53. Hoke JF, Muir KT, Glass PSA, Shlugman D, Rosow CE, Dershwitz M, et al. Pharmacokinetics of remifentanil and its metabolite (GR90291) in subjects with renal disease. Clin Pharmacol Ther, 1995;57:148.
54. Zaleski L, Abello D, Gold MI. Desflurane versus isoflurane in patients with chronic hepatic and renal disease. Anesth Analg, 1993;76(2):353-56.
55. Tsukamoto N, Hirabayashi Y, Shimizu R, Mitsuhata H. The effects of sevoflurane and isoflurane anesthesia on renal tubular function in patients with moderately impaired renal function. Anesth Analg, 1996;82(5):909-13.
56. Broyer M, Guest G, Crosnier H, Berard E. Recombinant growth hormone in children after renal transplantation. Lancet, 1994;343(8896):539-40.

Pain Management in Renal Transplantation

Nitin Sethi, Pradeep Jain

INTRODUCTION

Optimizing postoperative pain management is essential after all surgical procedures. Both kidney donors and recipients experience severe pain after surgery. Live donors are healthy individuals who undergo major surgical procedure without having any direct therapeutical benefit. Living kidney donors receive a 10–15 cm flank incision which can cause severe pain because of movement and if pain relief is inadequate atelectasis and lung infection can occur as patients avoid deep breathing and cough.[1] Laparoscopic approach for donor nephrectomy is associated with less pain and earlier discharge from hospital.

Kidney recipients usually receive a 20–25 cm incision from the anterior superior iliac spine to the pubic symphysis. Administration of systemic analgesics is difficult in these patients due to impaired renal function and risk of opioid induced respiratory complications.[2,3]

POSTOPERATIVE PAIN RELIEF AFTER DONOR NEPHRECTOMY

The various modalities of postoperative pain management in living kidney donors are:

1. Thoracic epidural analgesia
2. Intravenous patient controlled analgesia
3. Inter-pleural analgesia
4. Continuous wound infusion of local anesthetic
5. Paravertebral nerve block.

Thoracic Epidural Analgesia

A thoracic epidural injection blocks the noxious afferent stimuli from the surgical incision and also results in bilateral, selective thoracic sympathectomy.

The advantages of thoracic epidural analgesia are:

- Superior perioperative analgesia in comparison to systemic opioids.[4]
- Reduced pulmonary complications such as atelectasis, pulmonary infections and hypoxemia.[5, 6]
- Decrease in duration of postoperative ileus compared to systemic opioid therapy.[7, 8]
- Reduction in postoperative protein catabolism due to a reduction in postoperative nitrogen excretion, amino acid oxidation and decreased muscle protein synthesis.[9]
- Diminished postoperative sympathetic nervous system activity which protects against perioperative myocardial ischemia.[10]

A large proportion of patients given thoracic epidural analgesia after open donor neprectomy were found to be pain free in comparison to those given lumbar epidural analgesia with a significant number of patients given lumbar epidural analgesia having motor blockade. [11]

A combination of epidural opioids and local anesthetics uses lower doses of each agent, gives effective analgesia and reduces the side effects and problems associated with the use of individual drugs.[12]

Bupivacaine is the most widely used local anesthetic for postoperative analgesia, in concentrations of 0.0625% and 0.125%. A dilute solution of bupivacaine result in preferential blockage of sensory fibers with relative sparing of motor fibers however even a dilute solution can lead to some degree of motor and sympathetic blockade. Dilute ropivacaine solution in concentration of 0.1% provides equivalent analgesia as bupivacaine with little impact on motor function.

Fentanyl in concentration ranging from 2.5 μg/mL to 5 μg/mL and morphine in concentration of 0.05 mg/mL are the most commonly used opioids. At our institute patient controlled epidural analgesia with a background infusion of 0.062% bupivacaine and fentanyl 2.5 μg/mL and patient self-administered bolus dose is commonly used for providing postoperative analgesia. This allows patient self-titration and sparing of local anesthetic/opioid consumption.

Background infusion is usually given at 4 to 6 mL/hr, patient controlled bolus dose is 6 to 8 mL with a lockout interval of 20–30 minutes.

Intravenous Patient Controlled Analgesia

Opioids are the commonly used intravenous drugs to provide postoperative pain relief. Patient controlled analgesia (PCA) is the self-administration of the analgesic medication by the patients when they experience pain.

Intravenous PCA devices are microprocessor controlled pumps which are activated by depressing a button. When the patient experiences pain, a preset analgesic medication is delivered by depressing a button and when the pain is reduced no further demands are made thus a negative feedback loop exists.[13-15]

The quality of pain relief with a PCA pump is superior with a decreased opioid consumption and high patient satisfaction. Morphine and fentanyl are the commonly use opioids in intravenous PCA pump.[16] Morphine is used in a concentration of 0.5 mg/mL with a background infusion of 1 mL/hr, patient controlled bolus dose of 2 mL and a lockout interval of 8–10 minutes.

Fentanyl is commonly used in a concentration of 5 µg/mL with a background infusion of 1–2 mL/hr, patient controlled bolus dose of 4–5 mL and a lockout interval of 15–20 minutes.

Inter-Pleural Analgesia

There are mixed results regarding use of inter pleural analgesia, post-nephrectomy. [17,18,19]

In this technique the local anesthetic is injected between the parietal and visceral pleura. The drug reaches the intercostal nerves, splanchnic nerves and the sympathetic chain via retrograde diffusion. For pleural anesthesia the pleural catheter is positioned in the sixth intercostal space in the midaxillary line and 15 to 20 mL boluses of 0.125% to 0.25% bupivacaine are given every 6 hours. The analgesia usually extends from T5 to L1 dermatome.[20,21] Greif et al [21] concluded from their study conducted on patients undergoing elective nephrectomy that intra-pleural analgesia prolongs the time to first dose requirement of postoperative opioid and also significantly reduces the total intravenous opioid dose requirement.

Continuous Wound Infusion of Local Anesthetic

Surgical wound infiltration of local anesthetic is a useful adjunct to multimodal postoperative pain management.[22] Continuous wound infusion of local anesthetic blocks the nociceptive parietal afferent nerve fibers which may reduce the spinal cord dorsal horn neuron sensitization thus providing analgesia over the duration of wound infusion.[23] Wound infusion of local anesthetic not only provides pain relief but also increases the wound perfusion and oxygenation thus enhancing wound healing.[24] Continuous wound infusion is superior to single bolus injections of local anesthetics as it provides long duration of analgesia along with sparing of opioids use. Continuous surgical would infusion after open nephrectomy is provided by multiple holed soaker type catheters which are positioned by the surgeon towards the end of surgery between the transversus abdominis muscle and the internal oblique muscle.[25] Foastiere et al[25] have reported improved pain relief with a reduction in morphine consumption, early bowel recovery and a discharge in patient given continuous wound infusion of 0.5% ropivacaine at 4 m/hr in comparison to placebo.

Paravertebral Nerve Block

Paravertebral nerve block involves the blockade of the mixed spinal nerve as soon as it exits the intervertebral foramen.[26] Unilateral paravertebral nerve block is given for patients undergoing donor nephrectomy which results in minimal hemodynamic side effects in comparison to central neuraxial blockade.[27] Paravertebral block results in more intense blockade of nociceptive sensory fibers than epidural block with a reduction in postoperative opioid requirement.[28] In a pilot study[29], patients undergoing hand assisted laparoscopic donor nephrectomy received preoperative unilateral paravertebral block in T10 to L1 dermatome which resulted in excellent analgesia with significant opioid sparing. Continuous paravertebral nerve block results in superior pain relief than single blocks.[30] For continuous paravertebral nerve block after nephrectomy the catheter is placed in T7 paravertebral space. An initial bolus of 15 mL 0.5% ropivacaine is followed by continuous infusion of 5 to 10 mL/hr 0.2%, ropivacaine.[31]

POSTOPERATIVE PAIN RELIEF AFTER RENAL TRANSPLANT

Patients coming for renal transplant suffer from various comorbidities such as hypertension, coronary artery disease, diabetes mellitus, metabolic and electrolyte disturbances. There is also an alteration in the pharmacokinetics of various drugs including opioids, therefore a careful selection of the analgesic technique is essential.

The various modalities of pain relief in this group of patients are:

1. Intravenous patient controlled analgesia
2. Epidural analgesia
3. Peripheral nerve block.

Intravenous Patient Controlled Analgesia

Intravenous opioid, mainly fentanyl, and morphine has been used for providing postoperative analgesia after renal transplant without any major side-effects.[32] The main concern with use of morphine is that its active metabolite morphine-6-glucuronide is dependent on the kidney for its elimination. However the potent active metabolites may act in a negative feedback loop to limit the use of demand dose by the patient via the PCA pump.[32,33] Patients receiving intravenous opioids need to be closely monitored for any signs of respiratory depression or desaturation.

The PCA regimen for morphine is 0.5 to 1 mg demand dose with a lockout interval of 10 minutes and for fentanyl the demand dose is 15–20 μg with a lockout interval varying from 10 to 15 minutes.

Epidural Analgesia

Epidural analgesia has been reported to be safe and effective in kidney recipients.[34,35] A mixture of epidural local anesthetic plus opioids provide superior analgesia than either of the agents used alone. Theoretical concerns regarding the use of epidural analgesia in renal transplanted patients are presence of coagulation dysfunction predominantly due to platelet dysfunction, cardiovascular instability and resultant hypotension which can compromise graft function.

Peripheral Nerve Block

Peripheral nerve blocks are emerging as an alternative modality for pain relief after renal transplant as it does not involve systemic administration of opioids and can be administered safety even in patients with coagulation dysfunction.

Intercostal nerve blocks of the lower five intercostal nerves has been shown to reduce morphine requirements and improve pain relief in first 4 hours postoperatively but no overall change in the morphine consumption or pain relief in first 24 hours postoperatively.[36] There is also an inherent risk of developing pneumothorax while giving intercostal nerve block.

Shoeibi et al[37] combined an intercostal nerve block along with ilioinguinal nerve block for postoperative pain relief in kidney recepients and found a significant reduction in morphine consumption with improved pain relief in the first 24 hours postoperatively.

Transversus abdominis plane (TAP) block is gaining popularity as a modality for pain relief after abdominal surgery and has been shown to be very effective because of its opioid sparing action and improved patient satisfaction. TAP block involves the blockade of the anterior division of T7 to L1 nerves by depositing the local anesthetic in the plane between the internal oblique and the transversus abdominis muscle. Ultrasound is now commonly used for giving TAP block which improves the accuracy and outcome of the block.[38-41]

Administration of intraoperative TAP block has shown to reduce intraoperative and postoperative morphine requirements in a pilot study conducted on 20 patients undergoing renal transplant.[42] In order to prolong the duration of postoperative analgesia insertion of the catheter in the transversus abdominus plane has been described.[43]

CLINICAL PEARLS

- Adequate postoperative pain relief after donor nephrectomy and renal transplant surgery is vital.
- Several modalities such as central neuraxial and peripheral nerve blocks are available for providing pain relief.
- TAP block has been found to be effective in providing pain relief in kidney recepients.

REFERENCES

1. Ahmadnia H, Molaei M, Golparvar S. Effects of cryoanalgesia on post nephrectomy pain in kidney donors. Saudi J Kidney Dis Transpl, 2010;21:947-8.
2. Baker J, Yost CS, Niemann CU. Organ transplantation. In Miller RD, eds. Miller's Anesthesia. 6th edn. Phladelphia: Elsevier Churchill Livingstone, 2005:2239.
3. Dean M. Opioids in renal failure and dialysis patients. J Pain Symptom Manage, 2004;28:497-504.
4. Block BM, Liu SS, Rowlingson AJ, Cowan AR, Cowan JA Jr, Wu CL, Efficacy of postoperative epidural analgesia: A meta-analysis. JAMA, 2003;290:2455-63.
5. Ballantyne JC, Carr DB, deFerranti S, et al. The comparative effects of postoperative analgesic therapies on pulmonary outcome: cumulative meta-analyses of randomized, controlled trials. Anesth Analg, 1998 Mar;86(3):598-612.
6. Pöpping DM, Elia N, Marret E, Remy C, et al. Protective effects of epidural analgesia on pulmonary complications after abdominal and thoracic surgery: A meta-analysis. Arch Surg, 2008;143:990-9.
7. Liu SS, Wu CL. Effect of postoperative analgesia on major postoperative complications: A systematic update of the evidence. Anesth Analg, 2007;104:689-702.
8. Carli F, Trudel JL, Belliveau P. The effect of intraoperative thoracic epidural anesthesia and postoperative analgesia on bowel function after colorectal surgery: A prospective, randomized trial. Dis Colon Rectum, 2001;44:1083-9.
9. Lattermann R, Wykes L, Eberhart L, Carli F, Meterissian S, Schricker T. A randomized controlled trial of the anticatabolic effect of epidural analgesia and hypocaloric glucose. Reg Anesth Pain Med, 2007;32:227-32.
10. Bakhtiary F, Therapidis P, Dzemali O, et al. Impact of high thoracic epidural anesthesia on incidence of perioperative atrial fibrillation in off-pump coronary bypass grafting: A prospective randomized study. J Thorac Cardiovasc Surg, 2007;134:460-4.
11. Suarez-Sanchez L, Perales-Caldera E, Pelaez-Luna MC, et al. Postoperative outcome of open donor nephrectomy under epidural analgesia: a descriptive analysis. Transplant Proc, 2006;38:877-81.

12. Manion SC, Brennan TJ. Thoracic epidural analgesia and acute pain management. Anesthesiology, 2011;115(1):181-8.
13. Forrest W, Smcthurst PWR, Kienitz ME. Self administration of intravenous analgesics. Anesthesiology, 1970;33:363-65.
14. Sechzer PH. Studies in pain with the analgesic-demand system. Anesth Analg, 1971;50:1-10
15. Keeri-Szanto M. Apparatus for demand analgesia. Can J Anasth, 1971;18:581-82.
16. White PF. Use of patient controlled analgesia for management of acute pain. JAMA, 1988;259:243-47.
17. Murphy DF. Intercostal nerve blockade for fractured ribs and postoperative analgesia: description of a new technique. Reg Anesth, 1983;8:151-3.
18. Baude C, Long D, Chabrol B, et al. Postoperative analgesia for nephrectomy. Cah Anesthesiol, 1991;39:533-6.
19. Kaukinen S, Kaukinen L, Kataja J, et al. Interpleural analgesia for postoperative pain relief in renal surgery patients. Scand J Urol Nephrol, 1994;28:39-43.
20. Kreitzer JM, Reuben SS. Central nervous system toxicity in a patient receiving continuous intrapleural bupivacaine. J Clin Anesth, 1996;8:666-8.
21. Greif R, Wasinger T, Reiter K, et al. Pleural Bupivacaine for Pain Treatment After Nephrectomy. Anesth Analg, 1999;89:440-3.
22. White P. The changing role of non-opioid analgesic techniques in the management of postoperative pain. Anesth Analg, 2005; 101:S5-22.
23. Brennan T, Zahn P, Pogatsky-Zahn E. Mechanisms of incisional pain. Anesthesiol Clin North America, 2005;23:1-20.
24. Hopf HW, Hunt TK, West JM. Wound tissue oxygen tension predicts the risk of wound infection in surgical patients. Arch Surg, 1997;132:997-1005.
25. Forastiere F, Sofra M, Giannarelli D, Fabrizi L, Simone G. Effectiveness of continuous wound infusion of 0.5% ropivacaine by On-Q pain relief system for postoperative pain management after open nephrectomy.Br J Anaesth, 2008;101:841-7.
26. Coveney E, Weltz CR, Greengrass R, et al. Use of paravertebral block anesthesia in the surgical management of breast cancer: Experience in 156 cases. Ann Surg, 1998;227:496-501.
27. Davies RG, Myles PS, Graham JM. A comparison of the analgesic efficacy and side-effects of paravertebral vs epidural blockade for Thoracotomy–a systematic review and meta-analysis of randomized trials. Br J Anaesth, 2006;96:418-26.
28. Kairaluoma PM, Bachmann MS, Rosenberg PH, et al. Preincisional paravertebral block reduces the prevalence of chronic pain after breast surgery. Anesth Analg, 2006;103:703-8.
29. Clendenen SR, Wehle MJ, Rodriguez GA, et al. Paravertebral block provides significant opioid sparing after hand-assisted laparoscopic nephrectomy: An expanded case report of 30 patients. J Endour, 2009;23:1979-83.
30. Catala E, Casas JI, Unzueta MC, Diaz X, Aluaga L, Villar LJ. Continuous infusion is superior to bolus doses with thoracic paravertebral blocks after thoracotomies. J Cardiothoac Vasc Anesth, 1996;10:586-8.
31. Chelly JE, Ghisi D, Fanelli A. Continuous peripheral nerve blocks in acute pain management. Br J Anaesth, 2010;105:i86-i96.
32. Williams M, Milner QJ. Postoperative analgesia following renal transplantation-current practice in the UK. Anaesthesia, 2003 Jul;58(7):712-3.
33. Stein C, Schafer M, Machelska H. Why is morphine not the ultimate analhesic and what can we do to improve it? J Pain, 2000;1:51-6.
34. Solonynko I, Loba M, Orel J, et al. Renal transplantation–choice of anaesthesia. Wiad-Lek, 1997;50:1447-8.
35. Modi MP, Shah VR. Epidural infection of bupivacian with morphine for pain relief after renal transplantation: a comparison with PCA intravenous morphine. J anaesh Clin Pharmacol, 2009;25:277-80.
36. Knowles P, Hancox D, Letheren M, Eddlestone J. An evaluation of iintercostals nerve blockade for analgesia following renal transplantation. EUr J Anesthesiol, 1998;15:457-61.
37. Shoeibi G, Babakhani B, Mohammadi SS. The efficacy of llioinguinal-lliohypogastric and intercostal nerve co-blockade for postoperative pain relief in kidney recipients. Anesth Analg, 2009;108:330-3.
38. McDonnell JG, O'Donnell BD, Curley G, et al. Analgesic efficacy of transversus abdominal surgery: a prospective randomized controlled trial. Anesth Analg, 2007;104:193-7.
39. McDonnell JG, Curley G, Carney J, et al. The analgesic efficacy of transverses abdominis plane block after cesarean delivery: a randomized controlled trial. Anaesth Analg, 2008;106:186-91.
40. El-Dawlatly AA, Turkistani A, Kettner SC, et al. Ultrasound-guided transcerses abdominis plane block: description of a new technique and comparison with conventional systemic analgesia during laparoscopic choolecystectomy. BR. J Anaesth, 2009;102:763-7.
41. Niraj G, Searle A, Mathews M, et al. Analgesic efficacy of ultra-sound-guided transversus abdominis plane block in patients undergoing open appendicectomy. Br J Anaesth, 2009;103:601-5.
42. Mukhtar K, Khattak I. Transversus abdominis plane block for renal transplant recipients. Br J Anaesth, 2010 May;104(5): 663-4.
43. Jankovic ZB, Pollard SG, Nachiappan MM. Continuous transversus abdominis plane block for renal transplant recipients. Anesth Analg, 2009 Nov;109(5):1710-1.

8 CHAPTER Liver Transplantation

Natural History of Liver Disease

Anjali Gera, Shashank Pandey

INTRODUCTION

The liver is the only vital organ in adults that has the capacity to regenerate significantly after it has been injured. In addition to its role in recovery from injury, liver regeneration is also required to maintain day-to-day survival of organ because some liver cells undergo programmed death that is, apoptosis, everyday. Liver size remains constant because dead cells are replaced by proliferation of some of the remaining cells. When liver is injured, the rate of liver cell death increases as liver cells are killed by necrosis or apoptosis. This injury triggers a proliferative response in the surviving cells that allows eventual recovery to normal health. During regeneration, restoration of tissue integrity requires the balanced reconstitution of several liver cells (e.g. hepatocytes, biliary epithelial cells, endothelial cells, stellate cells, lymphocytes, and macrophages) and of the hepatic matrix that is scaffolding for these cells.

But, if the injury is chronic, i.e. not self limited, hepatic fibrosis or scarring develops, which leads to cirrhosis.

HEPATIC FIBROSIS

Fibrosis is a reversible scarring response that occurs in almost all patients with chronic liver injury. Fibrosis ultimately leads to cirrhosis, characterized by nodule formation and organ contraction. The causes of cirrhosis are multiple including congenital, metabolic, inflammatory and toxic liver disease.

It is important to understand the molecular basis of fibrosis because the fibrotic response underlies all the complications of endstage liver disease like portal hypertension, ascitis, encephalopathy, synthetic dysfunction and impaired metabolic capacity.

Thus fibrosis is deleterious both by its direct effects on cellular function and by its mechanical contribution to increased portal resistance.

BIOLOGICAL BASIS OF HEPATIC FIBROSIS

Hepatic fibrosis is a wound healing response in which damaged regions are encapsulated by extracellular matrix or scar. Extracellular matrix refers to the array of macromolecules comprising of scaffolding of normal and fibrotic liver. The components of hepatic extracellular matrix include-collagens, noncollagen glycoprotein, matrix bound growth factors, glycosaminoglycans, proteoglycans, and matricellular proteins.

The matrix composition of fibrotic liver differs both quantitatively and qualitatively from that of normal liver but these changes are similar regardless of the type of liver injury.

Fibrosis occurs earliest in regions where injury is most severe, especially in chronic inflammatory liver disease resulting from alcohol abuse or viral infection, e.g. pericentral injury is hallmark of alcoholic hepatitis and development of pericentral fibrosis (also k/a sclerosing hyaline necrosis or perivenular fibrosis) is an early marker of likely progression to panlobular cirrhosis.[1]

PROGRESSION AND REVERSIBILITY OF FIBROSIS

The rate of progression of fibrosis in an individual patient with CLD cannot be predicted with certainty. The development of fibrosis usually requires at least several months to years of ongoing insult. The only exception to this is venoocclusive disease (also k/a sinusoidal obstruction syndrome) and mechanical biliary obstruction in which, fibrosis progresses more rapidly. Mechanisms underlying these cases of fulminant fibrosis remain obscure but stellate cell activation and up—regulation of fibrogenic cytokines accompany these fibrotic states, as they do in the more common form of fibrosis.[2-4]

In hepatitis C infection, a median time to progression has been estimated to be 30 years, with a range of 18 to 42 years depending on presence of other risk factors.[5] In a cross sectional analysis of 2,235 French patients, independent risk factors for more rapid progression of fibrosis in hepatitis C included-alcohol abuse, older age at the time the infection was acquired and male gender.[5]

The severity of inflammation and injury usually correlates with the rate of progression as documented in studies of alcoholic liver disease and hepatitis C.[5]

Concurrent hepatic insult by more than one agent is synergistic for progression of fibrosis. This finding has been well documented in patient with hepatitis C and alcohol abuse.[5] It also applies to coinfection with hepatitis B, C and δ viruses[6] and to coinfection with hepatitis C and HIV virus.[7]

Iron overload, whether primary or secondary, is a risk factor for the progression of fibrosis. A relatively high iron content correlates with increased inflammation and fibrosis in hepatitis C[8] and exacerbates alcohol induced inflammation.[9] Increased steatosis is also associated with increased fibrosis in patients who have hepatitis C[10] or NASH. Other risk factors for fibrosis in patients with NASH include older age, obesity and presence of DM.[11]

The exact time when fibrosis becomes irreversible is not known. Dense cirrhosis with nodule formation and portal HT is generally considered irreversible. In alcoholic liver disease, significant liver injury and fibrosis can be reversed by abstinence. Remarkable reversibility is also seen in patients with hepatitis B who respond to antiviral compound lamivudine.[12] In patients with hepatitis C who have responded to interferon/ribavirin, short term regression of fibrosis has been observed even in patient in whom virus fails to clear in response to this regimen.[13] In mechanical biliary obstruction caused by chronic pancreatic disease, surgical decompression can also lead to reversal of fibrosis.[14]

The identification of host immune factors contributing to fibrosis could represent an impaired insight into the pathogenesis of fibrosis in humans.

In hepatitis C, predominant Th1 cytokine response has been correlated with relatively more severe liver injury and fibrosis.[15] The observed acceleration of fibrosis in patients with hep C who are co infected with the HIV further implicates the immune system in modulating fibrosis.

PORTAL HYPERTENSION

Portal hypertension is the most common and lethal complication of chronic liver disease. It is responsible for development of gastroesophageal varices, variceal hemorrhage, portal hypertensive gastropathy, ascitis, renal dysfunction, hepatic encephalopathy, arterial hypoxemia, disorders in metabolism of drugs or endogenous substances that are normally eliminated by liver, becteremia and hypersplenism.

Portal hypertension is defined by pathologic increase in portal venous pressure in which pressure gradient between the portal vein and inferior vena cava (portal pressure gradient or PPG) is increased above normal values (1–5 mm Hg). When PPG rises above 10–12 mm Hg complications of portal HT arise. PPG values between 6–10 mm Hg represent sub clinical portal HT.

The portal pressure is most commonly assessed clinically by measuring the hepatic venous pressure gradient (HVPG), which is the difference between the wedged hepatic venous pressure (WHVP) and free hepatic venous pressure (FHVP), at hepatic vein catheterization. The HVPG accurately reflects the portal pressure in both alcoholic and viral cirrhosis.

Portal HT can be caused by any disease interfering with blood flow at any level within the portal venous system. According to anatomic location, the disease causing portal HT is classified as prehepatic (diseases involving the splenic, mesentric or portal veins), intrahepatic (acute and chronic liver disease) or post hepatic (diseases interfering with venous outflow of the liver).

PATHOPHYSIOLOGY OF PORTAL HT

The PPG is the result of interaction between the portal blood flow and the vascular resistance to that flow. This relationship is defined by Ohm's law in the following equation.

$\Delta p = Q \times R$ in which ΔP is the PPG (the difference between the portal pressure and IVC pressure) Q is blood flow within the entire portal venous system (which in portal HT includes the portal systemic collaterals) and R is the vascular resistance of the entire portal venous system. This means portal pressure may be increased by an increase in portal blood flow, an increase in vascular resistance, or a combination of both. It is well estabilished that in cirrhosis the primary factor leading to portal hypertension is an increased resistance to portal blood flow (Flow chart 8.1).

Flow chart 8.1: Schematic representation of the pathophysiology of portal hypertention

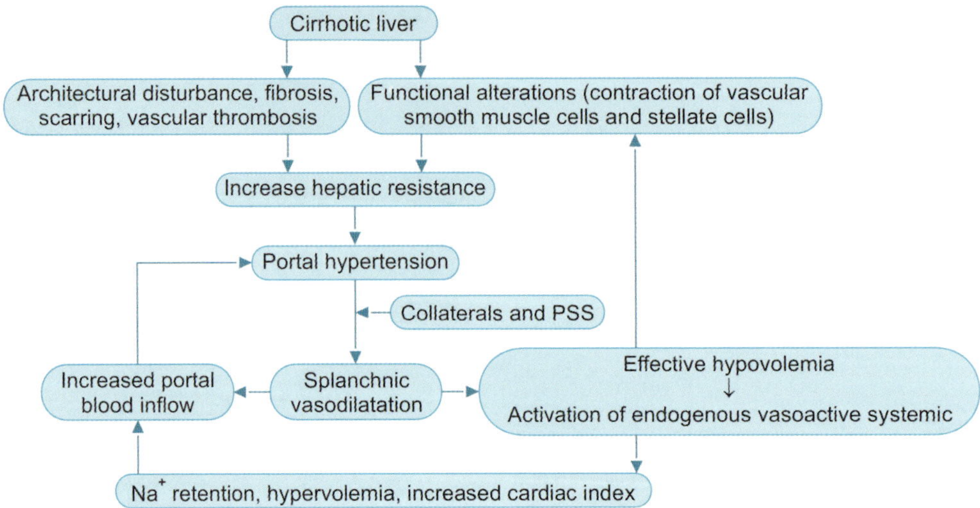

INCREASED VASCULAR RESISTANCE TO PORTAL BLOOD FLOW

In cirrhosis, increased intrahepatic vascular resistance is thought to be located mainly in the hepatic sinusoids. Earlier it was thought that the increased intrahepatic vascular resistance was a mechanical consequence of architectural distortion of hepatic microcirculation, by fibrosis, scarring and nodule formation. But studies have now suggested that thrombosis of medium and large portal and hepatic veins is a frequent occurrence in cirrhosis and that these events may be important in progression of cirrhosis and worsening of portal HT.[16]

In addition to these morphological changes of chronic liver disease, a dynamic component of increased resistance is present that represents active control of contractile elements in the liver. The contractile elements of the hepatic vascular bed are located at a sinusoidal level and at extra sinusoidal sites.[17-19]

They include smooth muscle cells of the intrahepatic vasculature and hepatic myofibroblasts which are abundant in the fibrous tissue in and around cirrhotic nodules. An insufficient release of hepatic vasodilators, an increased production of vasoconstrictors and an exaggerated response of the hepatic vascular bed to endogenous vasoconstrictors are all responsible for the dynamic component of increase intrahepatic resistance in cirrhosis (Table 8.1).

Endothelins are a family of homogenous 21 amino acid vasoactive peptides (ET-1, ET-2, ET-3) that are thought to play a major role in modulating hepatic vascular tone in cirrhosis.[20] Patients with cirrhosis have increased levels of ET-1 and ET-3.[20] Other vasoconstrictive factors that are involved in regulation of hepatic vascular tone are – norepinephrine, angiotensin II and vasopressin. The increased resistance promoted by norepinephrine is completely blunted by administration of alpha- adrenergic antagonists, such as prazosin. Cysteinyl leukotrienes are a group of highly potent vasoactive substances derived from the oxygenation and dehydration by 5-lipoxygenase of arachidonic acid.

Table 8.1: Factors modulating intrahepatic resistance in cirrhosis

Vasoconstrictors	*Vasodilators*
Endothelin	NO
Angiotensin	Carbon monoxide
Norepinephrine	
Vasopressin	
Leukotrienes	

Nitric oxide (NO) is a powerful endogenous vasodilator generated in several tissues by NO synthases from the amino acid, alpha arginine. NO has been identified as the endothelium derived relaxing factor. NO is the natural ligand for soluble guanylate cyclase and is responsible for an increase in cyclic guanosine monophosphate, the final agent responsible for the relaxation of vascular wall through the extrusion of cytosolic Ca^{2+}.

The decrease in NO generation is a major factor contributing to the increase in intrahepatic vascular resistance in cirrhosis. Because of insufficient release of NO which increases hepatic vascular tone and portal pressure, cirrhotic liver cannot accomodate volume overload (unlike normal liver), such as occurs after a meal. In normal conditions the vascular resistance of the liver decreases (through the release of NO) in response to increase in portal blood flow resulting from postprandial hyperemia, but it does not increase in cirrhotic liver so that an abrupt postprandial increase in portal pressure occurs, termed postprandial circulatory dysfunction.

Carbon monoxide, a byproduct of hemo group oxidation by heme oxygenesis is an important modulator of intrahepatic vascular tone. Although less potent than NO, carbon monoxide also activates guanylate cyclase and thereby promotes smooth muscle relaxation.

CONSEQUENCES OF PORTAL HYPERTENSION

Portal hypertension is responsible for many of the manifestations of advanced liver disease. Some of these complications are a direct consequence of portal hypertension, like gastrointestinal bleeding from ruptured gastroesophageal varices, portal hypertension gastropathy and colopathy hyperkinetic syndrome, hypersplenism and an increased availability of drugs and endogenous compounds with rapid hepatic uptake. Other complications in which portal hypertension plays a key role are ascites, abnormalities of renal function, hepatorenal syndrome, spontaneous bacterial peritonitis, hepatic pulmonary syndrome and hepatic encephalopathy.

Collateral Correlation

The most important clinical consequences of portal hypertension are related to formation of portal systemic collaterals. Collaterals develop in areas where anatomic connections exist between portal venous and systemic circulation. These are vascular channels that are functionally closed in normal conditions but become dilated in portal hypertension as a consequence of increased intravascular pressure and blood flow. The grossly dilated portal systemic collaterals characteristic of portal hypertension are not merely passively dilated vessels; a marked hypertrophy and hyperplasia of the collateral walls suggest that angiogenic factors activated in portal hypertension contribute to their formation.

The portal and systemic venous circulation are connected at several locations.[21] Gastroesophageal collaterals develop from connections between the short gastric and coronary veins and the esophageal, azygous and intercostal veins resulting in esophageal and gastric varices. Other collaterals develop as follows–between the superior hemorrhoidal and middle and inferior hemorrhoidal veins giving rise to anorectal varices; between the portal and epigastric veins through the reopening of the umbilical and paraumbilical veins forming a vascular net that is at times apparent on the abdominal wall as caput madusae and causing a murmur over umbilicus (Curveilheir Baumgarten syndrome); between the portal system and posterior abdominal wall through the liver capsule and diaphragm ; between the portal system and the left renal vein forming spontaneous splenorenal shunts. Ectopic varices may develop at other locations in the duodenum (primarily associated with extrahepatic portal hypertension), in colon and small intestine (most frequent in patients who have previously undergone abdominal surgery).

Lymph flow is also increased in portal HT. Enlargement of the hilar lymphatics and lymph nodes have been demonstrated. Increased lymph flow contributes to the formation of ascitis.

Esophageal Varices

When cirrhosis is diagnosed, varices are present in about 40% of compensated patients and in 60% of those who present with ascitis. Esophageal varices do not develop below the threshold HVPG value of 10–12 mm Hg. However not all patient with an HVPG above this threshold have esophageal varices and the relationship between the incidence of varices and an HVPG above this level is poorly understood. The HVPG frequently increases with worsening liver function and continued alcohol abuse and may decrease when liver function improves and alcohol is discontinued.[22] Therefore an increased HVPG is considered the most important risk factor for development of esophageal varices.

Once developed varices increase in size from small to large before they eventually rupture and bleed. Studies show variable rate of progression of varices ranging from 5% to 30% per year.[23] Considering all the studies, the median rate of progression varies from small to large and is about 12% per year during the first 2 years following the endoscopic diagnosis of small varices.

Improvement in liver function and abstinence from alcohol may result in regression or even disappearance of varices.[22] Changes in HVPG (either spontaneous or by drug therapy or TIPS) are usually accompanied by parallel changes in the size of esophageal varies, which are significantly reduced when HVPG decreases below 12 mm Hg or when it decreases more than 15% from the baseline value. An increased size of esophageal varices is associated with poor prognosis in cirrhosis.

The risk of bleeding increases with increase in size of varices. The risk is much lower (between 1% and 2%) in patients without varices at the first examination; it increases to about 5% per year in those with small varices and to 15%

per year in those with medium to large varices at diagnosis.[24] The risk for variceal bleeding is significantly associated with variceal size, the severity of liver dysfunction as expressed by the Child Pugh classification, and red weal marks (vessels newly formed on the variceal wall). The incidence of bleeding is significantly lower in Child Pugh class A patients than in class B or C patients.

Ruptured esophageal varices cause 60% to 70% of all episodes of gastrointestinal bleeding in patients with portal hypertension. Variceal bleeding is diagnosed at emergency endoscopy. Active treatment achieves control of bleeding within 24 hours of admission in nearly 80% of episodes.[25] Active bleeding on endoscopy, bacterial infections[26] and an HVPG above 20 mm Hg are significant prognostic indicators of failure to control bleeding. Immediate mortality from uncontrolled bleeding is in the range of 5% to 8%. Early rebleeding is significantly associated with a risk of death within 6 weeks. Active bleeding at emergency endoscopy, gastric varies, low albumin or high blood urea nitrogen level, and HVPG above 20 mm Hg have been reported as significant indicators of a risk for early re-bleeding.

Gastric Varices

Gastric varices may be found as continuation of esophageal varices along the lesser curve of stomach or in fundus; or rarely isolated gastric varices may be found in the fundus or in the rest of stomach. Gastric varices are commonly fed through the short or posterior gastric veins. They are frequently associated with a lower portal pressure than oesophageal varices and with large gastrosplenorenal shunt. The risk for bleeding in patients with gastric varices is lower than that of patients with esophageal varices, but the incidence of portal-systemic encephalopathy is higher in patients with gastric varices. Gastric varices are the source of 5% to 10% of all the episodes of upper gastrointestinal bleeding in patients with cirrhosis.

Portal Hypertensive Gastropathy

The gastric mucosal changes associated with portal HT are termed portal hypertensive gastropathy. The most frequently observed lesions of PHG are the mosaic pattern and cherry red spots. The mosaic pattern which consists of multiple erythematous areas outlined by a white reticular network is generally considered to be mild PHG. Cherry red spots are round, red lesions that are slightly raised over the surrounding hyperemic mucosa and carry a higher risk of bleeding and are considered to reflect "severe" PHG.

Patients with severe liver dysfunction and large esophageal varices are at higher risk for the development of PHG. The clinical course of PHG is characterized by overt or chronic gastric mucosal bleeding.

The PHG should be distinguished from gastric antral vascular ectasia (GAVE). This is a distinct entity that may be found in association with conditions other than cirrhosis such as scleroderma and chronic gastritis.

RENAL COMPLICATIONS IN CHRONIC LIVER DISEASE

Renal function impairment during the course of cirrhosis leads to inability to maintain the extracellular fluid volume within normal limits. This abnormal regulation of the extracellular fluid volume is a consequence of alterations in the splanchnic and systemic arterial circulation that causes functional renal abnormalities and sodium retention. The predominant abnormality of renal function is sodium retention and its clinical consequence is extracellular fluid accumulation as ascitis or edema. When sodium retention is severe, the ability to eliminate a regular water intake becomes impaired resulting in development of dilutional hyponatremia. As the disease progresses, renal vasoconstriction develops and results in renal hypoperfusion, reduction of GFR and eventually renal failure, the so-called hepato renal syndrome (Table 8.2).

Sodium retention is the first manifestation of renal impairment to develop. Sodium retention is caused by an increase in the renal tubular reabsorption of sodium in the proximal and distal tubules and it occurs in the presence of a normal or only moderately reduced GFR.[27,28] Although numerous mechanisms have been proposed to explain sodium retention in liver disorders, the two main systems responsible for sodium retention are Renin-Angiotensin-Aldosterone System (RAAS) and the Sympathetic Nervous System (SNS). These are activated as a homeostatic response to circulatory dysfunction. The two final products of RAAS system, angiotensin II and aldosterone, induce sodium retention by acting on the proximal tubules and collecting ducts respectively.[29] The SNS system stimulates sodium reabsorption in the proximal tubule, loop of Henle and distal and collecting tubules.[30]

Table 8.2: Functional renal abnormalities

Abnormality	*Clinical consequence*
Na^+ retention	Ascitis and edema
Water retention	Spontaneous delusional hypovabesia
Renal vasoconstriction	Hepatorenal syndrome

The pathogenesis of water retention in cirrhosis is related to 3 factors A) Reduced delivery of filtrate to ascending limb of loop of Henle (the diluting segment of the nephron), B) Reduced renal synthesis of prostaglandins, C) Increased secretion of arginine vasopressin (AVP) and the antiduretic hormone (Flow chart 8.2). The levels of AVP are high in cirrhosis because a non osmotic hypersecretion of AVP from the neurohypophysis occurs in response to a reduced effective intravascular volume, which is secondary to splanchnic vasodilation. The renal synthesis of prostaglandin E2 is increased in patients with cirrhosis to counteract the water retaining effects of AVP; that is why NSAIDs may impair the renal excretion of solute free water in this patients.[31]

The clinical consequence of impaired excretion of solute free water is the development of spontaneous hyponatremia. This type of hyponatremia is called as dilusional hyponatremia because it occurs in the setting of an increase in total body water and dilution of the extracullular fluid volume. Dilutional hyponatremia is associated with sodium retention and an increase in total body water. It should be distinguished from true hyponatremia. True hypovolemia is the sodium depletion that may develop in cirrhotic patients maintained on excessive diuretic treatment and sodium restriction after the complete disappearance of ascitis and edema.

PULMONARY MANIFESTATIONS OF CHRONIC LIVER DISEASE

Cirrhosis and portal hypertension are associated with pulmonary manifestations that affect the pleural space, lung parenchyma and pulmonary circulation (Table 8.3). Lung parenchyma is most commonly affected in primary biliary cirrhosis (PBC). Patients with advanced liver disease may experience the disinct pulmonary vascular problems which are recognized as hepatopulmonary syndrome (HPS) and portopulmonary hypertension (PPH).

Hepatic dysfunction can result in changes in pulmonary physiology that impair arterial oxygenation seriously alter cardiopulmonary hemodynamics. Successful liver transplantation has resulted in resolution of such pulmonary pathohysiologic conditions.

HYPOXEMIA OF LIVER DISEASE

Nonpulmonary causes of hypoxia include a decreased affinity of hemoglobin for oxygen saturation due to erythrocyte factors affected by hepatic dysfunction and the flow of venous blood bypassing the lungs through portal to pulmonary vein connections (extrapulmonary shunts) through perioesophageal and mediastinal vascular communications.

Flow chart 8.2: Pathogenesis of functional renal abnormalities in cirrhosis systemic vasoconstrictors- rennin angiotension system, sympathetic nervous system and arginine vasopressin

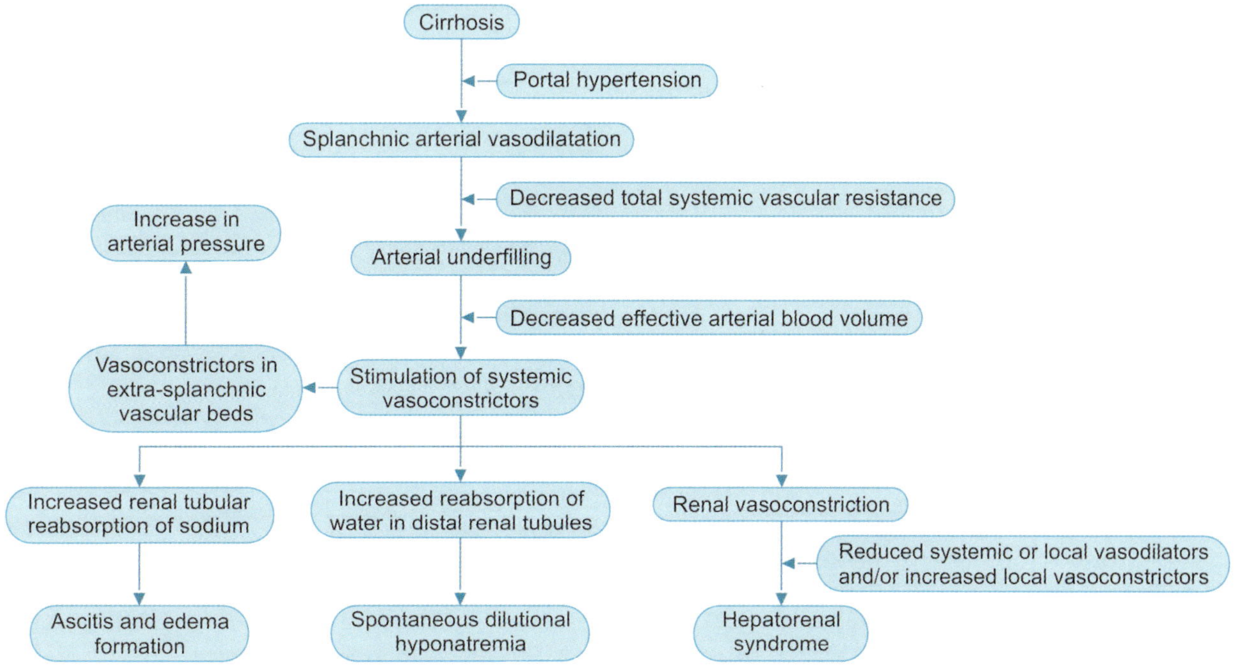

Table 8.3: Pulmonary manifestations of cirrhosis and portal HT

Pleural space
- Hepatic hydrothorax
- Elevated hemi diaphragm due to ascitis or hepatomegaly
- Chylothorax
- Thoracobiliary fistulae

Pulmonary parenchyma
- Interstitial lung disease
- Emphysema due to α1-antitrypsin disease

Pulmonary circulation
- Impaired hepatic vasoconstriction
- Hepatopulmonary syndrome
  - Precapillary/capillary vascular dilatation (type I)
  - Anatomic arteriovenous shunts (type II)
- Pulmonary hypertension
  - Hyperdynamic circulation
  - Volume excess
  - Portopulmonary hypertension
- Portopulmonary (mediastinal) vascular communications.

Pulmonary causes for arterial hypoxemia in patients with cirrhosis and portal hypertension are ventilation perfusion mismatch, diffusion limitation, physiologic and anatomic shunts and diffusion- perfusion defects.[32]

Ventilation perfusion mismatch can occur as a consequence of early small airway closure that occurs because of ascitis raising the hemidiaphragms, compression of the lungs by pleural effusion, dilation of blood vessels and airway inflammation. Diffusing abnormalities result from interstitial processes such as lymphocytic pneumonitis, fibrosing alveolitis (pulmonary fibrosis) diffuse granuloma and organizing pneumonitis. These diffusion limiting lesions are most commonly associated with interstitial lung disorders, such as those associated with PBC or chronic active hepatitis. Excess perfusion relative to ventilation (due to hyperdynamic circulation of liver disease) or reduced perfusion relative to ventilation (due to pulmonary hypertension) can also cause mismatch. Physiologic shunts due to noncardiogenic pulmonary edema have been found in both acute liver failure and deteriorating chronic liver failure. Anatomic shunts and diffusion perfusion abnormalities represent pathologic conditions that characterize HPS. Most cases of hypoxemia found in chronic liver disease are likely to be multifactorial with a predominant mechanism that can be identified.

Patients with severe hypoxemia (PaO_2 less than 50 mm Hg) should be considered to have HPS (arterial hypoxemia due to pulmonary vascular dilatation) until proved otherwise. In patients with severe pulmonary hypertension (mean pulmonary arterial pressure MPAP more than 50 mm Hg) may have minimal oxygenation abnormalities (PaO_2 is usually more than 60 mm Hg). Hypoxemia as a cause of dyspnea in patients with pleural effusion complicating liver disease is uncommon. Symptoms of dyspnea are caused by the mechanical effects of ascitis on hemidiaphragms as well as fluid causing direct compression of the lungs.

CONSEQUENCES OF LIVER DISEASE ON PLEURAL SPACE

The accumulation of fluid in pleural space (pleural effusion) as a consequence of hepatic disorders is known as hepatic hydrothorax.[33] The most common clinical symptom is dyspnea without chest pain. The pleural fluid accumulation associated with cirrhosis usually is right sided (66%), but it can be bilateral (17%) or left sided 17%.[33] Most cases of hepatic hydrothorax are associated with clinically evident ascitis. The peritoneal fluid can pass through small diaphragmatic defects that allow fluid to flow from the peritoneal to the pleural space with the help of a pressure gradient (increased intra abdominal to negative intrathoracic pressure).[32] Pleural fluid accumulation has been reported in patients with cirrhosis without clinical ascitis, perhaps because of the direct negative intrathoracic pressure effect. Hypolbuminemia, decreased colloid pressure and azygous hypertension also lead to formation of hepatic hydrothorax.

Bloody pleural effusions in the setting of liver disease are extremely uncommon and suggest metastasis from hepatocellular carcinoma, infarction following pulmonary emboli, or complications of esophageal sclerotherapy. Fluid of hepatic hydrothorax is usually serous and transudative (low protein) with a pH greater than 7.40, glucose levels similar to serum values, and protein levels slightly higher in pleural as compared to ascitic fluid. Amylase levels are generally low as are cell counts. Chylothorax is an uncommon subtype of hepatic hydrothorax, and contains increased levels of triglycerides. Thoracobiliary fistulae are rare and result in pleuritis, fever, dyspnea and the finding of bilioptysis (bilirubin in sputum).[34]

Therapy for hepatic hydrothorax includes—medical control of ascitis, therapeutic thoracocentesis, chest tube drainage of pleural fluid, pleural peritoneal shunt, pleural-central vein shunt, thoracoscopic repair of diaphragmatic defect and pleurodesis. Transjugular Intrahepatic Porto-systemic Shunting (TIPS) has been used successfully to manage the symptoms of hepatic hydrothorax in the

Table 8.4: Diagnostic criteria for HRS

- Fibrosing alveolitis (pulmonary fibrosis)
- Lymphocytic interstitial pneumonitis
- Non caseating granuloma
- Bronchiolitis obliterans with organizing pneumonitis
- Lymphocytic bronchiolitis
- Pulmonary hemorrhage

Flow chart 8.3: Spectrum of pulmonary vascular abnormalities in advanced liver disease

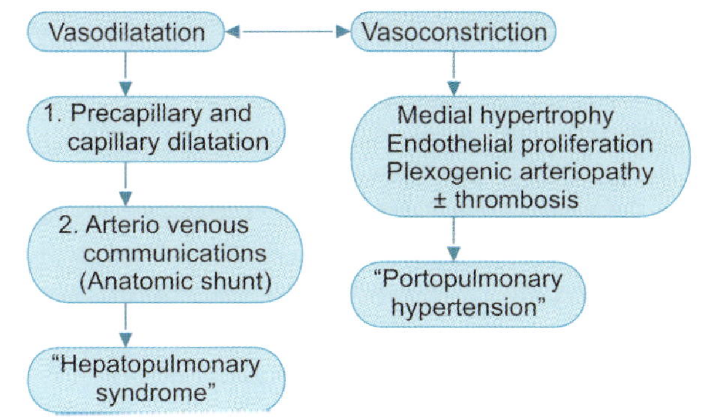

presence of marked ascitis.[35] Definitive management of refractory hepatic hydrothorax in the setting of ascitis is liver transplantation.

PULMONARY ABNORMALITIES

The two most common hepatic disorders associated with clinically important pulmonary parenchymal problems are PBC and α 1 antitrypsin deficiency. The pulmonary manifestations of PBC are summarized (Table 8.4).

Fibrosing alveolitis (also known as idiopathic pulmonary fibrosis) can be progressive and unresponsive to steroids or immunosuppressive therapy. Lymphocytic pneumonitis, noncaseating granuloma, and bronchiolitis obliterans with organizing pneumonitis (BOOP) may be associated with dense infiltrates, air bronchograms and patchy distributions that can be quite steroid responsive. There is no relation between the pathologic stage of PBC and the development of interstitial lung disease.

PULMONARY CIRCULATION

Chronic liver disease results in hyperdynamic circulation. In patients with advanced liver disease nitric oxide in the exhaled air has been detected which may contribute to cirrhosis-induced pulmonary vasodilatation.[36] In addition, pulmonary arterial bed constricts in the setting of hypoxia. Two district and clinically important process may evolve from this baseline hyperdynamic circulatory state, which complicates advanced liver disease (Flow chart 8.3).[37]

The loss of pulmonary vascular tone can evolve into anatomic vascular dilatation at the precapillarycapillary level and direct arteriovenous communications can develop. Significant hypoxemia may result owing to the inability of oxygen molecules to diffuse into the center of the dilated capillary bed or the flow of venous blood that directly bypasses the gas exchange alveolar units. Such vascular dilatation can occur also on the pleural surface. This pathophysiologic condition is called hepatopulmonary syndrome (HPS).

The factors that bypass normal hepatic metabolic pathways in the setting of portal hypertension and portosystemic shunts may interact with the pulmonary endothelium and produce an enhanced and prolonged vasoconstrictive-obliterative response. This progressive process can result in endothelial perforation, medial hypertrophy and if severe and uninterrupted, vascular obliteration with fibrosis, in situ thrombosis and the risk of severe increases in pulmonary arterial pressure. This pathologic condition has been called portopulmonary hypertension (PPH).

These pulmonary vascular abnormalities are clinically distinct. HPS is predominantly a gas exchange problem with severe hypoxemia as the predominant clinical manifestation. PPH is a pulmonary hemodynamic problem (with minimal oxygenation impairment) that can result in right heart failure due to severe pulmonary hypertension.

HEPATOPULMONARY SYNDROME (HPS)

The HPS is characterized clinically by the triad of pulmonary vascular dilatation causing hypoxemia in the setting of advanced liver disease. Hypoxemia is generally considered when PaO_2 is less than 70 mm Hg in patients with advanced liver disease. The severity of liver disease as quantified with the Childs Pugh Score does not appear to be related to the degree of hypoxemia.[38]

PORTOPULMONARY HYPERTENSION

An increase in pulmonary arterial pressure (mean pulmonary pressure more than 25 mm Hg at rest) occurs in as many as 20% of patients with advanced liver disease. Such pressure increases can result from increased pulmonary flow due to A) The hyperdynamic circulation of advanced liver disease; B) Excess volume with or without left ventricular dysfunction, or C) Vasoconstrictive–obliterative processes that characterize

Table 8.5: Pulmonary HT and hemodynamics

Type of pulmonary HT	MPAP	CO	PVR	PCWP
High flow, hyperdynamic circulation	↑	↑↑↑	↓	↓
Volume related	↑	↑	↑	↑
Vasoconstriction, obliteration (PPH)	↑↑↑	↑↓	↑↑↑	↓

the entity described as portopulmonary hypertension. The hemodynamic patterns that may distinguish these processes are shown in Table 8.5.

Other unusual causes of pulmonary hypertension include chronic thromboembolic disease possibly emanating from the inferior vena cava or portal system to pulmonary artery communications, tumor emboli from hepatocellular carcinoma and ova emboli from hepatic schistosomiasis.[39]

Vasoconstrictors such as angiotensin I and thrombaxene B_2 have been implicated in the pathogenesis of PPH.[40]

PORTOPULMONARY ANASTOMOSIS

In the setting of portal hypertension, continuous vascular communications from the portal axis through perioesophageal vessels to the superior vena cava and extra pulmonary veins may have clinical importance.[41] The superior vena cava connection may provide a pathway from thrombi, which form in such a tortous mediastinal venous plexus to be the source of chronic pulmonary thromboembolism and resultant pulmonary hypertension. Communication with the extrapulmonary veins provides a potential anatomic right to left shunt pathway in which venous blood bypasses the exchanges units of the lung with resultant hypoxemia. Pulmonary varices associated with portal hypertension have been described that can resemble a lung neoplasm. Complete resolution can follow successful liver transplantation.[42]

ADULT RESPIRATORY DISTRESS SYNDROME

Acute liver failure complications of cirrhosis and fulminant hepatic failure due to paracetamol poisoning can result in a rapid onset of dyspnea and severe hypoxemia due to the development of acute lung injury characterized by capillary leak.[43] Non cardiogenic pulmonary edema dominates the clinical manifestations, and diffuse alveolar damage is the principal histopathologic feature. In carefully selected patients (those without evidence of systemic infection), liver transplantation may result in resolution of such respiratory failure.

HEPATIC ENCEPHALOPATHY

Hepatic encephalopathy (HE) is defined as a disturbance in central nervous system function due to hepatic insufficiency or portosystemic circulation. The neurologic abnormalities are potentially reversible with correction of the liver disease or the abnormal portosystemic circulation. HE must be differentiated from the concurrence of neurologic symptoms and liver disease secondary to a common pathogenetic mechanism such as brain and liver damage caused by alcohol or copper (Wilson's disease).

The neurologic manifestations of HE are variable. The most distinctive presentation is acute episode of encephalopathy characterized by the sudden onset of an acute confusional state that can evolve into coma. Neuromuscular abnormalities like asterixis and pyramidal signs may be present. The term chronic hepatic encephalopathy is reserved for patients who have frequent episodes of encephalopathy or persistent cognitive (memory loss, confusion, disorientation) or neuromuscular disturbances (tremor, apraxia and in rare instances paraplegia). Minimal hepatic encephalopathy or subclinical hepatic encephalopathy corresponds to neurological manifestations not obvious at clinical examination but found with neuropsychological or neurophysiologic test.

Pathogenesis

Several hypotheses have been proposed to explain the changes in mental state that occur in HE. A common pathogenetic notion is that HE is caused by substances that under normal circumstances are efficiently metabolized by the liver, rather than by insufficient production of substrates that could be essential for neurologic function. Portosystemic shunting plays a crucial role, because the main impact of this circulatory disturbance is on the concentration of gut-derived substances that are cleansed by the liver.[44]

In patients with liver disease, the toxic substances reach the systemic circulation as a result of portosystemic shunting or reduced hepatic clearance and produce deleterious effects on brain function. Once the toxic substances are in neural tissue, a large number of neurochemical changes occur that affect multiple neurochemical pathways.

Hypothesis to explain changes in HE ranged from single unifying theories[45] to the notion of HE as multifactorial process.[46] GABA (γ-aminobutyric acid) theory explains the spectrum of HE through the direct effect of one toxin or a key aspect of neurologic function.[47] An alternative theory arises from the experimental observation that different toxins (fatty acids or mercaptans) enhance the negative effects of ammonia on consciousness (synergistic theory).[48] Current views emphasize the role of several toxins that affect neurologic function at different levels.

TOXINS

Ammonia

Ammonia is generated in different tissues from the breakdown of amino acids and other nitrogenous substances.[49] Under normal physiologic conditions, ammonia enters the portal circulation from the gastrointestinal tract. This ammonia is derived from the colonic bacteria and from deamidation of glutamine in the small intestine. After absorption by means of passive diffusion, ammonia reaches high first pass hepatic extraction (~ 80%). In the liver, ammonia is transformed in the periportal hepatocytes into urea (a high capacity and low affinity system) and in the centrivenular hepatocytes into glutamine (a low capacity and high affinity system). Urea is quantitatively the most important product of ammonia metabolism and elimination. Circulating urea diffuses into the intestine (~ 40%), where it undergoes hydrolysis into ammonia through ureases contained in colonic bacteria. Urinary elimination of urea is a route of ammonia disposal from the organism.

In addition to the intestine and the liver, kidney and muscle contribute to regulate arterial ammonia levels. In muscle, ammonia is transformed into glutamine through the action of glutamine synthetase. The ability of muscle to "fix" appreciable amounts of blood borne ammonia becomes important to regulate arterial ammonia in case of liver failure and highlights the importance of maintenance of adequate muscular mass by patients with HE. It is generally accepted that at rest skeletal muscle is an ammonia-consuming organ. During moderate to heavy exercise, the muscle releases ammonia.[50] The kidneys generate ammonia from the deamination of glutamine, a step involved in the regulation of arterial pH. The fraction of renal ammonia traditionally considered mild is released into the systemic circulation. The main factor resulting in the increase in blood ammonia that occurs in liver failure are a decrease in the capability of the liver to generate urea and glutamine and the bypass of first pass hepatic metabolism.

Patients with HE have increased diffusion of ammonia into the brain.[51] Variations in the passage of ammonia across the blood brain barrier may explain the poor relation between the level of ammonia and the degree of HE.

Glutamine in brain tissue, which is the product of ammonia metabolism and can be estimated with[1] H magnetic resonance spectroscopy, and glutamine in cerebrospinal fluid have a better relation to HE than does blood level of ammonia.[46] Ammonia has many deleterious effects on brain function and affects several neurotransmitter systems (Table 8.6).

Natural Benzodiazepines

Natural benzodiazepines are substances of non pharmacological origin which bind to GABA receptors. $GABA_A$ is a ligand-gated ion channel. The channel is surrounded by five peptide subunits (α,β,γ) that have four membrane spanning domains (M1, M2, M3, M4). The benzodiazepines binding domain is located in the M1 segment of α subunit. It has been proposed that natural benzodiazepines with agonist effects on GABA receptor induce a decrease of consciousness in HE. An alternative mechanism of action may be binding to peripheral type benzodiazepine receptors (PTBRs) which are present in mitochondria and activation of which results in the synthesis within astrocytes of neurosteroids, powerful inhibitors of neuronal GABA receptors.[52]

There are several theories in favor of a role for natural benzodiazepines in HE. The most relevant is the clinical observation of an improvement in mental state after the administration of flumazenil (a benzodiazepine receptor antagonist) in some patients with advanced stages of HE.[53] However the beneficial effects of flumazenil is mild and

Table 8.6: Effects of ammonia on nervous tissue

Effects	*Possible consequences*
Blocking of chloride channel	Impairment of postsynaptic inhibition
Increase in transport of neutral aminoacids and cerebral tryptophan	Interaction with serotonin related neurotransmitters
Enhancement of the synthesis of neurosteroids	Agonist effect on GABA neurotransmission
Modulation of GABA receptor	Agonist effect on GABA neurotransmission
Upregulation of benzodiazepine receptors	Agonist effect on GABA neurotransmission
Increase in brain glutamine	Brain edema
Increase in nitric oxide synthesis	Interaction with glutamatergic neurotransmission

transient and is seen in a subgroup of patients (~ 30%). A major limitation of this theory is lack of explanation of the mechanism by which levels of natural benzodiazepines increase in HE. An animal study showed generation in the intestinal flora of precursors of natural benzodiazepine.[54] These precursors would be transformed into natural benzodiazepines in the brain and accumulate secondary to liver failure.

Manganese

Manganese is involved in the development of parkinsonian manifestations of HE.[55] The concentration of manganese is elevated in the plasma of patients with cirrhosis and in the brain of patients who die with HE. Hypermagnesemia is the result of portosystemic shunting and a reduction in biliary excretion. Patients with cirrhosis typically have a hyperintense signal in the globus pallidum that has been attributed to the preferential accumulation of manganese in basal ganglia.[56]

OTHER COMPOUNDS

A group of potentially neurotoxic compounds of colonic origin include GABA, mercaptans and short-chain fatty acids.

CHANGES IN CENTRAL NERVOUS SYSTEM IN HE

Astrocytes

Astrocytes occupy one third of the volume of the cerebral cortex. Their foot processes surround brain capillaries, where they contribute to blood brain barrier function and neurons. This anatomic organization forms a syncitium, where critical metabolic supportive functions involved in the maintenance and regulation of the extracellular microenvironment, such as uptake of ions and neurotransmitters, influence neuronal excitability and neurotransmission. A specific astrocyte function is detoxification of ammonia through the amidation of glutamate to glutamine. Astrocyte swelling in HE arises from an increase in intracellular osmolality as a result of glutamine accumulation.[57] These findings have led to the proposal that HE is the clinical manifestation of a gliopathy,[58] in which neuronal dysfunction develops as a result of astrocytic abnormalities. The mechanisms by which abnormal glial cells influence neuronal function have been postulated as below.

a. Interaction with glutamate reuptake.[59] In experimental models, glial reuptake of glutamate released from presynaptic neurons is likely to be decreased. A decrease in reuptake will result in brain extra cellular glutamate with subsequent effects on glutamatergic neurotransmission.
b. Activation of PTBRs.[52] In increase in the number of PTBRs has been observed in the brain of patients who died with HE. Activation of PTBRs by different ligands, such as ammonia and diazepam binding inhibitor, results in an increase in the synthesis of neurosteoids (pregnenolone. dehydroepiandrosterone), ligands of the neuronal $GABA_A$ receptor thus affecting GABA-ergic neurotransmission.
c. Metabolic consequences of cellular swelling.[60] The cellular hydration state regulates cell function and gene expression. Swelling of astrocytes activates extracellular regulated protein kinases, elevates calcium concentration, and affects multiple ion channels and neurotransmitters, secondarily affecting glial- neuronal communication.

NEUROTRANSMITTER SYSTEMS

As with other forms of metabolic encephalopathy HE appears to occur as a result of abnormalities in neurotransmission. This hypothesis is supported by evidence of potential reversibility and by the lack of neuronal damage.

Brain Energy Abnormalities

The brain is the tissue with highest energy requirements of the body and depends entirely on the process of glycolysis and respiration within its own cells to synthesize its energy demands. In HE, a decrease in consumption of oxygen and glucose is accompanied by a parallel decrease in cerebral blood flow.[61] The decrease in energy consumption is secondary to the decrease in demand, as in other metabolic encephalopathies. Ammonia may impair glucolysis as it inhibits α-ketoglutarate dehydrogenase, the rate limiting enzyme of the tricarboxylic acid cycle.[46]

Brain Edema

Brain edema is a complication of fulminant hepatic failure and can progress to intracranial hypertension and death. Brain edema appears to originate from the accumulation of glutamine, the product of ammonia metabolism in astrocytes.[57] The osmotic effects of an acute increase in glutamine appear to overcome the compensatory capability of astrocytes, cells that are swollen in neuropathologic preparations. Other factors such as hyponatremia can enhance the effects of ammonia on brain swelling.[62]

In fulminant hepatic failure an additional factor that plays an important role in the development of intracranial hypertension is the presence of abnormalities of cerebral

Table 8.7: Precipitating factors for hepatic encephalopathy

Precipitating factor	*Possible effects*	*Mechanism of action*
Sepsis	▪ Increase in blood ammonia level ▪ Enhancement of the effects of putative toxins on CNS	Protein calabolism Activation of cytokins
GI bleeding	▪ Impairment in liver function ▪ Increase in blood ammonia level	Hepatic hypoperfusion Nitrogen load
Hypokalemia	Increase in blood ammonia level	Ammonia generation
Azolemia	Increase in blood ammonia level	Ammonia generation
Dehydration	Increase in blood ammonia level	Ammonia generation
Diuretics	Increase in blood ammonia level	Hypokalemia azotemia dehydration
Acute hepatitis	Impairment in liver function enhancement of effects on CNS	Liver injury activation of cytokines
Surgery	Impairment in liver function	Hepatic hypoperfusion
Constipation	Increase in blood ammonia level	Ammonia generation by intestinal flora
Large protein intake	Increase in blood ammonia level	Nitrogen load
Psychoactive drugs	Enhancement of effects on the CNS	Activation of inhibitory neurotransmission

circulation. Cerebral vasodilatation and antoregulation are characteristic findings in fulminant hepatic failure.[63]

Precipitating Factors for HE

Several factors are known to precipitate an episode of HE in patients with cirrhosis who are in stable condition (Table 8.7).

CLINICAL PEARLS

- Hepatic fibrosis is a reversible scarring process that underlies all the complications of end-stage liver disease.
- Portal hypertension is responsible for lethal consequences of advanced liver disease like formation of collaterals, variceal bleeding, gastropathy, hypersplenism, colopathy hyperkinetic syndrome.
- Cirrhosis and portal hypertension are associated with pulmonary manifestations that affect pleural space, lung parenchyma and pulmonary circulation.
- The neurological abnormalities in chronic liver disease are potentially reversible with correction of liver disease or the abnormal portosystemic circulation.

REFERENCES

1. Van Waes L, Lieber CS. Early perivenular sclerosis in alcoholic fatty liver: an index of progressive liver injury. Gastroenterology, 1977;73:646-50.
2. El-Youssef M, Mu Y, Huang L, et al. Increased expression of transforming growth factor-beta1 and thrombospondin-1 in congenital hepatic fibrosis: possible role of the hepatic stellate cell. J Pediatr Gastroenterol Nutr, 1999;28:386-92.
3. Sato Y, Asada Y, Hara S, et al. Hepatic stellate cells (Ito cells) in veno-occlusive disease of the liver alter allogeneic bone marrow transplantation. Histopathology, 1999;34:66-70.
4. DeLeve LD. Glutathione defense in non-parenchymal cells. Semin Liver Dis, 1998;18:403-13.
5. Poynard T, Bedossa P, Opolon P. Natural history of liver fibrosis progression in patients with chronic hepatitis C. Lancet, 1997;349:825-32.
6. Weltman MD, Brotodihardjo A, Crewe EB, et al. Coinfection with hepatitis B and C or B, C and delta viruses results in severe chronic liver disease and responds poorly to interferon-alpha treatment. J Viral Hepat, 1995;2:39-45.
7. Benhamou Y, Di Martino V, Bochet M, et al. Factors affecting liver fibrosis in human immunodeficiency virus-and hepatitis C virus-coinfected patients: impact of protease inhibitor therapy. Hepatology, 2001;34:283-7.
8. Beinker NK, Voigt MD, Arendse M, et al. Threshold effect of liver iron content on hepatic inflammation and fibrosis in hepatitis B and C. J Hepatol, 1996;25:633-8.
9. Tsukamoto H, Horne W, Kamimura S, et al. Experimental liver cirrhosis induced by alcohol and iron. J Clin Invest, 1995;96:620-30.
10. Wong VS, Wight DG, Palmer CR, Alexander GJ. Fibrosis and other histological features in chronic hepatitis C virus infection: a statistical model. J Clin Pathol, 1996;49:465-9.
11. Angulo P, Keach JC, Batts KP, Lindor KD. Independent predictors of liver fibrosis in patients with nonalcoholic steatohepatitis. Hepatology, 1999;30:1356-62.
12. Wanless IR, Nakashima E, Sherman M. Regression of human cirrhosis. Morphologic features and the genesis of incomplete septal cirrhosis. Arch Pathol Lab Med, 2000;124:1599-607.
13. Shiratori Y, Imazeki F, Moriyama M, et al. Histologic improvement of fibrosis in patients with hepatitis C who have sustained response to interferon therapy. Ann Intern Med, 2000;132:517-24.
14. Hammel P, Couvelard A, O'Toole D, et al. Regression of liver fibrosis after biliary drainage in patients with chronic pancreatitis and stenosis of the common bile duct. N Engl J Med, 2001;344:418-23.

15. Napoli J, Bishop GA, McGuinness PH, et al. Progressive liver injury in chronic hepatitis C infection correlates with increased intrahepatic expression of Th1-associated cytokines. Hepatology, 1996;24:759-65.
16. Wanless IR, Wong F, Blendis LM, et al. Hepatic and portal vein thrombosis in cirrhosis: possible role in development of parenchymal extinction and portal hypertension. Hepatology, 1995;21:1238-47.
17. Kaneda K, Ekataksin W, Sogawa M, et al. Endothelin-1-induced vasoconstriction causes a significant increase in portal pressure of rat liver: localized constrictive effect on the distal segment of preterminal portal venules as revealed by light and electron microscopy and serial reconstruction. Hepatology, 1998;27: 735-47.
18. Zhang JX, Pegoli W Jr, Clemens MG. Endothelin-1 induces direct constriction of hepatic sinusoids. Am J Physiol, 1994;266:G624-32.
19. Kawada N, Tran-Thi TA, Klein H, Decker K. The contraction of hepatic stellate (Ito) cells stimulated with vasoactive substances. Possible involvement of endothelin 1 and nitric oxide in the regulation of the sinusoidal tonus. Eur J Biochem, 1993;213:815-23.
20. Møller S, Gülberg V, Henriksen JH, Gerbes AL. Endothelin-1 and endothelin-3 in cirrhosis: relations to systemic and splanchnic haemodynamics. J Hepatol, 1995;23:135-44.
21. Bosch J, Navasa M, Garcia-Pagán JC, et al. Portal hypertension. Med Clin North Am, 1989;73:931-53.
22. Vorobioff J, Groszmann RJ, Picabea E, et al. Prognostic value of hepatic venous pressure gradient measurements in alcoholic cirrhosis: a 10-year prospective study. Gastroenterology, 1996; 111:701-9.
23. D'Amico G, Garcia-Tsao G, Cales P, et al. Diagnosis of portal hypertension. How and when? In: DeFranchis ed Portal Hypertension III. Proceedings of the third Bareno International consensus workshop on definitions methodology and therapeutic strategies. Oxford: Blackwell Science, 2001:36-63.
24. D'Amico G PL. The clinical course of portal hypertension in liver cirrhosis. In: Rossi P ed. Diagnostic imaging and imaging-guided therapy. Berlin: Soringer Verlag, 2000:15-24.
25. Ben-Ari Z, Cardin F, McCormick AP, et al. A predictive model for failure to control bleeding during acute variceal haemorrhage. J Hepatol, 1999;31:443-50.
26. Goulis J, Armonis A, Patch D, et al. Bacterial infection is independently associated with failure to control bleeding in cirrhotic patients with gastrointestinal hemorrhage. Hepatology, 1998;27:1207-12.
27. Chaimovitz C, Szylman P, Alroy G, Better OS. Mechanism of increased renal tubular sodium reabsorption in cirrhosis. Am J Med, 1972;52:198-202.
28. Angeli P, Gatta A, Caregaro L, et al. Tubular site of renal sodium retention in ascitic liver cirrhosis evaluated by lithium clearance. Eur J Clin Invest, 1990;20:111-7.
29. Bernadi M, Trevisani F, Caraceni P. The renin-angiotensin-aldosterone system in cirrhosis. Malden, MA: Blackwell Science, 1999:175-197.
30. DiBona GF. Neural control of the kidney: functionally specific renal sympathetic nerve fibers. Am J Physiol Regul Integr Comp Physiol, 2000;279:R1517-24.
31. Pérez-Ayuso RM, Arroyo V, Camps J, et al. Evidence that renal prostaglandins are involved in renal water metabolism in cirrhosis. Kidney Int, 1984;26:72-80.
32. Krowka MJ, Cortese DA. Pulmonary aspects of liver disease and liver transplantation. Clin Chest Med, 1989;10:593-616.
33. Alberts WM, Salem AJ, Solomon DA, Boyce G. Hepatic hydrothorax. Cause and management. Arch Intern Med, 1991; 151:2383-8.
34. Johnson MM, Chin R Jr, Haponik EF. Thoracobiliary fistula. South Med J, 1996;89(3):335-9.
35. Strauss RM, Martin LG, Kaufman SL, Boyer TD. Transjugular intrahepatic portal systemic shunt for the management of symptomatic cirrhotic hydrothorax. Am J Gastroenterol, 1994;89:1520-2.
36. Sogni P, Garnier P, Gadano A, et al. Endogenous pulmonary nitric oxide production measured from exhaled air is increased in patients with severe cirrhosis. J Hepatol, 1995;23:471-3.
37. Agustí AG, Rodriguez-Roisin R. Effect of pulmonary hypertension on gas exchange. Eur Respir J, 1993;6:1371-7.
38. Krowka MJ, Wiseman GA, Burnett OL, et al. Hepatopulmonary syndrome: a prospective study of relationships between severity of liver disease, PaO(2) response to 100% oxygen, and brain uptake after (99m)Tc MAA lung scanning. Chest, 2000;118: 615-24.
39. Crawford AB, Regnis J, Laks L, et al. Pulmonary vascular dilatation and diffusion-dependent impairment of gas exchange in liver cirrhosis. Eur Respir J, 1995;8:2015-21.
40. Tokiwa K, Iwai N, Nakamura K, et al. Pulmonary hypertension as a fatal complication of extrahepatic portal hypertension. Eur J Pediatr Surg, 1993;3:373-5.
41. Mantz FA Jr, Craige E. Portal axis thrombosis with spontaneous portacaval shunt and resultant cor pulmonale. AMA Arch Pathol, 1951;52:91-7.
42. Man KM, Keeffe EB, Brown CR, et al. Pulmonary varices presenting as a solitary lung mass in a patient with end-stage liver disease. Chest, 1994;106:294-6.
43. Matuschak GM, Rinaldo JE, Pinsky MR, et al. Effect of end-stage liver failure on the incidence and resolution of the adult respiratory distress syndrome. J Crit Care, 1987;2:162-173.
44. Conn HO. Portal-systemic shunting and portal-systemic encephalopathy: a predictable relationship. Hepatology, 1995;22: 365-7.
45. Fischer JE, Baldessarini RJ. False neurotransmitters and hepatic failure. Lancet, 1971;2:75-80.
46. Butterworth RF. The neurobiology of hepatic encephalopathy. Semin Liver Dis, 1996;16:235-44.
47. Schafer DF, Jones EA. Hepatic encephalopathy and the gamma-aminobutyric-acid neurotransmitter system. Lancet, 1982;1:18-20.
48. Zieve L, Doizaki WM, Zieve J. Synergism between mercaptans and ammonia or fatty acids in the production of coma: a possible role for mercaptans in the pathogenesis of hepatic coma. J Lab Clin Med, 1974;83:16-28.
49. Cooper AJ, Plum F. Biochemistry and physiology of brain ammonia. Physiol Rev, 1987;67:440-519.
50. Dietrich R, Bachmann C, Lauterburg BH. Exercise-induced hyperammonemia in patients with compensated chronic liver disease. Scand J Gastroenterol, 1990;25:329-34.
51. Lockwood AH, Yap EW, Wong WH. Cerebral ammonia metabolism in patients with severe liver disease and minimal hepatic encephalopathy. J Cereb Blood Flow Metab, 1991;11:337-41.
52. Norenberg MD. Astrocytic-ammonia interactions in hepatic encephalopathy. Semin Liver Dis, 1996;16:245-53.
53. Barbaro G, Di Lorenzo G, Soldini M, et al. Flumazenil for hepatic encephalopathy grade III and IVa in patients with cirrhosis: an Italian multicenter double-blind, placebo-controlled, cross-over study. Hepatology, 1998;28:374-8.

54. Yurdaydin C, Walsh TJ, Engler HD, et al. Gut bacteria provide precursors of benzodiazepine receptor ligands in a rat model of hepatic encephalopathy. Brain Res, 1995;679:42-8.
55. Krieger S, Jauss M, Jansen O, et al. Neuropsychiatric profile and hyperintense globus pallidus on T1-weighted magnetic resonance images in liver cirrhosis. Gastroenterology, 1996;111:147-55.
56. Butterworth RF, Spahr L, Fontaine S, Layrargues GP. Manganese toxicity, dopaminergic dysfunction and hepatic encephalopathy. Metab Brain Dis, 1995;10:259-67.
57. Cordoba J, Blei AT. Brain edema and hepatic encephalopathy. Semin Liver Dis, 1996;16:271-80.
58. Norenberg MD. The role of astrocytes in hepatic encephalopathy. Neurochem Pathol, 1987;6:13-33.
59. Butterworth RF. Hepatic encephalopathy and brain edema in acute hepatic failure: does glutamate play a role? Hepatology, 1997; 25:1032-4.
60. Häussinger D, Kircheis G, Fischer R, et al. Hepatic encephalopathy in chronic liver disease: a clinical manifestation of strocyte swelling and low-grade cerebral edema? J Hepatol, 2000;32:1035-8.
61. Lockwood AH, Yap EW, Rhoades HM, Wong WH. Altered cerebral blood flow and glucose metabolism in patients with liver disease and minimal encephalopathy. J Cereb Blood Flow Metab, 1991;11:331-6.
62. Córdoba J, Gottstein J, Blei AT. Chronic hyponatremia exacerbates ammonia-induced brain edema in rats after portacaval anastomosis. J Hepatol, 1998;29:589-94.
63. Larsen FS. Cerebral circulation in liver failure: Ohm's law in force. Semin Liver Dis, 1996;16:281-92.

Acute Liver Failure

Bhuwan Chand Panday, Shashank Pandey

INTRODUCTION

Acute liver failure (ALF) is a rapidly progressive liver disease with severe liver dysfunction.[1,2] It is suspected when the onset of jaundice progresses to encephalopathy with coagulation disorder in a short period of time. The term acute liver failure has been further divided into three subcategories, according to the development of encephalopathy from the first evidence of jaundice; hyperacute (within 7 days of jaundice), acute (8–28 days of jaundice), subacute (28 days -14 weeks of jaundice).[3] There are many complications of ALF which involve almost all the systems of the body along with the abnormal coagulation cascade, CNS involvement being the most important. In the central nervous system, cerebral edema and increased intracranial pressure (ICP) is due to high ammonia levels, which can lead to hepatic encephalopathy, coma and death. Though the overall incidence of ALF is low, the mortality rate is high. ALF occurs worldwide however predominant causes may vary according to the geographical region, e.g. western world has the predominance of drug induced liver injury while viral infection induced hepatocyte injury is common in developing countries.[1] Management of ALF requires well equipped centre along with trained staff. Advancement in liver transplant and intensive care management has increased the survival rate significantly.[4] Liver transplant has very encouraging results; however the cost involved becomes a limiting factor. Prior to liver transplant the mortality rate of ALF patients was aproximately 80%.[2] Early diagnosis, regular monitoring, optimal management and prevention of further deterioration may have a better outcome.

Pathophysiology

The main cause of morbidity and mortality in ALF is alteration of central nervous system (cerebral edema, encephalopathy). ALF occurs when there is rapid death of enormous number of hepatocytes, and this number exceeds the regeneration. It can lead to multiorgan failure, coma and death. The pathophysiology of ALF is still not fully understood but most of the studies have reported hyperammonemia to be the main cause of CNS dysfunction. Hyperammonemia leads to increased glutamine synthesis. Increased glutamine level causes the astrocytes swelling and later cerebral edema, which in turn leads to intracranial hypertension. This can worsen to encephalopathy, coma and eventually lead to death. Piyush R, et al. in their study used conventional and diffusion-weighted magnetic resonance imaging on fulminant hepatic failure patients and concluded that the nature of cerebral edema is predominantly cytotoxic. This cytotoxic edema is mainly due to increased ammonia concentration.[5] Altered cerebral metabolism on one hand alters the blood brain barrier and on the other hand increases cerebral blood flow. Neuronal membrane fluidity, expression of neurotransmitter and its activation is altered in hepatic encephalopathy. Alteration of CNS (Cerebral edema, encephalopathy) is the predominant cause of morbidity and mortality in ALF patients.

Clinical Features

Acute liver failure is seen globally, though the predominant causes may vary from place to place. It most commonly affects the younger population. The common presenting symptoms are sudden onset of malaise, fatigue, loss of appetite and in a few patients, abdominal pain. Few patients may present with bradycardia, hypertension, pappilloedema, altered consciousness and coma.

Careful physical examination may show signs of jaundice, hepatomegaly, right upper quadrant tenderness and altered neurological status. Prothrombin time should be assessed in all patients with moderate to severe acute hepatitis. Hospital admission should be considered in case of altered mental status or coagulopathy. ALF affects almost all the systems of the body, though the CNS manifestations are most important and carry prognostic value. Grading of hepatic encephalopathy should always be done as it plays an important role in the management (Table 8.8). Hepatic encephalopathy (Grade 3 and 4) frequently progress to intracranial hypertension and herniation. Therefore early diagnosis and intensive care management is the mainstay of decreasing morbidity and mortality.

GENERAL MANAGEMENT OF ACUTE LIVER FAILURE

1. The patients must be kept in isolation, as they are vulnerable to an increase in ICP and herniation. Even a

Table 8.8: Grading of hepatic encephalopathy[6]

Grade	Level of Consciousness	Personality and Intellect	Neurologic Signs	Electroencephalogram (EEG) Abnormalities
0	Normal	Normal	None	None
Subclinical	Normal	Normal	Abnormalities only on psychometric testing	None
1	Day/night sleep reversal, restlessness	Forgetfulness, mild confusion, agitation, irritability	Tremor, apraxia, incoordination, impaired handwriting	Triphasic waves (5 Hz)
2	Lethargy, slowed responses	Disorientation to time, loss of inhibition, inappropriate behavior	Asterixis, dysarthria, ataxia, hypoactive reflexes	Triphasic waves (5 Hz)
3	Somnolence, confusion	Disorientation to place, aggressive behavior	Asterixis, muscular rigidity, hyperactive reflexes, Babinski signs	Triphasic waves (5 Hz)
4	Coma	None	Decerebration	Delta/slow wave activity

mild stimulus can worsen the already raised ICP and cause cerebral herniation.

2. Any position which can increase ICP should be avoided. A head up position upto 30° may be beneficial but adequate cerebral perfusion pressure (CPP) should be ensured.[7]
3. Adequate sedation and analgesia is required in the ICU to avoid increase in intracranial pressure, however any long acting sedative should be avoided as it may hinder the assessment of neurological status.[7] ICP monitoring done in ALF patients have reported no significant change in the outcome of both monitored and unmonitored ICP in the liver transplant patient.[8]
4. Patients on ventilatory support should be kept on controlled hyperventilation to improve the autoregulation of cerebral blood flow.[9]
5. Decreasing whole body temperature decreases the metabolism and systemic production of ammonia hence decreasing ammonia uptake. Moderate hypothermia (32°C) restores cerebral blood flow autoregulation.[10] Fever should strictly be avoided, as it can worsen the ICP. Cold air or fluid can be used, but NSAIDs should be avoided.
6. Lactulose (a semisynthetic disaccharide) solution, 20 gm three times a day (lactulose 10 gm/15 mL of solution) is recommended to reduce ammonia levels.[11] Tracheal intubation should always be considered prior to lactulose as there is a risk of pulmonary aspiration. Rectal lactulose has also been mentioned in some studies but its efficacy is not well defined (300 mL of lactulose solution is mixed with 700 mL of water and should be retained for 30–60 min, can be repeated 4–6 hourly). Regular abdominal girth measurement is important as lactulose can cause abdominal distension.
7. Correction of coagulopathy is needed whenever there is hemorrhage or any invasive procedure planned. Vitamin K and fresh frozen plasma can be administered for correction.
8. Oral, non absorbable antibiotics are recommended in hepatic encephalopathy. These drugs decrease the ammonia level by affecting the intestinal flora. Neomycin, 1–3 grams orally, 6 hourly for six days can be given. In patients with renal dysfunction, ototoxicity and nephrotoxicity have been reported. Rifaximin is another drug of this group, given 400 mg thrice a day for seven days. Though it has been used for longer duration in some studies. Rifaximin reduces ammonia level significantly with minimal adverse effect.[12,13]
9. Probiotic regimens may be beneficial in patines with hepatic encephalopathy. Acarbose enhances carbohydrates and glucose passage in the colon and has shown to improve their absorption.
10. Serum zinc which is required in the urea cycle is usually depressed in patients of hepatic encephalopathy. Administration of zinc for long term may improve hepatic encephalopathy by increasing the urea formation from ammonia and amino acid. Antioxidant action of zinc might also be the contributing factor for the beneficial effects of zinc.[14]

ETIOLOGY BASED MANAGEMENT OF ALF

Besides general management the treatment of specific cause has an equally important treatment role in the management of ALF (Table 8.9).

ROLE OF LIVER TRANSPLANT IN ALF

Advancement of liver transplant surgery has come as a boon for certain group of patients. Liver transplant is required in

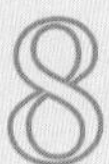

Table 8.9: Recommended treatment of acute liver failure according to etiology[15]

Cause of ALF	Treatment
Acetaminophen toxicity	Check for acetaminophen toxicity, if present N-acetylcystine to be given : **Oral** Loading 140 mg/kg (with 5% DW) Thereafter 70 mg/kg 4 hourly Total of 17 doses can be given. **Intravenous** Loading 150 mg/kg (with 5% DW) in 15 min, After 4 hours 50 mg/kg , Followed by 100 mg/kg in next 16 hours.
Mushroom poisoning	Penicillin G, Silymarin, consider liver transplant
Drug induced	Enquire about prescribed and non prescribed medications Discontinue all except needed medications
Wilsons disease	Immediate liver transplant
Autoimmune hepatitis	Corticosteroids (prednisolone 40–60 mg/kg) Consider liver transplant
HELLP	Obstetrician consultation Expedite delivery
Acute ischemic injury	Cardiovascular support
Budd chiari syndrome	Exclude malignancy Hepatic vein thrombosis with hepatic failure Consider liver transplant
Malignant infiltration	Biopsy

acute LF patient who fail to recover spontaneously.[16] The most commonly used criteria for liver transplantation in ALF patients are King's College Criteria (Table 8.10). It has markedly decreased the mortality rate and improved the prognosis in ALF patients. A successful liver transplant requires adequate infrastructure, team of trained staff, a compatible donor and appropriate fund.

Table 8.10 King's College Criteria for liver transplantation in fulminant hepatic failure

Acetaminophen-induced	Other causes
Arterial pH < 7.3 Or Grade III or IV encephalopathy and INR > 6.5 and Serum creatinine > 3.4 mg/dL	INR > 6.5 Or Any three of the following variables - ▪ Age <10 years or > 40 years ▪ Non A, non B hepatitis, halothane hepatitis, idiosyncratic drug reactions ▪ INR >3.5 ▪ Serum Bilirrubin > 17.5 mg/dL ▪ Duration of jaundice before onset of encephalopathy > 7days

PROGNOSIS

Several prognostic models like actin-free Gc-Globulin,[17] serum Gc-Globulin,[18] arterial blood lactate,[19] serum phosphorus,[20] arterial blood ammonia,[21] serum alfa-feto-protein,[22] etc. have been described but serum actin-free Gc-Globulin has a positive predictive value of 68% and a negative predictive value of 67%.[17] Its level has been found to be significantly higher in spontaneous survivors patients rather than those who underwent liver transplant or who could not survive.

The ALF due to toxic etiology carry the best prognosis as there is no fibrosis and chronic pulmonary hypertension. Earlier the mortality rate of ALF patients was very high.[2] The survival rate has increased to more than 60%, with the advancement in skill of liver transplant and intensive care management.[4] Though liver transplant has encouraging results, it is not a feasible option for all patients due to non availability of donor, lack of adequate infrastructure or due to monitory concerns. Liver support system along with cerebral resuscitation in the intensive care setting can decrease the morbidity and mortality in acute liver failure patients.

CLINICAL PEARLS

- Jaundice, encephalopathy and coagulopathy are the salient features in acute liver failure.
- It worsens the condition rapidly and affects almost all the organs of the body.
- Early diagnosis and timely intervention (medical or surgical) can improve the morbidity and mortality in such patients.

REFERENCES

1. Bernal W, Auzinger G, Dhawan A, Wendon J. Acute liver failure. Lancet, 2010:376:190-201.
2. Hernan I. Vargas, Hepatobiliary disease, Chapter 34, Current Critical Care Diagnosis and Treatment, 2nd Edition, 768-776.
3. O'Grady JG, Schalm SW, Williams R. Acute liver failure: redefining the syndromes. Lancet, 1993;342:273-5.
4. Ostapowicz GA, Fontana RJ, Schiodt FV, et al. Results of a prospective study of acute liver failure at 17 tertiary care centers in United States. Ann Intern Med, 2002;137:947-954.
5. Ranjan P, Mishra AM, Kale R, Saraswat VA, Gupta RK. Cytotoxic Edema Is Responsible for Raised Intracranial Pressure in Fulminant Hepatic Failure: In Vivo Demonstration Using Diffusion-Weighted MRI in Human Subjects, Metabolic Brain Disease 2005;20.
6. Sood GK. Emedicine for webmed, Acute Liver Failure, available at: http://www.emedicine.medscape.com, updated on march 29,2011 accessed on 6th august 2012.
7. Trotter JF. Practical management of acute liver failure in the Intensive Care Unit. Curr Opin Crit Care, 2009;15:163-7.
8. Bernuau J, Durand F. Intracranial pressure monitoring in patients with acute liver failure: a questionable invasive surveillance. Hepatology, 2006;44:502-4.
9. Strauss G, Hansen BA, Knudsen GM, Larsen FS. Hyperventilation restores cerebral blood flow autoregulation in patients with acute liver failure. J Hepatol, 1998;28:199-203.
10. Jalan R, Olde Damink SW, Deutz NE, Hayes PC, Lee A. Restoration of cerebral blood flow autoregulation and reactivity to carbon dioxide in acute liver failure by moderate hypothermia. Hepatology, 2001;34:50-4.
11. Tripathi KD. Essentials of Medical Pharmacology, 6th Edition, Chapter 48, Drugs for constipation and diarrhea, 651-664.
12. Sundaram V, Shaikh OS. Hepatic Encephalopathy: Pathophysiology and emerging therapy. Medical Clin North America, 2009;93:819 -836.
13. Maclayton DO, Rifaximin for the treatment of hepatic encephalopathy. Annals Pharmacotherapy, 2009;43:77-84.
14. Marchesini G, Fabbri A, Bianchi G, Brizi M, Zoli M. Zinc Supplementation and Amino Acid With Advanced Cirrhosis. Hepatology, 1996;23:1084-92.
15. Polson J, Lee WM. AASLD Position paper: The management of acute liver failure. Hepatology, 2005;41:1179-1197.
16. Steadman RH, Van Rensburg A, Kramer DJ. Transplantation for acute liver failure: perioperative management. Curr Opin Organ Transplant, 2010;15:368-373.
17. Schiødt FV, Bangert K, Shakil AO, McCashland T,Muray N, Hay JE, et al. Acute Liver Failure Study Group, Predictive value of actin-free Gc-Globulin in acute liver failure. Liver Transpl, 2007 Sep;13(9):1324-9.
18. Schiødt FV, Rossaro L, Stravitz RT, Shakil AO, Chung RT, Lee WM, Acute Liver Failure Study Group, Gc-Globulin and prognosis in acute liver failure. Liver Transpl, 2005 Oct;11(10):1223-9.
19. William Bernal, Nora Donaldson, Duncan Wyncoll, Julia Wendon, Blood lactate as an early predictor of outcome in paracetamol induced acute liver failure: a cohort study, Lancet, 2002;359:558-63.
20. Chung PY, Sitrin MD, Te HS, Serum phosphorus levels predict clinical outcome in fulminant hepatic failure. Liver Transpl, 2003 Mar;9(3):248-53.
21. Bhatia V, Singh R, Acharya SK, Predictive value of arterial ammonia for complications and outcome in acute liver failure. Gut, 2006 January;55(1):98-104.
22. Yang SS, Cheng KS, Lai YC, Wu CH, ChenTK, Lee CL, et al. Decreasing serum alpha-fetoprotein levels in predicting poor prognosis of acute hepatic failure in patients with chronic hepatitis B, J Gastroenterol, 2002;37(8):626-32.

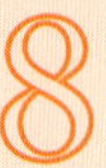

Coagulation Abnormalities Associated with Chronic Liver Disease

Anjeleena Kumar Gupta, Shashank Pandey

INTRODUCTION

Liver plays a key role in blood coagulation. Clotting is a dynamic process involving formation of a platelet plug, propagation of coagulation cascade and termination of coagulation to limit clot size. This process involves a delicate balance of procoagulants and anticoagulants factors which get disturbed in patients with liver disease resulting in bleeding or thrombotic tendency. All coagulation factors and their inhibitors are synthesized by the liver except the von Willebrand factor (vWF)[1] which is synthesized by the endothelial cells. Recently, it has been shown that this balance might be reset to a lower level in cases of chronic liver disease so that these patients do not display any sign of anticoagulation in stable condition but in the event of additional insults, like infection they may exhibit bleeding.[2] Once end stage liver disease occurs, liver transplantation is the only treatment to restore normal coagulation and correct genetic clotting defects such as hemophilia or factor V Leiden mutation.

Overview of Hemostasis

Normal hemostasis involves an interplay of procoagulant, anticoagulant and fibrinolytic systems. Vessel wall injury initiates the coagulation cascade. Once tissue injury occurs the platelets attach to endothelial collagen releasing many enzymatic substances. Formation of platelet plug and its stabilization by vWF blocks the injury site. After initial control, the intrinsic and extrinsic system activation ultimately stabilizes the clot (Flow charts 8.4 to 8.6). Fibrinolytic system and the natural anticoagulant pathway (Flow chart 8.7) ultimately limits the clot size.

Coagulation abnormalities in liver disease predispose to increased risk of bleeding or thrombosis.

Bleeding Tendency

It is secondary to decreased production of clotting factors, thrombocytopenia, altered platelet function, inhibition of platelets by nitric oxide, hypofibrinogenemia and decreased thrombin activable fibrinolysis inhibitor (TAFI).

Flow chart 8.4: Extrinsic pathway for initiating blood clotting

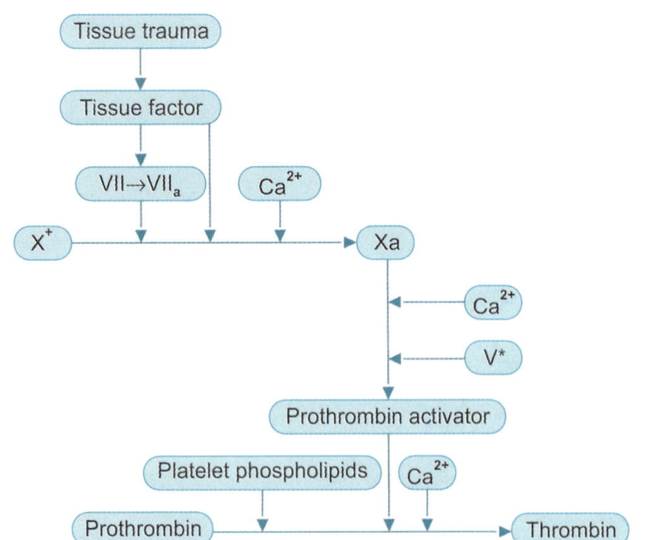

Flow chart 8.5: Intrinsic pathway for intiating blood clothing

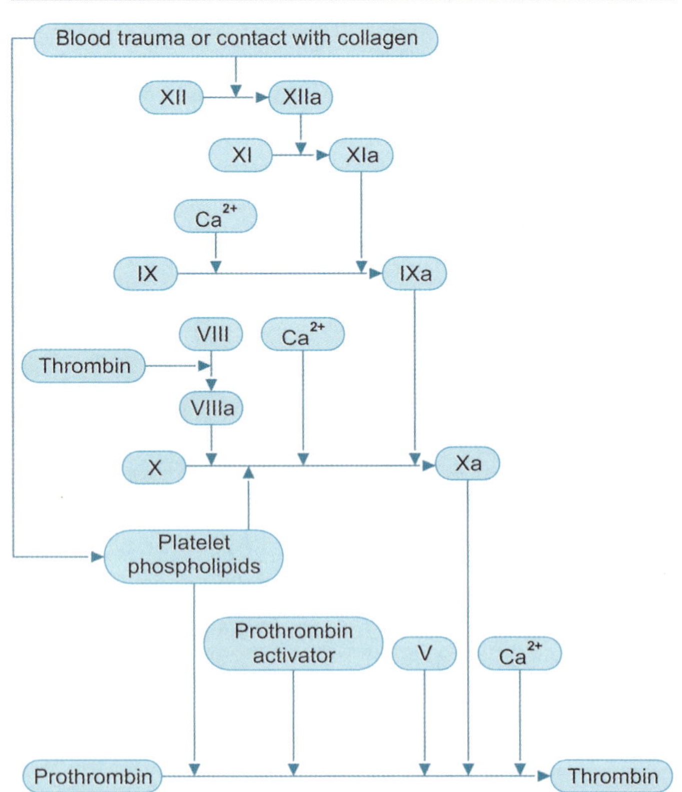

Flow chart 8.6: Scheme for conversion of prothrombin to thrombin and polymerization of fibrinogen–fibrin fibers

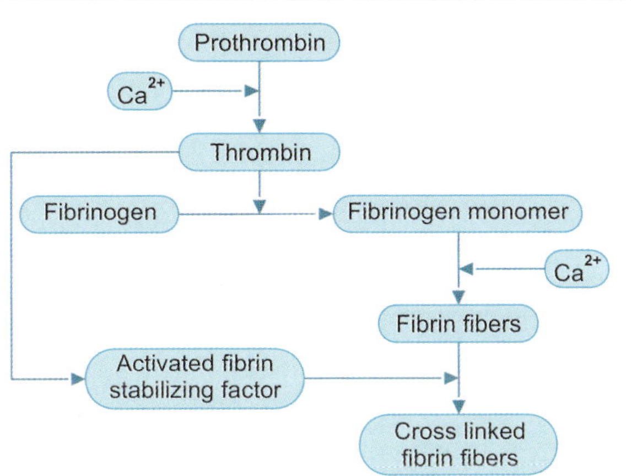

Thrombotic Tendency

It is secondary to decreased synthesis of anticoagulants protein C and S, decreased antithrombin levels, decreased plasminogen and increased levels of factor VIII and vWF.

Problems Encountered in Cirrhotic Patients

Hypocoagulability

Increased bleeding risk is related to decreased production of vitamin K dependent coagulation factors (II, VII, IX and X), fibrinogen, factor V, XI XII, prekallikrein, kininogen and plasminogen.[3] However, prediction of risk of bleeding on the basis of factor levels or prothrombin time (PT) is difficult due to the additional effect of factors promoting thrombosis or presence of superimposed infection.

Thrombocytopenia in liver disease is attributable to decreased thrombopoietin levels,[4] splenic sequestration of platelets secondary to portal hypertension,[5,6] destruction of platelets by auto antibodies[7] and bone marrow suppression.[8] Coagulation is dependent not only on the platelet number but also their function. Defective interaction between platelets and endothelium affects clot formation which is correctable by adding recombinant factor VIIa in an in vitro model.

Platelet dysfunction can also be secondary to renal dysfunction in liver disease (hepatorenal syndrome) leading to uremia and changes in vessel wall endothelial function. Platelet function in such cases is correctable by effective dialysis. In cirrhosis, platelet number even affects thrombin generation by potentiating clotting cascade.[9] Platelet counts above $50 \times 10^3/\mu L$ are known to be associated with adequate thrombin production, however, levels above $100 \times 10^3/\mu L$ are desirable.

In cirrhotics, overt sepsis can affect platelet function, production and adhesion. Infection is associated with increased production of endogenous heparinoids (heparan sulfate and dermatan sulfate) secondary to changes in nitric oxide metabolism.[10] These heparinoids thereby prevent clot formation and facilitate blood flow within a vessel.

Hyperfibrinolysis is detectable in 30–46% of patients with chronic liver disease. However, incidence of clinically

Flow chart 8.7: Fibrinolytic and anticoagulant pathway

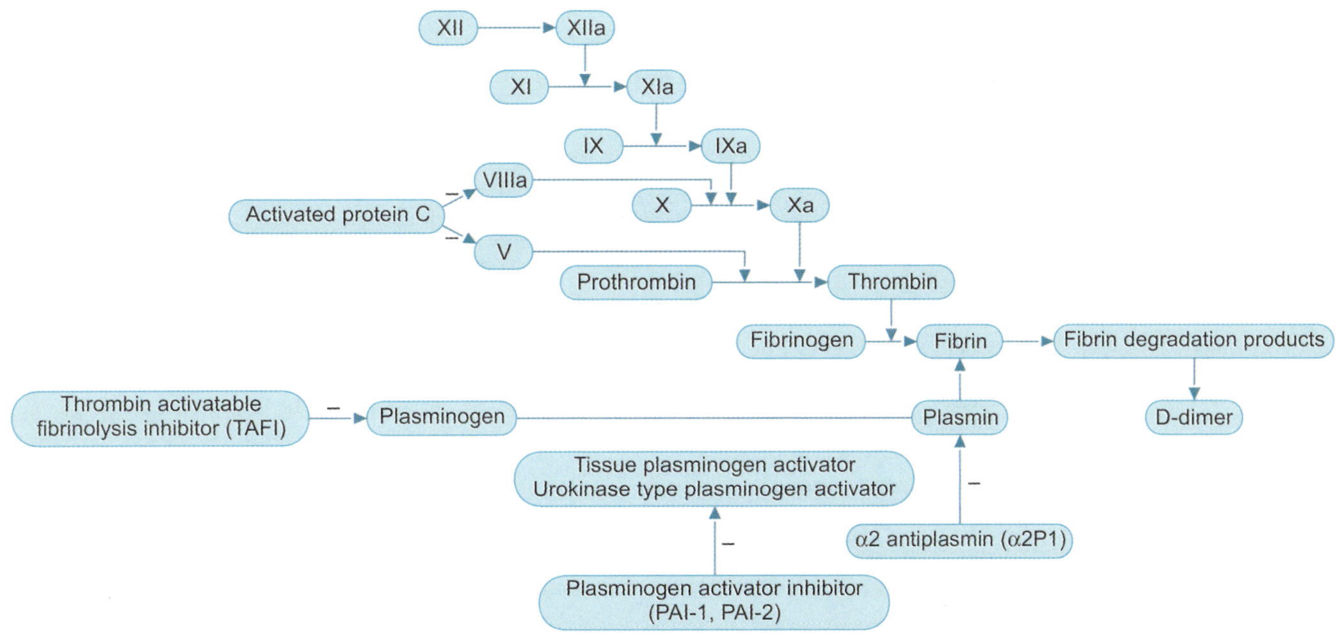

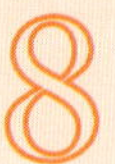

significant hyperfibrinolysis is about 5–10% of those with decompensated cirrhosis.[11] Accelerated intravascular coagulation and fibrinolysis is a clinical condition seen in cirrhotics resembling disseminated intravascular coagulation, associated with intractable bleeding following puncture marks and dental extractions. Hyperfibrinolysis in this condition promotes premature dissolution of clot, consumption of clotting factors and decreased platelet aggregation due to degradation of vWF and fibrinogen platelet receptors.[12] There is also dysregulation of tPA, PAI-1 and TAF1.

Only TAF1 is synthesized in liver but the clearance of the other two is altered in cirrhosis. Role of hyperfibrinolysis may be implicated in several other clinical situations as well:

- Hemostatic plug formed by primary hemostasis may disrupt leading to variceal bleeding.
- Bleeding following dental extractions may be the result of increased fibrinolysis in saliva. Fibrinolysis in other body cavities may result in bleeding from biliary tree and urinary bladder.
- Systemic hyperfibrinolysis could be secondary to ascitic fluid fibrinolytic activity due to increased thoracic duct delivery of ascitic fluid to the systemic circulation.[13]
- During liver transplantation, hyperfibrinolysis may be the result of increased levels of tPA in the recipient.

Hypercoagulability

In cirrhosis, hypercoagulability is often underestimated due to lack of proper measurement tools and reliance on clinical endpoints, e.g. deep vein thrombosis (DVT) and portal vein thrombosis. A study by Northup et al[14] demonstrated a 0.5% incidence of DVT despite a "coagulopathic profile" by conventional tools in patients with liver disease. In another study by Gatt et al[15] in vitro assays demonstrated increased thrombin generation in subjects with cirrhosis, when compared with normal controls. These observations disprove the old dogma of 'auto-anticoagulation' in liver disease.

In cirrhosis, apart from reduced synthesis of non-endothelial derived cloting factors there is also a significant decrease of natural anticoagulants particularly protein C and antithrombin III (AT III).[16]

AT III is a non vitamin K dependent glycoprotein synthesized by liver and endothelium.[17] Its concentration falls due to reduced synthesis and/or increased consumption secondary to hyperfibrinolysis resulting in thrombotic complications. Protein C and protein S (vitamin K dependent glycoproteins) are synthesized by hepatocytes.[18] The plasma levels of protein C and S fall by tissue damage due to their enhanced binding to the acute phase proteins (including compliment C4).

Increased levels of endothelial derived factor VIII (prothrombotic) and vWF (favor platelet adhesion) seen in cirrhotics favor thombosis. Traditionally, one treats thrombotic predisposition by warfarin, based on international normalized ratio (INR) measurements but this is not suitable in cirrhotics.[19] The increased INR levels secondary to deficiency of procoagulant factors may be offset by similar or enhanced deficiency of anticoagulant factors (not titrable by INR measurements). Therapy has to be individualized to treat thrombotic complications (DVT, portal vein thrombosis (PVT) and pulmonary embolism) in cirrhotics. In PVT though anticoagulation has reduced postoperative complications in patients awaiting liver transplantation, but it can also increase the risk of portal hypertensive bleeding.[20]

Problems Encountered in Acute Liver Failure

During acute liver failure plasma concentrations of factor V and VII decrease first, due to their short half lives (12 hours and 4–6 hours respectively) followed by factors II, VII and X. Even the high concentration of cytokines activates mononuclear cells and increases the expression of tissue factors thereby activating factor II, V, VII, X whereas any thrombin generated is inhibited by AT III preventing activation of factors VIII, IX and consequently XI, thus preserving their plasma levels.[21]

Progressive hepatic necrosis depletes factor V and VII and results in prolongation of PT and INR. Since spontaneous bleeding is relatively rare in acute liver failure despite prolongation of above parameters, the effect may be offset by liver synthesized anticoagulants as seen in cirrhotics. Although iatrogenic bleeding by invasive procedures may occur in the face of prolonged PT and INR one tends to correct it by transfusing fresh frozen plasma (FFP). Large volumes of FFP required for the correction of INR may be detrimental by worsening of body edema and intracranial hypertension.

In order to limit the volume replacement of FFP required to correct laboratory value of INR, recombinant activated factor VII (rFVIIa) is used. Correction of INR especially prior to placing an intracranial pressure monitor is recommended.[22]

Abnormalities in Liver Transplant

Patients undergoing liver transplantation may have severe bleeding due to preoperative coagulopathy secondary to underlying liver disease or coagulation abnormalities related to transplantation by the activation of fibrinolytic system. However, it contributes to blood loss in pre anhepatic phase in only 10–20% patients.[23] In the pre anhepatic stage, coagulation abnormalities are mild related to etiology of liver disease with baseline hypocoagulable state[24] and surgical technique. This stage involves adhesiolysis and transection of collateral vessels.

Patients of hepatocellular carcinoma and cholestatic cirrhosis demonstrate a hypercoagulable state and less fibrinolytic activity during transplantation as opposed to those with other etiologies.[25] Anhepatic phase involves clamping of appropriate vessels so surgical blood loss is minimal. Despite impairment of synthetic and clearance function, dramatic changes in PT and activated thromboplastin time (APTT) have not been seen. However hyperfibrinolysis occurs due to intense release of tPA and absence of its clearance due to lack of liver at that time. This is demonstrable by decreased α-antiplasmin and plasminogen activity and increase in fibrin and fibrin degradation products (FDPs).[26] However in primary biliary cirrhosis (PBC) as compared with other types of cirrhosis there is less fibrinolytic activity with a preserved capacity to generate thrombin. Reperfusion of liver may result in severe coagulopathy secondary to trapping of platelets in the graft, local thrombin generation on the damaged graft endothelium, platelet extravasation, increased phagocytosis by Kupffer cells and increased fibrinolysis. Even hypothermia after revascularization enhances splanchnic platelet dysfunction and prolongs coagulation reaction time by reducing enzymatic activity.[27] Release of heparin and heparin like substances from damaged ischemic endothelium has been shown in 25–95% of cases.[28] Hemodilution secondary to intraoperative fluids and preservation of solution from donor liver can additionally decrease plasma levels of coagulation factors.

Laboratory Testing for Coagulation Defects

A peripheral blood smear, platelet count, PT, APTT, thrombin time (TT) and fibrinogen level are done routinely, but in selected cases D-dimer test, reptilase time (RT), euglobulin clot lysis time, bleeding time, FDPs and estimation of individual clotting factors should also be done.

Coagulation abnormalities may not be evident till the clotting factors fall to less than 30–40% of normal. Prothrombin time is used to assess the extrinsic coagulation pathway comprising of tissue factor, factor VII and factors of common pathway (II, V, X and fibrinogen). Initially in mild liver disease, PT is prolonged but with the progression of disease APTT levels also get prolonged. However, this prolongation may be blunted in compensated cirrhosis due to high factor VIII levels. In chronic liver disease fibrinogen levels may be normal or increased but in decompensated cirrhosis hypofibrinogenemia results in prolongation of PT, APTT, TT and RT. In cirrhosis, platelet count may be decreased due to hypersplenism, bone marrow depression and changes in thrombopoietin metabolism. Bleeding risk in these patients is not only assessed by INR levels but also by the specific levels of circulating platelets. It has been demonstrated that adequate thrombin production occurs with platelet count above 50,000/micro L and optimal thrombin production with levels close to 100,000/micro L. Thus, these values are used as targets for low-moderate risk and high risk procedures. During liver transplant, decreased PAI-I, decreased α_2P1 and increased tPA result with shortened euglobulin lysis time. Marked increase in D-dimer, low fibrinogen and normal factor VIII may points towards DIC. Individual factor levels may also give useful information. Proportional decrease in factor V and VII points towards liver failure while reduction of factor VII more than factor V favor vitamin K deficiency. Fibrinogen rich cryoprecipitate may be used if fibrinogen level falls below 120 mg/dL since it is associated with diminished clot formation and resistance to recombinant factor VIIa. Thromboelastography plays an important role in assessing coagulation abnormalities during liver transplant. It allows rapid onsite assessment of the functional clotting status and as a guide to replacement of blood components. Thromboelastometry is similar to thromboelastography but involves a stationary cup and rotating pin. Sonorheometry is a novel method which utilizes ultrasound waves to measure clot formation. This technique is under investigation.[29]

Management strategies to control bleeding involve blood components (red cells, fresh frozen plasma (FFP), cryoprecipitate), vitamin K, desmopressin acetate, platelets, antifibrinolytic agents (tranexamic acid, aprotinin), thrombopoietin, rFVIIa and cell salvage (auto-transfusion).

FFP contains all the clotting factors and can correct elevated PT effectively but the correction is short lived (24–48 hours) depending on half life of clotting factors, especially factor VII.[30] A common indication is presence of bleeding with INR> 2 or PT longer than 4 seconds beyond that of control.[31]

FFP is the main therapy in patients of liver disease with coagulopathy. It is generally recommended in the dose of 10–15 mL/kg. The transfusion of FFP may have to be repeated depending on repeat coagulation tests. To increase the activity of clotting factors by 1–2%, a dose of 10–15 mL/kg of FFP is necessary during massive blood transfusion. To avoid dilutional decrease of clotting factors, for every 2 units of blood, 1unit of FFP is typically given.[32] It can lead to volume overload, intracranial hypertension, transmission of blood borne infections, transfusion related acute lung injury (TRALI) and allergic, febrile or hemolytic reactions. Thus, due to uncertainty of risk benefit ratio in cirrhotics, caution should be advised in their use.

Cryoprecipitate is indicated in severe coagulation abnormality and hypofibrogenemia (< 100 mg/dL) or dysfibrinogenemia. Cryoprecipitate contains the cold insoluble residue that remains on thawing FFP to 4°C. Cryoprecipitate is rich in fibrinogen, factor VIII, vWF, XIII and fibronectin. Each bag of cryoprecipitate contains 80–100 IU/mL factor VIII and at least 140 mg of fibrinogen.[33]

In cirrhotic bleeding, fibrinogen levels must be measured and substituted if low (<120 mg/dL). Recommended dosage is 1 bag of cryoprecipitate per 10 kg body weight.

Vitamin K deficiency may be treated with one dose of intravenous (10 mg) vitamin K. It is indicated in patients with severe acute liver disease, primary biliary cirrhosis, chronic liver disease, patients on broad spectrum antibiotics and poor nutritional intake.

Desmopressin acetate 1 desamino-8-d-arginine vasopressin (DDAVP) is a synthetic analogue of antidiuretic hormone that raises plasma levels of factor VIII and vWF and enhances adherence of platelets to vessel wall. It is administered as 0.3 µg/kg intravenous infusion over 20–30 minutes. It shortens or normalizes prolonged bleeding time in liver disease.[34] DDAVP has comparable results to FFP or platelets but is more convenient, better tolerated and less expensive compared to the use of blood products.[3] Side effects are mild such as facial flushing, headache, hypertension and hyponatremia.

Platelets may be indicated in patients showing active bleeding or with a platelet count below 50,000/m^3 or history of platelet dysfunction. Platelet count may not increase even after platelet transfusion in splenomegaly, disseminated intravascular coagulation (DIC), severe infection and autoimmunization. Transfusion of platelets increases the platelet count immediately with a maximal effect seen at one hour after completion of transfusion. Generally a six pack of pooled platelets or one unit of apheresis platelets should increase the platelet count by 30,000/micro L. It is reasonable to aim for levels above 50,000/m^3 for moderate risk procedures and above 100,000/m^3 for high risk procedures.[35]

Antifibrinolytic agents (tranexamic acid and aprotinin) inhibit plasmin generation and decrease bleeding associated with fibrinolysis in chronic liver disease.[36] It decreases intraoperative blood loss and transfusion requirements during liver transplantation.[37-39] Hyperfibrinolysis is difficult to diagnose by testing but must be suspected in case of delayed bleeding after a procedure of intractable oozing from puncture wound. Antifibrinolytics should be considered in cirrhotics with bleeding from peritoneal sources or dental extractions. *Aprotinin* is a serine protease inhibitor which antagonizes various proteases[40] and Kallikrein inactivator, inflammatory and antioxidant effects which might be of benefit. Besides these advantages it poses problems with a high risk of anaphylactic reactions, renal dysfunction and stroke.[41] *Epsilon aminocaproic acid (EACA)* inhibits conversion of plasminogen to plasmin by interfering binding of plasminogen to fibrin. Statistically its use has not been shown to be of benefit.[42] *Tranexamic* acid, more potent than EACA, also inhibits fibrinolysis. Recent trials show decreased fibrinolysis and blood loss with its use. Tranexamic acid is administered intravenously at a loading dose of 10 mg/kg and repeated 3–4 times per day for 2–8 days. However different doses used in other studies are without clear cut effects.[43-46] These agents are contraindicated in DIC.

Recombinant factor VIIa is genetically engineered concentrate of human coagulation factor VIIa which is similar to plasma derived factor VIIa. It rapidly normalizes elevated prothrombin time in cirrhotics but the risk of reducing bleeding is unclear. The effect on INR is evident for at least one to two hours. It enables a stable fibrin clot and has been approved by food and drug administration (FDA) for treatment of hemophilia A and B. Administration in doses 5 to 80 mg/kg IV for at least two doses have demonstrated decreased bleeding in patients of acute and chronic liver failure.[47] It should be used with caution in DIC, coronary artery disease and severe sepsis because of the risk of thrombosis.[48, 49]

Thrombopoietin stimulates megakaryocyte growth and maturation in-vitro and is a potent in-vivo thrombopoietic growth factor. It may be useful for thrombocytopenia seen in liver disease[50] but is not FDA approved.

Prothrombin complex concentrates (PCCs)—These concentrates contain human derived concentrated vitamin K dependent factors (II, IX, X), variable amounts of factor VII in an inactive form and natural anticoagulants as protein C and protein S. Very little data suggests its efficacy in cirrhosis related bleeding but the theoretical advantage is use of low infused volume as opposed to FFP in active bleeding.

CLINICAL PEARLS

- Chronic liver disease resets the hemostatic balance resulting in increased bleeding or thrombosis. The definite treatment to restore normal coagulation is liver transplantation.
- Coagulation abnormalities are secondary to fall in clotting factors or decreased platelet count which can be assessed onsite by thromboelastography.

- One must aim for platelet levels above $50\times10^3/m^3$ and $100\times10^3/m^3$ for moderate and high risk procedures respectively.

REFERENCES

1. Rapaport SI. Coagulation problems in liver disease. Blood Coagul Fibrinolysis, 2000;11 Suppl 1:S69-S74.
2. Goulis J, Armonis A, Patch D, Sabin C, Greenslade L, Burroughs AK. Bacterial infection is independently associated with failure to control bleeding in cirrhotic patients with gastrointestinal hemorrhage. Hepatology, 1998;27:1207-12.
3. Wada H, Usui M, Sakuragawa N. Hemostatic abnormalities and liver diseases. Semin Thromb Hemost, 2008;34:772.
4. Liebman HA, McGehee WG, Patch MJ, Feinstein DI. Severe depression of antithrombin III associated with disseminated intravascular coagulation in women with fatty liver of pregnancy. Ann Intern Med, 1983;98:330-3.
5. Noguchi H, Hirai K, Aoki Y, Sakata K, Tanikawa K. Changes in platelet kinetics after a partial splenic arterial embolization in cirrhotic patients with hypersplenism. Hepatology, 1995;22:1682-88.
6. Yanaga K, Tzakis AG, Shimada M, Campbell WE, Marsh JW, Stieber AC, et al. Reversal of hypersplenism following orthotopic liver transplantation. Ann Surg, 1989;210:180-3.
7. Kajihara M, Okazaki Y, Kato S, et al. Evaluation of platelet kinetics in patients with liver cirrhosis: similarity to idiopathic thrombocytopenic purpura. J Gastroenterol Hepatol, 2007;22:112.
8. Peck-Radosavljevic M. Thrombocytopenia in liver disease. Can J Gastroenterol, 2000;14 Suppl D:60D-66D.
9. Tripodi A, Primignani M, Chantarangkul V, et al. Thrombin generation in patients with cirrhosis: the role of platelets. Hepatology, 2006;44:440.
10. Senzolo M, Coppell J, Cholongitas E, et al. The effects of glycosaminoglycans on coagulation: a thromboelastographic study. Blood Coagul Fibrinolysis, 2007;18:227.
11. Kujovich JL. Hemostatic defects in end stage liver disease. Crit Care Clin, 2005;21:563.
12. Ferro D, Celestini A, Violi F. Hyperfibrinolysis in liver disease. Clin Liver Dis, 2009;13:21.
13. Agarwal S, Joyner KA Jr, Swaim MW. Ascites fluid as a possible origin for hyperfibrinolysis in advanced liver disease. Am J Gastroenterol, 2000;95:3218.
14. Northup PG, McMahon MM, Ruhl AP, et al. Coagulopathy does not fully protect hospitalized cirrhosis patients from peripheral venous thromboembolism. Am J Gastroenterol, 2006;101:1524.
15. Gatt A, Riddell A, Calvaruso V, et al. Enhanced thrombin generation in patients with cirrhosis-induced coagulopathy. J Thromb Haemost, 2010.
16. Van Thiel DH, George M, Fareed J (2001) Low levels of thrombin activatable fibrinolysis inhibitor (TAFI) in patients with chronic liver disease. Thromb Haemost, 85(4),667-70.
17. Schipper HG, ten Cate JW. Antithrombin III transfusion in patients with hepatic cirrhosis. Br J Haematol, 1982;52:25-33.
18. Fair DS, Marlar RA. Biosynthesis and secretion of factor VII, protein C, protein S, and the protein C inhibitor from a human hepatoma cell line. Blood, 1986;67:64-70.
19. Mammen EF. Coagulation abnormalities in liver disease. Hematol Oncol Clin North Am, 1992;6:1247.
20. Francoz C, Belghiti J, Vilgrain V, et al. Splanchnic vein thrombosis in candidates for liver transplantation: usefulness of screening and anticoagulation. Gut, 2005;54:691.
21. Hollestelle MJ, Thinnes T, Crain K, Stiko A, Kruijt JK, van Berkel TJ, et al. Tissue distribution of factor VIII gene expression in vivo--a closer look. Thromb Haemost, 2001;86:855-61.
22. Stravitz RT, Kramer AH, Davern T, et al. Intensive care of patients with acute liver failure: recommendations of the US Acute Liver Failure Study Group. Crit Care Med, 2007;35:2498.
23. Kang Y. Coagulation and liver transplantation: current concepts. Liver Transpl Surg, 1997;3:465-67.
24. Kirby RM, McMaster P, Clements D, Hubscher SG, Angrisani L, Sealey M, et al. Orthotopic liver transplantation: postoperative complications and their management. Br J Surg, 1987;74:3-11.
25. Palareti G, Legnani C, Maccaferri M, Gozzetti G, Mazziotti A, Martinelli G, et al. Coagulation and fibrinolysis in orthotopic liver transplantation: role of the recipient's disease and use of antithrombin III concentrates. S. Orsola Working Group on Liver Transplantation. Haemostasis, 1991;21:68-76.
26. Emeis JJ, van den Hoogen CM, Jense D. Hepatic clearance of tissue-type plasminogen activator in rats. Thromb Haemost, 1985;54:661-664.
27. Himmelreich G, Hundt K, Neuhaus P, et al. (1992) Decreased platelet aggregation after reperfusion in orthotopic liver transplantation. Transplantation, 53(3),582-6.
28. Moriau M, Kestens PJ, Masure R. Heparin and antifibrinolytic agents during experimental hepatectomy and liver transplantation. Pathol Eur, 1969;4:172-182.
29. Viola F, Mauldin FW Jr, Lin-Schmidt X, et al. A novel ultrasound-based method to evaluate hemostatic function of whole blood. Clin Chim Acta, 2010;411:106
30. Amitrano L, Guardascione MA, Brancaccio V, Balzano A. Coagulation disorders in liver disease. Semin Liver Dis, 2002;22:83-96.
31. Everson GT. A hepatologist's perspective on the management of coagulation disorders before liver transplantation. Liver Transpl Surg, 1997;3:646-52.
32. Martin DJ, Lucas CE, Ledgerwood AM, Hoschner J, McGonigal MD, Grabow D. Fresh frozen plasma supplement to massive red blood cell transfusion. Ann Surg, 1985;202:505-11.
33. O'Shaughnessy DF, Atterbury C, Bolton Maggs P, et al. Guidelines for the use of fresh-frozen plasma, cryoprecipitate and cryosupernatant. Br J Haematol, 2004;126(1):11-28.
34. Grant A, Neuberger J. Guidelines on the use of liver biopsy in clinical practice. British Society of Gastroenterology. Gut, 1999;45,IV1–IV11.
35. Argo CK, Balogun RA. Blood products, volume control, and renal support in the coagulopathy of liver disease. Clin Liver Dis, 2009; 13:73.
36. Hu KQ, Yu AS, Tiyyagura L, et al. Hyperfibrinolytic activity in hospitalized cirrhotic patients in a referral liver unit. Am J Gastroenterol, 2001;96(5):1581-86.
37. Kahl BS, Schwartz BS, Mosher DF. Profound imbalance of pro-fibrinolytic and anti-fibrinolytic factors (tissue plasminogen activator and plasminogen activator inhibitor type 1) and severe bleeding diathesis in a patient with cirrhosis: correction by liver transplantation. Blood Coagul Fibrinolysis, 2003;14(8):741-44.
38. Boylan JF, Klinck JR, Sandler AN, et al. Tranexamic acid reduces blood loss, transfusion requirements, and coagulation factor use in primary orthotopic liver transplantation. Anesthesiology, 1996; 85(5), 1043-1048; discussion 30A-31A.
39. Neuhaus P, Bechstein WO, Lefebre B, et al. Effect of aprotinin on intraoperative bleeding and fibrinolysis in liver transplantation. Lancet, 1989;2(8668): 924-5.
40. Shore-Lesserson L. Point-of-care coagulation monitoring for cardiovascular patients: past and present. J Cardiothorac Vasc Anesth, 2002;16:99-106.

41. Vater Y, Levy A, Martay K, Hunter C, Weinbroum AA. Adjuvant drugs for end-stage liver failure and transplantation. Med Sci Monit, 2004;10:RA77-RA88.
42. Kang Y, Lewis JH, Navalgund A, Russell MW, Bontempo FA, Niren LS, et al. Epsilon-aminocaproic acid for treatment of fi brinolysis during liver transplantation. Anesthesiology, 1987;66: 766-73.
43. Dalmau A, Sabate A, Acosta F, Garcia-Huete L, Koo M, Sansano R, et al. Tranexamic acid reduces red cell transfusion better than epsilon-aminocaproic acid or placebo in liver transplantation. Anesth Analg. 2000;91:29-34.
44. Dalmau A, Sabate A, Acosta F, Garcia-Huete L, Koo M, Reche M, et al. Comparative study of antifibrinolytic drugs in orthotopic liver transplantation. Transplant Proc, 1999;31:2361-2.
45. Dalmau A, Sabate A, Koo M, Rafecas A, Figueras J, Jaurrieta E. Prophylactic use of tranexamic acid and incidence of arterial thrombosis in liver transplantation. Anesth Analg, 2001;93:516.
46. Dalmau A, Sabate A, Koo M, Bartolome C, Rafecas A, Figueras J, et al. The prophylactic use of tranexamic acid and aprotinin in orthotopic liver transplantation: a comparative study. Liver Transpl, 2004;10:279-84.
47. Ejlersen E, Melsen T, Ingerslev J, et al. Recombinant activated factor VII (rFVIIa) acutely normalizes prothrombin time in patients with cirrhosis during bleeding from oesophageal varices. Scand J Gastroenterol, 2001;36(10):1081-5.
48. O'Connell KA, Wood JJ, Wise RP, et al. Thromboembolic adverse events after use of recombinant human coagulation factor VIIa. JAMA, 2006;295(3):293-8.
49. Ramsey G. Treating coagulopathy in liver disease with plasma transfusions or recombinant factor VIIa: an evidence-based review. Best Pract Res Clin Haematol, 2006;19(1):113-26.
50. Fernandes-Costa F, Metz J. Vitamin B12 binders (transcobalamins) in serum. Crit Rev Clin Lab Sci. 1982;18:1-30.

Hepatorenal Syndrome

Anjeleena Kumar Gupta, Anjali Gera, Bhuwan Chand Panday, Shashank Pandey

INTRODUCTION

The definition of hepatorenal syndrome (HRS) as proposed by the International Ascitis Club is the most widely accepted—it states "Hepatorenal syndrome, is a clinical condition that develops in patients with chronic liver disease and advanced hepatic failure and portal hypertension characterized by impaired renal function and marked abnormalities in the arterial circulation and activity of endogenous vasoactive systems."

Renal dysfunction occurs in absence of intrinsic renal disease. Risk of developing HRS in patients with cirrhosis is 18% at 1 year, increasing to 39%, at 5 years.[1] Gonwa et al noted that it is a fatal condition, unless liver transplantation is performed after which renal function shows a significant improvement post-transplantation.[2] Renal dysfunction associated with HRS not only affects overall survival but also influences outcome and survival in patients undergoing liver transplantation.[3-7]

Pathophysiology

Hepatorenal syndrome (HRS) commonly occurs in patients with cirrhosis, ascitis, portal hypertension, severe alcoholic hepatitis or fulminant hepatic failure. It may be triggered by infection, gastrointestinal bleeding, diuretic overdosing or severe diarrhea secondary to lactulose use. The major hemodynamic derangement in HRS is renal vasoconstriction. Deterioration in liver function poses increased resistance to portal flow triggering changes in intestinal microcirculation which result in splanchnic vasodilatation. Nitric oxide,[8] prostaglandins[9, 10] and other vasoactive substances[9] have been hypothesized as mediators of splanchnic vasodilatation. There is a compensatory increase in plasma volume and cardiac output in the presence of reduced peripheral vascular resistance, giving rise to hyperdynamic circulation as seen in cirrhosis. Increasing splanchnic arteriolar vasodilatation results in severe arterial hypotension and decline in 'effective' arterial blood volume which is sensed by juxtaglomerular apparatus. This results in secretion of renin which in turn stimulates renin angiotensin aldosterone system. Increased antidiuretic hormone secretion, however produces renal vasoconstriction, a prominent decrease in renal perfusion and glomerular filtration rate (GFR) and progressive azotemia. This 'underfill' theory results in renal failure.[5] Many vasoactive chemicals such as atrial natriuretic factor,[11] prostacyclin, thromboxane A2[12] and endotoxin[13] are hypothesized in mediating systemic hemodynamic changes. Medications to counteract splanchnic vasodilatation (ornipressin, terlipressin, octreotide) have shown to improve GFR in patients with HRS. This evidence supports splanchnic vasodilatation as a key factor in producing HRS (Flow chart 8.8). Renal failure in HRS is a consequence of blood flow changes rather than direct damage to kidneys. Kidneys appear normal to naked eye and function normally when placed in an environment of healthy liver following liver transplantation. Evidence points towards 'underfill' theory as a better explanation for development of HRS.

Another theory proposes that renal vasoconstriction is a result of either a deficiency in the synthesis of a vasodilatory factor or a "Hepatorenal reflex.'

The predictive factors associated with greater risk for the development of HRS have been described in cirrhotic patients with ascitis (Table 8.11).[1]

No specific test or marker for the diagnosis of HRS is available. The diagnosis is based on the demonstration of a

Flow chart 8.8: Pathophysiology of hepatorenal syndrome

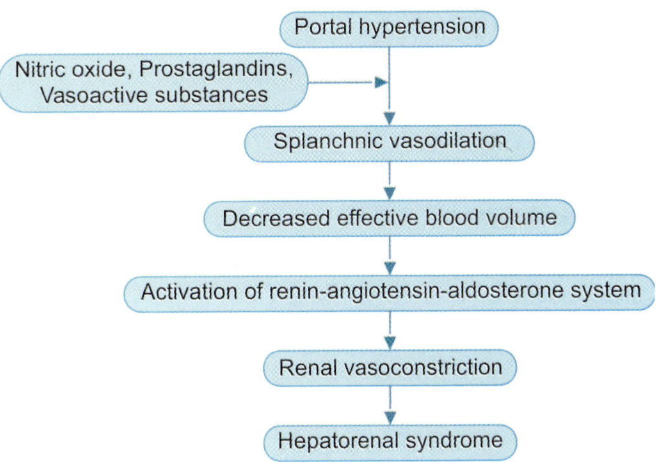

Table 8.11: Parameters associated with higher risk for development of hepatorenal syndrome in cirrhotic patients with ascitis

▪ Previous episode of ascitis
▪ Absence of hepatomegaly
▪ Poor nutritional status
▪ Moderately increased BUN
▪ Moderately increased serum creatinine
▪ Low serum sodium
▪ High serum potassium
▪ Low urinary sodium excretion
▪ Low baseline plasma osmolality
▪ High baseline urine osmolality
▪ High plasma renin activity
▪ Low arterial pressure
▪ Reduced solute free water excretion after water load
▪ Increased plasma norepinephrine
▪ Presence of esophageal varices

reduced GFR in the absence of data suggesting other causes for renal failure.

Classification

The HRS has been categorized into two forms. The renal dysfunction in either form has the same pathophysiology and manifestations but the deterioration in renal function is dependent on creatinine clearance or rise in blood creatinine levels. The outcome of the two forms is different.

Type 1 HRS is characterized by a rapidly progressive renal impairment usually precipitated by spontaneous bacterial peritonitis (SBP). The serum creatinine level usually doubles to greater than 221 µmol/L (2.5mg/L) or creatinine clearance halves to less than 20 mL/min over a period less than two weeks. Type 1 HRS usually develops secondary to acute deterioration in circulating function resulting in rapid impairment of liver function and encephalopathy. These patients are usually hypertensive on inotropic or vasopressor support. These patients usually have a model for end-stage liver disease (MELD) score of 20 or higher and a Child score of 12 or higher. Without treatment the median survival of these patients is 2 weeks.[14] These patients need to be hospitalized. Studies have shown a favorable outcome in patients treated with vasopressin analogues (terlipressin, octapressin) and transjugular intrahepatic portosystemic shunt (TIPS). However, the ideal treatment for these patients is liver transplantation.

Type 2 HRS is characterized by slow and stable reduction in the GFR. There is an increase in serum creatinine level to > 133 umol/L (1.5 mg/dL) or decrease in creatinine clearance to less than 40 mL/min with a urine sodium < 10 µmol/L. The spectrum of illness involves portal hypertension and diuretic resistant ascitis prior to deterioration in kidney function. The median survival of these patients is approximately six months,[1] unless patient undergoes liver transplantation. These patients benefit with peritoneo-venous shunting and can be managed as outpatients.

Causes

Major risk factors for development of HRS are hypotension (mean arterial blood pressure < 80 mm Hg), dilutional hyponatremia and severe urinary sodium retention (urine sodium <5 mEq/L). Besides these, SBP, acute alcoholic cirrhosis, large volume paracentesis without albumin replacement, diarrhea secondary to lactulose use and aggressive use of diuretic medications may precipitate HRS.

Signs and Symptoms

The HRS is diagnosed on the basis of altered laboratory tests as symptoms are not specific and may occur late in the course of the disease. As most people with HRS have cirrhosis, signs and symptoms may include features of chronic liver disease including palmar erythema, asterixis, clubbing, muscle wasting, jaundice, spider nevi, fetor hepaticus, xanthelasma, gynecomastia, caput medusa, bruits, atrophic testis, ascitis, hepatosplenomegaly and altered mental status.

Diagnosis

Several diagnostic criteria have been proposed by different consensus groups to diagnose HRS but in a patient of liver disease other causes of renal failure need to be excluded.

A. **Diagnostic Criteria, Consensus Conference, Chicago (1994)**
   - Hepatic failure and portal hypertension
   - Serum creatinine > 1.5 mg/dL (132 µmol/L) or GFR < 40 mL/min
   - No improvement after diuretic withdrawal and IV saline infusion (1500 mL)
   - No shock, no ongoing bacterial infection, nephrotoxic agents or fluid losses
   - Proteinuria < 500 mg/dL, normal renal ultrasonography.

B. **Diagnostic Criteria (of HRS proposed by) International Ascites Club (1996)**
   - Low GFR, as indicated by serum creatinine levels greater than 1.5 mg/dL or 132 µmol/L or 24 hour creatinine clearance < 40 mL/min.

- Absence of shock, volume depletion and use of nephrotoxic drugs (NSAIDs)
- No improvement in serum creatinine level despite stopping use of diuretics for atleast 4 to 5 days and volume repletion with 40 g intravenous albumin
- Absence of
  - Proteinuria
  - Sonographic evidence of obstructive uropathy
  - Parenchymal renal disease
  - Pre-renal failure secondary to volume depletion
  - Acute tubular necrosis (ATN) secondary to shock
  - Drug-induced renal failure
  - Glomerulopathies in cirrhotic patients due to alcohol or hepatic viruses.

Additional Criteria

1. Urine volume lower than 500 mL/day
2. Urine sodium lower than 10 mEq/L
3. Urine osmolality greater than plasma osmolality
4. Fewer than 50 urine red blood cells per high-power field
5. Serum sodium concentration lower than 130 mEq/L

C. New Diagnostic Criteria, San Francisco (2005)

- Cirrhosis with ascites
- Serum creatinine > 1.5 mg/dL
- No improvement after diuretic withdrawal and IV albumin infusion (1 g/kg/d) for 48 h
- Absence of shock
- No recent nephrotoxic agents
- Proteinuria < 500 mg/day, microhematuria (< 50 RBC/field), normal renal ultrasonography.

All the major criteria must be fulfilled for diagnosis of HRS but the minor criteria are not necessary for diagnosis, they only provide supportive evidence. It is essential to exclude pre-renal failure which involves low plasma sodium concentration, high urine sodium measurements and hyaline casts in the urine on microscopy.

Treatment

Although, definitive treatment for HRS is orthotopic liver transplantation but long waiting lists in transplant centers require medical therapy to act as bridges prior to transplantation. Mortality in such patients after transplantation may be as high as 25% within the first month.[15] Nephrotoxic drugs like tacrolimus and cyclosporine may worsen the renal function in the initial stages after liver transplantation in patients with HRS but in the long-term there is usually a recovery in kidney function.

The HRS patients should be daily monitored for pulse, blood pressure, body weight, input and output. The investigations should include not only complete blood count, liver and kidney function tests but also serum albumin and coagulation studies. 24 hours urinary volume should be tested for urinary sodium, sediment and culture. Abdominal ultrasound should be done to rule out any parenchymal nephropathy, mass lesion or obstructive uropathy. Spontaneous bacterial peritonitis should be ruled out by a diagnostic paracentesis.

A. Medical treatment

Supportive treatment like salt restricted diet, discontinuation of diuretics, fluid restriction to 1L/day in presence of dilutional hyponatremia and nutritional support should be given. Drugs producing vasoconstriction of the splanchnic circulation or volume expansion seem to show beneficial effects.

1. Albumin: Improvement in renal function in HRS has been shown following expansion of plasma volume by albumin. Various regimes for administration have been proposed. One such regime involves a bolus dose of 1 gm/kg/day albumin on 1st day followed by 20 to 40 grams daily subsequently. Most studies show the use of albumin along with other medical or surgical therapy.
2. Vasopressin analogues: Improved results have been seen in patients with HRS following therapy with agonists of vasopressin V_1 receptors such as ornipressin and terlipressin, which act as vasoconstrictors to the splanchnic circulation.

   Ornipressin showed improvement in renal function (increase in renal plasma flow (RPF) and GFR) in HRS in number of studies[16,17] but it can cause severe ischemia to major organs.[15] Deterioration in renal function following discontinuation of treatment with ornipressin has also been observed. In view of these adverse effects another vasopressin analogue terlipressin was used. It has its effect more on V_1 than on V_2 receptors. It has been used along with albumin. This combination resulted in improvement in blood pressure and renal function without any ischemic side effects, so much so, that discontinuation of the drug did not even result in HRS. Terlipressin is given as an intravenous dose of 0.5 mg/4 hr and later increased to a maximum dose of 2 mg/4 hr. The beneficial effect of the drug may take several days for action. In one study, the serum creatinine levels reduced to less than 1.5 mg/dL in 60–75% patients with type I HRS. Cochrane review in 2006 included six randomized trials for the treatment of type 1 and 2 HRS which showed reduced mortality and improved renal function with terlipression. Albumin and fresh frozen plasma also played an important role in the improvement. However, large studies were required for definite conclusions.[18] Unavailability of this drug in many countries becomes its major limitation. Yet another vasopressin analogue, octapressin, had been used in type 1 HRS in which RPF and GFR showed improvement though patient died of sepsis, gastrointestinal bleeding or liver failure.

3. Somatostatin analogues and alpha agonist: Octreotide, a somatostatin analogue regulates the tone of splanchnic blood vessel. It inhibits splanchnic vasodilatation. They have not been found to be useful in HRS.[9,19] Midodrine, an alpha agonist results in systemic vasoconstriction. Few studies have shown an improvement in HRS when treated with oral midodrine and subcutaneous octreotide.[20,21] Angeli et al showed improved renal function in type I HRS following administration of midodrine, octreotide and albumin.[20]
4. Dopamine: It is frequently used in low doses to improve renal blood flow by its vasodilatory properties but many studies including those by Bellomo et al have demonstrated no significant benefit in GFR, RPF or urine output in HRS patients.[22] These studies had the disadvantage of small sample size and absence of control groups.
5. Misoprostol: A synthetic analogue of prostaglandin E has been used in treatment of HRS[23, 24] as these patients have low urinary vasodilatory prostaglandins. But, their use has not shown improvement in HRS patients. A study by Fevery et al demonstrated reversal of HRS in four patients but it was accompanied by administration of large doses of colloids which may have played a dominant role.[25]
6. Saralasin: An angiotensin II receptor antagonist used to reverse renal vasoconstriction also did not prove to be beneficial in HRS. On the other hand it inhibited the homeostatic response to hypotension seen in cirrhotics leading to worsening of renal function. Other agents used in HRS include norepinephrine, pentoxifylline and acetylcysteine.

B. Surgical treatment

1. Peritoneo-venous shunting: It has been used for treating refractory ascitis in type 2 HRS. It results in plasma volume expansion and thereby improvement in circulatory function. It has no role in type 1 HRS.
2. Transjugular intrahepatic portosystemic shunt (TIPS):[26,27] A small stent is placed between the portal and hepatic vein thereby decompressing the high portal pressures.A catheter is placed in the hepatic vein under radiologic guidance, through the internal jugular vein or femoral vein. It shows improvement in renal function and GFR as well as reduces the activity of sympathetic and renin angiotensin aldosterone system in cirrhotic patients[28-30] with 60–70% success rate. Complications include worsening of hepatic encephalopathy, inability to adequately reduce portal pressure and bleeding.[32,33] There is an increased risk of mortality in patients with Child score > 12. Recently, vasoconstrictors with TIPS are used in type 1 HRS to achieve a completely normalized renal function.
3. Liver dialysis: It involves extracorporeal dialysis to remove toxins (bilirubin and creatinine) from circulation, through addition of a second dialysis circuit containing albumin bound membrane. It is not routinely recommended in HRS. Indications include severe volume load, metabolic acidosis, no response to vasoconstrictors, TIPS, albumin or refractory hyperkalemia. This system results in improvement in sodium levels, urine volume, mean arterial blood pressure and decreased mortality.[31,32]
4. Molecular adsorbents recirculation system (MARS): It acts as a bridge to liver transplantation in HRS patients but the technique is still in very early stages.[33]
5. Liver transplantation: It is the ideal treatment for HRS but is limited by the availability of donors. Survival rate at 1 and 3 years is 85 and 73% respectively after liver transplantation. Patients with HRS have higher morbidity, mortality and hospitalization. Gonwa et al demonstrated requirement of hemodialysis in one third of patients postoperatively with only 5% requiring long-term hemodialysis.[2] In initial few days avoidance of nephrotoxic immunosuppressants have been recommended till recovery of renal function. Generally, the GFR improves by sixth postoperative week and systemic and neurohormonal abnormalities resolve by first postoperative month.

Transplantation for type 1 HRS is limited as most patients die prior to transplantation as a result of short survival rate and long waiting periods. In such scenarios liver transplantation is a good option. In addition, the duration of pretransplant creatinine elevation is a good predictor to determine post transplant renal function as demonstrated by Campbell et al.[33]

CLINICAL PEARLS

- HRS involves renal dysfunction (in absence of intrinsic renal disease) in patients with end stage liver disease.
- HRS is classified as type I and type 2 depending on creatinine clearance or rise in blood creatinine levels.
- Definitive treatment for HRS is orthotopic liver transplantation. However, medical therapy and surgical treatment act as bridges prior to transplantation.

REFERENCES

1. Ginés A, Escorsell A, Ginés P, et al. Incidence, predictive factors, and prognosis of hepatorenal syndrome in cirrhosis. Gastroenterology, 1993;105:229-36.
2. Gonwa T, Morris C, Goldstein R, et al. Long term survival and renal function following liver transplantation in patients with and without hepatorenal syndrome–Experience in 300 patients. Transplantation, 1991;51:428-30.
3. Davis C, Gonwa T, Wilkinson A. Pathophysiology of renal disease associated with liver disorders: implications for liver transplantation. Liver Transplant, 2002;8:91.
4. Pham PTT, Pham PCT, Rastogi A, et al. Review article. Current management of renal dysfunction in the cirrhotic patient. Aliment Pharm Therapy, 2005;21:949.
5. Schrier RW, Arroyo V, Bermardi M, et al. Peripheral arterial vasodilation hypothesis. A proposal for the initiation of renal sodium and water retention in cirrhosis. Hepatology, 1998;8:1151.
6. Platt JF, Ellis JH, Rubin JM, et al. Renal duplex doppler ultrasonography: a noninvasive predictor of kidney dysfunction and hepatorenal, failure in liver disease. Hepatology, 1994;20(2):362-9.
7. Gonwa T, Klintmalm G, Levy M, et al. Impact of pretransplantation renal function on survival after liver transplantation. Transplantation, 1995;59:361.
8. Martin PY, Ginès P, Schrier RW. Nitric oxide as a mediator of hemodynamic abnormalities and sodium and water retention in cirrhosis. N Engl J Med, 1988;339(8):533-41.
9. Ginès P, Arroyo V. Hepatorenal Syndrome. J Am Soc Nephrol, 1999;10(8):1833-9.
10. Epstein M. Hepatorenal Syndrome: Emerging perspectives of pathophysiology and therapy. J Am Soc Nephrol, 1994;4(10): 1735-53.
11. Lenz K, Hörtnagl H, Druml W, et al. Ornipressin in the treatment of functional renal failure in decompensated liver cirrhosis. Effects on renal hemodynamics and atrial natriuretic factor. Gastroenterology, 1991;101(4):1060-7.
12. Moore K, Ward PS, Taylor GW, Williams R. Systemic and renal production of thromboxane A2 and prostacyclin in decompensated liver disease and hepatorenal syndrome. Gastroenterology, 1991; 100(4):1069-77.
13. Arroyo V, Guevara M, Ginès P. Hepatorenal syndrome in cirrhosis: pathogenesis and treatment. Gastroenterology, 2002; 122(6):1658-76.
14. Sherman DS, Fish DN, Teitelbaum I. Assessing renal function in cirrhotic patients: problems and pitfalls. Am J Kidney Dis, 2003; 41(2):269-78.
15. Xu X, Ling Q, Zhang M, et al. Outcome of patients with hepatorenal syndrome type 1 after liver transplantation: Hangzhou experience. Transplantation, 2009;87(10):1514-9.
16. Guevara M, Ginès P, Fernández-Esparrach G, et al. Reversibility of hepatorenal syndrome by prolonged administration of ornipressin and plasma volume expansion. Hepatology, 1998;27(1):35-41.
17. Gülberg V, Bilzer M, Gerbes AL. Long-term therapy and retreatment of hepatorenal syndrome type 1 with ornipressin and dopamine. Hepatology, 1999;30(4):870-5.
18. Gluud LL, Kjaer MS, Christensen E. Terlipressin for hepatorenal syndrome. Cochrane Database Syst Rev, 2006;18(4):CD005162.
19. Pomier-Layrargues G, Paquin SC, Hassoun Z, Lafortune M, Tran A. Octreotide in hepatorenal syndrome: a randomized, double-blind, placebo-controlled, crossover study. Hepatology, 2003;38 (1):238-43.
20. Angeli P, Volpin R, Gerunda G, et al. Reversal of type 1 hepatorenal syndrome with the administration of midodrine and octreotide. Hepatology, 1999;29(6):1690-7.
21. Esrailian E, Pantangco ER, Kyulo NL, Hu KQ, Runyon BA. Octreotide/Midodrine therapy significantly improves renal function and 30-day survival in patients with type 1 hepatorenal syndrome. Dig Dis Sci, 2007;52(3):742-8.
22. Bellomo R, Chapman M, Finfer S, Hickling K, Myburgh J. Low-dose dopamine in patients with early renal dysfunction: a placebo-controlled randomized trial. Australian and New Zealand Intensive Care Society (ANZICS) Clinical Trials Group. Lancet, 2000;356: 2139-43.
23. Ng CK, Chan MH, Tai MH, Lam CW. Hepatorenal syndrome. Clin Biochem Rev, 2007;28(1):11-7.
24. Clewell JD, Walker-Renard P. Prostaglandins for the treatment of hepatorenal syndrome. Ann Pharmacother, 1994;28(1):54-5.
25. Fevery J, Van Cutsem E, Nevens F, Van Steenbergen W, Verberckmoes R, De Groote J. Reversal of hepatorenal syndrome in four patients by per oral misoprostol (prostaglandin E1 analogue) and albumin administration. J Hepatol, 1990;11(2):153-8.
26. Wong F, Pantea L, Sniderman K. Midodrine, octreotide, albumin, and TIPS in selected patients with cirrhosis and type 1 hepatorenal syndrome. Hepatology, 2004;40:55-64.
27. Guevara M, Gines P, Bandi JC, et al. Transjugular intrahepatic portosystemic shunt in hepatorenal syndrome: Effects on renal function and vasoactive systems. Hepatology, 1998;28:416-22.
28. Brensing KA, Textor J, Perz J, et al. Long-term outcome after transjugular intrahepatic portosystemic shunt in nontransplant cirrhotics with hepatorenal syndrome: A phase II study. Gut, 2000;47:288-95.
29. Testino G, Ferro C, Sumberaz, A, et al. Type-2 hepatorenal syndrome and refractory ascites: Role of transjugular intrahepatic portosystemic shunt in eighteen patients with advanced cirrhosis awaiting orthotopic liver transplantation. Hepatogastroenterology, 2003;50:1753-5.
30. Blendis L, Wong F. The natural history and management of hepatorenal disorders: from pre-ascites to hepatorenal syndrome. Clin Med, 2003;3(2):154-9.
31. Mitzer SR, Stange L Klammt S, et al. Improvement of hepatorenal syndrome with extracorporeal albumin dialysis MARS. Results of a prospective, randomized, controlled clinical trial. Liver Transpl, 2000;6:277-86.
32. Rifai K, Ernst T, Kretschmer U, et al. The Prometheus device for extra corporeal support of combined liver and renal failure. Blood Purif, 2005;23:298-302.
33. Campbell MS, KoUyar OS, Brensinger CM, et al. Renal function after orthotopic liver transplantation is predicted by duration of pretransplantation creatinine elevation. Liver Transpl, 2005;11: 1048-55.

Hepatopulmonary Syndrome

Anjeleena Kumar Gupta, Anjali Gera, Shashank Pandey

INTRODUCTION

Presence of hypoxaemia in patients with liver disease in absence of any cardiorespiratory disorder prompts one to consider the presence of hepatopulmonary syndrome (HPS). It is characterized by the presence of hypoxia, liver disease, increased $AaDO_2$ in room air and intrapulmonary vascular dilatation. Incidence varies from 4% to 47% depending on the diagnostic criteria and method used.[1-3] Mild hypoxemia is commonly seen in cirrhotic patients but severe hypoxemia affects the morbidity and mortality among patients waiting for liver transplant. HPS may occur not only in patients with advanced liver disease and portal hypertension but also in absence of chronic liver disease. It may also be seen in Budd Chiari syndrome, prehepatic portal hypertension, acute or chronic inflammatory liver disease and Abernathy syndrome.

PATHOGENESIS

Presence of abnormal intrapulmonary vascular dilatation (IPVD) is the hallmark of HPS. Although, the pulmonary parenchyma seems normal but there is dilatation of pulmonary vasculature at precapillary and capillary level leading to intrapulmonary shunts. The diameter of these vessels may increase from the normal (<15 μm) to upto 80 μm[4] secondary to portal hypertension which may affect the perfusion of the bowel resulting in enhanced enteral translocation of gram negative bacteria and endotoxins. This process may release vasoactive mediators like tumor necrosis factor α (TNFα), nitric oxide (NO) and hem-oxygenase derived carbon monoxide.[5-7] The constitutive and the inducible isoforms of nitric oxide synthase[5,8-11] and increased expression of endothelial type B endothelin receptors[12-14] have been implicated in this process. Clearance of NO is also decreased secondary to portosystemic shunting and decreased reticuloendothelial cell function in cirrhosis.[15]

Structurally, the pulmonary parenchyma is normal but histological examination reveals dilated intrapulmonary arterioles and capillaries and vasculature between pulmonary arteries and veins which are seen as spider nevi on the pleura.

SYMPTOMS AND SIGNS

Clinical features of 80% patients of HPS are those of chronic liver disease and the rest may have dyspnea as the presenting symptom. Dyspnea may be either progressive in nature resulting in cyanosis or may even be life threatening.

Hyperdynamic circulation with increased cardiac output, decreased systemic and pulmonary vascular resistance and decreased arterial mixed venous oxygen content difference is observed in HPS. Impaired arterial oxygenation is the hallmark of HPS. It is the result of ventilation perfusion mismatch, intrapulmonary shunting and limitation of oxygen diffusion. An arterial partial pressure of oxygen lower than 60 mm Hg should prompt to rule out HPS.[16]

Dyspnea may be accompanied by platypnea and orthodeoxia. Platypnea is defined as the increase in dyspnea in upright posture which is relieved on lying down. Orthodeoxia is defined as the worsening of arterial oxyhemoglobin saturation in upright position but better on lying down. This is due to preferential perfusion of intrapulmonary vascular dilatations in lung bases in upright position.

Some patients develop digital clubbing, cyanosis, cutaneous telangiectasias (spider nevi) due to chronic hypoxemia while others may have features of systemic arterioembolization leading to stroke, cerebral hemorrhage or brain abscess.[16, 17] Severe hypoxia results in diffusely dilated pulmonary circulation with development of right to left shunts, loss of hypoxic pulmonary vasoconstriction and over perfusion of low ventilation units. Intrapulmonary vascular dilatations do not act as true anatomic shunts as partial improvement in the oxygenation is seen in such patients when breathing 100 percent oxygen. The capillaries in an intrapulmonary vascular dilatation have an expanded diameter such that oxygen molecules from adjacent alveoli are unable to diffuse and oxygenate the hemoglobin present in the red blood cells in the center of the venous blood but on breathing 100 percent oxygen, the driving diffusion pressure overcomes this perfusion defect and improvement occurs.

Recent data suggests 50% mortality within 41 months of diagnosis of HPS.[18] However, severity of liver disease does not influence the outcome of HPS.[19]

DIAGNOSIS

Once HPS is suspected in patients with chronic liver disease, hypoxemia should be documented by pulse oximetry and arterial blood gas analysis (ABG). ABG should be done not only in supine and erect position but also while patient is breathing 100% oxygen to assess the amount of right to left shunting. Assessment of shunt fraction is done by measuring PaO_2 while patient wears a nose clip and breathes 100% oxygen through a tightly fitting mouthpiece for 20 minutes. The following formula is used to calculate shunt fraction:

$$Qs/Qt = [(PAO_2\text{-}PaO_2), 0.003]/[([PAO_2\text{-}PaO_2], 0.003)+5]$$

Qs = shunt flow, Qt = total flow, PAO_2 = alveolar partial pressure of oxygen, PaO_2 = arterial partial pressure of oxygen

Shunt fraction generally increases 5 percent for every 100 mm Hg drop in PaO_2 below 600 mm Hg. Limitation of this formula is assumption of normal, rather than increased, cardiac output at baseline.

Chest X-ray may demonstrate bilateral interstitial markings in lower lobes reflecting arterial vasodilation. Pulmonary function tests may demonstrate low diffusion capacity for carbon monoxide but it is not diagnostic of HPS. A SpO_2 <97% (PaO_2 ≤80 mm Hg) and a $DAaO_2$ value >15 mm Hg have been proposed as a criteria for further diagnostic evaluation.[20] All such patients require tests to demonstrate presence of intrapulmonary vascular dilatation. Commonly used tests are contrast enhanced echocardiography and technetium (Tc) –99m labelled macroaggregated albumin perfusion scanning.

Contrast enhanced echocardiography involves intravenous injection of either indocyanine green or agitated saline to produce microbubbles (60–150 microns diameter). Under normal circumstances these bubbles are unable to traverse pulmonary circulation and do not appear in left atrium but their presence in three to five beats after the appearance of contrast in right side of heart indicates pulmonary vasodilatation. This can be distinguished from intracardiac right to left shunt in which case the bubbles will appear within first three beats following injection. In HPS, transthoracic approach is found to be superior than transoesophageal echocardiography.[21,22] This technique is more sensitive in standing position as compared to recumbent position due to increased number and size of shunts.[23] Increased left atrial volume seen on echocardiography may discriminate patients with HPS from those who have cirrhosis but not HPS. A volume greater than 50 mL predicts HPS with a sensitivity and specificity of 86 and 81 percent respectively.[24] Contrast echocardiography is not an accurate tool for diagnosis in presence of other pulmonary abnormalities like hydrothorax or obstructive disease.[4] An alternative to contrast echocardiography is scintigraphic perfusion scanning. Under normal circumstances, 99m Tc albumin macroaggregates exceeding 20 microns in diameter get trapped in the pulmonary capillary bed but in presence of cardiac right to left shunt or pulmonary vasodilatation, the uptake of 99m Tc albumin macroaggregate is seen in brain, spleen or kidney. Under normal circumstances, less than 6% of total counts can be detected on brain scanning but more than 6% brain uptake (positive scan) shows correlation with hypoxemia (PaO_2 < 60 mm Hg) and degree of shunting. This technique thus helps in diagnosis and quantification of magnitude of shunt.[25] Pulmonary angiography is not a standard diagnostic tool and is generally reserved for excluding alternative causes of hypoxemia such as pulmonary emboli or pulmonary hypertension. It is done in patients with focal arteriovenous malformations which may be amenable to embolization.[26] Krowka et al demonstrated two radiographic patterns which had clinical correlation[27] with Type 1 pattern demonstrating diffuse spidery abnormalities associated with severe hypoxemia, orthodeoxia with a good response to 100 percent oxygen while Type 2 pattern demonstrating localized arteriovenous communications with poor response to supplemental oxygen.

TREATMENT

Multiple treatment options have been proposed to correct hypoxemia and improve gas exchange in HPS but liver transplantation is the treatment of choice. Attempts have been made to obliterate intrapulmonary vascular dilatations and oppose circulating vasodilators. Treatment modalities include the use of phenylephrine, methylene blue, aspirin, indomethacin, somatostatin analogues, antioxidants,[28] almitrine and plasma exchange. Case reports have documented successful use of inhaled N(G)nitro-L-arginine methyl ester (L-NAME), an inhibitor of nitric oxide synthesis.[29] On the other hand, inhalation of NO after pediatric liver transplantation improved oxygenation among severely hypoxemic patients.[30-32] NO reached the better ventilated portions of lungs leading to dilatation of local capillary blood vessels and improving ventilation perfusion ratio.[4] Taniai et al demonstrated relief in HPS with inhaled NO in early postoperative period.[33] Hypoxia impairs wound healing and makes one susceptible to bacterial infection.[33] Oxygen supplementation helps to reduce hypoxemia in HPS so it should be continued for atleast 2 weeks or until patient achieves stable condition after liver transplantation. Reduction in portal pressure seems to be an effective approach. Transjugular intrahepatic portosystemic shunts

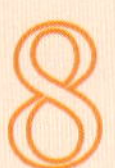

(TIPS) has also been used in small number of patients with HPS awaiting liver transplant.[34-38] Variability of results does not promise its routine use in HPS. β-blockers and nitrates which are used in chronic portal hypertension exert no beneficial effect in HPS.

Liver transplantation is the treatment of choice in HPS, although it was once considered a contraindication to transplant. HPS is associated with greater mortality in candidates awaiting transplant. Rodriguez et al suggested screening of patients for HPS in all those awaiting liver transplantation.[39] Schenk et al[19] reported an average survival time four times less in patients with HPS than those without it. No randomized trials have been done to assess the benefit of liver transplantation in HPS. But, studies[40] have demonstrated significant improvement in oxygenation following transplantation in HPS. Some studies demonstrate improvement within days while others may show a delayed resolution occurring over 2 to 14 months.[41-45] Kim et al[46] demonstrated similar results in patients with and without HPS even though liver decompensation was greater in the former group of patients.

Increased mortality after liver transplantation is often due to respiratory complications[47] but other causes may be portal venous thrombosis, intracranial events or multiorgan failure.[21] Bottari et al[48] proposed a simple scoring system to predict risk of mortality in cirrhotic patients with HPS. Child Pugh A, B and C are scored as 1,2 and 3 while PaO_2 80–70, 70–60 and 60–50 mm Hg are scored as 1,2 and 3 respectively. Individual score of both parameters is summed for a total score ranging from 2–6. Mortality risk is low, moderate and high if total score is 2–3, 4–5 and 6 respectively.

Patients whose hypoxemia fails to improve after transplantation should be reassessed for spontaneous recurrence of HPS or development of pulmonary hypertension.[49,50]

Novel treatment options include antibiotics that aim to reduce enteral bacterial translocation. Animal models suggest their effectiveness in preventing the development of HPS but longstanding clinical effects remain to be shown.[51]

CLINICAL PEARLS

- HPS is characterized by hypoxemia in patients with liver disease in absence of cardiorespiratory disorder.
- HPS is diagnosed by contrast enhanced echocardiography and technetium 99m labelled macro aggregated albumin perfusion scanning.
- Liver transplantation is the treatment of choice in HPS, besides symptomatic treatment with phenylephrine, nitric oxide, plasma exchange and TIPS.

REFERENCES

1. Krowka MJ, Cortese DA. Hepatopulmonary syndrome. Current concepts in diagnostic and therapeutic considerations. Chest, 1994;105:1528.
2. Stoller JK, Lange PA, Westveer MK, et al. Prevalence and reversibility of the hepatopulmonary syndrome after liver transplantation. The Cleveland Clinic experience. West J Med, 1995;163:133.
3. Hopkins WE, Waggoner AD, Barzilai B. Frequency and significance of intrapulmonary right-to-left shunting in end-stage hepatic disease. Am J Cardiol, 1992;70:516.
4. M Passarells, MB Fallon, SM Kawut. Portopulmonary Hypertension. Clin Liver Dis, 2006;10:653-63.
5. Nunes H, Lebrec D, Mazmanian M, et al. Role of nitric oxide in hepatopulmonary syndrome in cirrhotic rats. Am J Respir Crit Care Med, 2001;164:879-85.
6. Carter EP, Hartsfield CL, Miyazono M, Jakkula M, Morris KG Jr, McMurtry IF. Regulation of heme oxygenase-1 by nitric oxide during hepatopulmonary syndrome. Am J Physiol Lung Cell Mol Physiol, 2002;283:L346-53.
7. Strassburg CP. Shock liver. Best Pract Res Clin Gastroenterol, 2003;17:369-81.
8. Fallon MB, Abrams GA, Luo B, Hou Z, Dai J, Ku DD. The role of endothelial nitric oxide synthase in the pathogenesis of a rat model of hepatopulmonary syndrome. Gastroenterology, 1997;113:606-14.
9. Liu L, Zhang M, Luo B, Abrams GA, Fallon MB. Biliary cyst fluid from common bile duct-ligated rats stimulates endothelial nitric oxide synthase in pulmonary artery endothelial cells: a potential role in hepatopulmonary syndrome. Hepatology, 2001;33:722-7.
10. Rolla G, Brussino L, Colagrande P, et al. Exhaled nitric oxide and impaired oxygenation in cirrhotic patients before and after liver transplantation. Ann Intern Med, 1998;129:375-8.
11. Schroeder RA, Ewing CA, Sitzmann JV, Kuo PC. Pulmonary expression of iNOS and HO-1 protein is upregulated in a rat model of prehepatic portal hypertension. Dig Dis Sci, 2000;45:2405-10.
12. Ooi H, Colucci WS, Givertz MM. Endothelin mediates increased pulmonary vascular tone in patients with heart failure: demonstration by direct intrapulmonary infusion of sitaxsentan. Circulation, 2002;106:1618-21.
13. Giaid A, Yanagisawa M, Langleben Dea. Expression of endothelin-1 in the lungs of patients with pulmonary hypertension. N Engl J Med, 1993;328:1732-39.
14. Davie N, Haleen SJ, Upton PD, et al. ET(A) and ET(B) receptors modulate the proliferation of human pulmonary artery smooth muscle cells. Am J Respir Crit Care Med, 2002;165:398-405.
15. Zhang HY, Han DW, Zhao ZF, et al. Multiple pathogenic factor-induced complications of cirrhosis in rats: a new model of hepatopulmonary syndrome with intestinal endotoxemia. World J Gastroenterol, 2007;13:3500.
16. Schenk P, Fuhrmann V, Madl C, et al. Hepatopulmonary syndrome: prevalence and predictive value of various cut offs for arterial oxygenation and their clinical consequences. Gut, 2002;51: 853-59.
17. Abrams GA, Rose K, Fallon MB, et al. Hepatopulmonary syndrome and venous emboli causing intracerebral hemorrhages after liver transplantation: a case report. Transplantation, 1999;68:1809-11.
18. Abrams GA, Sanders M, Fallon MB. Utility of pulse oximetry in the detection of arterial hypoxemia in liver transplant candidates. Liver Transpl, 2002;8:391.
19. Schenk P, Schoniger-Hekele M, Fuhrmann V, et al. Prognostic significance of the hepatopulmonary syndrome in patients with cirrhosis. Gastroenterology, 2003;125:1042.

20. Hansoti RC, Shah NJ. Cirrhosis of liver simulating congenital cyanotic heart disease. Circulation, 1996;33:71.
21. Martinez C, Barbera JA, Navasa M, et al. Hepatopulmonsry syndrome associated with cardiorespiratory disease. J Hepatol, 1999;30:882.
22. Aller R, Moys JL, Moreira V, et al. Diagnosis of hepatopulmonary syndrome with contrast transesophageal echocardiography: advantages over contrast transthoracic echocardiography. Dig Dis Sci, 1999;44:1243.
23. Lenci I, Alvior A, Manzia TM, et al. Saline contrast echocardiography in patients with hepatopulmonary syndrome awaiting liver transplantation. J Am Soc Echocardiogr, 2009;22:89.
24. Zamirian M, Aslani A, Shahrzad S. Left atrial volume: a novel predictor of hepatopulmonary syndrome. Am J Gastroenterol, 2007;102:1392.
25. Krowka MJ, Wiseman GA, Burnett OL, et al. Hepatopulmonary syndrome: a prospective study of relationships between severity of liver disease, PaO(2) response to 100% oxygen, and brain uptake after (99m)Tc MAA lung scanning. Chest, 2000;118:615-24.
26. Castro M, Krowka MJ. Hepatopulmonary syndrome: a pulmonary vascular complication of liver disease. Clin Chest Med, 1996;17: 35-48.
27. Krowka MJ, Dickson ER, Cortese DA. Hepatopulmonary syndrome. Clinical observations and lack of therapeutic response to somatostatin analogue. Chest, 1993;104:515.
28. Tieppo J, Cuevas MJ, Vercelino R, et al. Quercetin administration ameliorates pulmonary complications of cirrhosis in rats. J Nutr, 2009;139:1339.
29. Brussino L, Bucca C, Morello M, et al. Effect on dyspnoea and hypoxaemia of inhaled N(G)-nitro-L-arginine methyl ester in hepatopulmonary syndrome. Lancet, 2003;362:43.
30. Egawa H, Kasahara M, Inomata Y, et al. Long-term outcome of living related liver transplantation for patients with intrapulmonary shunting and strategy for complications. Transplantation, 1999;67: 712.
31. Alexander J, Greenough A, Baker A et al. Nitric oxide treatment of severe hypoxemia after liver transplantation in hepatopulmonary syndrome: case report. Liver Transpl Surg, 1997;3:54.
32. Durand P, Baujard C, Grosse AL. Reversal of hypoxemia by inhaled nitric oxide in children with severe hepatopulmonary syndrome, type 1, during and after liver transplantation. Transplantation, 1998;65:437-9.
33. Taniai N, Onda M, Tajiri T, et al. Reversal of hypoxemia by inhaled nitric oxide in a child with hepatopulmonary syndrome after living-related liver transplantation. Transplant Proceed, 2002;34:2791-92.
34. Chevallier P, Novelli L, Motamedi JP, et al. Hepatopulmonary syndrome successfully treated with transjugular intrahepatic portosystemic shunt: a three-year follow-up. J Vasc Interv Radiol, 2004;15:647.
35. Paramesh AS, Husain SZ, Shneider B, et al. Improvement of hepatopulmonary syndrome after transjugular intrahepatic portosystemic shunting: case report and review of literature. Pediatr Transplant, 2003;7:157.
36. Lasch HM, Fried MW, Zacks SL, et al. Use of transjugular intrahepatic portosystemic shunt as a bridge to liver transplantation in a patient with severe hepatopulmonary syndrome. Liver Transpl, 2001;7:147.
37. Selim KM, Akriviadis EA, Zuckerman E, et al. Transjugular intrahepatic portosystemic shunt: a successful treatment for hepatopulmonary syndrome. Am J Gastroenterol, 1998;93:455.
38. Benitez C, Arrese M, Jorquera J, et al. Successful treatment of severe hepatopulmonary syndrome with a sequential use of TIPS placement and liver transplantation. Ann Hepatol, 2009;8:71.
39. Rodriguez-Roisin R, Krowka MJ, Hervê F, et al. ERS Task Force Pulmonary-Hepatic Vascular Disorders (PHD) Scientific Committee. Pulmonary-hepatic vascular disorders (PHD). Eur Respir J, 2004;24:861.
40. Battaglia SE, Pretto JJ, Irving LB, et al. Resolution of gas exchange abnormalities and intrapulmonary shunting following liver transplantation. Hepatology, 1997;25:1228.
41. Swanson KL, Wiesner RH, Krowka MJ. Natural history of hepatopulmonary syndrome: impact of liver transplantation. Hepatology, 2005;41:1122.
42. Starzl TE, Groth CG, Brettschneider L, et al. Extended survival in 3 cases of orthotopic homotransplantation of the human liver. Surgery, 1968;63:549.
43. Schwarzenberg SJ, Freese DK, Regelmann WE, et al. Resolution of severe intrapulmonary shunting after liver transplantation. Chest, 1993;103:1271.
44. Lange PA, Stoller JK. The hepatopulmonary syndrome. Effect of liver transplantation. Clin Chest Med, 1996;17:115.
45. Al-Hussaini A, Taylor RM, Samyn M, et al. Long-term outcome and management of hepatopulmonary syndrome in children. Pediatr Transplant, 2010;14:276.
46. Kim HY, Choi MS, Lee SC, Park SW, Lee JH, Koh KC, et al. Outcomes in patients with Hepotopulmonary Syndrome undergoing Liver Transplantation. Transplant Proceed, 2004;36: 2762-63.
47. Mazzeo AT, Lucanto T, Santamaria LB. Hepatopulmonary syndrome: a concern for the anesthetist? Preoperative evaluation of hypoxemic patients with liver disease. Acta Anaesthesiol Scand, 2004;48:178.
48. Bottari G, Mazzeo AT, and Santamaria LB. The importance of predicting the prognosis in patients with hepatopulmonary syndrome: a simple scoring system. Transplantation Proceed, 2006;38:795-97.
49. Aucejo F, Miller C, Vogt D, et al. Pulmonary hypertension after liver transplantation in patients with antecedent hepatopulmonary syndrome: a report of 2 cases and review of the literature. Liver Transpl, 2006;12:1278.
50. Koch DG, Caplan M, Reuben A. Pulmonary hypertension after liver transplantation: case presentation and review of the literature. Liver Transpl, 2009;15:407.
51. Rabiller A, Nunes H, Lebrec D, et al. Prevention of gram-negative translocation reduces the severity of hepatopulmonary syndrome. Am J Respir Crit Care Med, 2002;166:514-17.

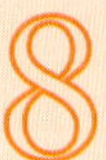

Porto-pulmonary Hypertension

Anjeleena Kumar Gupta, Anjali Gera, Shashank Pandey

INTRODUCTION

Porto-pulmonary hypertension (PPHT) as the name suggests is pulmonary arterial hypertension in presence of portal hypertension. Pulmonary arterial hypertension (PAH) is defined on the findings of right heart catheterization by a mean pulmonary vascular resistance > 240 dyn·s·cm−5, pulmonary arterial pressure > 25 mm Hg at rest and > 30 mm Hg during exercise along with mean pulmonary capillary wedge pressure < 15 mm Hg. Pulmonary hypertension is classified as idiopathic pulmonary arterial hypertension (primary pulmonary hypertension) or secondary pulmonary hypertension. Presently, World Health Organization (WHO) has reclassified it into five groups,[1] of which, only first group is considered pulmonary arterial hypertension and the rest four groups as pulmonary hypertension. First group of PAH not only includes PPHT but also idiopathic PAH and PAH secondary to connective tissue disorders, congenital heart disease, chronic hemolytic anemia, etc.[1] Portal hypertension could be secondary to cirrhosis, portal vein thrombosis, congenital anomalies of portal circulation, sclerosis of hepatic vein or periportal fibrosis in absence of cirrhosis.[2,3] Prevalence of PPHT varies between 3–5% in patients with advanced liver disease. Risk of development of PPHT is 2–10% in patients with cirrhosis. In autopsy studies, histological evidence of pulmonary hypertension is seen in 0.73% patients with cirrhosis. Pulmonary hypertension can occur secondary to portal hypertension even in absence of liver disease.

PATHOGENESIS

Numerous theories have been postulated for the development of PPHT viz humoral, genetic, hyperkinetic circulation, left ventricular dysfunction or vascular obstruction. Humoral substances like interleukin-1, serotonin, glucagon, vasoactive intestinal peptide, endothelin-1, secretin are normally metabolized by liver. In absence of this metabolic function, portosystemic collaterals allow them to reach pulmonary circulation resulting in PPHT.

A gene located in locus 2q33 of chromosome 2 and defective function of bone morphogenetic protein receptor type II[4-6] has been shown to be the causative agent of familial PAH. Patients of hereditary hemorrhagic telangiectasia having pulmonary hypertension demonstrate mutations in ALK-1, a member of growth factor receptor family.[7] Hyperkinetic circulation is evident in almost all cases of advanced liver disease. High cardiac output increases the amount of stress on the vessels of pulmonary circulation. If the pulmonary vascular resistance is low then there would be distension of arterial vessels resulting in hepatopulmonary syndrome. By contrast, increased pulmonary vascular resistance secondary to proliferation of endothelial cells and smooth muscle cells would result in PAH. In early stages of liver disease the medial hypertrophy that occurs is reversible but as disease advances it becomes a component of pulmonary arteriopathy. Pulmonary arteriopathy may be plexogenic (medial hypertrophy, intimal fibrosis and lesions involving the entire vessel wall) or thrombotic (medial hypertrophy, thrombosis and eccentric non-laminar intimal fibrosis). The resultant vascular obstruction may even lead to increased pulmonary vascular resistance.

SYMPTOMATOLOGY

Most patients with PPHT have symptoms and signs of portal and pulmonary hypertension. Symptomatology of portal hypertension generally precedes that of PAH by two to fifteen years.[8,9]

Patients with mild PPHT may not have any symptoms or signs of pulmonary vascular disease but they need to be monitored as progression of disease may pose a threat to these patients. In most patients dyspnea on exertion is the primary complaint. Other presenting symptoms are fatigue, palpitations, syncope, hemoptysis and orthopnea.[8]

Common physical signs include raised jugular venous pulse, accentuated pulmonic component of second heart sound, a systolic murmur of tricuspid regurgitation along the left sternal border (accentuates on inspiration) and dependent pitting edema indicating right heart failure or decompensated cirrhosis.

DIAGNOSIS

One should clinically examine the patients looking for specific signs like an accentuated P2 heart sound. Radiographic features of PPHT demonstrate an enlarged cardiac silhouette with pulmonary arterial prominence. Electrocardiogram shows right ventricular hypertrophy and right bundle branch block which are specific but not sensitive for PPHT. The pulmonary function tests demonstrate normal lung volumes and air flow rates but decreased diffusion capacity for carbon monoxide, decreased arterial partial pressure of oxygen (PaO_2) and decreased alveolar–arterial oxygen gradient ($AaDO_2$) [but not as low as hepatopulmonary syndrome (HPS)].

The diagnosis requires the presence of raised pulmonary arterial pressure and pulmonary vascular resistance. Echocardiography usually provides the first sign towards diagnosis. Transthoracic doppler echocardiography is a useful screening tool for PPHT but it generally overestimates right ventricular pressure producing false positive results as evidenced by the pressures estimated at subsequent cardiac catheterization. Right ventricular systolic pressures > 5 mm Hg on echocardiography should be confirmed by right heart catheterization. Prior to confirming PPHT all other causes of PAH viz left heart disease, obstructive lung disease should be excluded.

Once diagnosis of PPHT is confirmed, one should establish the severity of the disease for prognosis and treatment. PPHT is classified into mild, moderate and severe depending on New York Heart Association class, mean pulmonary arterial pressure, cardiac index, pulmonary vascular resistance and right arterial pressure (Table 8.12). In mild to moderate PPHT cardiac output is normal or high along with slightly raised pulmonary vascular resistance. However, pulmonary vascular resistance is markedly raised with low cardiac output in severe PPHT. Prognosis of severe PPHT is grave.

TREATMENT

Although specific treatment is available but is expensive, so the individual should be assessed in relation to the severity of underlying liver disease, risk factors and adherence of patients to the treatment schedules. One should assess the reversibility of pulmonary vascular constriction with vasodilators such as nifedipine and prostacyclin. Even a 20% reduction in pulmonary vascular pressure is considered responsiveness to treatment. Effective management of PPHT aims to reduce pulmonary arterial pressure, unloading the right heart and allowing time for remodelling of pulmonary vasculature so that the candidates who were earlier not suitable for liver transplant now become potential recipients. Liver transplant in patients with mean pulmonary artery pressure > 35 mm Hg have increased mortality approaching 50%. So such high pressures become a relative contraindication to liver transplantation. How much should the pulmonary artery pressure be reduced and for how long prior to liver transplantation is currently unclear. Pure vasodilators in PPHT can cause significant hypotension secondary to systemic vasodilatation and decreased right ventricular filling.

Mostly IV Epoprostenol (prostacyclin, flolan) a pulmonary vasodilator has been used to reduce pulmonary arterial pressure. Although the safety and efficacy of the drug has not been proven in randomized controlled studies but it has shown to improve the hemodynamic and exercise capacity of such patients.[10-12] Side effects of therapy include jaw pain, diarrhea, arthralgia and high cardiac output states.[13,14] Long-term treatment with the drug can lead to splenomegaly.

Table 8.12: Frequency of visits based on MELD Score

	Normal	*Mild*	*Moderate*	*Severe*
NYHA class	–	I, II	II, III	III, IV
Mean pulmonary arterial pressure (mm Hg)	15–24	25–34	35–44	>45
Cardiac index (L min^{-1} m^{-2})	2.5–4.0	>2.5	>2.5	>2.0
Pulmonary vascular resistance (dyne s^{-1} cm^{-2})	<240*	240–500	500–800	>800
Right arterial pressure (mm Hg)	0–5	0–5	5–8	>8
Prognosis	–	Favourable	Questionable	Poor
Specific treatment required†	–	No	Questionable	Yes
Reversibility after liver transplantation	–	Yes	Questionable	No

NYHA, New York Heart Association. Not all factors indicate same degree of severity in individual patients; distinction between mild, moderate, and severe portopulmonary hypertension must be based on combination of several factors viewed in clinical context. *Some workers deem pulmonary vascular rate 120 dyne S^{-1} cm^{-2} upper limit of normal in patients with liver disease; † specific treatment—i.e., intravenous epoprostenon, other prostanoids, or endothelin-receptor antagonists in highly selected cases—may be necessary in patients with mild to moderate portopulmonary hypertension who require liver transplantation or other manor surgery.

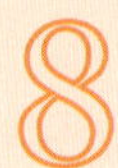

Furthermore, the administration of the drug requires a continuous delivery of the drug by permanent central venous access and infusion delivery system which adds to the risk of infection, thrombosis, infusion pump failure and rebound pulmonary hypertension by interruption of infusion.

Difficult logistics of epoprostenol drug delivery have led to the availability of other prostanoids that can be administered orally (Beraprost sodium),[15] subcutaneously (Trepostinil),[16] and as aerosol (Iloprost).[17,18] These drugs have limited effectiveness in reducing pulmonary arterial pressure. Reduction in pressure has also been tried with the use of nitric oxide, a selective pulmonary artery vasodilator. It is a useful diagnostic tool during right heart catheterization as it allows assessment of pulmonary arterial pressure response to vasodilators.

Bosentan, a dual endothelin receptor antagonist[19,20] administered orally has benefited patients with idiopathic pulmonary artery hypertension. In patients with liver disease this drug was not included in the initial trials because of its potential towards hepatotoxic effect as evidenced by a rise in aminotransferase activity. Bosentan impairs the activity of bile salt transporters leading to hepatocellular bile salt accumulation.[21]

Sitaxsentan, a novel selective inhibitor of type A endothelin receptors has been associated with severe liver injury.[22]

Sildenafil, a phosphodiesterase-5 inhibitor blocks degradation of cyclic guanosine monophosphate the second messenger of nitric oxide. It is a selective pulmonary vasodilator used orally for treatment of pulmonary hypertension,[23,24] but controlled data in patients of PPHT is not yet available.

Anticoagulation has also been recommended in patients of primary pulmonary hypertension but its efficacy in clinical trials of PPHT has not been proven. Most patients do not receive anticoagulation because it can increase the risk of hemorrhage in patients with esophageal or gastric varices and also the coagulopathy can be compounded by the additional failure of synthesis of coagulation factors by liver.

Liver transplantation is thought to benefit a selected group of patients with mild to moderate PPHT. These patients should be managed in transplant centers which have the required expertise. Pulmonary hypertension in such cases in generally reversible,[25-27] but caution should be exercised in severe PPHT. Mortality rates are often high in patients with severe PPHT following liver transplantation. In mild to moderate PPHT liver transplantation should be preceeded by pulmonary vasodilator therapy for an improved outcome.[12,30] In severe PPHT there is a risk of graft dysfunction secondary to hepatic venous congestion caused by decreased right ventricular function post liver transplantation. These cases may benefit by combined liver and lung transplantation or heart-lung-liver transplantation.[29,30]

CLINICAL PEARLS

- Pulmonary arterial hypertension secondary to portal hypertension results in portopulmonary hypertension.
- PAH is diagnosed on the findings of right heart catheterization with raised pulmonary arterial pressure and pulmonary vascular resistance.
- Treatment options of PPHT involve pulmonary vasodilators, prostanoids, endothelin receptor antagonists, phosphodiesterase-5 inhibitor, anticoagulation and liver transplantation.

REFERENCES

1. Simonneau G, Robbins IM, Beghetti M, et al. Updated clinical classification of pulmonary hypertension. J Am Coll Cardiol, 2009; 54:S43.
2. Mandell MS, Groves BM. Pulmonary hypertension in chronic liver disease. Clin Chest Med, 1996;17:17.
3. Cohen MD, Rubin LJ, Taylor WE, Cuthbert JA. Primary pulmonary hypertension: an unusual case associated with extrahepatic portal hypertension. Hepatology, 1983;3:588.
4. Nichols WC, Koller DL, Slovis B, et al. Localization of the gene for familial primary pulmonary hypertension to chromosome 2q31-32. Nat Genet, 1997;15:277.
5. Deng Z, Haghighi F, Helleby L, et al. Fine mapping of PPH1, a gene for familial primary pulmonary hypertension, to a 3-cM region on chromosome 2q33. Am J Respir Crit Care Med, 2000; 161:1055.
6. Deng Z, Morse JH, Slager SL, et al. Familial primary pulmonary hypertension (gene PPH1) is caused by mutations in the bone morphogenetic protein receptor-II gene. Am J Hum Genet, 2000; 67:737.
7. Trembath RC, Thomson JR, Machado RD, et al. Clinical and molecular genetic features of pulmonary hypertension in patients with hereditary hemorrhagic telangiectasia. N Engl J Med, 2001; 345:325-34.
8. Robalino BD, Moodie DS. Association between primary pulmonary hypertension and portal hypertension: analysis of its pathophysiology and clinical, laboratory and hemodynamic manifestations. J Am Coll Cardiol, 1991;17:492.
9. Lebrec D, Capron JP, Dhumeaux D, Benhamou JP. Pulmonary hypertension complicating portal hypertension. Am Rev Respir Dis, 1979;120:849.
10. Krowka MJ, Frantz RP, McGoon MD, Severson C, Plevak DJ, Wiesner RH. Improvement in pulmonary hemodynamics during intravenous epoprostenol (prostacyclin): a study of 15 patients with moderate to severe portopulmonary hypertension. Hepatology, 1999;30:641-48.
11. Kuo PC, Johnson LB, Plotkin JS, Howell CD, Bartlett ST, Rubin LJ. Continuous intravenous infusion of epoprostenol for the treatment of portopulmonary hypertension. Transplantation, 1997;63:604-06.

12. Plotkin JS, Kuo PC, Rubin LJ, et al. Successful use of chronic epoprostenol as a bridge to liver transplantation in severe portopulmonary hypertension. Transplantation, 1998;65:457-59.
13. Rubin LJ. Primary pulmonary hypertension. N Engl J Med, 1997; 336:111.
14. Rich S, McLaughlin VV. The effects of chronic prostacyclin therapy on cardiac output and symptoms in primary pulmonary hypertension. J Am Coll Cardiol, 1999;34:1184.
15. Galie N, Humbert M, Vachiery JL, et al. Effects of beraprost sodium, an oral prostacyclin analogue, in patients with pulmonary arterial hypertension: a randomized, double-blind, placebo-controlled trial. J Am Coll Cardiol, 2002;39:1496-502.
16. Simonneau G, Barst RJ, Galie N, et al. Continuous subcutaneous infusion of treprostinil, a prostacyclin analogue, in patients with pulmonary arterial hypertension: a double-blind, randomized, placebo-controlled trial. Am J Respir Crit Care Med, 2002;165: 800-04.
17. Hoeper MM, Schwarze M, Ehlerding S, et al. Long-term treatment of primary pulmonary hypertension with aerosolized iloprost, a prostacyclin analogue. N Engl J Med, 2000;342:1866-70.
18. Olschewski H, Simonneau G, Galie N, et al. Inhaled iloprost for severe pulmonary hypertension. N Engl J Med, 2002;347: 322-29.
19. Halank M, Miehlke S, Hoeffken G, et al. Use of oral endothelin-receptor antagonist bosentan in the treatment of portopulmonary hypertension. Transplantation, 2004;77:1775.
20. Grander W, Eller P, Fuschelberger R, Tilg H. Bosentan treatment of portopulmonary hypertension related to liver cirrhosis owing to hepatitis C. Eur J Clin Invest, 2006;36(S3):67.
21. Fattinger K, Funk C, Pantze M, et al. The endothelin antagonist bosentan inhibits the canalicular bile salt export pump: a potential mechanism for hepatic adverse reactions. Clin Pharmacol Ther, 2001;69:223-31.
22. Barst RJ, Rich S, Widlitz A, Horn EM, McLaughlin V, McFarlin J. Clinical efficacy of sitaxsentan, an endothelin-A receptor antagonist, in patients with pulmonary arterial hypertension: open-label pilot study. Chest, 2002;121:1860-68.
23. Chua R, Keogh A, Miyashita M. Novel use of sildenafil in the treatment of portopulmonary hypertension. J Heart Lung Transplant, 2005;24:498.
24. Lodato RF. Viagra for impotence of pulmonary vasodilator therapy. Am J Respir Crit Care Med, 2001;163:312-13.
25. Taura P, Garcia-Valdecasas JC, Beltran J, et al. Moderate primary pulmonary hypertension in patients undergoing liver transplantation. Cardiovasc Anesth, 1996;83:675-80.
26. Schott R, Chaouat A, Launoy A, Pottecher T, Weitzenblum E. Improvement of pulmonary hypertension after liver transplantation. Chest, 1999;115:1748-49.
27. Scott A, De Wolf A, Kang Y, et al. Reversibility of pulmonary hypertension after liver transplantation: a case report. Transplant Proc, 1993;25:1789-90.
28. Kuo PC, Plotkin JS, Gaine SP, et al. Portopulmonary hypertension and the liver transplant candidate. Transplantation, 1999;67:1087-93.
29. Dennis CM, McNeil KD, Dunning J, et al. Heart-lung-liver transplantation. J Heart Lung Transplant, 1996;15:536-38.
30. Wallwork J, Williams R, Calne RY. Transplantation of liver, heart, and lungs for primary biliary cirrhosis and primary pulmonary hypertension. Lancet, 1987;2:182-85.

Preoperative Assessment and Management of a Living Donor for Liver Transplant

Ranju Gandhi, Shashank Pandey

INTRODUCTION

Liver transplant (LTP) is now well recognized as modality of choice in acute and chronic end stage liver disease (ESLD). The gap between available livers for transplantation and requests for transplantation is ever widening. Living donor liver transplant (LDLT) could partly help alleviate the current organ shortage and reduce the number of patients dying while awaiting cadaveric LTP. With the option of LDLT, transplant is no longer confined to the sickest patients, a necessary triage that governs liver allocation for recipients of cadaveric LTP. In India and some other Asian countries like Korea, China and Japan, LDLT is the predominant type of LTP in view of traditional, religious, emotional and historical barriers to deceased donor liver transplant (DDLT). However, in countries with well established deceased donor organ allocation, LDLT comprises less than 10% of all liver transplants.[1,2] The data from USA shows that LDLT comprises less than 3% of liver transplants. The concept of partial liver allograft for LTP in children was proposed by Smith in 1969 and was first successfully performed by Raia in 1989.[3,4] The success of paediatric LDLT and the growing waiting times and waitlist mortality and morbidity was the driving force to extend the use of living donation to adult recipients. Most of the series show the outcomes of adult LDLT to be favourable.[5-12] Ensuring donor safety is of paramount importance in any living donor transplant program. Since the introduction of living donor liver transplant (LDLT) in 1989, more than 7000 LDLTs have been performed in USA. Living donor hepatectomy is a major procedure with standard surgical and anesthetic risks. The major impedent to LDLT are reports of donor morbidity and mortality.[13] It has been a contributory factor in suspension of living liver transplantation program in some centres as in France.[14]

Numerous series have confirmed the safety of donors in LDLT.[5-12] Published data of donor deaths from 1989 to February 2006 showed the rate of donor death definitely or possibly related to the donor surgery to be 0.20%.[13] The most common cause of deaths related to donor hepatectomy was sepsis, liver failure, unknown, myocardial infarction, cerebral haemorrhage, pulmonary embolism and peptic ulcer disease. Some of the donor deaths may have not been reported at centres where mandatory reporting systems to record outcomes for all living donors are not stringently applied. Reporting of donor morbidity and mortality will not only facilitate better estimation of donor risk but also prevent these complications and potentially improve outcomes. Fatal gas gangrene and complications of multiple myeloma are other unusual causes of donor death reported in literature.[14,15]

ANATOMICAL CONSIDERATIONS

Precise estimation of hepatic anatomy is indispensable for donor safety. Chisuwa et al reported that of 203 potential donors screened, 19% were excluded.[16] There is considerable variation in the hepatic hilar anatomy, specially in the hepatic artery and biliary tree. Couinaud first described the anatomical classification of liver which was refined by Bismuth.[17,18] This is used worldwide to describe allografts by the transplant community. The four anatomical allografts utilized for LDLT include

1. The entire right liver lobe (Couinaud segments V-VIII)
2. The entire left liver lobe (Couinaud segments II-IV)
3. The left lateral segment (Couinaud segments II and III)
4. The extended right liver or "trisegment" allograft (Couinaud segments IV-VIII)

The right lobe allograft, which accounts for greater than 60% of the donor's liver mass is the most commonly employed allograft for adult LDLT.

ETHICAL ISSUES

In context of living donor surgery higher than usual standard responsibility and accountability is required among all members of the liver transplant team. The donor does not stand to gain substantial benefit for self except of psychological benefit with high sense of self–esteem and contribution to saving of another's life. Trotter et al reported that donors had significantly higher scores for physical functioning, social functioning, and mental health than the normal US population.[19]

DONOR SELECTION

The LDLT is inevitably linked with risks to formerly healthy in dividuals. It requires responsible proceeding, implementation of standards for indications, evaluation of donors, informed consent, and technical procedures.[20] The donor selection process plays a pivotal role in preventing complications.

Strict donor selection criteria that seek to absolutely minimize donor risk should be developed (Tables 8.13 and 8.14). Donor risk must be balanced against recipient benefit, a situation referred to as "double equipoise". Caution should be exercised to restrict adult LDLT to situations in which the recipient has a high likelihood of a long term benefit based on published data. Minimum standards have been defined for UNOS (United Network for Organ Sharing) certification of live liver donor transplant programs.

The concept of combination of factors that determine graft and recipient survival is defined as donor/recipient match.[21] It includes donor, intraoperative and recipient factors. Approximately 50% of eligible liver recipients have an identifiable voluntary liver donor. In SGRH about 100% have an identifiable voluntary liver donor. In a few cases there may be multiple criteria for selecting a donor among multiple candidates in a family. In India, The transplantation of Human organs Act which came into force in February 1995 has been amended to better regulate and curb commercial transactions in organ transplant.[22]

In the transplantation of human organs (amendment) bill 2009 "near relative" has been expanded to include grandfather, grandmother, grandson or granddaughter to spouse, son, daughter, father, mother, brother and sister.[23] When the donor or the recipient being near relative is a foreign national, prior approval of the Authorization committee is required before planning organ removal. If it is found that there is preparation or submission of false documents including false affidavits to establish that the donor is making the donation as a near relative or by reason of affection or attachment towards the recipient, punishment for 5–10 years and fine of 5–20 lakhs can be levied on the defaulter.

Table 8.13: Requirements for candidates for living donor liver transplant (LDLT)/living donor evaluation criteria

- Healthy and willing ASA 1 and 2 adult patients aged between 18–45 years.
- Family member within 3 degrees of consanguinity.
- Absence of active systemic disease.
- No patent foramen ovale.
- Normal organ function including absence of coagulopathy, diabetes mellitus, mitral valve prolapse, arrhythmias, neuromuscular disorders, hiatal hernia with significant reflux or airway abnormalities.
- The body mass index should be less than 30.
- Stable cardiopulmonary function, no renal disease and normal liver function.
- No graft-transmittable infections (HIV, hepatitis viruses (A, B,C), CMV, syphilis, Epstein-Barr virus).
- No malignant diseases, including past history.
- Not a habitual drinker or history of substance abuse.
- The volume of the remnant liver in the donor should be atleast 30%.
- Liver should have less than 30% steatosis as assessed on plain CT scan.

Table 8.14: Contraindications for candidates for living donor liver transplant (LDLT)

- Smoking, obesity and oral contraceptive drugs (relative)
- Coagulation disorders heterozygous factor V deficiency (Leiden mutation), protein C and S deficiency (absolute)
- Psychologically unstable

DONOR EVALUATION

1. Medical
2. Surgical
3. Psychological.

The family is educated about the nature of liver disease and the need for transplantation and possibility of living donation introduced systematically as part of the informational material about transplantation. Donor evaluation process proceeds in phases and is coordinated with evaluation of the recipient. At the initial phase I, preliminary conditions such as age, relationship to the recipient, ABO blood matching and history of any disease can be identified during initial screening. Genetic relatedness is no longer mandatory because of improved results of immunosuppression for non-related transplants. There is widespread acceptance of the appropriateness of emotionally related donors, most commonly between spouses.

In phase II, a comprehensive medical and psychosocial evaluation is conducted. Psychosocial assessment is done by transplant coordinator, psychiatrist, and social worker to evaluate the donor and recipient as individuals as well as in the context of their relationship. Financial incentive and coercion for donation should not be present either directly or indirectly, overt or concealed. Detection and elimination of undue coercion extended by recipient or extended family is one of the prime responsibility of the liver transplant team. In case of living donor liver transplantation, where risks are greater than other living donations, recipient should be informed of the donor risks and be allowed the final decision of rejecting the option of living liver donation. After full consent is given, medical tests start. Such tests include comprehensive history and physical examination. Presence of smoking, use of oral contraceptive pills, or obesity (BMI >30) in prospective donor are possible risk factors for postoperative pulmonary embolism which pose a serious threat to donor safety. LDLT offers the advantages of possibility of diet modification and cessation of smoking. If BMI >30, weight loss is advised or an alternative donor selected. ABO typing should be identical or compatible. Increasing donor age has a negative impact on the outcomes of the recipients in LDLT.[21,24,25] However, Kuramitsu et al. reported that right lobe donors aged more than 60 years showed a similar survival compared with younger donors.[26]

LABORATORY EVALUATION

Donors are evaluated as for any major surgery. Laboratory investigations include:

- Hematology includes complete blood count (CBC) Serum chemistry (Blood Sugar)
- Liver function tests (Bilirubin, SGOT, SGPT, ALP, Total protein, Albumin, GGT)
- Kidney function tests (BUN, creatinine, sodium, potassium, phosphorus, chloride)
- Clotting studies (prothrombin time, activated partial thromboplastin time)
- Serology for viral hepatitis B (HBsAg), Hepatitis C, HIV 1 and 2 and CMV IgG, IgM
- ECG (electrocardiogram), PFTS (pulmonary function tests) echocardiography.

Ultrasound of abdomen and Doppler ultrasound is performed for evaluation of hepatic artery vascular anatomy and to detect any gross pathologic conditions.

In some countries, screening is done for hepatitis A and Epstein Barr Virus VCA IgG. Dobutamine stress echocardiography is obtained in selected donors if indicated by ECG abnormalities. For hypercoaguable donors, coaguable protein and homocysteine levels are done. Institutional guidelines can vary. Some centres practice individual coagulation factor assays for all donors. A study conducted in Korea compared anti-hepatitis B core antibody-positive (anti-HBc-positive) donors with anti-hepatitis B core antibody-negative donors for living-donor liver transplantation.[27] The authors found anti-HBc-positive to have the same risk for donor operation as anti-HBc-negative donors.

Second line of screening is endoscopy of upper GIT in presence of hemorrhoids, blood tests to check for tumor markers (alpha fetoprotein, CEA, CA 125, CA19.9), and an imaging study of liver by CT scan.

IMAGING OF LIVER

In LDLT, the preoperative imaging study of donor liver plays an important role in donor selection, surgical planning and to maximize the success of safe surgical procedures in both donor and recipient. Computed tomography (CT) is the most commonly employed technique for imaging of liver and segmental volume quantification. CT angiography has replaced conventional angiography for mapping hepatic artery, portal vein and hepatic vein. An unenhanced CT is performed to assess the degree of steatosis in potential donors by means of a liver attenuation index (LAI), a simple, prospective CT based grading system. LAI at unenhaned CT (CTL-S, defined as mean hepatic attenuation minus splenic attenuation) if >-10 Hounsfield units (Hu) indicate >30% macrovesicular steatosis, CTL-S between -10–5 Hu 6–30% steatosis (mild steatosis) and CTL-S > 5 Hu 0–5% (no steatosis). If steatosis >20%, then liver biopsy is indicated for accurate quantification and characterization of microvesicular steatosis. At our centre we accept <20% steatosis in right and upto 30% in left lobe grafts. Macrosteatosis greater than 30% is judged to be a contraindication for liver donation. If LAI > 5, graft assessment is done by triphasic CT scan or MR scan. Volumetry documents adequate liver volume, and defines hepatic vascular anatomy. It predicts the remnant liver volume for the donor and adequacy of graft for the recipient. Though a graft-to-body weight ratio of 1.5% is considered ideal, the required graft size-to-recipient body weight ratio of atleast 0.8% is required to achieve graft and patient survival of 90%. There is considerable challenge to procure an allograft with sufficient liver volume to meet the metabolic needs of the recipient as well at the same time leave enough for the donor.

Livers with inadequate volume, detectable pathology (focal leisons or diffuse hepatic disease), or anatomic variations like significant or isolated crossover supply MRCP or remnant segmental duct arising intrahepatically from graft hepatic duct which might jeopardize donor outcome are not selected for LRLT.

Evaluation of hepatic vascular anatomy is indispensible for optimal surgical planning. There can be considerable variation in hepatic arterial anatomy with a reported incidence of 24–45% in different series. Variation in portal venous anatomy is less common being reported in 20% of cases. It may require more than one anastomosis in the recipient.

BILIARY ANATOMY EVALUATION

Anatomical variation of the biliary system is well known. Preoperative mapping of donor biliary anatomy is essential for optimal donor selection and planning surgical technique to avoid postoperative biliary complications. Preoperatively, Magnetic resonance cholangiopancreatography (MRCP) is done to delineate biliary anatomy. In addition, a cholangiogram is performed intraoperatively. Huang et al. Classified variants of right lobe ductal drainage into five types as follows[28]

1. Normal bifurcation (62.6% of normal population).
2. Trifurcation variant (confluence of the right posterior, right anterior, and left anterior to the common hepatic duct, 19%).
3. Aberrant drainage of the right posterior duct into the left main duct (11%).
4. Low lying drainage of the right posterior duct into the common hepatic duct (5.8%).
5. Low lying drainage of the right posterior duct into the cystic duct (1.6%).

PREANESTHETIC ASSESSMENT OF LIVER DONOR

Donors undergo preanesthetic assessment while being assessed by the multidisciplinary liver transplant team and reassessed the day before donor hepatectomy. On the preoperative visit, anesthesiologist should establish a rapport and reassure of his/her presence throughout the perioperative period. All the preoperative fears and anxiety of donors should be addressed and allayed. Details of anesthesia care are discussed. Options about postoperative pain-relief via intravenous or epidural route are discussed. The use of patient controlled analgesia (PCA) device is explained. Donors should be given a logical explanation as to what to expect in the postoperative period. Unrealistic underplay of the procedure should be avoided. They can be told that from existing reports/literature, there can be minor problems like wound pain, wound scar sensation, or upper abdominal pain. Most return to their usual activities within 3–4 months. No long-term liver donor outcome data exists as it is a relatively newer procedure. List of allergies and medications are recorded. Donors are assessed for the adequacy of vascular access including central line placement and modified Allen's test.

Some centres practice preoperative phlebotomy for intra-operative blood product usage.

Selective centres (France) used to practice prophylaxis against thromboembolic disease with low molecular weight heparin night before hepatectomy.

Prospective donor is kept nil per oral for 6–8 hours before surgery. 10% dextrose at the rate of 1 mL/kg/hour is given. Prophylactic antibiotics are given intravenously two hours before surgery including third generation cephalosporin and metronidazole. H2 blocker or proton pump inhibitor and benzodiazepine like alprazolam can be given night before and morning of surgery. Blood and blood products are crossmatched.

EXTENDED CRITERIA LIVER DONORS (ECLD)

In a living donor-based program, after a thorough preoperative assessment more than half of the family donors are rejected thus reducing the donor pool. Extended criteria for selection of liver donor are used in exceptional circumstances to utilize liver donors that initially appear unsuitable without compromising donor safety or recipient survival. Common reasons for donor rejection are mismatched blood groups, hepatic steatosis, small or large-for-size grafts, deranged liver function tests and anatomical anamolies of the donor liver. Some of the methods employed in ECLD are swap donation, dual lobe transplant, weight modification in donor or the recipient. This has helped to optimize the donor pool. At SGRH, the outcome of donors with extended criteria is good.

DONOR EVALUATION IN FULMINANT HEPATIC FAILURE/EMERGENCY LDLT

In patients admitted with fulminant hepatic failure or stage 3 or 4 hepatic coma who may progress to herniation within 24–48 hours, donor evaluation may have to be compressed to an overnight process and proceed with transplantation within 24–36 hours of admission. Such a situation is inherently coercive. Family can be given the option of waiting for cadaveric donor, ultimately making a collaborative decision with the family to proceed with LDLT if it seems unsafe to wait. It is a challenging situation as donor evaluation has to be expeditious yet thorough. Informed consent has to be obtained without coercion and there has to be provision of an adequate graft volume while minimizing donor morbidity.

In this scenario, as there is insufficient time to truly embrace the risks and benefits, it is reported that the donors tolerate the failure of a transplantation done in an urgent situation poorly from psychological viewpoint.

RECENT ADVANCES IN LIVING LTP

Laparoscopic live donor hepatectomy or laparoscopy-assisted approach for right donor hepatectomy is the technical advancement in LTP practiced at some centres. It may

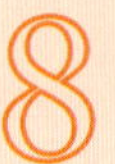

offer benefits of a smaller incision, shorter hospital stay and increased willingness to donate as has been seen with kidney transplantation.

CLINICAL PEARLS

- Donor safety is of paramount importance for the success of LDLT.

REFERENCES

1. Hayashi pH, trotter JF. Review article:adult-to-adult right hepatic lobe living donor liver transplantation. Aliment Pharmacol Ther, 2002;16:1833-41.
2. German Foundation of organ transplantation (Deutsche Stiftung fur organ transsplantation) Available at http://www.dso.de. Accessed: August 16, 2006.
3. Smith B. Segmental liver transplantation from a living donor. J Pediatr Surg, 1969;4:126-132.
4. Raia S, nery J, Mies S. Liver transplantation from live donors. Lancet, 1989;2:497.
5. Malago M, et a1. Living related liver transplantation: 36 cases at the university of Hamburg. Transpl Proc, 1994;26(6):3620-1.
6. Strong RW. Whither living donor liver transplantation? Liver Transpl Surg, 1999;5(6):536-8.
7. Russo M, et a1. Impact of adult living donor liver transplantation on waiting time survival in candidates listed for liver transplantation. Am J Transpl, 2004;4(3):427-31.
8. Marcos A, et al. Right lobe living donor liver transplantation. Transplantation, 1999;68(6):798-803.
9. Boillot o, et al. Initial French experience in adult-to-adult living donor liver transplantation. Transpl Proc, 2003;35:962-3.
10. Gautier S. Living donor liver transplantation in Russia. Transpl Proc, 2003;35:957.
11. Todo S, et al. Living donor liver transplantation in adults: outcome in Japan. Liver Transpl, 2000;6:S66-S72.
12. Chen C, et al. Living-donor liver transplantation: 12 years of experience in Asia. Transplantation, 2003;75:S6-S11.
13. Trotter JF, Adam R, Lo CM, Kenison J. Documented deaths of hepatic lobe donors for living donor liver transplantation. Liver Transplantation, 2006;12:1485-8.
14. Melloul E, Dondero F, Burtz Cp, Bouadma L, Arnulf B, Belghiti J. Living liver donor death related to complications of myeloma. Liver Transpl, 2009;15:326-9.
15. Miller C, Florman S, Kim-Schluger L, Lento p, De La garza J, Wu J, et al. Fulminant and fatal gas gangrene of the stomach in a healthy live liver donor. Liver Transpl, 2004;10:1315-9.
16. Chisuwa H, Hashikura Y, Mita A, Miyagawa S, terada M, Ikegami t, et al. Living liver donation: preoperative assessment, anatomic considerations, and long-term outcome. transplantation, 2003;75(10):1625-6.
17. Couinaud C. Le Foie: Etudes Anatomiques et Chirurgicales. 1957; Paris: Masson.
18. Bismuth H. Surgical anatomy and anatomical surgery of the liver. World J Surg, 1982;6:3-9.
19. Trotter JF, talamantes M, McClure M, Wachs M, Bak T, Troullot T, et al. Right hepatic lobe donation for living donor liver transplantation: Impact on donor quality of life. Liver Transpl, 2001;7:485-93.
20. Pascher A, Sauer IM, Walter M, Haeninnen EL, Theruvath T, Spinelli A, et al. Donor evaluation, donor risks, donor outcome, and donor quality of life in adult-adult living donor liver transplantation. Liver transplantation, 2003;8(9):829-37.
21. Yoshizumi T, Taketomi A, Soejima Y, et al. Impact of donor age and recipient status on left-lobe graft for living donor adult liver transplantation. Transpl Int, 2008;21;81-8.
22. The transplantation of Human organs Act,1994.
23. The transplantation of Human organs (Ammendment) Bill, 2009.
24. Morioka D, Egawa H, Kasahara M, et al. Outcomes of adult-to-adult living donor adult liver transplantation: a single institution's experience with 335 consecutive cases. Ann Surg, 2007;245:315-25.
25. Yoshida R, Iwamoto T, Yagi T, Sato D, Umeda Y, et al. Preoperative assessment of the risk factors that help to predict the prognosis after living donor liver transplantation. World J Surg, 2008;32:2414-24.
26. Kuramitsu K, Egawa H, Keeffe EB, et al. Impact of age older than 60 years in living donor liver transplantation. Transplantation, 2007;84:166-72.
27. Hwang S, Moon DB, Lee Sg, park KM, Kim KH, Ahn CS, Lee yJ, Chu CW, yang HS, Cho SH, oh KB, Ha ty, Min pC. Safety of anti-hepatitis B core antibody-positive donors for living-donor liver transplantation. Transplantation, 2003;75(3Suppl):S45-8.
28. Huang TL, Cheng YF, Chen CL, et al. Variants of the bile ducts : Clinical application in the potential donor of living-related hepatic transplantation. Transplant Proc, 1996;28:1669-70.

Selection and Preparation of a Patient for Liver Transplant

Shikha Sharma

FUNCTIONS OF THE LIVER

The liver performs more than 500 functions in the body. An understanding of some important functions will help us in understanding the pathophysiology of patients with liver disease (Acute or Chronic) leading to hepatic failure.[1] Hepatic failure is the manifestion of failure of various functions of the liver, which lead to the complications encountered in patients of liver disease.

Some important functions are:[2]

a. Protein synthesis and large part of amino acid synthesis.
b. Production of coagulation factors 1 (fibrinogen), prothrombin, V,VII, IX, X and XI, protein C, protein S and antithrombin.
c. Major site of thrombopoietin production which regulates the production of platelets by the bone marrow.
d. Synthesis of albumin.
e. Synthesis of angiotensinogen, an enzyme, which is activated by renin (released from kidneys) and raises blood pressure.
f. Drug metabolism and conversion of ammonia to urea.
g. Storage of glucose, vit A, vit D, vit B_{12}, iron and copper.

Disease of the liver is the disease of the synthetic and metabolic functions of the liver.

Patients developing various diseases of the liver may develop end-stage liver disease (ESLD) and become candidates for liver transplant.

Indications for Liver Transplant

The diagnosis indicating potential candidacy are:[3]

1. Primary biliary cirrhosis
2. Primary sclerosing cholangitis
3. Autoimmune hepatitis
4. Chronic hepatitis C
5. Drug induced liver disease
6. Cryptogenic cirrhosis
7. Hemochromatosis
8. Wilson's disease
9. Alpha-1-antitrypsin deficiency
10. Alcoholic cirrhosis of liver
11. Neoplasm of liver or biliary passages
12. Congential factor VIII/IX deficiency.

Uncommon Indications

1. Budd-Chiari syndrome
2. Metabolic liver disease–e.g. Crigler Najjar Syndrome, Type1 Primary hyperoxalurea
3. Alagille syndrome
4. Polycystic kidney disease-may require combined liver and kidney transplant
5. Hepatic trauma
6. Systemic diseases-amyloidosis, sarcoidosis

Apart from these indications, the patient should be able to provide for the costs of liver transplant, post-transplant care and also be willing to comply with follow up care.

In most transplant centers, a selection committee composed of transplant surgeons, hepatologists, psychiatrists, anesthesiologists, nurse coordinators and social workers is involved into determining the suitability of transplant candidates and their priority for transplantation.

Controversial Indications[3,4]

Certain conditions leading to liver decompensation like alcoholic liver disease, chronic hepatitis-B and primary hepatic malignancies raise concerns regarding the usefulness of liver transplantation due to recurrent nature of the disease, especially hepatitis B and malignancy. Also, long term survival is substantially reduced in these patients when compared with other transplant recipients. The least controversial is alcoholic liver disease but a selection criteria is often desirable.

Alcoholic Liver Disease Requires a Special Mention

The major concern in these patients is the likelihood of their returning to alcoholism after transplantation. In countries where deceased donor transplantation programs are carried out, there has been controversy regarding the allotment of donor organs to these patients. To remove bias certain criteria have been employed to assign these patients into risk groups for recidinism and noncompliance (Table 8.15).

Table 8.15: Criteria employed to assign patients with alcoholism into risk groups for recidinism and noncompliance

Low-risk patients
▪ Long documented period of abstinence (>6 months)
▪ No previous failure at alcohol rehabilitation
▪ Good social support system
▪ No psychiatric disorder
Moderate-risk patients
▪ Intermediate period of abstinence (1–6 months)
▪ One or more previous failure at alcohol rehabilitation
▪ Willing to enter alcohol rehabilitation program (if medically fit)
▪ Minimal social support system
▪ Relative psychiatric contraindication to liver transplantation
High-risk patients
▪ Undocumented or short period of abstinence (<1 month)
▪ Multiple failures to remain abstinent inspite of medical complications of liver disease
▪ Poor or absent social support system
▪ Absolute psychiatric contraindication to liver transplantation

In countries where living donor liver transplantation programs are functioning, a specific period of abstinence is a pre-requisite, which varies from 3 to 6 months.

Chronic Hepatitis B[8]

Historically, patients with hepatitis B surface antigen were regarded as poor candidates for liver transplant as their survival was 25–30% less than survival in patients following liver transplantation from other etiologies.

Patients with chronic HBV infection develop graft reinfection, which may range from carrier state (more common) to hepatitis to cirrhosis to liver failure.[5] Highest risk of recurrence is in patients with HBV cirrhosis (67%) and that too in those with HBV DNA positive than those with HBV DNA and HbsAg negative. Patients with fulminant hepatitis B however have a low rate of reinfection.

Use of hepatitis B immunoglobulin minimizes the risk of reinfection.[6] Anti hepatitis B antigen level of more than 100–200 IU/mL are to be maintained. Lamivudine, ganciclovir and famciclovir potentially inhibit HBV replication.[7]

Hepatic Malignancy

Hepatocellular carcinoma and cholangiocarcinoma are primary hepatic tumors for which liver transplantation has been performed.[8]

Due to poor results of liver transplantation for cholangiocarcinoma, many transplant centers consider it to be an absolute contraindication.

However, patients with primary sclerosing cholangitis who are at risk for development of superimposing cholangiocarcinoma, should be offered transplantation early because survival after development of cholangiocarcinoma is very poor.

In patients with hepatocellular carcinoma, the tumor must be confined to the liver (confirmed by CT scans of pelvis, chest, abdomen and bone scan). Patients with unresectable tumors and significant cirrhosis should be considered for liver transplantation.

Hepatocellular Carcinoma (HCC)

Liver transplantation should be viewed as treatment of choice for patients who have an unresectable tumor or if the malignancy is confined to liver.[8]

The tumor should be single and 2cm or larger but less than 5cm or no more than three lesions,[9] should be present, where the largest lesion is less than 3 cm with no radiographic evidence of extrahepatic disease.

For optimal results the patient should receive transplantation within 6 months of listing. The 5-year survival in these patients is approximately 61%.

The number of patients suffering from these diseases may be enormous but only a small percentage of them would require liver transplant. Liver transplantation is an accepted therapeutic modality in patients with acute or chronic liver failure who do not respond to conventional therapy. Apart from this, other criteria are also used to determine the need for transplantation.

Patients with the following complications of ESLD require liver transplant:

- Recurrent variceal bleed
- Intractable ascites
- Spontaneous bacterial peritonitis
- Refractory encephalopathy
- Severe jaundice
- Exacerbated synthetic dysfunction and fulminant hepatic failure.

Contraindications to Liver Transplant

The absolute contraindication to liver transplant is

- Spontaneous bacterial peritonitis (till infection is cleared)
- Active infection anywhere in the body
- Advanced cardiopulmonary disease
- Extrahepatic malignancies (as tumor recurrence occurs with immunosuppression) with the exception of carcinoid tumors.

- Established anatomical porto-pulmonary hypertension (PASP ≥ 50 mm Hg, mean peak airway pressure ≥ 35 mm Hg)

Relative Contraindications to Liver Transplant

While no single relative contraindication may prevent a patient from receiving liver transplantation these conditions when presenting in a high risk recipient or if presenting in multiples may prevent liver transplant. These are:

- Chronic renal failure (combined liver-kidney transplant may be required)
- Advanced cachexia
- Large hepatocellular carcinoma (more advanced than stage II)
- Medication resistant hepatitis B virus (HBV) cirrhosis
- Portal and mesenteric vein thrombosis
- History of prior malignancy not meeting American Joint Committee on Cancer (AJCC) criteria
- Multisystem organ failure state.

LISTING FOR LIVER TRANSPLANTATION

Any prospective candidate for transplantation requires routine evaluation with hematologic and blood bank studies, blood chemistry profile, viral serology (HBV, HCV, HIV, CMV), chest radiography, CT scan and ultrasound of abdomen, ECG, pulmonary function testing, renal function assessment by creatinine clearance, examination of blood flow in hepatic vessels, echocardiography with stress studies, dental and psychiatric evaluation, cancer screening with Papanicolaou test, mammography and CA125 studies.

Based on these tests and clinical condition of the patient, quantitative risk stratification schemes are used to estimate perioperative risk of the patients with cirrhosis. These are

(a) *Child-Turcotte-Pugh (CTP) scoring system* to assess severity of liver disease[10]

Points	1	2	3
Encephalopathy (grade)*	None	1 and 2	3 and 4
Ascites	Absent	Slight	Moderate
Bilirubin (mg/dL)	1–2	2–3	>3
Albumin (g/dL)	3.5	2.8–3.5	<2.8
Prothrombin time (seconds prolonged)	1–4	4–6	>6
or			
INR	<1.7	1.7–2.3	>2.3
For primary biliary cirrhosis: bilirubin (mg/dL)	1–4	4–10	>10

*According to grading of trey, burns, and saunders (1996)

Patients with child-turcotte pugh (CTP) score of 5–6 (class A) have 90% chance of surviving more than 5 years without transplantation, while patients with CTP score of 7 to 9 (class B) have 80% chance of surviving 5 years without transplantation whereas more than 35% patients with CTP score of 10 or more can be expected to die within 1 year without transplantation.

(b) *Model for End-stage Liver Disease* (MELD score)

The MELD score is based on a patient's serum bilirubin, serum creatinine and international normalized ratio (INR) for prothrombin time and is calculated from a validated predictive equation as:[11]

(3.8 × In. bilirubin value) + (11.2 × In. INR) + (9.6 × In. creatinine value) where bilirubin and creatinine values are in mg/dL and In. represents natural logarithm. The United Network for Organ Sharing (UNOS) provides an online calculator available as UNOS MELD calculator.[12] UNOS made following modifications to the score:[13]

- If patient has been dialyzed in last 7 days then serum creatinine is taken as 4.0.
- Any value less than 1 is given a value of 1.

MELD model assigns patients score from 6 to 40 which helps in predicting survival of patients both in the waiting list as well as the risk of postoperative mortality.[10,14]

(c) *The Milan Criteria* for listing of patients with HCC

The patients with hepatocellular carcinoma have specific criteria which are[15]

<5 cm single lesion or multiple lesions involving no more than 3 lesions with the largest lesion measuring ≤3 cm with no extrahepatic manifestation and no vascular manifestation.

Based on UNOS rules these patients are awarded extra points (22) to their MELD score.

The liver transplant group at University of California at San Francisco (UCSF) have advocated a *modification in Milan Criteria* which is: [16]

- Single lesion ≤ 6.5 cm
- Multiple lesions ≤ 3 cm
- Largest tumor diameter, if multiple, ≤ 4.5 cm
- Total tumor diameter, if multiple, ≤ 8 cm

BIOCHEMICAL AND CLINICAL INDICATIONS FOR LIVER TRANSPLANTATION

A major challenge is to identify potential candidates for liver transplantation at a time when survival longer than 1–2 years is unlikely but when major complications which increase

Table 8.16: Indications for liver transplantation in chronic liver disease[17]

- Cholestatic liver disease
  - Bilirubin >10 mg/dL
  - Intractable pruritis
  - Progressive bone disease
  - Recurrent bacterial cholangitis
- Hepatocellular liver disease
  - Serum albumin <3g/dL
  - Prothrombin time >3 seconds above control
- Both cholestatic and hepatocellular liver disease
  - Recurrent or severe hepatic encephalopathy
  - Refractory ascites
  - Spontaneous bacterial peritonitis
  - Recurrent portal hypertensive bleeding
  - Progressive malnutrition
  - Chronic fatigue and weakness
  - Development of hepatorenal syndrome
  - Detection of small hepatocellular carcinoma

the risk of perioperative mortality have not yet occurred (Table 8.16).

Ideally, patients should undergo transplantation prior to the development of these biochemical and clinical manifestations which predict a poor outcome.

Acute Liver Failure (Fulminant Hepatic Failure)

Fulminant hepatic failure defines the presence of acute liver failure with superimposed hepatic encephalopathy developing within two weeks of the onset of jaundice. Subfulminant hepatic failure defines hepatic encephalopathy occurring from 2 weeks to 3 months. Cerebral edema is common in patients with fulminant hepatic failure where as portal hypertensive complications occur in subfulminant patients.

King's College, London (Table 8.17) and Paris group, at Villejuif (Table 8.18) have proposed criteria for liver transplantation in fulminant hepatic failure.

Aggressive supportive therapy is necessary to treat and prevent complications of bleeding, infection, cerebral edema, renal failure and respiratory failure. Specific contraindications to liver transplantation in patients with fulminant hepatic failure are uncontrolled sepsis, brainstem dysfunction and refractory hypotension.

Care of Patients Before Liver Transplantation

Patients of liver failure require general medical care and may even require life saving procedures while they are waiting for liver transplantation. The Model for End-stage Liver Disease (MELD) is a useful tool to estimate risk of mortality in patients of liver failure waiting for liver transplantation. A score of 40 predicts 100% mortality in 3 months.[13] MELD score also determines the frequency with which a patient should be monitored before liver transplantation (Table 8.19).[18]

Table 8.17: Criteria of King's College, London

- Acetaminophen toxicity patients
  - pH < 7.3 or
  - Prothrombin time > 6.5 (INR) and serum creatinine levels > 3.4 mg/dL
- Other patients
  - Prothrombin time > 6.5 (INR)
  - Any three of the following variables:
    - Age <10 years or >40 years
    - Etiology: non-A, non-B hepatitis, halothane hepatitis, idiosyncratic drug reaction
    - Duration of jaundice before encephalopathy > 7 days
    - Prothrombin time >3.5 (INR)
    - Serum bilirubin level > 17.6 mg/dL

Table 8.18: Criteria of Hopital Paul-Brousse, Villejuif

Hepatic encephalopathy and
- Factor V level <20% in patients younger than 30 years
- Factor V level <30% in patients 30 years or older

Table 8.19: Frequency of visits based on MELD Score

MELD Score	*Visits*
>25	Weekly
19–24	Monthly
11–18	Three months
≤ 10	Six months to yearly

These visits require assessment of electrolytes, complete blood count and coagulation profile and updating of MELD score. Also assessment of portosystemic encephalopathy, ascites and edema are done and medicines adjusted for systemic comorbidities. Screening for HCC is done in patients with hepatitis B and C, hemochromatosis and alcoholic liver disease as they have an increased risk for developing HCC.

Vaccinations for hepatitis B and hepatitis A, influenza and pneumococci are done.

End stage liver disease impacts almost all the organs of the body manifesting as various signs and symptoms of the disease.

a. Central nervous system: Chronic liver failure is associated with cerebral edema and encephalopathy. The failure of hepatic clearance of toxins leads to the accumulation of ammonia, manganese and also alteration in endogenous neurotransmitters and messengers like γ-aminobutyric acid (GABA), glutamate and nitric oxide.
b. Cardiovascular system: End stage liver disease leads to a state of hyperdynamic circulation, in majority of patients, with elevated cardiac output and arteriolar vasodilatation. It may be caused by the release of toxic substances from the damaged liver and also due to vasoactive substances, which bypass hepatic metabolism. The hyperdynamic circulatory state resolves after liver transplant but in some cases may persist for many years post-transplant.
c. Pulmonary system: The pulmonary complications of liver failure are pulmonary hypertension, ventilation-perfusion abnormalities and restrictive lung disease. Hypoxemia in the absence of intrinsic lung disease or ascites, is due to intrapulmonary shunting or diffusion defects. Restrictive lung disease most commonly results from ascites and/or pleural effusion and often responds to fluid removal.
d. Renal system: End stage liver disease can also cause renal failure. Primary renal disease, proteinuria, and hypovolemia as a cause of renal hypoperfusion should be ruled out before a diagnosis of hepatorenal syndrome is made.
e. Gastrointestinal system: Patients develop ascites, portal hypertension and esophageal varices.
f. Hematological and coagulation system: Coagulation defects occur due to decreased synthesis of all clotting factors except factor VIII and fibrinogen. Anemia is common due to malnutrition and bleeding. The number of circulating platelets is reduced due to splenic sequestration. Platelets also have functional defect. Fibrinolysis occurs due to low levels of antiplasmin and inadequate clearance of tissue plasminogen activators.

   The action of opioids, propranolol, lignocaine and other drugs is prolonged due to increased volume of distribution and decreased metabolism.

LIVER SPECIFIC COMPLICATIONS AND MANAGEMENT

Patients waiting for liver transplantation may have following complications and their optimization is requested prior to transplantation.

Portal Hypertension

Portal hypertension is the main complication of cirrhosis. It is responsible for the most life threatening complications of cirrhosis, i.e. gastrointestinal bleed from esophageal varices, hepatorenal syndrome and hepatic encephalopathy.[19]

Portal hypertension occurs in cirrhosis due to change in liver structure secondary to fibrous tissue and intrahepatic vasoconstriction which accounts for 20–30% increase in intrahepatic resistance. It then leads to the formation of porto-systemic collaterals. However, inspite of formation of collaterals, portal hypertension persists because collaterals (1) lead to increase in portal venous inflow and (2) have higher resistance than normal liver so decompression does not occur.[20]

Varices and Variceal Bleeding

Gastroesophageal varices are present in nearly 50% patients of cirrhosis and their presence correlates with the severity of liver disease. Patients with hepatic venous pressure gradient (HVPG) >10 mm Hg have increased chances of developing varices.[21]

Patients with HVPG >20 mm Hg have increased chances of rebleeding and a reduction in HVPG to <20 mm Hg has shown that bleeding does not occur in these patients. These patients also have a lower risk of developing ascites, spontaneous bacterial peritonitis and thereby death due to these complications.[21]

Esophageal Variceal Bleeding

The mortality rate from esophageal variceal bleeding remains high inspite of advancements in diagnosis and treatment. Patients with gastric varices, alcohol induced cirrhosis and advanced age have increased risk of variceal bleeding.

PRIMARY PROPHYLAXIS

Pharmacotherapy: Non selective β-blockers are used to decrease the risk of variceal bleed. β-blockers decrease cardiac output which decreases the portal pressure and also collateral flow. The unopposed α-mediated splanchnic vasoconstriction decreases the splanchnic flow too. β-blockers should be titrated so that the heart rate is not less than 55 beats/min and systolic blood pressure is decreased by 20%.[22] β-blockers decrease the risk of bleeding by 50% and maximum benefits are seen in patients with child A or B cirrhosis. Long acting nitrates can be added to β-blockers in patients who do not respond to β-blockers alone.[23]

Endoscopic therapy: Endoscopic variceal sclerotherapy has been used in primary prophylaxis of variceal bleeding. However, poor results compared with pharmacotherapy have led to its discontinuation. Variceal band ligation has been shown to be safer and more effective than β-blockers for primary prevention of variceal bleeding.[23]

Secondary prophylaxis: Patients who have had one episode of bleeding have 70% chance of rebleeding within six weeks. Transjugular intrahepatic portosystemic shunt (TIPS) remains the most effective method of rescue especially in patients with failed pharmacological and endoscopic treatment. However, hepatic encephalopathy remains a problem and may lead to mortality in these patients.[23,24]

Gastric Variceal Bleeding

Gastric varices are less prevalent than esophageal varices and are categorized into:

Type 1: Which are along lesser curvature and an extension of esophageal varices

Type 2: Which occur along the fundus
Isolated gastric varices also occur in absence of esophageal varices.

Treatment modalities include:

- Endoscopic ablation with tissue adhesives (can cause cerebral emboli)
- Locally administered thrombin
- TIPS.

The TIPS is very effective with a success rate of 90% and 20% chances of rebleeding and that too due to sclerosis or ulcer formation secondary to banding.[24]

Acute Variceal Bleeding and its Management

Patient presenting with acute variceal bleeding should be managed by protection of airway, insertion of large bore intravenous cannula and blood volume resuscitation. Fresh frozen plasma and platelets transfusions are required to correct coagulopathy and when platelets are less than 30,000/mm3. The plasma volume should not be over-expanded as it may increase portal pressure and thereby increase the variceal bleeding.[25,26]

- Pharmacotherapy[25–27]
  - Somatostatin: It is used for immediate control of bleeding. Somatostatin is given as an initial intravenous bolus of 250 μg followed by an infusion of 250–500 μg/hr. It has fewer side effects.
  - Vasopressin and terlipressin: Vasopressin and terlipressin have been used to arrest variceal bleeding. Vasopressin can cause side effects like coronary artery vasoconstriction leading to myocardial infarction, arrythmias, bowel ischemia, cerebrovascular ischemia and peripheral tissue necrosis. To avoid these complications a combination of vasopressin and nitroglycerin is used.

    Terlipressin is a longer acting analogue of vasopressin and has fewer side effects.
- Endoscopic therapy[27]

  Endoscopic sclerotherapy can control bleeding in 80–90% of patients. A combination of sclerotherapy with somatostatin is superior to sclerotherapy alone. Endoscopic band ligation is a superior option but it requires an expert endoscopist as the field of vision is decreased in active bleeding.
- Balloon tamponade

  Balloon tamponade can be used to control bleeding till a definitive procedure is planned as nearly 50% patients have rebleeding when balloon is deflated.

TIPS or shunt surgery is advocated in patients in whom bleeding cannot be controlled with two endoscopic therapeutic procedures within 24 hours.[26,27]

Shunt surgery is planned in child's class A cirrhosis while TIPS is preferred in child's class B and C cirrhosis.[26, 27]

Hepatic Encephalopathy

Hepatic insufficiency leads to short-term memory loss, lack of concentration and irritability in early stages and more advanced disease leads to lethargy, stupor or coma.

Decreased hepatic function or portosystemic shunts cause nitrogenous substances from the gut to enter systemic circulation and adversely affect the brain.

The nitrogenous compounds cause alteration in glutamenergic, serotoninergic, GABA ergic and catecholamine pathways.[28]

Ammonia is a key factor in hepatic encephalopathy. In fulminant hepatic failure, >200 mg/dL of ammonia may be seen which can increase the risk of cerebral herniation.

The common precipitating factors include gastrointestinal bleeding, electrolyte abnormalities, renal failure, infection, recent placement of TIPS and use of sedatives.

Treatment Goals

The treatment goals are supportive care, removal of precipitating factors and reduction of nitrogenous load from the gut.

Nutritional Management

Due to increased catabolic state in patients with hepatic insufficiency 1–1.5 g/day of protein is recommended. In the urea cycle, enzyme cofactor may be deficient in cirrhotic patients and supplementation may be required.[29]

Lowering of ammonia load

Lactulose is used to lower ammonia production in the gut. It incorporates ammonia into the gut bacteria and thereby facilitates increased nitrogen excretion in the feces.[29]

Lactulose decreases the pH in the cecum which alters bacterial metabolism favoring uptake of ammonia.

Antibiotics such as neomycin also lower blood ammonia. Normally, ammonia is removed by the body from formation of urea in periportal hepatocytes and glutamine synthesis in perivenous hepatocytes, brain and skeletal muscles. In patients with cirrhosis, urea cycle enzymes and glutamine synthetase activity is decreased.[30]

L-ornithine-L-aspartate (OA) has been tried for lowering ammonia levels. Benzoate is also effective in lowering ammonia levels.

Ascites

Ascites is the most common complication of portal hypertension. A patient presenting with ascites requires physical examination and abdominal paracentesis along with ascitic fluid analysis.

Analysis for ascitic cell count and serum : ascites albumin gradient is estimated. If the cell count is more than 250 cell/mm^3 then culture is warranted.

The treatment of ascites includes[31]

- Dietary sodium restriction (2000 mg/dL)
- Oral diuretic therapy.

1. Chronic hyponatremia is common in cirrhotic patients. Severe hyponatremia (serum sodium <120 mmol/L) requires fluid restriction. However, cirrhotic patients do not develop symptoms of hyponatremia until sodium level is less than 100 mmol/L or the decline in sodium level is very rapid. Hyponatremia needs to be corrected slowly as rapid correction can result in central pontine myelinolysis.[32]
2. Diuretic therapy: A combination of spironolactone (100 mg) and frusemide (40 mg) in a single morning dose is recommended. This combination maintains normokalemia.

If in encephalopathy, serum sodium level less than 120 mmol/L despite fluid restriction and serum creatinine greater than 2 mg/dL occurs, then diuretic therapy is stopped and re-evaluation of patient is done.

Refractory ascites: Ascites which does not respond to diuretic therapy and sodium restricted diet can be treated with therapeutic paracentesis approximately every two weeks. Post paracentesis albumin infusion of 5 to 8g/L of ascitic fluid removed is recommended.[32,33]

Peritoneovenous shunt: has been used for control of ascites but they do not improve survival and have high complication rate.[33]
Transjugular intrahepatic portosystemic shunt: TIPS is superior to medical therapy for ascites but does not improve survival.[34]

Spontaneous Bacterial Peritonitis

Presence of infection is a contraindication for liver transplant till infection is cleared. A cell count of more than 250 polymorphonuclear cells and/or a positive bacterial culture of ascitic fluid gives the diagnosis of SBP. These patients should receive broad spectrum antibiotics, e.g. cefotaxime or ofloxacin. A sterile culture or a decrease in PMN count is an important result in repeated paracentesis after antibiotic treatment.[21]

Short-term inpatient quinolone should be considered in prevention of bacterial infections in patients with low protein (<1g/dL), ascites, variceal hemorrhage and prior SBP.[20]

Hepatorenal Syndrome (HRS)

Functional renal failure can occur in patients of cirrhosis and ascites at the rate of 18% after one year and 39% at five years.[27] Portal hypertension causes release of endogenous vasodilators which cause peripheral arterial vasodilatation, especially in splanchnic circulation.

The hallmarks of HRS are reversible renal constriction and mild systemic hypotension. The kidneys are structurally normal at least in early stages and tubular function intact.

HEPATORENAL SYNDROME

Hepatorenal syndrome involves development of renal failure in patients with severe liver disease.

Diagnostic Criteria of Hepatorenal Syndrome[28]

Major Criteria[35]

- Chronic or acute liver disease with advanced hepatic failure and portal hypertension
- Low GFR: Serum creatinine >133 μmol/L or 24h creatinine clearance <40 mL/min
- Absence of shock, ongoing bacterial infection or treatment with nephrotoxic drugs
- Absence of gastrointestinal or renal fluid losses
- No sustained improvement in renal function following diuretic withdrawal and expansion of plasma volume with 1.5 L of isotonic saline

- Proteinuria <0.5 g/day and no ultrasonographic evidence of obstructive uropathy or parenchymal renal disease.

Additional Criteria[35]

- Urine volume <0.5 L/day
- Urine sodium <10 mmol/L
- Urine osmolality > plasma osmolality
- Urine red blood cells <50 high power field
- Serum sodium concentration <130 mmol/L.

Clinically HRS can be divided into Type 1 and 2. Type 1 HRS is characterized by rapid and progressive impairment of renal function defined as doubling of initial serum creatinine to higher than 221/mmol/L in less than 2 weeks and GFR below 20 mL/min. Patients have mean survival of less than 2 weeks. Type 2 HRS is characterized by increase in initial serum creatinine level less than 221/mmol/L. The main clinical consequence of type 2 HRS is diuretic-resistant ascites. Patients have longer median survival time of approximately 6 months.[36]

Treatment: Medical therapy is used to temporarily improve renal function while patient awaits liver transplantation.

Vasoconstrictors, such as vasopressin analogues, ornipressin and terlipressin and the alpha 1-adrenergic agonists like vasopressin have shown promising results by acting on V1 vasopressin receptors in vascular smooth muscle cells causing splanchnic vasoconstriction and increase in systemic and renal perfusion.

Patients given terlipressin have a 50–75% response rate defined as improved GFR to more than 40 mL/min but typically remains below normal. It acts as a bridge to liver transplant and improves prognosis after transplantation.[37]

Hemodialysis is not tolerated well by patients of HRS and is recommended only for medically resistant hyperkalemia or severe fluid overload. CRRT is also an option in these patients. Surgical options are TIPS and liver transplantation.[34]

Diet: Low sodium diet and fluid restriction are recommended

Medication: Vasoconstrictor agents, e.g. vasopressin analogs (e.g. ornipressin, terlipressin) or α_1 adrenergic agonists (e.g. norepinephrine, nidodrine) are used.[36]

HEPATOPULMONARY SYNDROME (TABLE 8.20)

The liver controls pulmonary vascular tone by releasing vasoactive substances. In severe liver failure, the imbalance between vasodilator and vasoconstrictive mediators leads to alteration of the respiratory function. A significant decrease of pulmonary vascular resistance occurs with development of intrapulmonary vascular dilatations and portopulmonary hypertension when vasoconstriction prevails with an increase of pulmonary vascular resistance.[38,39]

The clinical symptoms consist of dyspnea and hypoxemia. PaO_2 on ABG is <60 mm Hg.[38] Dyspnea develops on lying flat. Hypoxemia worsens on sitting up and improves when lying flat.

Platypnea and orthodeoxia occur because the pulmonary AVMs occur predominantly in the bases of lung causing blood to pool in bases when sitting up or standing.

Treatment: Supplemental oxygen is required for treatment of symptoms. Other therapies, such as somatostatin to inhibit vasodilatation are of modest benefit. Inhaled nitric oxide synthesis inhibitors may be a future treatment option.[41] HPS regresses after liver transplant.

HEPATIC HYDROTHORAX

Hepatic hydrothorax is defined as presence of pleural fluid (usually >500 mL) in patients with cirrhosis in the absence of primary cardiac or pulmonary disease. It occurs in 5–10% of cirrhotic patients.[42]

Due to capacitance of peritoneal cavity large volume of ascites is usually well tolerated but even 1–2 liters of fluid within pleural cavity can lead to shortness of breath, cough and hypoxemia. Chest tube drainage of pleural effusion is not recommended due to the possibility of volume loss and renal failure.

Pleural effusion in patients with chronic liver disease requires evaluation and also treatment which is similar to treatment of ascites

The recommended steps of evaluation and treatment are shown in Flow chart 8.9.

Table 8.20: Hepatopulmonary syndrome vs portopulmonary hypertension (HPS v/s PPHTN)[40]

	HPS	*PPHTN*
Pathophysiology	AV shunting in lungs particularly at bases	Intense pulmonary vasoconstriction and thickened pulmonary vasculature
Symptoms	Platypnea	Dyspnea on exertion, syncope, orthopnea
Physical findings	Hypoxemia, orthodeoxia	Loud P2, TR murmur, normal SpO_2 at rest
Echocardiogram	Positive bubble study	Elevated pulmonary artery systolic pressure
Treatment	Liver transplant	Same as primary pulmonary HTN, if mean PAP <40 mm Hg
		Can safely undergo liver transplant

Proposed Mechanisms for the Development of Hepatic Hydrothorax[43,45]

- Azygous vein hypertension causing formation of collateral anastomoses between portal and azygous systems.
- Transfer of peritoneal fluid into the pleural space via diaphragmatic defects and transdiaphragmatic lymphatics.
- Hypoalbuminemia resulting in decreased colloid osmotic pressure.
- Lymphatic leakage from the thoracic duct.

Clinical and Laboratory Features of Hepatic Hydrothorax[43]

Location

- Right sided (85%)
- Left sided (13%)
- Bilateral (2%)

No pericardial effusion

Flow chart 8.9: Evaluation and treatment of hepatic hydrothorax

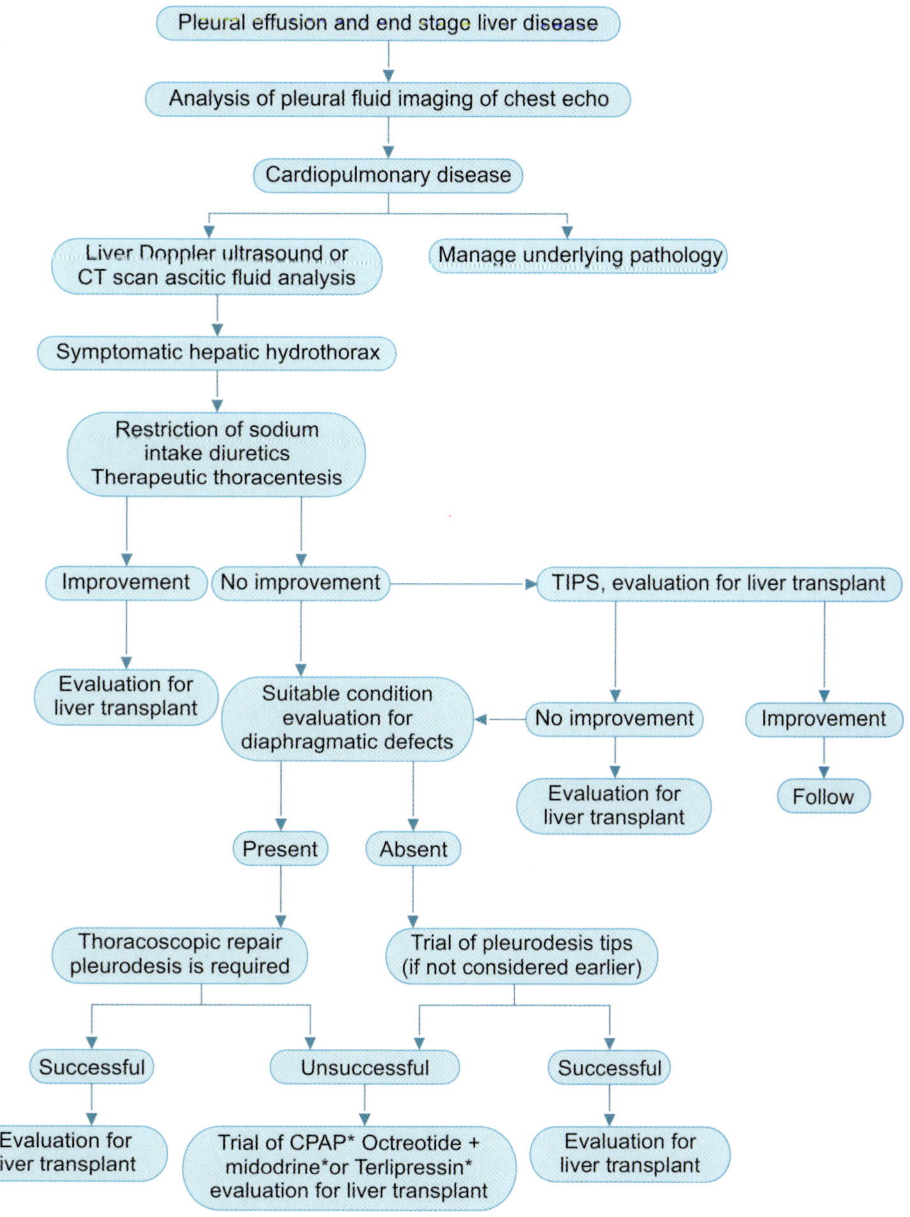

Laboratory Features[44]

- Cell count < 500 cells/mm^3
- Total protein concentration < 2.5 g/dL
- Total protein pleural fluid to serum ratio < 0.5
- Lactate dehydrogenase pleural fluid to serum ratio < 0.5
- Serum to pleural fluid albumin gradient > 1.1 g/dL
- Pleural fluid amylase concentration < serum amylase concentration
- pH 7.40 to 7.55.

Coagulation Disorders

Patients with ESLD show hemostatic defects. They have impaired coagulation due to reduced synthesis of clotting factors and vitamin K deficiency, systemic fibrinolysis due to reduced synthesis of α_2 antitrypsin and thrombin activatable fibrinolysis inhibitor, thrombocytopenia due to sequestration due to splenomegaly, impaired synthesis of thrombopoietin and immune destruction.[46] These patients also have platelet dysfunction due to circulating platelet inhibitors, excess nitric oxide production and deficiency of platelet glycoprotein receptors.[46, 47]

Disseminated intravascular coagulation can occur due to release of procoagulants from injured hepatocytes, impaired clearance of activated clotting factors and reduced synthesis of coagulation inhibitors.[46, 48]

Patients of ESLD show thrombotic complications. Hepatic vein thrombosis is common in cirrhotic patients.[49] Portal vein thrombosis occurs in 9–20% of patients with cirrhosis, and is more frequent in those with advanced disease.[49] These patients have antithrombin, protein C and protein S levels in range of 30–65% of normal. The high level of procoagulant factors (VWF, fibrinogen and FVIII) may contribute to hypercoaguability.[50,51]

Treatment: The hemostatic defects need to be corrected in patients who are actively bleeding, require surgery or an invasive procedure. The aim of therapy is to achieve hemostatic competence rather than complete correction of abnormal laboratory values.[46]

Patients with INR > 2.0 (with normal aPTT or aPTT >1.3 × control) may require fresh frozen plasma. If fibrinogen levels are <125 mg/dL, cryoprecipitate may be required and in patients with platelet count <50,000–75,000/mL, platelet transfusion may be considered[46] (for invasive procedure). A platelet count of 10,000/mL is a common trigger for platelet transfusion.

Osteopenia and Osteoporosis

Osteoporosis and fractures are common in patients of CLD. It is common in patients with primary biliary cirrhosis, primary sclerosing cholangitis, chronic hepatitis C and alcoholic cirrhosis.[52]

Oral daily intake of 800/IU of vitamin D and 1–2g of elemental calcium is recommended. The guidelines for management of osteoporosis in patients with chronic liver failure recommend a baseline bone mineral densitometry. If T-score is more than –1.5 or between –1.5 to –2.5 no treatment is recommended. Patients with BMD less than –2.5 should have thyroid function test, serum calcium, phosphate, estradiol, follicle stimulating hormone, leutinizing hormone, testosterone and sex hormone binding globulin levels.[52]

Premenopausal women can be given hormone replacement therapy with estrogen and progesterone and transdermal testosterone in hypogonadal men. Patients intolerant to HRT/ testosterone or bisphosphonates can be given calcitriol or calcitonin.

Malnutrition

Severe malnutrition is associated with an increased need for packed red blood cells, FFP and cryoprecipitate during liver transplantation.

In patients with end stage liver disease, parenteral and enteral nutrition should be started. High carbohydrate and/ or high-lipid supplements with decreased amino acid content are recommended. Patients with alcoholic liver disease and Wernicke encephalopathy benefit from preoperative vitamin B supplementation.[53]

CLINICAL PEARLS

Recommendations as proposed by American Association of Study of Liver Disease (AASLD) are:[54]

- Patients with cirrhosis should be referred for transplantation when they develop evidence of hepatic dysfunction (CTP > 7 and MELD > 10) or when they experience their first major complication (ascites, variceal bleeding, or hepatic encephalopathy).
- Children with chronic liver disease should be referred when they deviate from normal growth curves or develop evidence of hepatic dysfunction or portal hypertension.
- Patients with type I hepatorenal syndrome should have an expedited referral for liver transplantation.
- Chronic smokers, patients over the age of 50, and those with a clinical or family history of heart disease or diabetes should undergo evaluation for coronary artery disease.

- All patients undergoing evaluation for potential liver transplantation should undergo screening for pulmonary hypertension.
- Patients with severe pulmonary hypertension should be considered for liver transplantation only if the condition can be effectively controlled with medical therapy.
- Morbid obesity should be considered a contraindication to liver transplantation.
- The presence of renal insufficiency is an important predictor of postoperative renal failure and mortality after liver transplantation, and hence a thorough pretransplantation evaluation of renal function is important.
- Selected patients with chronic renal and liver disease should be considered for combined liver-kidney transplantation.
- All patients with chronic liver disease should be screened for osteoporosis during evaluation for liver transplantation.
- Patients with clinically decompensated cirrhosis from chronic hepatitis C infection should be referred for consideration of liver transplantation.
- Patients with decompensated cirrhosis secondary to chronic hepatitis B should be considered for treatment with antiviral therapy in coordination with the transplant center.
- The posttransplantation care of patients with HBV should include antiviral therapy.
- Liver transplantation should be considered in decompensated patients with autoimmune hepatitis who are unable to undergo or be salvaged by medical therapy.
- Transplantation should be delayed for a minimum of 3 to 6 months of abstinence from alcohol to avoid exposing patients who may not need transplantation to the risk of unnecessary surgery.
- Liver transplantation is the only effective treatment for liver failure secondary to primary biliary cirrhosis and for decompensated cirrhosis secondary to primary sclerosing cholangitis.
- Because of the high incidence of colon cancer, regularly scheduled colonoscopies should be performed both before and after transplantation in all patients who have inflammatory bowel disease.
- Careful assessment for lung disease should be performed before transplantation in patients with cirrhosis secondary to α-1-antitrypsin deficiency, although coexistent disease in uncommon.
- Urgent liver transplantation is the only effective option for patients with fulminant hepatic failure resulting from Wilson disease.
- Liver transplantation should be considered for selected patients with decompensated cirrhosis secondary to non-alcoholic steatohepatitis (NASH) cryptogenic cirrhosis. The posttransplantation care of these patients should include metabolic monitoring.
- Liver transplantation should be viewed as the treatment of choice for selected patients with hepatocellular carcinoma who are not candidates for surgical resection and in whom malignancy is confined to the liver.
- Optimal results following transplantation are achieved in patients with a single lesion 2 cm or larger and less than 5 cm, or no more than three lesions, the largest of which is less than 3 cm, and no radiographic evidence of extrahepatic disease.
- Liver retransplantation, which is the only means of prolonging life in patients whose initial graft has failed, makes an important contribution to overall survival and should be considered in selected patients with primary graft failure, hepatic artery thrombosis, severe rejection, or recurrent disease. However, retransplantation is associated with diminished survival and increased costs compared with primary transplantation. Retransplantation should be considered before patients develop severe hepatic and renal failure.

REFERENCES

1. Sherwood, Lauralee. Human Physiology. From Cells to Systems. 3rd edn. Boston: Wadsworth 1997.
2. Liver a Vital Organ 24 April, 2002 http:/1www.liverfoundation.org/html.
3. Saab S, Han SH, Martin P. Liver transplantation. Selection, listing criteria and preoperative management. Clin Liver Dis Aug, 2000; 4(3):513-32 (Medline).
4. Neuberger J, Schulz KH, Day C, et al. Transplantation for alcoholic liver disease: does it matter? J Hepatol, 2003;38:629-34 (Pubmed).
5. Roche B, Feray C, Gigon M, et al. HBV DNA persistence 10 years after liver transplantation. Hepatology, 2003;38:86-95.
6. Villamil FG. Prophylaxis with anti-HBs immune globulins and nucleoside analogues after liver transplantation for HBV infection. J Hepatol, 2003;38:86-95 (Pubmed).
7. Ben Ari-Z, Mor E, Tur-Kaspa R. Experience with lamivudine therapy for hepatitis B virus infection in liver transplantation recipient. J Intern Med, 2003;253(5):544-52.
8. Varela M, Sala M, Llovet JM, Bruix J. Treatment of hepatocellular carcinoma: is there an optimal strategy? Cancer Treat Rev, 2003; 29:99-104.
9. Mazzaferro V, Regalia E, Doci R, et al. Liver transplantation for treatment of small hepatocellular carcinoma in patients with cirrhosis. N Engl J Med, 1996;334:693-9.
10. Pugh RN, Murray-Lyon IM, Dawson JL, Pietronic MC, Williams R. Transection of esophagus for bleeding esophageal varices. The British Journal of Surgery, 1973;60(8):646-9.
11. Malinchoc M, Kamath PS, Gordon FD, et al. A model to predict poor survival in patients undergoing transjugular intrahepatic portosystemic shunts. Hepatology, 2000;31(4):864-71.

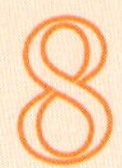

12. Kamath PS, Wiesner RH, Malinchoc M, Kremers W, et al. A model to predict survival in patients with end-stage liver disease. Hepatology, 2001;33(2):464-70.
13. UNOS: MELD/PELD calculator documentation. 2009.
14. Wiesner, et al. Model for end-stage liver disease (MELD) and allocation of donor livers. Gastroenterology, 2003;124(1):91-6.
15. http/www.scribd.com/doc/The-Milan-Criteria-for-HCC.
16. Yao FY, Bass NM, et al. Liver transplantation for hepatocellular carcinoma: expansion of the tumor size limits doesnot adversely impact survival. Hepatology, 2001;33:1394-1403.
17. Cosme Manzarbeitia, Julian Katz, et al. Liver Transplantation. Medscape reference: 2012.
18. Dells SG, Bakoyiannis A, Biliatis I, et al. Model for end-stage liver disease (MELD) score as a prognostic factor for postoperative morbidity and mortality in cirrhotic patients. HPB (Oxford), 2009; 11(4):351-7.
19. Child CG, Turcott JG. Surgery and portal hypertension. Major Prob/Clin Surg, 1964;1:1-85 (Medline).
20. Joel J, Heidelbaugh MD, et al. Am Fam Physician, 2006;74(5):767-76.
21. De Franchis R, Primignani M. Why do varices bleed? Gastroenterol Clin N Am, 1992;21:81-101.
22. Friedman S. Alcoholic liver disease, cirrhosis and its major sequaelae. In: Goldman L, Benett JC, eds. Textbook of Medicine 21st edn. Philadelphia Pa: Saunders, 2000;804-12.
23. Jutabha R, Jensen DM, et al. Randomized study comparing banding and propranolol to prevent initial variceal haemorrhage in cirrhotics with high risk esophageal varices. Gastroenterology, 2005;128:870-81.
24. Carbonell N, Pauwells A, Serfaty L, et al. Improved survival after variceal bleeding in patients with cirrhosis over the past two decades. Hepatology, 2004;40:652-9.
25. Rossle M, Richter GM. New non operative treatment for variceal haemorrhage. Lancet, 1989;2(8655):153.
26. David Patch, Lucy Dagher. Acute variceal bleeding: General management. World J Gastroentero, 2001;7(4):456-75.
27. Garcia-Tsao, Sanyal AJ. Practice Guidelines Committee of Association for study of liver diseases: Prevention and management of gastroesophageal varices and variceal haemorrhage in cirrhosis. Am J Gastroenter, 2007;102:2086-2102.
28. Fitz JG. Hepatic encephalopathy, hepatopulmonary syndrome, hepatorenal syndrome, coagulopathy and endocrine complications of liver disease. In: Feldman M, Friedman LS, Sleisenger MH, eds. Sleisenger and Fordtran's Gastrointestinal and liver disease: Pathophysiology, Diagnosis, Management. 7th edn. Philadelphia Pa: Saunders, 2002;1543-54.
29. Strauss E, Tramote R, Silva EP, et al. Double blind randomized trial comparing neomycin and placebo in treatment of hepatic encephalopathy. Hepatogastroenterology, 1992;39:542-5.
30. Cash WJ, McConville P, Mc Dermott E, et al. Current concepts in assessment and treatment of hepatic encephalopathy QJM, 2010; 103(1):9-16.
31. Runyon BA. Care of patients with ascites. N Eng J Med, 1994;330: 337-42.
32. Runyon BA. Management of adult patients with ascites caused by cirrhosis. Hepatology, 1998;27:264-72.
33. Gines P, Arroyo V, Vargas V, et al. Paracentesis with intravenous infusion of albumin as compared with peritoneovenous shunting in cirrhosis with refractory ascites. N Engl J Med, 1991;325: 829-35.
34. Ochs A, Rossle M, Haag K, et al. The transjugular intrahepatic portosystemic shunt procedure for refractory ascites. N Eng J Med, 1995;332:1192-97.
35. Arroyo V, Gines P, Gerbes AL, et al. Definition and diagnostic criteria of refractory ascites and hepatorenal syndrome in cirrhosis. International Ascites Club. Hepatology, 1996;23:164-76.
36. Moreau R. Hepatorenal syndrome in patients with cirrhosis. J Gastroenterol Hepatol, 2002;17:739-47.
37. Ortega R, Gines P, Uriz J, et al. Terlipressin therapy with and without albumin for patients with hepatorenal syndrome. Results of a prospective, nonrandomized study. Hepatology, 2002;36:941-48.
38. Krovoka MJ. Hepatopulmonary syndrome. In: Plenak D SL, edn. Critical care Issues in Liver transplantation. The American Association for Study of Liver Diseases and the International Liver Transplantation Society, 1999;58-65.
39. Herve P, Lebrec D, Brenot. Pulmonary vascular disorders in portal hypertension. Eur Respir J, 1998;11:1153-66.
40. Budhiraja R, Hassoun PM. Portopulmonary hypertension: a tale of two circulations. Chest, 2003;123(2):562-76.
41. Krowka M. Hepatopulmonary syndrome and liver transplantation. Liver Transpl, 2001;6:113-15.
42. Alberts WM, Salem AJ, Soloman DA, et al. Hepatic hydrothorax. Cause and Management. Arch Intern Medicine, 1991;151:2383-388.
43. Garcia N Jr, Mihas AA. Hepatic hydrothorax: Pathophysiology diagnosis and management. Clin Gastroenterol, 2004;38:52-8.
44. Gur C, Ilan Y, Shibolet O. Hepatic hydrothorax – pathophysiology, diagnosis, treatment–review of literature. Liver Int, 2004;24:281-4.
45. Camron Kaifar, Nooman Gilani. Hepatic hydrothorax current concepts of pathophysiology and treatment options. Annals of Hepatology, 2008;7(4):313-20.
46. Jody L Kujovich. Hemostatic defects in end-stage liver disease. Crit Care Clin, 2005;21:563-587.
47. Escolar G, Cases A, Vinas M, et al. Evaluation of acquired platelet dysfunction in uremio and cirrhotic patients using platelet function analyser (PFA-100). Haematologica, 1999;84:614-9.
48. Bakker CM, Knot CA, Stibbe J, et al. Disseminated intravascular coagulation in liver cirrhosis. J Hepatol, 1992;15:330-35.
49. Wanless IR,Wong F, Blenddis LM, et al. Hepatic and portal vein thrombosis in cirrhosis: possible role in development of parenchymal extinction and portal hypertension. Hepatology, 1995;21:1238-47.
50. Koster T, Blann AD, Briet E, et al. Role of clotting factor VIII in effect of von Willebrand factor on occurance of deep vein thrombosis. Lancet, 1995;345:152-5.
51. Amitrano L, Guardascione MA, Brancaccio V, et al. Risk factors and clinical presentation of portal vein thrombosis in patients with liver cirrhosis. J Hepatol, 2004;40:736-41.
52. Collier JD, Ninkovic M, Compston JE. Guidelines on the management of osteoporosis associated with chronic liver disease. Gut, 2002;50(suppl 1):1-9.
53. Muller MJ. Malnutrition in cirrhosis. J Hepatol, 1995;23(suppl 1): 31-35.
54. Karen F Murray, Robert L, Carithers Jr. AASLD practice guidelines: Evaluation of the patient for liver transplantation. Hepatology, 2005;41(6):1-26.

Surgical Technique in Liver Transplantation

Naimish Mehta, Vibha Varma, Vinay Kumaran

INTRODUCTION

Liver transplantation (LT) is a lifesaving procedure for patients who have end-stage liver disease. Liver failure can be either acute (fulminant or subfulminant failure) or chronic (decompensated cirrhosis). Dr Thomas Starzl attempted the first human LT in 1963, but a successful LT was not achieved until 1967. Initial outcomes were modest but with refinements in surgical techniques, a better understanding of donor and recipient management and the discovery of immunosuppressive drugs like cyclosporine and tacrolimus led to significant improvement in the transplant outcomes. All these advances established liver transplantation as an excellent treatment modality for end stage liver disease, with current 1-year patient survival rate of 85–90% and 5-year survival rate of 75%. Approximately 10,000 transplants are performed annually worldwide, and despite this most centers are reporting an increase in waiting list mortality. The main impairment to wider application of liver transplantation is the shortage of donor organs. Living-donor liver transplantation (LDLT) was introduced as a logical extension of reduced size liver transplantation. The advantages include selection of an ideal donor, ability to schedule the case electively, maximal time to prepare the recipient, and relatively short cold ischemia time. However, while living-donor transplantation increases the number of livers available for the pediatric and adult recipient pools, donor safety remains an important concern. Approximately 5–10% of orthotopic LT in Europe and the USA are living related grafts, as opposed to a vast majority being living donor grafts in Asian countries (Japan, Korea, Hong Kong), as well as in India where deceased donor organ donation is less frequent.

INDICATIONS FOR LIVER TRANSPLANTATION

A patient suffering from end stage liver disease is a potential candidate for liver transplantation with an overall goal of prolonging and improving the quality of life. The liver could be damaged due to various reasons as listed in Table 8.21. However presence of cirrhosis alone is not sufficient to warrant transplantation. Patients are considered for transplantation when they develop evidence of irreversible hepatic decompensation (variceal bleeding, ascites, bacterial peritonitis, encephalopathy, hepatorenal syndrome, hepato-pulmonary syndrome, cancer) or severely impaired quality of life due to associated disease.

Liver Transplantation for Acute Liver Failure (ALF)

The ALF is defined as sudden onset of jaundice, encephalopathy, coagulopathy <8 weeks (fulminant hepatic failure) or progressive liver failure of less than 26 weeks duration (subfulminant) with no pre-existing liver disease. ALF accounts for approximately 5% to 6% of all liver transplantations. Acetaminophen drug overdose is the leading cause of ALF in western countries, whereas cryptogenic and Wilson's disease

Table 8.21: Indications for liver transplantation

Acute/Fulminant liver failure:
- Seronegative hepatitis (sporadic non A non B hepatitis)
- Drugs (paracetamol, isoniazid)
- Viral (hepatitis B)
- Metabolic (neonatal hemochromatosis, Wilson's disease)

Chronic liver disease:
- Viral hepatitis B,C
- Autoimmune hepatitis
- Cholestatic disorders (Primary sclerosing cholangitis, Primary biliary cirrhosis
- Extrahepatic biliary atresia
- Alcoholic liver disease (ALD)
- Budd-Chiari syndrome
- Veno-occlusive disease
- Non alcoholic steatohepatitis (NASH)
- Cryptogenic cirrhosis

Malignancy:
- Hepatocellular carcinoma
- Primary neuro-endocrine tumor

Metabolic disorders:
- Wilson's disease
- Hemochromatosis
- Alpha-1 antitrypsin deficiency
- Primary oxalosis, familial amyloid polyneuropathy
- Crigler-Najjar syndrome Type I

Miscellaneous:
- Polycystic liver disease

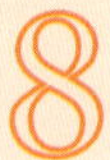

were leading causes in our series at Sir Ganga Ram Hospital, New Delhi. Indications for LT in patients with ALF are based on selection criteria based on King's College criteria.

King's College criteria for Nonacetaminophen etiology
INR >6.5 irrespective of degree of encephalopathy
Or
Any three of the following five criteria
Age <10 years or >40 years
Unfavorable etiology (sero-negative hepatitis or drug reaction)
Jaundice to encephalopathy interval of >7 days
INR >3.5 or PT>50sec
Serum bilirubin >17.5 mg/dL.

The ALF typically affects young individuals who had previously been in good health, with a mortality rate of 80% to 90%. Advent of LT has saved many such young lives with a success rate of more than 90%. However timely referral to a specialist center for liver transplantation is of paramount importance, because death from sepsis and cerebral edema may occur within days of the onset of stage 3 or 4 hepatic encephalopathy.

Timing of Referral

Selection and timing of patient referral for liver transplant evaluation is important to achieve optimal outcomes. The severity of liver disease is graded from A to C on the basis of child-Pugh scoring system. Usually all grade C and most patients with grade B are candidates for liver transplantation. In USA, the United Network for Organ Sharing (UNOS) adopted a system called the Model for End Stage Liver Disease (MELD) to prioritise candidates waiting for liver transplants based on a mathematical formula found to be useful for predicting mortality in patients listed for LT. Many transplant centers would consider a Child-Pugh score of 7 as appropriate for referral whereas others use a MELD score of 10 or above as an indication to list for liver transplantation.

RECIPIENT EVALUATION

The LDLT involves comprehensive preoperative workup, extensive planning, a complex operation, close monitoring and meticulous care in post-operative period and in the long-term. Patients would be listed for transplantation after a complete assessment by a multi-disciplinary team comprising of transplant surgeons, hepatologists, intensivists, anesthesiologists, psychiatrists, transplant coordinators, social workers and dieticians. Various investigations performed are listed in Table 8.22. These are done to ascertain the functioning of other body organs as end stage liver disease can have harmful effects on them.

Table 8.22: Recipient evaluation tests

Laboratory investigations
- Complete blood count, PT, aPTT
- Complete biochemistry, liver function tests
- Hepatitis (A, B, C), HIV, CMV, EBV, HSV serology
- Autoimmune hepatitis tests (ANA, AMA, SMA, immunoglobulins)
- Serum ceruloplasmin, ferritin, TIBC
- Serum alpha-1 antitrypsin
- Tumor markers
- Lipid profile, thyroid function tests
- Urinalysis
- Drug and alcohol blood level

Radiology
- Chest X-ray
- Liver ultrasound (U/S) and portal vein (PV), Doppler study
- Abdominal computed tomography (CT) scan—triphasic

Cardiovascular and pulmonary evaluation
- Echocardiography (ECG) and stress echocardiography
- Pulmonary function tests and arterial blood gases

Table 8.23: Blood group compatibility chart

Blood group	*Can donate liver for*	*Can receive a liver from*
O	O, A, B, AB	O
A	A, AB	A, O
B	B, AB	B, O
AB	AB	A, B, AB, O

DONOR EVALUATION

Who can be a Donor?

Donor needs to be from the family—mother, father, son, daughter, sister, brother, spouse (first degree relative). Donor should be healthy and blood group compatible (Table 8.23), who is willing to donate, in sound state of mind and, between 18–55 years of age.

Blood Group Compatibility Chart

Irrespective of the Rh factor, blood group compatibility is as mentioned in the Table. Rh+ or – does not make any difference.

Donor should not be pregnant or overweight, and should preferably have a BMI (body mass index) < 30. Those consuming alcohol on regular basis are not suitable; smokers should stop smoking ideally 6 weeks before surgery. Donor is counselled adequately both before and after the evaluation is completed.

Part of the Liver to be Removed and Regeneration

In a person having a normal functioning liver, 60–70% of liver can be safely removed. In an adult patient generally right lobe is taken as the graft and it constitutes 60% of the liver volume, while the left lobe which is 40% of whole liver volume is generally used as graft in small size adults or in larger children, the left lateral segment which constitutes 25% of the liver volume is sufficient for pediatric recipients. About 40–60% of liver is removed from living donor. Thirty percent of liver as remnant is adequate for the donor and this is what is left behind after donor hepatectomy, depending upon the volume required for the patient. Liver has a unique capacity to regenerate and hence the liver left behind in the donor grows back to normal size in 2–3 months and so does the grafted liver donated and implanted in the patient. This process of regeneration starts immediately following donor hepatectomy and liver transplantation, however full regeneration takes 2–3 months from the time of surgery.

Once a donor is identified, he/she is thoroughly investigated and cleared by various allied specialties before being taken up for surgery. As mentioned earlier donor is again counselled and explained about the surgery and the postoperative recovery.

Donor assessment involves three steps:

1. First step—Basic screening

   This involves blood grouping, complete blood count, and serum creatinine so that the next step of evaluation, triphasic CT scan can be performed. Viral markers for hepatitis B and C virus infection, liver function tests and plain CT-scan of the abdomen are also performed. Plain CT of the abdomen gives information about the fat content in the liver by calculating the liver attenuation index (LAI). Donor who is found to have fatty liver at this level would go either for biopsy or would be rejected depending on the value of liver attenuation index (LAI). Any LAI ≥6 is acceptable; those with LAI between 0 to 5 undergoes a liver biopsy to account for the fat content in the liver, if the patient does not have another donor. Any LAI < 0 is not accepted.
2. *Second step—Triphasic CT scan:* Once the basic screening is satisfactory, this imaging is done to look for the volume of the whole liver, volume of the part to be removed and that of the remnant liver. The right or left lobe of the liver is removed as the graft for the patient depending upon whether the volume of that part of the liver is at least 0.8–1% of the patient's body weight. At the same time the remnant liver volume in the donor should be at least 30% of the whole volume of the liver.

   Liver biopsy is done if the LAI is < 5 and more than 0, when there is no other live donor. If the body mass index (BMI) is > 30, the donor is asked to reduce weight; liver biopsy is done after the BMI has reduced to < 30. Any fat content >20% is not acceptable, between 15–20% is acceptable once the final volume is adequate after taking into account for the fat content. Apart from giving information about the volume it also gives information about the vascular anatomy of the liver. This guides the donor surgery and also helps in planning the implantation of the new liver into the patient.
3. *Third step-advanced work-up:* Once the liver is found to be fat free and of adequate volume, the remaining investigations are guided towards ruling out any overt abnormalities in other systems of the body and also for fitness before a major surgical procedure. Chest physician, cardiologist, hepatologist, gynecologist (in case of female donors), psychiatrist (to assess donors mental fitness and willingness to donate to ensure that donation is voluntary and without any coercion) and anesthesiologist's clearance is obtained before surgery. This requires various investigations pertaining to the different organ systems.
4. Donor and recipient have an authorization committee clearance before transplantation to ensure related organ donation and to prevent donation with ulterior motives. Relation is established through documentary evidences/ affidavits and tissue matching by HLA testing.

SURGICAL PROCEDURE

The recipient operation involves 3 steps:

Recipient Hepatectomy

Position and Incision

The patient is placed in the supine position with both arms abducted. A 'Mercedes-Benz' incision is made.

Mobilization of the Right and Left Lobe

The falciform ligament is divided with the help of diathermy till the groove between right and middle hepatic vein is identified. Self-retaining retractors (Omnitract) are then placed to allow for wider exposure (Figs 8.1A and B). Wet abdominal sponges are then placed to keep the bowels at bay. The left triangular ligament is then divided till the edge of left

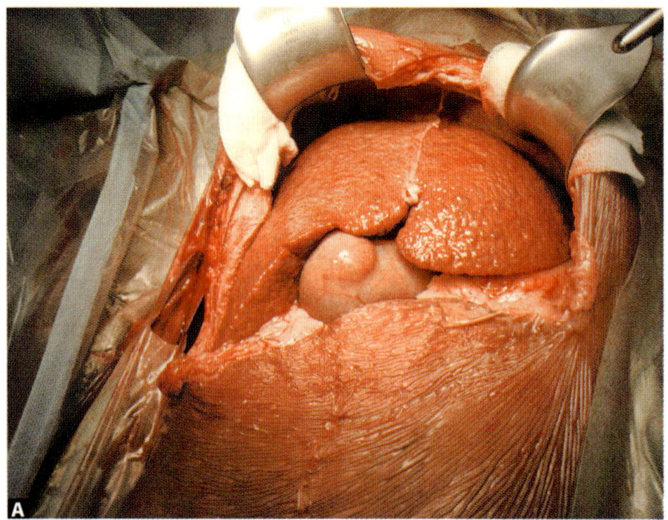

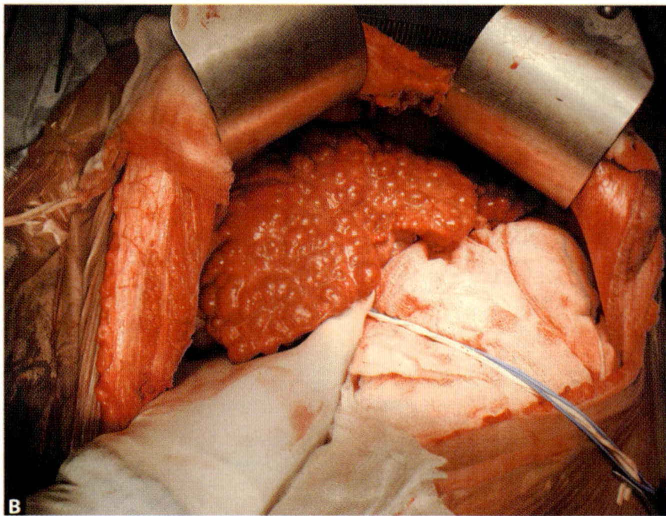

Figs 8.1A and B: (A) Wide exposure with self-retaining retractor (Recipient); (B) Grossly cirrhotic liver

hepatic vein is seen. The gastrohepatic omentum is serially clamped, cut and ligated with appropriate care being taken to dissect for any accessory or replaced left hepatic artery (LHA). The right triangular and coronary ligaments are divided and right lobe mobilized from the retroperitoneum till the edge of right hepatic vein (RHV). The right lobe is cautiously freed of any adhesions inferiorly, since there is high incidence of bleeding due to portal hypertension.

Posterior Caval Dissection

Right adrenal vein needs to be carefully dissected, clamped, cut and doubly ligated to allow access for looping the inferior vena cava (IVC). This gives good control in the eventuality of excessive bleeding which is not uncommon and this also allows space for clamping the IVC at the caudal end during implantation. The IVC is then dissected off the retroperitoneum with Lahey's right angled dissector and the intervening tissues are carefully tied with 2-0 silk sutures.

Dissection of the Porta

The differentiating point in preparation of the recipient for receiving deceased donor graft and living donor graft lies in 'high hilar dissection' thereby preserving adequate length of hepatic artery, portal vein and the bile duct for anastomoses. Portal dissection is commenced with identification of cystic artery and duct, which are ligated and divided. The common bile duct (CBD) is looped while preserving its vascular supply. Left hepatic artery is identified and dissected till its origin from the common hepatic artery. Dissection is further carried on the right hepatic artery (RHA) till its anterior and posterior divisions. In doing so, small branches supplying the bile duct are cut between ligatures. Segment 4 hepatic artery is also dissected till its entry point into the liver. We ligate the artery after the donor team has completed partial transection of the liver and identified the course of middle hepatic vein (MHV). The bile duct is further dissected up into the hilum so as to get secondary divisions of the duct. This enables duct to duct and tension-free anastomoses of the bile duct especially if the graft has more than a single duct. Portal vein lying posterior to the common bile duct and the artery is isolated and looped. Rest of the structures in the porta are divided between ligatures or with diathermy. The portal vein is dissected proximally till supra-pancreatic portion and distally until the bifurcation.

Anterior Caval Dissection

The liver and the right lobe are rotated to the left, allowing for anterior caval dissection, and liver/caudate lobe is mobilized from IVC after dividing the retrohepatic veins. The dissection on anterior IVC is continued till the RHV is looped (Fig. 8.2).

Division of Portal Structures

At this stage portal vein clamping is performed to allow division of the bile duct high onto the hilar plate. A vascular clamp is placed on the proximal end of the duct to avoid obscuring the field due to bleeding. Portal vein is divided just below the bifurcation and distal end is sutured with 4–0 prolene (Fig. 8.3). The portal vein of the explant liver will

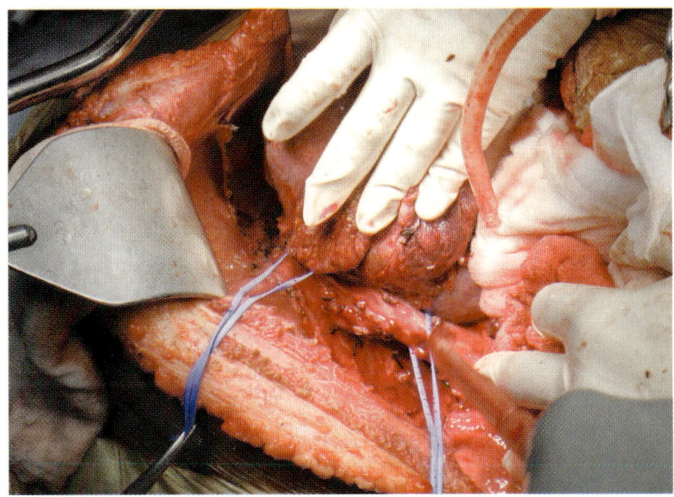

Fig. 8.2: Anterior caval dissection with looping of right hepatic vein and inferior vena cava

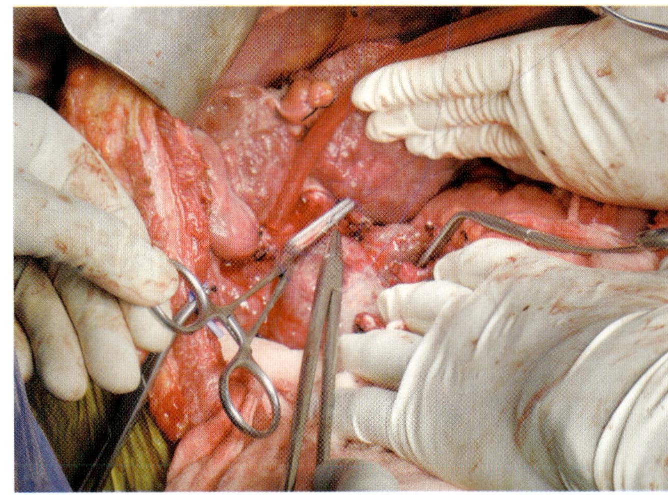

Fig. 8.3: Division of portal vein

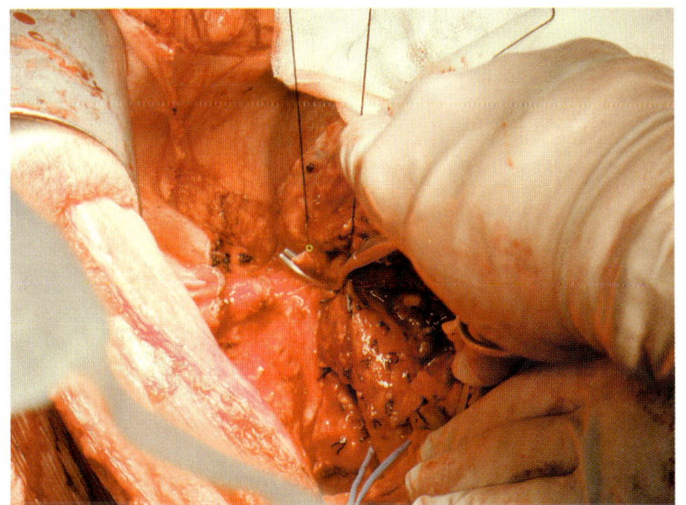
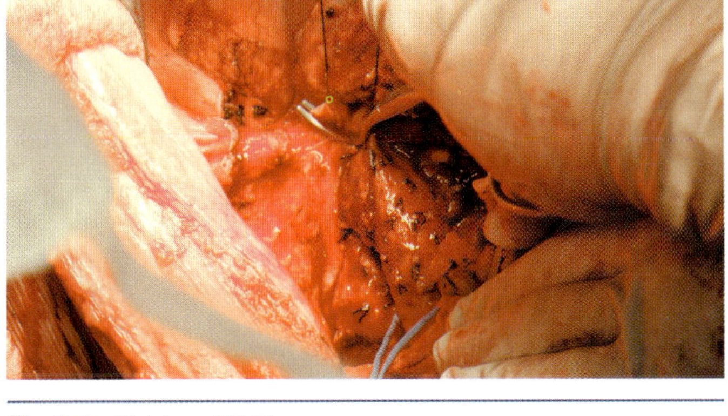

Fig. 8.4: Division of RHV

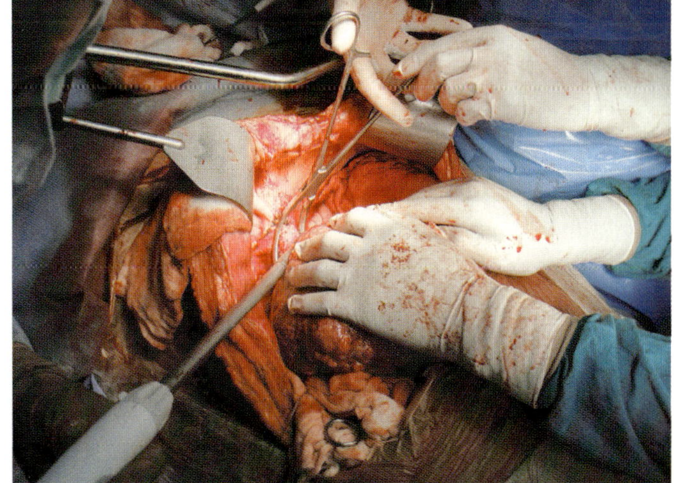

Fig. 8.5: Division of MHV and LHV

be retrieved on bench for the graft 'Middle hepatic venous reconstruction'.

Division of Hepatic Veins

Right hepatic vein is then clamped, cut and sutured with 4–0 prolene continuous suture (Fig. 8.4). Retro-hepatic cava is further dissected till the MHV and LHV are the only structures holding the liver back. To facilitate this, liver is retracted towards right and operating table is given a left upper tilt. The MHV and LHV are divided with the use of stapler 45 mm vascular stapler and liver explanted (Fig. 8.5). The surface of the IVC and the retroperitoneum are carefully examined and hemostasis is achieved.

The process of implantation is different for the graft from a living donor and that from the deceased donor.

Perioperative Instructions/Prophylaxis

Donor is kept fasting as for any other major procedure under general anesthesia for 6 hours. Intravenous antibiotics are administered at induction of anesthesia, sequential compression devices are applied prior to induction as a prophylaxis for deep venous thrombosis. Warming blankets are used intra-operatively to prevent hypothermia. Nasogastric tube is placed at the time of surgery, which is generally kept till the first postoperative day. It is important to have low central venous pressure during parenchymal transection.

Donor Hepatectomy in Living Donor

Donor hepatectomy is more challenging than the same surgery performed for a tumor because of important facts such as: (1) Liver must be harvested with all the vessels, and any inferior hepatic veins of caliber greater than 5 mm must be preserved in case of right lobe, (2) A precise line of parenchymal transection must be marked, (3) The biliary radicals must be well vascularized and (4) The parenchymal transection must be performed with full perfusion of the liver. The steps of surgery which follow elaborate this concept.

Position: Supine with the left arm by the side of the patient.

Incision: Bilateral subcostal with midline extension. For the right lobe graft, the extent of subcostal incision on the left side is limited.

Laparotomy: A quick exploration of the abdomen rules out any gross abnormality which might have been missed on preoperative evaluation, for example: tubercles on the visceral or parietal peritoneum, any abnormal lesions, fatty liver, etc. If the liver appears fatty, a biopsy is performed and frozen section report is requested. This is to rule out macrosteatosis in the graft (>20%).

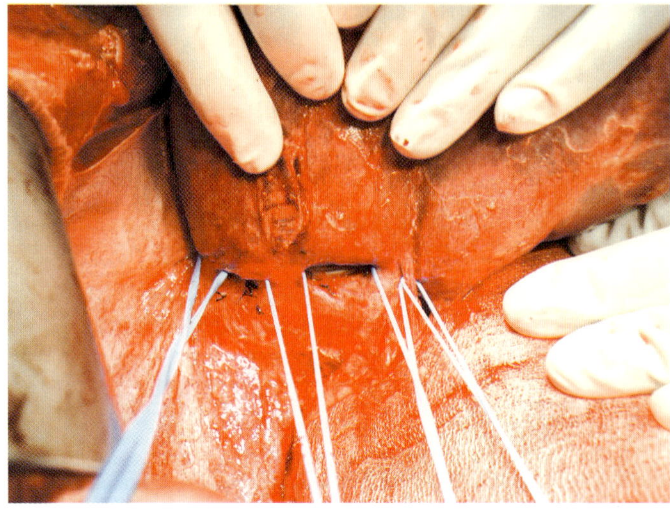

Fig. 8.6: Looping of RHA and right inferior hepatic veins 1 and 2

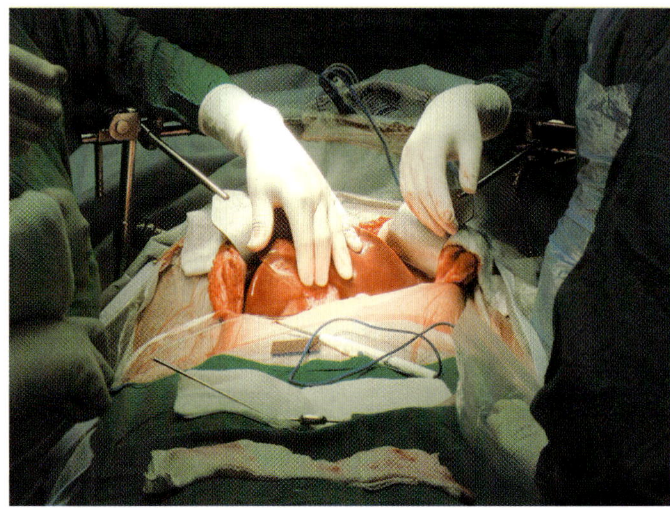

Fig. 8.7: Wide exposure with self-retaining retractor (Donor)

Right Lobe Graft

Mobilization

The falciform ligament is divided till it divides into the right and left triangular ligament and the IVC is identified and the groove between RHV and MHV is identified. The right lobe is mobilized further by dividing the triangular ligament and the right edge of RHV is identified. The right lobe is then mobilized so that the IVC is exposed and any short hepatic veins smaller than 5 mm are ligated while those more than or equal to 5 mm are preserved for implantation into the recipient. This ensures proper venous drainage of all the segments of the graft. The retrohepatic-cava is dissected to the extent that the line between the RHV and MHV down to the midportion of the caudate process is cleared. The RHV is dissected and looped before starting the portal dissection (Fig. 8.6).

Hilar Dissection

Peritoneum over the hepatoduodenal ligament is divided to identify the important vascular biliary anatomy. The side of liver to be removed guides the decision for the limits of dissection of the vascular and biliary radicals. Gall bladder is dissected off the liver bed carefully so that the capsule of the liver is not breached. Cystic duct is identified, cannulated with infant feeding tube for intra-operative cholangiogram (IOC), prior to which the patient is given amikacin injection and the cystic duct is divided towards the gall bladder; the cystic artery is also identified and divided well towards the gall bladder (Fig. 8.7). IOC is then performed. Contrast is injected into the infant feeding tube which has been primed earlier with saline to remove any air bubbles which would interfere with the interpretation of the biliary anatomy. About 5 mL of contrast is injected into the cystic duct and while doing so the lower end of bile duct is closed by pinching it between the left thumb and index finger so that the dye does not go down into the duodenum. IOC thus performed is studied to find out the biliary anatomy, it adds to the information obtained from the prior MRCP (Fig. 8.8). Additional information about the biliary anatomy especially regarding any anomalous biliary

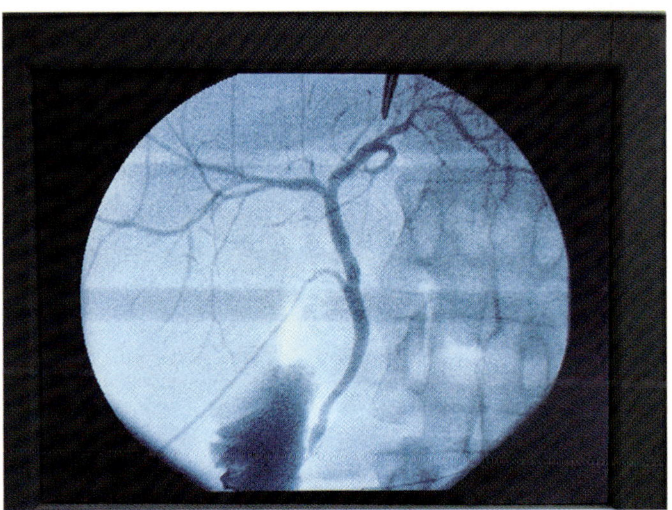

Fig. 8.8: Intraoperative cholangiogram for biliary anatomy

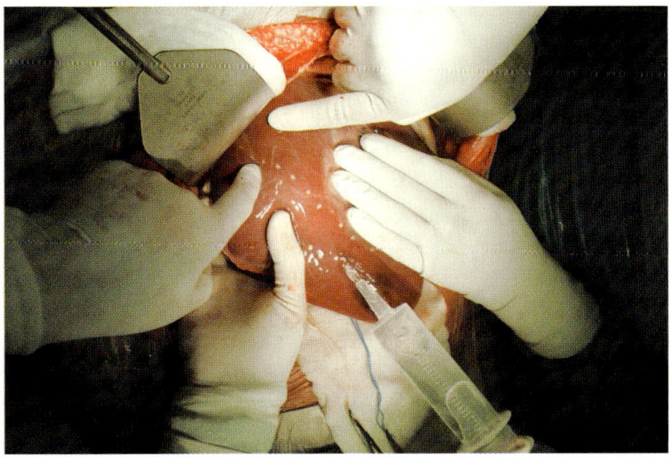

Fig. 8.10: Line of transection between right and left lobes after temporary clamping of RHA and RPV

radicals crossing from the right to the left or vice versa is identified and taken care of during parenchymal transection and division of the bile duct.

Porta hepatis dissection is then resumed. The cystic artery is followed proximally to identify the right hepatic artery. If the segment-4 artery is arising from the RHA, the division of the right hepatic is distal to the segment-4 artery. For the right sided graft, left lobe is not mobilized and similarly the vascular and biliary radicals are not dissected. However the LHA is identified. The right artery is dissected carefully without handling the adventitia too much and is dissected off the right hepatic duct. The RPV is identified and is dissected all around before looping and any caudate tributaries are divided between ligatures (Fig. 8.9).

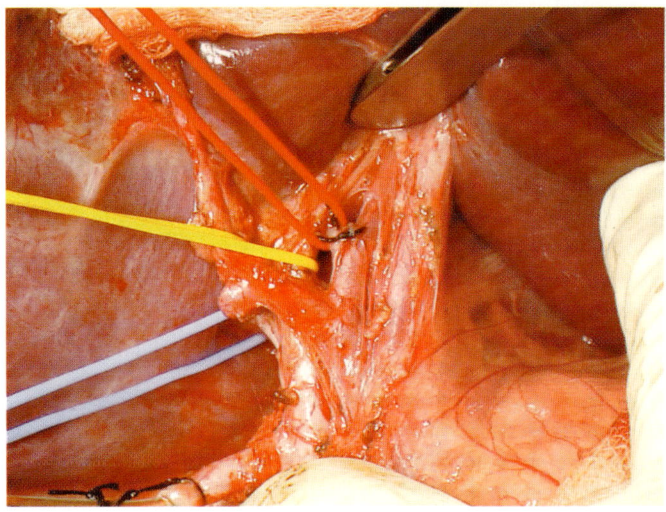

Fig. 8.9: Looping of right side hilar structures, right hepatic artery and right portal vein

Parenchymal Transection

The RHA and RPV so identified are temporarily clamped with vascular bulldog clamps to identify the line of demarcation between the right and left lobe of liver. This line is marked with a diathermy and the clamps are then taken off (Fig. 8.10). The line of transection is from the groove in between the RHV and MHV on the antero-superior surface of liver to the midportion of gall bladder bed and inferiorly till it reaches the hilar plate. Parenchymal transection is done using a combination of CUSA (cavitron ultrasonic suction and aspiration device), bipolar cautery with saline irrigation and monopolar cautery. The parenchymal transection is started from the inferior border of the liver (gallbladder bed) and the aim is to identify the formation of MHV by following the segment 4b and segment 5 tributaries. Once the MHV is identified it is followed carefully without injuring it and the transection line is very close to it, in other words it is cored out of the left lobe so that the segment 4 and the segment 4b/fissural vein is left intact. This ensures proper venous drainage of the remnant. The MHV is followed up proximally till the segment 8 tributaries have joined it and the segment 4b vein is identified. Depending upon the presence or absence of segment 4b/fissural vein, and the point at which the segment-8 vein drains, the graft is taken with subtotal or partial MHV. Once the junction of segment 8 and MHV is identified, it is looped. The RHV is also dissected superiorly all around so that the vascular clamp can be applied later, before it is divided. The last bit of parenchymal transection is done using the 'hanging maneuver' whereby a number 12 Fr Ryles tube is passed above in the groove between the RHV

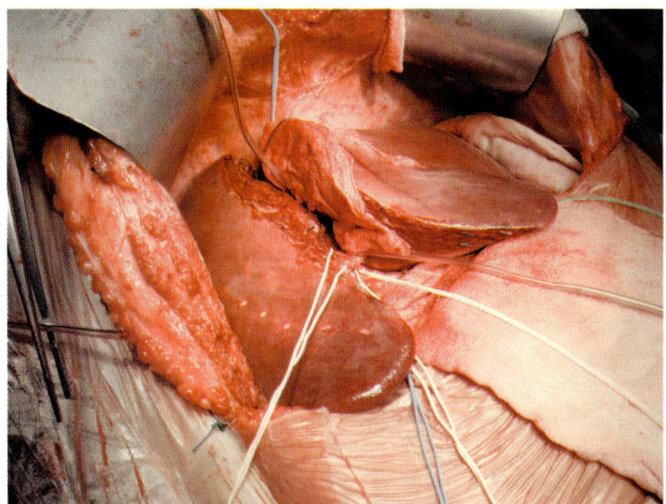

Fig. 8.11: Hanging maneuver

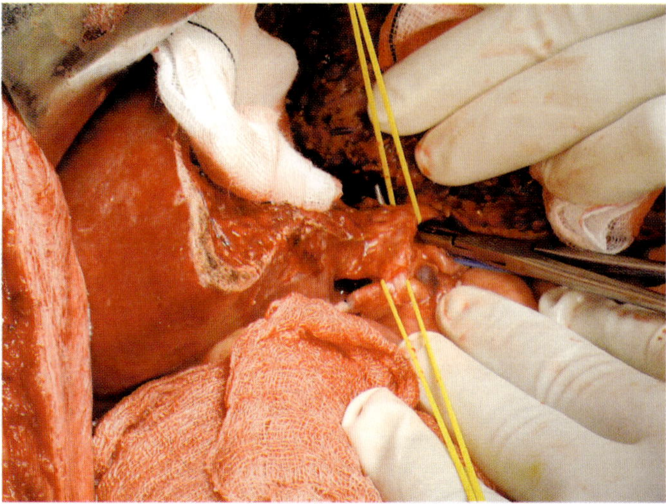

Fig. 8.12: Looping of bile duct for donor hepatectomy

and MHV and is guided inferiorly above the midportion of the caudate process (the right half of which is transected), and above the RPV, RHA and the hilar plate with the right hepatic duct. The tube is lifted to facilitate transection of the last bit of parenchyma (Fig. 8.11).

Division of Structures at the Porta

The hilar plate around the bile duct confluence is cleared by dissecting it from the adjacent liver parenchyma. The hepatic artery and portal vein are well separated from the hilar plate by this time. Hilar plate contains the peribiliary plexus of vessels which supplies the bile ducts and which is very important for prevention of any biliary complications both in the donor and the recipient. The bile duct is looped on the corresponding side of the graft and is divided sharply more towards the periphery so that the confluence or the left hepatic duct is not compromised (Fig. 8.12). Donor is given 5,000 units of heparin intravenously, 3 minutes following which the vascular divisions are performed (Fig. 8.13). The MHV is divided using the linear stapler 45 mm, following which the RHA is divided after clamping the donor RHA proximal to the site of division. The portal vein is clamped proximal to the confluence on the right side and RPV is divided. The RHV is divided with a cuff of cava after clamping it proximally. Right inferior hepatic vein, if any is taken with a cuff of cava and ligated with a marker which is removed at the time flushing in the back bench. Graft is removed from the donor and placed in the basin containing sterile bags with ice all around. It is transferred to the back bench for preparing the graft before it is implanted into the recipient. Stump of RHV is closed with 3–0 prolene continuous sutures; stump of RPV is closed with continuous 4-0 prolene sutures and the RHA stump is closed with continuous 4-0 prolene. The bile duct is closed with 6-0 polydioxanone (PDS) sutures. Dye test is done through the cystic duct to look for any leak from the cut surface. Cholangiogram is done to confirm that the biliary confluence is not compromised and the cystic duct is then ligated with 2-0 silk. Left lobe is anchored back to the falciform ligament to prevent any rotation and congestion of the remnant. Hemostasis is achieved and wound is closed over an abdominal drain (28 Fr) placed in the subhepatic space. Postoperatively donor trachea is extubated and the patient shifted to intensive care unit for observation. Blood transfusion is generally not required in donor hepatectomy.

Left Lobe Graft

The first left lobe live donor liver transplant was reported by Strong et al in 1989[1] in a pediatric recipient. The first left lobe live donor liver transplant in an adult patient was reported in 1994 by Hashikura.[2]

Incision and Exploration

It is similar to what is done in a right lobe graft, the left extent of the incision might be extended more to the left (beyond the left extent of rectus muscle).

Mobilization of the Liver

The falciform is divided till the bifurcation into triangular ligaments. The left triangular ligament is divided till the left border of LHV is exposed and the IVC is identified superiorly.

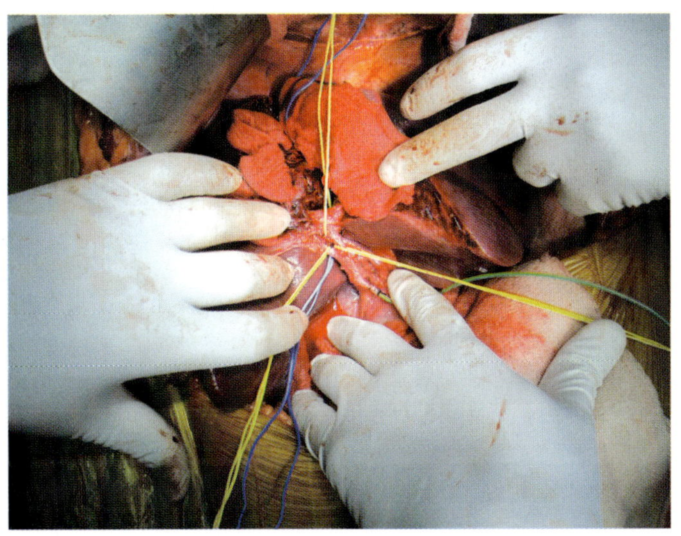

Fig. 8.13: Vascular divisions performed after injecting heparin

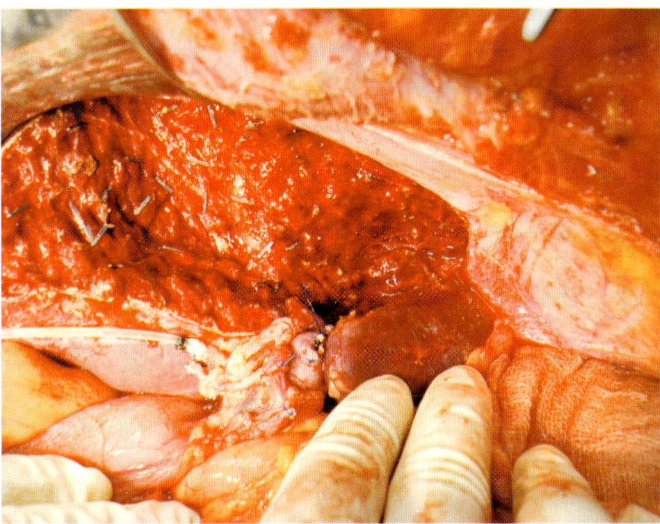

Fig. 8.14: Stump closure of vascular structures, demarcation of MHV groove on left lobe (Remnant), MHV retrieved with right lobe graft

The lesser omentum is inspected and palpated for the presence of accessory/replaced left hepatic artery; this would be known on the preoperative triphasic CT scan of the donor. If present left accessory or replaced LHA from the left gastric is preserved. The caudate is exposed and reflected laterally to identify the IVC posteriorly.

Hilar Dissection

Cystic duct is similarly identified; cannulated and intra-operative cholangiogram is performed to confirm the biliary anatomy. Cholecystectomy is then performed. The biliary anatomy is very important especially in situations where the right posterior sectoral duct drains into the left where the left duct is to be divided distal to the posterior sectoral ductal drainage. The LHA and left portal vein is then identified and common bile duct is dissected all around and looped. The portal vein is looped after dividing the caudate tributaries, if any. The LHA, if accessory or replaced from the left gastric artery, is dissected down to the left gastric artery and any gastric branches encountered might require ligation. Segment 4 artery, if arising from the RHA, is taken separately for double anastomosis in the recipient.

Hepatic Vein Dissection

The common trunk of LHV and MHV is dissected all around as far as possible; looping of the trunk can be done after the parenchymal transection.

Parenchymal Transection

The line of transection is marked by temporarily clamping the LHA and the left portal vein. This line generally extends from the right of MHV to the gall bladder fossa and the hilum. If the caudate is included in the left lobe, the line of transection goes down to the left of IVC. If the caudate is not included in the left lobe, the line of transection after reaching the hilum goes along the ligamentum venosum laterally. If the left lateral lobe is taken, the line of transection is taken to the right of falciform ligament and the MHV is actually left in the right lobe remnant (the segment-4 artery is spared and hence only the left lateral segmental artery is clamped for defining the line of transection). The line of transection after reaching the hilum again goes along the ligamentum venosum leaving behind the caudate lobe. Parenchymal transection is done as is done for right lobe graft.

Division of the Hilar Structures and Removal of the Graft

The bile duct is looped after completion of the parenchymal transection and the left hepatic duct is transected with scissors well away from the confluence so that the right duct and confluence is not compromised. The LHA (left lateral segmental artery in case of left lateral segmentectomy) is divided after clamping it proximally. The left portal vein is then clamped beyond the confluence and divided followed by clamping and division of the LHV and MHV trunk. Graft is then transferred to the basin containing preservative solution and taken to the back-bench for preparing the graft for implantation. Stump of LHA, LPV, LHV-MHV, and LHD are sutured as is done after removal of right graft (Fig. 8.14). Dye test is done through the cystic duct following which a completion cholangiogram is done. These tests rule out bile leak and any compromise of the confluence of the bile duct. Hemostasis is achieved and drain is placed in the subhepatic space.

Right or Left Lobe

Generally the right lobe is adequate for adult recipients and left lateral lobe for pediatric patients. Left lobe is adequate for small size adult recipients and pediatric patients who are big. The aim is to accept a graft size which is at least 0.8 to 1% of recipient weight and in pediatric patients it should not be more than 5%.

Timing of Vascular Clamping and Removal of Graft

In the living donor program it is important to synchronise the steps of vascular clamping and division with the steps in the recipient so that the anhepatic phase and the cold ischemia time can be minimized.

Variants of the Graft

Left lobe graft—when the left lobe graft volume is adequate for the patient (Graft Recipient Weight Ratio-GRWR between 0.8–1.0), it is preferable to take the left lobe compared to the right lobe. This is so because it is technically simpler to take the left lobe compared to the right and the remnant liver volume is not a problem (it is adequate for the donor).

Postoperative Care

Donor is started on liquid diet on 1st postoperative day (POD), which is progressively increased to normal diet by the 3rd to 4th day. Doppler examination of the remnant liver is performed once on the 1st POD. The abdominal drain is generally removed on the 3rd–4th POD. Liver function tests generally normalize in 5–6 days. Donor is discharged home by 6th POD.

Morbidity and Mortality Associated with Donor Hepatectomy

Morbidity of donor hepatectomy is seen in 10–15% of donors. These can be in the form of pleural effusion, ascites, bile leak from the raw surface of liver and rarely biliary stricture. Generally these can be managed conservatively; rarely a percutaneous drainage or a biliary stenting may be required. Very rarely surgical intervention is required. No surgical procedure is without any risk and donor hepatectomy is also associated with a mortality of 0.2–0.5%.

Organ Procurement from a Deceased Donor

Brain Death

The majority of organ transplants the world over are from deceased donors. For heart it is the only option. The recognition that a person whose brain is dead but whose other organs continue to work because of medical support is truly dead, paved the way for development of solid organ transplants into a routine, life-saving modality.[3,4]

Death is an irreversible biological event that consists of permanent cessation of the critical functions of the organism as a whole[4]. Brain death, comprising permanent cessation of cerebral and brainstem function meets the criteria. The commonest causes of brain death in reported series are head injuries and intra-cranial bleeds.[5,6,7]

Diagnosis of brain death: The diagnosis of brain death can be made clinically by the bedside.[7] Before the tests for brain death are administered, the following prerequisites must be met:

1. Clinical or imaging evidence of brain damage. The cause of brain death should be known
2. Medical conditions that may confound clinical assessment should be excluded or corrected such as electrolyte imbalance, acid-base imbalance and endocrine insufficiencies
3. There should be no drug or other intoxication which may confound the diagnosis
4. The core temperature should be more than 36°C
5. The systolic blood pressure should be more than 100 mm Hg

Neurologic examination: All the following signs must be present

1. Coma
2. Absent motor response including response to pain stimulus above the neck
3. Absent papillary light reflex, pupils in midposition or dilated
4. Absent corneal reflex
5. Absent oculo-vestibular reflexes (cold caloric test)
6. Absent jaw jerk
7. Absent gag reflex
8. Absent cough with tracheal suctioning
9. Absent sucking or rooting reflexes
10. Apnea as demonstrated by the apnea test.

Movements originating from the spinal cord or peripheral nerves may occur after brain death in as many as 75% of cadavers.[5]

Management of the Deceased Donor

Brain death causes a number of physiological changes which may damage the organs to be transplanted, if not managed appropriately. At the time of brain death, the dead brain tissue releases a storm of cytokines and toxic metabolites which may cause refractory hypotension. Hypotension is also caused by lack of sympathetic tone, diabetes insipidus, adrenal insufficiency, and possibly by deliberate volume restriction.[8]

Interventions that improve the function of one organ may be harmful for another. Adequate fluid resuscitation to ensure a good diuresis to preserve the kidneys may result in water-logged lungs and congested liver which might compromise the chances of using them. Management of hypotension requires a judicious use of fluid resuscitation and pressors. High doses of pressors which reduce renal and splanchnic blood flow should be avoided.

Diabetes insipidus may result in production of large volumes of dilute urine (sometimes more than 1000 mL per hour) with hypernatremia. It can be managed with a combination of fluid replacement and nasal desmopressin or intravenous vasopressin. Adrenal insufficiency can be managed with intravenous hydrocortisone. Some centers have a protocol of using intravenous tri-iodothyronine in all organ procurements.

Organ Procurement

The organ procurement operation, particularly when multiple organs are being procured, requires coordination between the different teams. Typically there is a thoracic team to procure the heart and lungs and a team to procure the abdominal organs. Usually the liver team would procure the kidneys as well, but sometimes there is a separate kidney team. The teams should discuss the sequence of steps before beginning the procurement.

The anesthesiologist is responsible for maintaining hemodynamic stability and tissue oxygenation during the procurement. Access for administering fluids as well as for monitoring blood pressure should be in the upper extremities as the lower extremities would be cut off when the aortic cannula is placed.

The basic principle of organ procurement is to maintain perfusion and oxygenation until the organ is ready to be removed and then to rapidly cool it to a temperature of 4°C with preservative solution until it is ready to be implanted into the recipient. Although the sequence of steps varies, the basic principles remain the same.

The patient is cleaned and draped from chin to mid-thigh (Fig. 8.15). Drapes with plastic bags are preferred so that the perfusion fluid does not run on to the floor and the surgeon's feet. An incision is made from the supra-sternal notch to the symphysis pubis. Some surgeons prefer to make a cruciate incision but this is not essential.

A sternotomy may be performed at this time but many surgeons prefer to do it after establishing control of the infra-renal aorta (Fig. 8.16).

The abdominal part of the operation begins with an inspection of the abdominal viscera to assess the quality of the organs as well as to rule out any unsuspected pathology. Unexpected malignancies may be found in as many as 5% of donors[9]. The right colon and the duodenum are mobilized to expose the vena cava and the aorta (Cattel-Braasch maneuver). The aorta is slung just above its division into the common iliac arteries and mobilized for a short length. Two slings (usually umbilical tape) are passed around it.

If the chest was not opened earlier, it is opened now. The pericardium is opened. If the thoracic organs are not to be procured then the descending aorta should be slung in the

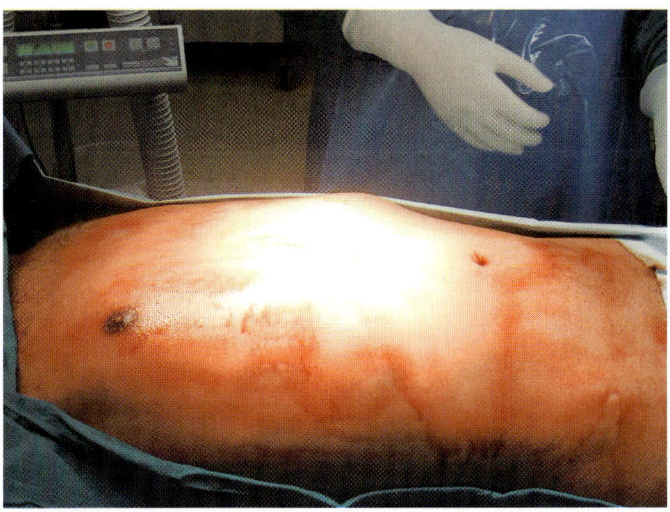

Fig. 8.15: Surgical exposure for multiorgan procurement

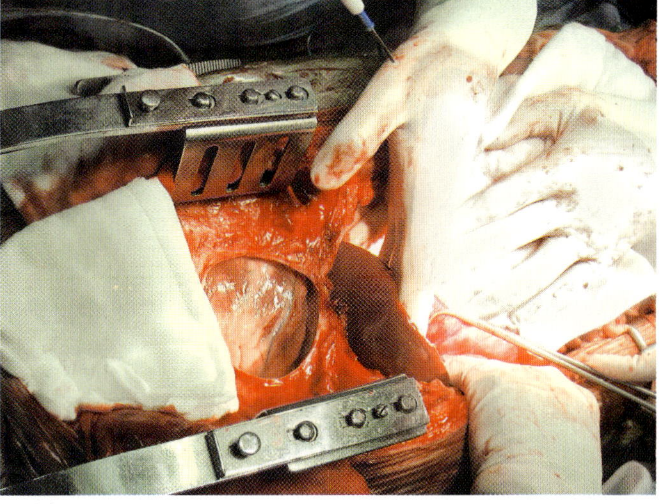

Fig. 8.16: Sternotomy with midline abdominal incision for wide exposure

chest above the diaphragm. If the thoracic organs are being procured and the heart and lung team is not comfortable with this then the supraceliac aorta is slung in the abdomen. This requires mobilization of the left lobe of the liver and the gastrohepatic omentum taking care not to damage any replaced or accessory LHA.

If the donor is hemodynamically unstable then the organs can be cold flushed now and further dissection done afterwards but with a stable patient it is preferable to perform more dissection and prepare the organs for recovery.

The duodenojejunal flexure is mobilized and the inferior mesenteric vein identified on its left side. It is cannulated for the portal flush. Some centers do not do a portal flush in situ. If the pancreas is being procured then it is preferable not perform this step. The cannula can sometimes damage the splenic vein. A portal flush under pressure can cause swelling in the pancreas and possibly pancreatitis in the graft.

The liver is mobilized, taking down the falciform as well as the right and left triangular ligaments. Dissection at the porta hepatis is begun. The porta is palpated between the fingers to identify a replaced or accessory RHA coming from the superior mesenteric artery. The bile duct is slung and divided, tying the duodenal side. The gall bladder is opened and the biliary system is flushed with cold saline or lactated Ringers solution. Bile is toxic to the biliary epithelium in the cold and should be washed out as thoroughly as possible. The hepatic arteries are identified. The gastroduodenal artery can be divided after clamping to confirm adequate flow in the hepatic arteries. The common hepatic artery is followed proximally to its origin from the celiac axis. The pancreas along with the spleen is mobilized. The superior mesenteric artery is identified as it arises from the aorta. If there is a replaced or accessory RHA it should be identified and care taken not to damage it.

The organ is now ready for procurement. The lower sling on the aorta is tied and the aorta cannulated. The upper sling is tied around the aortic cannula. Gravity flush with cold University of Wisconsin (UW) or HTK (Histidine Tryptophan Ketoglutarate) Custodiol solution is begun. The vena cava is divided above the diaphragm to allow outflow and the aorta is clamped above the celiac axis to prevent the preservative solution being wasted perfusing the head and neck and upper extremities. If UW solution is used 2–3 liters suffices while 7–10 liters of HTK are required (it is less viscous). Cold ice slush is placed around the organs to be procured and the flush continued until the outflow is clear. Now the procurement begins by opening the aorta between the superior mesenteric artery and the take-off of the renal arteries. The ostia of the renal arteries can be visualized from inside the aortic lumen and damage avoided. A patch of the aorta with both celiac axis and superior mesenteric artery is detached. The superior mesenteric artery is divided distal to any possible replaced or accessory right hepatic artery. The left gastric artery is followed up to the lesser curve of the stomach and detached from it taking to preserve any replaced or accessory LHA. The vena cava is transected between the liver and the renal veins. The adrenal gland is a useful landmark and cutting through the adrenal gland ensures that neither the renal vein nor any caudate vein is damaged. Finally, the liver is detached along with a cuff of the diaphragm and removed for benching. The liver is packed in two sterile isolation bags with enough preservative solution to prevent contact with the ice. The bag is packed in enough ice to keep it cool until implantation.

Removal of the kidneys begins by identifying the ureters at the pelvic brim as they cross the iliac vessels and dividing them as low as possible. They are lifted off the retroperitoneum up to the renal hilum. The vena cava is divided just above its formation and lifted off the retroperitoneum, as is the aorta. Both kidneys are removed en bloc with the aorta and vena cava and separated on the bench.

Benching

Living Donor Graft

This involves preparation of the donor graft before implanting into the recipient.

Perfusion

Graft liver removed from the donor is quickly transferred to the back bench where it is flushed with cold histidine tryptophan ketoglutarate (HTK) solution via the RPV/LPV till the effluent from the RHV and MHV/LHV is clear. The graft is perfused with three times the estimated volume of the graft (Fig. 8.17).

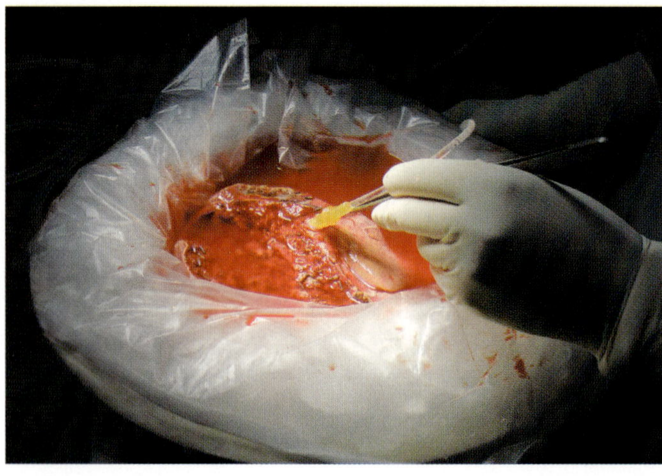

Fig. 8.17: Flushing of right lobe liver graft with HTK solution

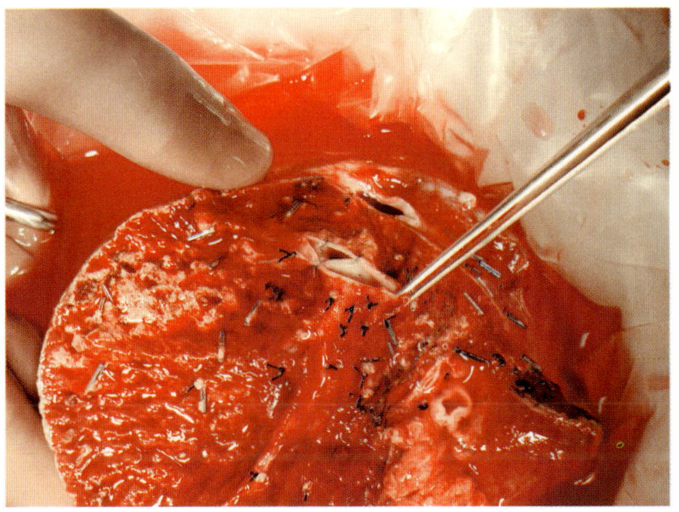

Fig. 8.18: Seg VIII and MHV venous ostia before extension

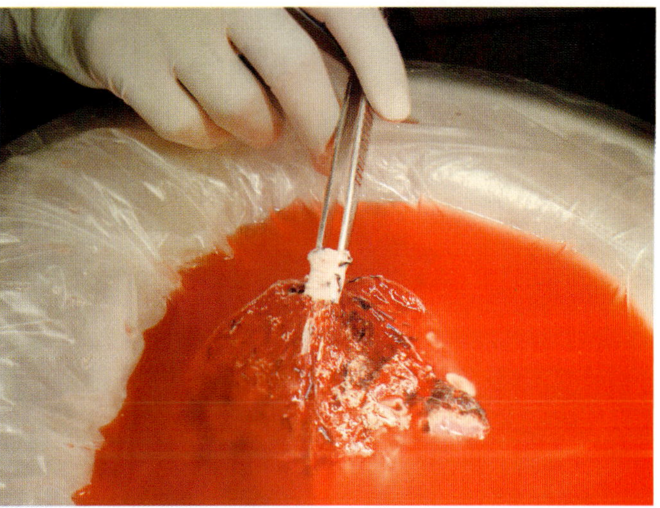

Fig. 8.19: Neo-MHV created by an extension graft on Seg VIII and MHV

Graft is then weighed to make sure that the graft volume is adequate for the recipient (GRWR of 0.8–1 is acceptable).

Venoplasty and Extension

Hepatic venoplasty: The donor graft will come with either a complete or partial middle hepatic vein (MHV) based on segment IV drainage. In case of partial MHV retrieval-segment VIII vein is joined with MHV with 6–0 prolene sutures (Fig. 8.18).

The MHV extension: depending upon the lie of the segment 8 vein, the MHV extension is done with either straight or Y graft (autologous or cryopreserved vein), (Fig. 8.19).

Portal vein is extended with the help of straight or Y graft depending upon the type of portal vein in the donor.

Hepatic artery is also prepared for implantation by cutting back the edges and removing excessive tissue around the artery, if any. A conduit is used in case of double arterial inflow, if required.

Caudate lobe bile duct is oversewn with 6–0 PDS. If the ducts are more than one however in the same hilar sheath, then these are brought together by sutures taken in the hilar plate.

Deceased Donor Graft

The liver needs to be prepared for implantation into the recipient. Without going into the technical details, the quality of the liver is re-assessed. Fatty livers tend to be more firm in the cold with rounded edges while fibrotic livers tend to be hard with sharp edges. A liver biopsy can be done at this stage and a frozen section assessed for steatosis and fibrosis. The vessels are cleared of extraneous tissue, their anatomy assessed and the ends freshened for anastomosis. Accessory arteries may require reconstruction on the bench to ensure a single inflow. Any open ends and rents in the vessels are dealt with to avoid bleeding from the liver after reperfusion. The liver is now ready for implantation.

Implantation

Living Donor Graft (Right or Left lobe)

IVC Clamping

Before implantation is attempted, a trial clamping of IVC is done and the hemodynamic response is checked. Then IVC is clamped distally as well as above the opening of hepatic veins (Fig. 8.20). The right/middle and left hepatic venous sutures are removed and the opening extended onto the IVC based on the size of the donor RHV/MHV+LHV.

Hepatic Venous Anastomoses

Donor RHV/MHV+ LHV is anastomosed with the extended opening in the IVC with 4–0 prolene sutures (Fig. 8.21). The extended MHV in case of right lobe graft is anastomosed directly onto IVC with 5–0 prolene sutures; the sutures are kept loose providing an outlet while the donor liver would be flushed before reperfusion (Fig. 8.22). Any accessory or inferior RHV in the graft is also anastomosed to the IVC.

Portal Venous Anastomosis

The portal vein is anastomosed end to end with 6–0 prolene and the liver is flushed first with 500 mL of gelofusin followed by blood (half volume of the actual

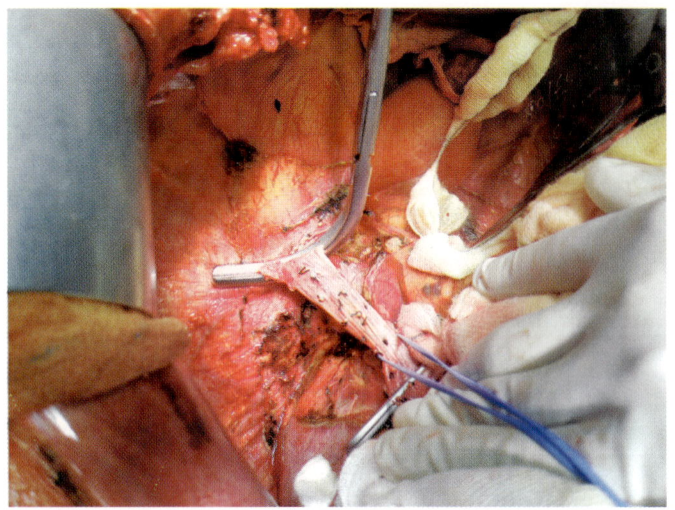

Fig. 8.20: Complete inferior vena caval camping for implantation

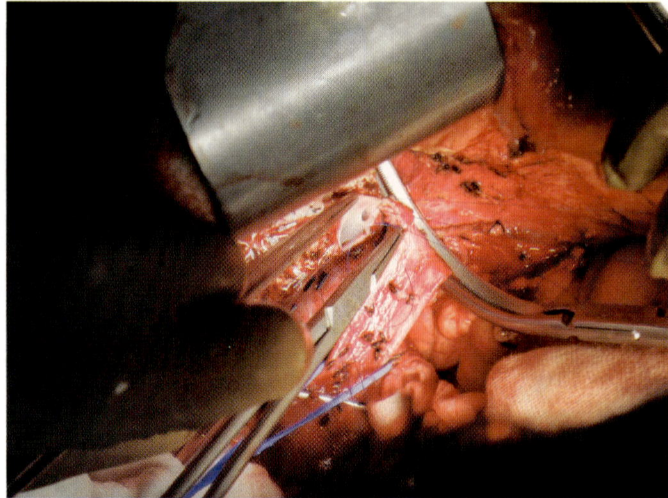

Fig. 8.21: Right hepatic vein being anastomosed to IVC

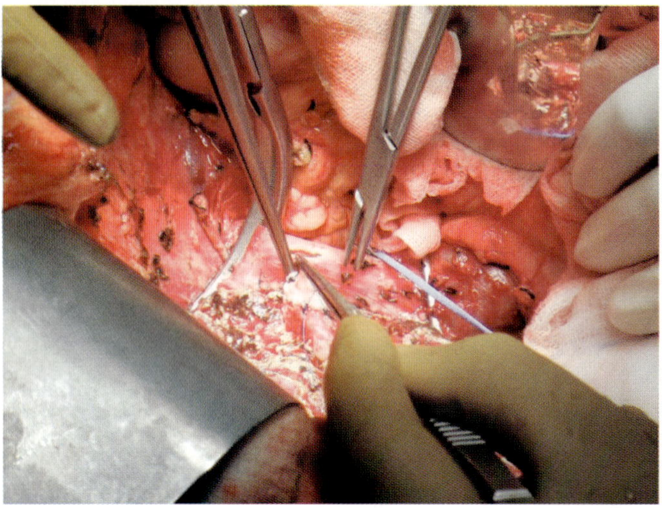

Fig. 8.22: Flushing of graft with Gelofusin through portal vein anastomosis and venting through MHV-IVC anastomosis

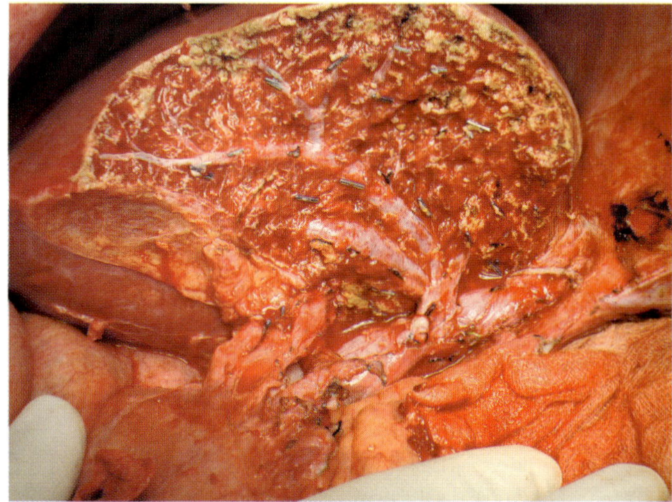

Fig. 8.23: Reperfused right lobe liver graft

donor graft weight. After the flush both the portal (with a 'growth factor provided') and MHV, in case of right lobe graft, and MHV+LHV anastomoses, in left lobe graft, are tightened.

Reperfusion

Now all the clamps will be removed in serial fashion starting with supra-hepatic IVC followed by infra-hepatic IVC and then lastly portal vein (Fig. 8.23). Hemostasis is confirmed and if required additional sutures are taken.

Arterial and Biliary Anastomoses

Arterial anastomosis is then performed end to end with 7–0 prolene sutures under 2.5 loupe magnification followed by biliary anastomoses (either duct to duct or Roux-en-Y hepaticojejunostomy) with 6–0 PDS. Abdomen is closed over an abdominal drain, in monolayer with no. 1 nylon after checking hemostasis, swab and instrument counts.

Deceased Donor Graft

In case of deceased donor retrieval it would be full graft. The steps of implantation would be little different as compared to, in living donor graft.

The IVC of the graft is anastomosed to recipient IVC either end to side or side to side with 3–0 prolene sutures. Graft main portal vein is anastomosed to the recipient main portal vein. Similarly, graft coelic axis trunk is anastomosed to

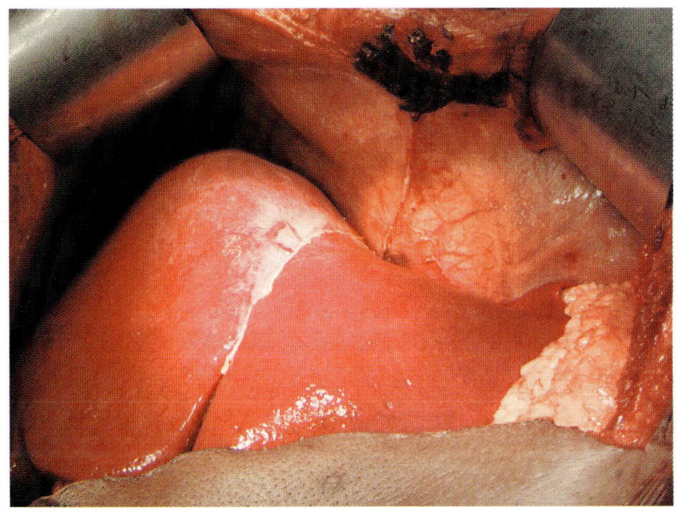

Fig. 8.24: Reperfused deceased donor graft

the 'hepatic artery proper' of the recipient (Fig. 8.24). Biliary anastomosis is duct to duct with 5–0 PDS sutures. Drains are placed and abdomen is closed in monolayer after checking for hemostasis and swabs and instrument count.

Postoperative Care

The patient is then shifted to intensive care unit where continuous monitoring is done. The patient's trachea is usually extubated on the next day based on the arterial blood gases and clinical condition. Immunosuppressive therapy is instituted after 24–36 hours based on liver and renal functions. Protocol doppler ultrasound is performed for first 5 postoperative days. The patient is then shifted to the ward once the condition is stable.

CLINICAL PEARLS

- **Liver transplantation is a life saving procedure for both chronic and acute liver failure of varied etiology.** Proper selection of patients after extensive pretransplant evaluation is the key to success following liver transplantation.
- **Deceased donors are rare in Asian countries and hence LDLT is the major contributor to the donor pool.** Living donor should undergo stepwise evaluation before the procedure so that the best suitable donor is selected (non fatty liver with graft recipient weight ratio of at least 0.8).
- **Donor safety is of utmost importance in a living donor liver transplantation program.** Graft retrieval in living donor involves technical expertise. It is to ensure a good quality graft and a well perfused, adequate remnant liver volume in the donor.
- **In living donor liver transplantation, the donor and the recipient have the surgery simultaneously so that the cold ischemia time is shortened.** Implantation in the recipient mandates a good outflow, proper inflow tract, and a well vascularised biliary anastomosis. This ensures a good graft function and minimizes the rates of postoperative complications.
- **Understanding of brain death, declaration of the same, maintenance of the donor for organ retrieval (once the donor family agrees for organ donation), recognition of a good deceased donor graft, and the actual retrieval process is important for a successful DDLT program.**

REFERENCES

1. Strong RW, Lynch SV, Ong TH, et al. Successful liver transplantation from a living donor to her son. N Engl J Med, 1990;322:1505-7.
2. Hashikura Y, Makuuchi M, Kawasaki S, et al. Successful living related partial liver transplantation to an adult patient. Lancet, 1994;343:1233-4.
3. Wijdicks EFM. Brain Death. Lippincott, Williams and Wilkins, Philadelphia, 2001:175.
4. Bernat JL. Ethical issues in the perioperative management of neurologic patients. Neurol Clin, 2004;22:457-71.
5. Saposnik G, Bueri JA, Mauricio J, Saizar R, Garretto NS. Spontaneous and reflex movements in brain death. Neurology, 2000;54:221-23.
6. Goudreau JL, Wijdicks EF, Emery SF. Complications during apnea testing in the determination of brain death: predisposing factors. Neurology, 2000;55:1045-8.
7. Wijdicks EJ, Rabinstein AA, Manno EM, Atkinson JD. Pronouncing brain death: contemporary practice and safety of the apnea test. Neurology, 2008;71:1240-4.
8. Wood KE, Becker BN, McCartney JG, D'Allesandro AM, Coursin DB. Care of the potential organ donor. N Engl J Med, 2004;351:2730-9.
9. Boggi U, Vistoli F, Del Chiaro M, et.al. A simplified technique for the en bloc procurement of abdominal organs that is suitable for pancreas and small-bowel transplantation. Surgery, 2004;135:629-41.

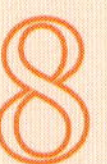

Anesthetic Management of Liver Donor

Nitin Sethi, Shashank Pandey

INTRODUCTION

Living donor transplantation has emerged as an excellent option for patients awaiting liver transplantation who are unlikely to receive a deceased donor liver. Cultural problems with cadaveric donation, has made living donation programs popular in Asia, where most transplants are from living donors. The first successful living donor liver transplant was performed using the left lobe in a pediatric patient in 1989.[1] Earlier living donation was reserved mostly for children, in whom the left hepatic lobe or one or more segments were used. The first adult to adult right hepatic lobe transplantation was performed in 1994 in Japan.[2]

The advantages of living organ donation over deceased organ donation are:

1. Living donors are always hemodynamically stable and the procedure can be planned electively.
2. Cold ischemia time of the organ can be reduced from 10 or more hours to less than 1 hour with a decrease in associated markers of inflammation seen after reperfusion.
3. Significant reduction in time spent on the waiting list to receive an organ from a deceased donor.

The estimated donor mortality for living donor liver transplantation (LDLT) is about 0.2%. Mortality for left lobe donation is 0.05–0.21%, compared to 0.23–0.5% for right lobe donation.[3]

The donor being essentially a healthy individual, minimizing complications and reducing the impact of donation on the donor quality of life is extremely important.

Preoperative Evaluation

Donor evaluation is essential for the safety of the donor and recipient. Two important considerations for donor selection are:

1. Donors with normal liver function and normal anatomy
2. Donors without any systemic diseases or abnormalities

During the initial phase of evaluation, patient age (ideally between 20–60 years), relationship to the recipient, ABO blood matching and detailed history of any disease, including physical and psychological examination, is done.

Postoperative pulmonary embolism is a genuine threat to the donor. Smoking, routine use of birth control pills or obesity should be considered as possible risk factors for this complication. A BMI > 30 kg/m^2 should be corrected or an alternative donor should be selected out of concern for donor's safety.[4,5]

After consent for donation has been made medical tests are done. Medical tests include a blood count, coagulation profile, liver and renal function tests, serological tests for hepatitis B, hepatitis C and human immunodeficiency virus (HIV), chest radiography, electrocardiography and echocardiography.

The imaging study of the donor liver is very important to ensure safe surgical procedures in both the donor and recipient.

Doppler ultrasound is performed for evaluation of hepatic artery vascular anatomy and to detect any gross pathologic condition.

Computed tomography (CT) and magnetic resonance imaging (MRI) is used to define the donor's vascular anatomy and graft volume. A graft to recipient body weight ratio of at least 0.8 should be the aim to avoid post transplantation liver graft dysfunction.[7]

Monitoring (Table 8.24)

In addition to the American Society of Anaesthesiologists (ASA) standards for monitoring, an arterial line and central

Table 8.24: Monitoring for living donor hepatectomy

1. ASA standard monitoring: pulse oximetry, non invasive blood pressure, $EtCO_2$, ECG
2. Neuromuscular monitor
3. Bispectral index monitoring (BIS)
4. Temperature
5. Urine output
6. Invasive arterial blood pressure
7. Central venous pressure
8. Laboratory estimations
   a. Hemoglobin
   b. Serum electrolytes
   c. Arterial blood gases
   d. Blood sugar

venous access is essential. A large bore peripheral venous access is also obtained in addition to the central venous access for fluid administration. An arterial line is useful for early recognition of hypotension and for obtaining samples for blood gas analysis.

Central venous pressure monitoring is useful to ensure a low CVP at the time of hepatic resection as elevated CVP has been considered by some authors as a prime determinant of bleeding during resection.[8]

Induction and Maintenance of Anesthesia

Prior to induction of anesthesia, placement of a thoracic epidural catheter for providing intraoperative and postoperative analgesia is a common practice at our center however, some centers use only patient controlled analgesia for postoperative pain management. Avoidance of epidural catheter placement based on concerns of postoperative coagulopathy from extensive hepatectomy does not seem to be justified.

Large hepatic resection may produce transient hepatic dysfunction, therefore choosing drugs whose elimination is not completely dependent on hepatic metabolism may be preferable.[9]

For induction of anesthesia any of the intravenous induction agents such as thiopentone, propofol or etomidate can be used. Single intravenous boluses of hypnotic agents cause only minimal alterations in liver function.[10]

Tracheal intubation can be performed using non-depolarizing muscle relaxants such as vecuronium, rocuronium, atracurium and cis-atracurium.

Under general anesthesia, radial artery, central venous catheter, nasogastric tube and a urinary bladder catheter is placed. The patient is placed in the supine position with both arms tucked at the side.

All patients are positioned carefully to avoid compression or stretch injury. A gel ring is placed under the head and a gel pad placed under the arms. An intermittent pneumatic compression device and padded boots are placed on the lower extremities. Patient warming is important to maintain adequate clotting and to minimize the risk of surgical site infection. This is achieved with a convective heating blanket, an intravenous fluid warmer and an adjustable ambient room temperature.

Maintenance of anesthesia is achieved using a volatile anesthetic agent and intravenous narcotics such as fentanyl 1–2 µg/kg/hr or remifentanil 0.1–0.5 µg/kg/min.

Various volatile anesthetics, including isoflurane, sevoflurane and desflurane are used in living donor liver transplant. According to data from animal and human studies most of the currently available volatile anesthetics have been shown to preserve hepatic blood flow and function.[11-14]

Isoflurane, a potent peripheral vasodilator with relatively mild cardiodepressive effects, decreases total hepatic blood flow but oxygen delivery to the liver is well preserved.[15]

Animal studies have shown that desflurane preserves total hepatic blood flow better than halothane or isoflurane.[13,16] Desflurane is unique among the class of volatile anesthetics in that it is highly stable and undergoes very little degradation yielding minimal excretion of organic or inorganic fluoride. It has been found to be safe in patients with renal failure.[17] Ko et al[18] compared the effects of desflurane and total intravenous anesthesia with propofol-remifentanil on postoperative hepatic and renal function after right hepatectomy in liver donor and concluded that living donors for liver transplant may have a better outcome following anesthesia with desflurane.

Non-depolarizing muscle relaxants are administered as a continuous infusion, with the degree of muscle relaxation being monitored with a neuromuscular monitor. A continuous epidural infusion of 0.125%–0.25% bupivacaine at the rate of 5–7 mL/hr is also given throughout the intraoperative period, this provides significant analgesia during general anesthesia with minimal hemodynamic effects.

Drugs such as cisatracurium, atracurium and remifentanil may be ideal for maintenance of anesthesia as they are more reliably eliminated than drugs that depend on hepatic hydrolysis and/or conjugation for termination of their effects.

Intraoperative Hemodynamics

Major changes in the intraoperative hemodynamics during donor hepatectomy are as follows:

1. Manipulation of the liver can occasionally twist the liver on its vascular pedicle or compress the vena cava, leading to decrease in venous return with consequent brief episodes of hypotension.[19,20]
2. After right hepatectomy, donors have been shown to have a significantly higher cardiac output (CO) and a significantly lower, systemic vascular resistance (SVR) and an increased heart rate as compared to before resection.[21] There is evidence in literature that splanchnic mediators such as endotoxins released during liver surgery, may have an important role.[22] Levels of nitric oxide, a potent vasodilator, have been shown to be elevated in response to endotoxin and cytokine release.[23,24] Hemodynamic changes occurring during hepatectomy may be due to an early increase in nitric oxide production.

Table 8.20: Techniques for maintaining low CVP

1. Adjust fluid therapy to maintain urine output 0.5–1 mL/kg/hr
2. Continuous intraoperative epidural infusion of bupivacaine
3. Use of nitroglycerine, when liver distension or excessive oozing is observed

Role of Low Central Venous Pressure (CVP)

Healthy donors undergoing right hepatectomies lose about 600 mL to 900 mL of blood on an average.[26]

Maintaining a low CVP has been regarded as a simple and effective way to reduce blood loss during liver resection. Maintaining a CVP between 2 and 5 mm Hg results in low pressure in the hepatic veins and sinusoids thus limiting distension, favoring less blood loss and allowing easier control of inadvertent venous injury (Table 8.20).[25-27]

The risk of severe air embolism is increased under low central venous pressure and the anesthesiologist should be highly vigilant for such an event.

Low central venous pressure is safe with regards to renal function, provided a good renal perfusion pressure (> 60 mm Hg) and renal blood flow is maintained throughout surgery.[28]

Several issues complicate assessment of an accurate CVP, such as tilt of the operating table during transection, positive end expiratory pressure, intrathoracic pressure, use of surgical retractors and liver manipulation. Various authors have failed to find a correlation between blood loss during transection and CVP.[24,29]

Jawan et al[30] have concluded from their study that autologous donation of 250–300 mL blood 2–3 days before donor hepatectomy does not seem to affect the intraoperative CVP and has no favorable effect in reducing blood loss during liver resection.

Lutz et al[24] have recommended the use of intraoperative cell salvage, preoperative autologous donation and intraoperative hemodilution as measures to avoid transfusion of banked blood to the patients.

Fluid Management

Metabolic acidosis commonly seen during hepatic resection is primarily due to lactic acidosis. Elevation in lactate levels is thought to be due to decreased hepatic blood flow and impaired hepatic function due to extensive hepatic resection. Hyperchloremic metabolic acidosis due to normal saline administration also contributes to this observed acidotic state.[31] Lactate containing crystalloid solutions are specifically avoided to minimize lactate load in the presence of potential hepatic dysfunction.

For fluid replacement, lactate free solutions such as 0.9% normal saline or plasmalyte (Baxter healthcare Corporation, Deerfied, USA) can be used. At our center, 0.9% normal saline is the primary intravenous fluid used during hepatectomy. Sodium bicarbonate (50 meq in every liter 0.9% normal saline) is added to prevent metabolic acidosis.

Although there are several negative effects of sodium bicarbonate administration, it has certain positive effects such as improved diaphragmatic and myocardial function. Because of potential worsening of liver functions, metabolic acidosis should be aggressively corrected in the initial stages itself.[32]

Utilization of albumin for fluid management in the perioperative period is a controversial issue. Albumin has been shown to modulate cellular apoptosis and decrease neutrophil activation and complications associated with its use are rare.[33,34]

We commonly administer 200 mL, 20%, salt poor albumin (100 mL, 20% albumin added to 1000 mL, 0.9% normal saline) to our patients immediately following completion of resection.

Albumin is given to increase plasma oncotic pressure and to compensate for potentially reduced hepatic synthetic function. Other colloid solutions such as hetastarch can also be used for volume expansion immediately following resection. Fluid administration is limited to maintain central venous pressure (CPV) less than 5 mm Hg throughout the parenchyma dissection in an effort to reduce blood loss.[24] Urine output is maintained at greater than or equal to 0.5 mL/kg/hr.

At the end of liver resection 50 μ/kg heparin is administered IV to prevent clotting in the remaining liver following interruption of the vasculature.[18,19] Infusions of muscle relaxants and narcotics are discontinued at the initiation of abdominal closure. The trachea is extubated when the TOF ratio > 0.9, the patient is breathing spontaneously, fully awake and able to follow commands. Almost all patients are extubated in the operating room provided that at the end of surgery, pH and electrolytes are normal, there has been no massive transfusion or overt blood loss and there have been no hemodynamic or respiratory abnormalities.

Postoperative Care

Since donor hepatectomy is a major surgical procedure the patients are kept in the intensive care unit for one or two days.

Postoperative pain following donor hepatectomy is significant as all donors are healthy individuals with no previous exposure to major surgical procedures. In our center all patients are attached with a programmable PCEA pump containing 0.125% bupivacaine in the immediate postoperative period. Opioids are added to the PCEA pump from the 2nd postoperative day onwards.

Aggressive pulmonary recruitment maneuvers are initiated in all our patients. Patients are encouraged to do incentive spirometry and are also given chest physiotherapy.

Postoperative Outcome

Large hepatic resections lead to alteration in postoperative liver function, particularly hemostasis and drug metabolism. A direct relationship exists between the prolongation of prothrombin time and the extent of liver resection because major liver resection leads to impaired synthesis of clotting factors, inhibition of regulatory proteins and decreased clearance of activated clotting factors and plasminogen activator.[14,28,35-37] A prolonged prothrombin time is a common finding after major hepatic resection.[35,38-40] Borromeo et al[35] have found that prothrombin time requires 3–6 days to return to normal values after right donor hepatectomy. Sensitivity of the central nervous system to the depressant effects of systemic opioids has been noted in some patients possibly due reduced hepatic opioid metabolism.[40] Table 8.25 lists the postoperative complications seen after living donor liver transplant.
Regenerative ability of the liver is remarkable and the residual, otherwise healthy, liver is expected to double in size within the first week following resection.[38]

In a study done by Kwon et al[41] the donor liver regenerated upto 88.5% of preoperative volume with full recovery of liver function at postoperative day 30.

Table 8.25: Postoperative complications in living donor

Anesthetic Complications	*Surgical Complications*
Sore throat	Small bowel obstruction
Arrhythmias	Cholestasis
Incisional pain	Portal vein thrombosis
Phlebitis	Bile leak
Transient neuropraxia	Biliary stricture
Intraoperative pressure sore	Wound infection
Pleural effusion	Prolonged ileus
Atelectasis	Acute gastritis
Pneumonia	Fluid collection between lung and liver
Pneumothorax	Blood clot
Pulmonary edema	Fever/elevated white blood cell count
Encephalopathy	Incisional hernia

A hyperdynamic state with increased cardiac index and augmented splanchnic blood flow has been shown to presist for at least 3 days following hepatic resection.[42]

CLINICAL PEARLS

- Living donor transplant decreases the cold ischemia time of the organ from 10 or more hours to less than 1 hour with a decrease in associated markers of inflammation seen after reperfusion.
- Important considerations for living donor selection are donor with normal liver function and anatomy, and without any systemic disease or abnormalities.
- Drugs such as cisatracurium, atracurium and remifentanil may be ideal for maintenance of anesthesia as they are more reliably eliminated than drugs that depend on hepatic hydrolysis and/or conjugation for termination of their effects.
- Maintaining a low central venous pressure (CVP) is an effective way to reduce blood loss during liver resection.
- Risk of severe air embolism is increased under low central venous pressure and the anesthesiologist should be highly vigilant.
- Lactate containing crystalloid solutions are avoided to minimize lactate load in the presence of potential hepatic dysfunction.
- Postoperative pain is significant after donor hepatectomy as all donors are healthy individuals with no previous exposure to major surgical procedures.
- A prolonged prothrombin time is a common finding after major hepatic resection and is proportional to the extent of liver resection.

REFERENCES

1. Strong RW, Lynch SV, Ong TH, Matsunami H, Koido Y, Balderson GA. Successful liver transplantation from a living donor to her son. N Engl J Med, 1990;322:1505-07.
2. Yamaoka Y, Washida M, Honda K, Tanaka K, Mori K, Shimahara Y, et al. Liver transplantation using a right lobe graft from a living related donor. Transplantation, 1994;57:1127-30.
3. Middleton PF, Duffield M, Lynch SV, Padbury RT, House T, Stanton P, et al. Living donor liver transplantation–Adult donor outcomes: A systematic review. Liver Transpl, 2006;12:24-30.
4. Hashikura Y, Kawasaki S, Miyagawa S, Terada M, Ikegami T, Nakazawa Y, et al. Donor selection for living-related liver transplantation. Transplant Proc, 1997;29:3410-11.
5. Beavers KL, Sandler RS, Fair JH, Johnson MW, Shrestha R. The living donor experience: donor health assessment and outcomes after living donor liver transplantation. Liver Transpl, 2001;7: 943-7.

6. Chisuwa H, Hashikura Y, Mita A, Miyagawa S, Terada M, Ikegami T, et al. Living liver donation: preoperative assessment, anatomic considerations, and long-term outcome. Transplantation, 2003; 75:1670-6.
7. Inomata Y, Uemoto S, Asonuma K, Egawa H, Kiuchi T, Fujita S, et al. Right lobe graft in living donor liver transplantation. Transplantation, 2000;69:258-64.
8. Jones RM, Moulton CE, Hardy KJ. Central venous pressure and its effect on blood loss during liver resection. Br J Surg, 1998;85:1058-60.
9. Schumann R, Zabala L, Angelis M, Bonney I, Tighiouart H, Carr DB. Altered hematologic profiles following donor right hepatectomy and implications for perioperative analgesic management. Liver Transpl, 2004;10:363-368.
10. Sear JW. Toxicity of i. v. anaesthetics. Br J Anaesth, 1987;59:24-45.
11. Sandberg E, Raines DE. Anaesthesia for liver surgery and transplantation. In: Longnecker DE, Brown DL, Newman MF, Zapol WM, (eds). Anaesthesiology McGraw Hill Co, 2008;1338-77.
12. Chibber A, Dziak J, Kolano J, Norton JR, Lustik S. Anaesthesia care for adult liver donor hepatectomy: our experience with 100 cases. Liver Transpl, 2007;13:537-42.
13. Hartman JC, Pagel PS, Proctor LT, Kampine JP, Schmeling WT, Warltier DC. Influence of desflurane, isoflurane and halothane on regional tissue perfusion in dogs. Can J Anaesth, 1992;39: 877-87.
14. O'Riordan J, O'Beirne HA, Young Y, Bellomy MC. Effects of desflurane and isoflurane on splanchnic microcirculation during major surgery. Br J Anaesth, 1997;78:95-96.
15. Cammu G, Troisi R, Cuomo O, Hemptinne Bde, Florio E Di, Mortier E. Anaesthetic management and outcome in right lobe living liver donor surgery. Eur J Anaesth, 2002;19:93-98.
16. Weiskopf RB, Eger EI II, Jonescu P, Yasuda N, Cahalan MK, Freire B, et al. Desflurane does not produce hepatic or renal injury in human volunteers. Anesth Analg, 1992;74:570-4.
17. Koblin DD, Eger EI II, Johnson BH, Konopka K, Wasbell L. I-653 resists degradation in rats. Anesth Analg, 1988;67:534-8.
18. Ko JS, Gwak MS, Choi SI, Kim IA, Yang M, et al. The effects of desflurane and propofol remifentanil on postoperative hepatic and renal function after right hepatectomy in liver donor. Liver Transpl, 2008;41:1150-58.
19. Pomfret EA, Pomposelli JJ, Jenkins RL. Live donor liver transplantation. J Hepatol, 2001;34:613-24.
20. Pomfret EA, Pomposelli JJ, Lewis D, Gordon FD, Burns DL, Lally A, et al. Live donor adult liver transplantation using right lobe grafts: donor evaluation and surgical outcome. Arch Surg, 2001;136:425-33.
21. Niemann CU, Roborts JP, Ascher NL, Yost CY. Intraoperative hemodynamics and liver function in adult to adult living liver donors. Liver Transpl, 2002;8:1126-32.
22. Boermeester MA, Straatsburg JH, Hoadijk AT, Meyer C, Frederikks WM, Wesdorp RI, et al. Endotoxin and interleukin–I related hepatic inflammatory response promotes liver failure after portial hepatectomy. Hepatology, 1995;22:1499-06.
23. Moncada S, Higgs EA. Molecular mechanisms and therapeutic strategies related to nitric oxide. FASEB J, 1995;9:1319-30.
24. Palmer RK. The discovery of nitric oxide in the vessel wall. A unifying concept in the pathogenesis of sepsis. Arch surg, 1993; 128:396-01.
25. Lutz RM, Gamazo CV, Görlinger K, Malagó M, Peters J. Blood-transfusion requirements and blood salvage in donors undergoing right hepatectomy for living related liver transplantation. Anesth Analg, 2003;96:351-5.
26. Chan AC, Blumgart LH, Wuest DL, Melendez JA, Fong Y. Use of preoperative autologous blood donation in liver resections for colorectal metastases. Am J Surg, 1998;175:461-5.
27. Itamoto T, Katayama K, Nakahara H, Tashiro H, Asahara T. Autologous blood storage before hepatectomy for hepatocellular carcinoma with underlying liver disease. Br J Surg, 2003;90:23-8.
28. Redai I, Edmond J, Brentjens T. Anesthetic considerations during liver surgery. Surg Clin North Am, 2004;84:401-11.
29. Chen CL, Chen YS, de Villa VH, Wang CC, Lin CL, Goto S, et al. Minimal blood loss living donor hepatectomy. Transplantation, 2000;69:2580-6.
30. Jawan B, Cheng YF, Tseng CC, Chen YS, Wang CC, Huang TL, et al. Effect of autologous blood donation on the central venous pressure, blood loss and blood transfusion during living donor left hepatectomy. World J Gastroenterol, 2005;11:4233-36.
31. Waters JH, Gottlieb A, Schoenwald P, Popovich MJ, Sprung J, Nelson DR. Normal saline versus lactated ringer's solution for intraoperative fluid management in patients undergoing abdominal aortic aneurysm repair: An Outcome Study. Anesth Analg, 2001;93:817-22.
32. Dell RB, Winters RW. Acid-base effects of hypertonic sodium bicarbonate solutions: A commentary. J Pediatr, 1972;80:681-2.
33. Zoellner H, Hofler M, Beckmann R, Hufnagl P, Vanyek E, Bielek E, et al. Serum albumin is a specific inhibitor of apoptosis in human endothelial cells. J Cell Sci, 1996;109:2571-80.
34. Dubois MJ, Vincent JL. Use of albumin in the intensive care unit. Curr Opin Crit Care, 2002;8:299-01.
35. Borromeo CJ, Stix MS, Lally A, Pomfrer EA. Epidural catheter and increased prothrombin time after right lobe hepatectomy for living donor transplantation. Anesth Analg, 2000;91:1139-41.
36. Young BH, Tsui SL, Leung CC, Lo CM, Liu CL, Fan ST, et al. Management of postoperative analgesia in living liver donors. Transplant Proc, 2000;32:2110.
37. Fan ST, Lo CM, Liu CL, Yong BH, Chan JK, Mg IO. Safety of donors in live donor liver transplantation using right lobe grafts. Arch Surg, 2000;135:336-40.
38. Habib N, Zografos G, Dalla Scrra G, Greco L, Bean A. Liver resection with total vascular occlusion for malignant tumours. Br J Surg, 1994;81:1181-4.
39. Schumann R, Zabala L, Angelis M, Bonney I, Tighiouort H, Corr DB. Altered hematologic profiles following donor right hepatectomy and implications for perioperative analgesia management. Liver transpl, 2004;10:363-8.
40. Siniscalchi A, Begliomini B, Pietri LD Braglia V, Gazzi M, Masetti M, et al. Increased prothrombin time and platelet counts in living donor right hepatectomy: Implications for epidural anaesthesia. Liver transplant, 2004;10:1144-9.
41. Kwon KH, Kim YM, Kim S, Kim HS, Lee WJ, Choi JS. Postoperative liver regeneration and complication in live liver donor after partial hepatectomy for living donor liver transplantation. Yonesi Med J, 2003;44:1069-77.
42. Thasler WE, Bein T, Jauch KH. Postoperative effects of hepatic resection surgery on hemodynamic pulmonary fluid balance and indocyanine green clearance. Arch Surg, 2002;(387)271-75.

Anesthetic Management of Patients for Liver Transplantation

Vijay Vohra

Liver transplantation has become a viable option for patients with advanced liver disease to prolong life with improved quality. Advances in anesthesia and perioperative care, improvement in immunosuppression and surgical techniques have all contributed to this reality. The anesthetic management of these patients still remains complex and challenging. Preoperative evaluation aims to identify patients who need to be optimized before surgery. The results of liver transplant surgery have improved throughout the 1990s but major bleeding, coagulopathy, electrolyte disturbances and cardiovascular instability still occur more frequently than in any other routine surgical procedure.

Liver Donor and Deceased Donor Liver Transplant

The number of available cadaveric donors is limited and the number of the patients on the waiting list for orthotopic liver transplantation continues to grow. This is a major issue in Asian countries where availability of cadaveric organs is limited due to social and cultural reasons. This has led to development live donor liver transplant programs, which form the major share of organ transplanted.

The advantage of Live Donor (LDLT) and Deceased Donor Liver Transplant (DDLT) is that the liver harvested from a healthy individual is of predictable good quality. The timing of the transplantation is planned and the potential good tissue matching. The reduced waiting period for a living donor organ may decrease the risks of decompensation or death before transplantation. The surgical procedures for LDLT are technically more challenging and LDLT requires a full understanding of the hepatobiliary anatomy. A wide range of complication rates is reported in the literature in the donors after LDLT. The main drawback with LDLT is the risk to healthy donors undergoing major surgery who is otherwise well. This modality has a potential psychological burden on the donor but on the other hand could give a great sense of having done something noble and fulfilling. Psychological assessment is essential for the donors to see the suitability for this major step of liver donation. The donor is made aware that the liver grows up to 85% of its normal size within a period of weeks.

Donor safety is of paramount importance in living donor transplants and only donors who have no significant comorbid condition are taken up for organ donation. The number of LDLT in Asia as a whole has continued to increase with cadaveric transplants contributing to the overall numbers in very small way. On the other hand in USA, LDLT accounted for less than 5% of liver transplants and cadaveric transplants remain the mainstay of liver transplant program. The overall number of LDLT procedures performed in Asian countries and areas with well-established programs (Japan, Korea, India, China and Hong Kong) has steadily increased over years. In India, both live donor and deceased donor program are operational but well-established transplant centers are practicing more of live donor transplants. At our center at Medanta, The Medicity Hospital in Gurgaon, India its mainly LDLT with sporadic cases of cadaveric transplants. The main reason is that the awareness about cadaveric organ donation is still lacking besides the religious beliefs, which are hindrances in the way of organ donation after brain death is pronounced. Cardiac standstill is still practiced as death of an individual, unless there is possibility of organ donation.

In India therefore there are both cadaveric liver transplant program as well as living donor liver transplant, the former being more in the southern part of India.

For DDLT, organ allocation is based on Child-Turcotte-Pugh score, which is the widely used method of assessing severity of liver disease. It has a number of fallacies including subjective nature of assessment of encephalopathy and ascites besides the score is discontinuous in nature. There is a ceiling for the objective variables as well, if INR becomes more than 2.3, bilirubin > 3 mg% and albumin < 2.5 gm%. This has led to change in the allocation policy which is not based on the duration, the patient is on the waiting list. The new organ allocation policy as practiced in United States of America gives preference to patients who are sicker and are likely to die sooner without transplantation. They have devised a new method which uses Model for End Stage Liver Disease (MELD) score as a predictor of mortality on the waiting list for liver transplantation.[1,2]

Preoperative Evaluation Plan, Necessary Investigation and Risk Stratification

Preanesthetic Evaluation

Preoperative evaluation is performed in two stages. In the first stage, all the listed transplant candidates examined and evaluated. The second stage evaluation is performed 1 or 2 days before the surgery. The aim of the assessment is firstly to identify prohibitive risks, which must be addressed before attempting transplant, e.g. significant pulmonary hypertension, gross hyponatremia. Assessing any neurologic deterioration since the initial first stage evaluation is necessary and signs of progressive metabolic acidosis, infection or sepsis should be sought. Cardiovascular instability, pulmonary infection, coagulopathy, should be corrected and treated. It is ensured that patient is in the best condition for surgery. Packed red cells can be infused to build up preoperative hemoglobin, aiming for 10 gm% but fresh frozen plasma, cryoprecipitate and platelets, are infused only if there are bleeding tendencies. Relevant investigations—Hb, total counts, arterial blood gases, urea, creatinine, liver function test (LFT), liver enzymes and electrolytes including coagulogram be repeated as they serve as a baseline reference.

Preoperative assessment of renal function is critical in the perioperative management of these patients. Poor preoperative renal function is likely to predict poor prognosis and these are at a higher risk for intraoperative blood loss, postoperative need for dialysis, perioperative morbidity and mortality.[3] Serum creatinine is not a sensitive index of renal function in these cases and creatinine clearance is used as a preferred indicator for renal function. Hepatorenal syndrome (HRS) should always be suspected as the cause of renal failure and treated aggressively. Vasopressin analogues, terlipressin in the dose of 0.5 to 1 mg three times a day along with albumin infusion has been seen to improve renal function with improvement of serum creatinine levels and creatinine clearance.

Cardiovascular assessment is done with electrocardiography and echocardiography. Patients of chronic liver disease can easily develop fluid overload and functional tricuspid regurgitation might be visible on echocardiography. Cardiomyopathy is known to exist in alcoholic liver disease, which is revealed on echocardiography or on stress testing. End stage liver disease is associated with low systemic vascular resistance and high cardiac output and may precipitate ischemic event in patients with compromised coronary vasculature.

Ascites of portal hypertension is sometimes accompanied with hydrothorax. Hydrothorax is normally left alone unless it causes respiratory compromise in which event therapeutic drainage is done. If there is doubt of underlying pathology, computerized tomography of the chest is done to rule out consolidation underlying the hydrothorax. In the Indian subcontinent pulmonary tuberculosis should be ruled out in presence of fluid in the chest.

Risk Stratification

The disease severity scoring of these patients is based on Child Pugh classification which was modified to Child Turcotte Pugh and this is based on two clinical and three laboratory parameters (Table 8.26).

Although CTP score gives a fair estimate of severity of the disease, it does not correlate very well with the outcome of the patient following liver transplantation.

Modifications in CTP Score

There have been attempts to modify CTP score as it has a few drawbacks. The major drawback of having parameters which are subjective in nature, has been taken care of by MELD score. There have been attempts to incorporate serum creatinine in the CTP score, in the score suggested by Samiullah et al.[4] They found usefulness of creatinine modified CTP score only in patients in CTP class B only.

Model for End-stage Liver Disease

This was first used in reference to patients of portal hypertension undergoing trans jugular intrahepatic porto-systemic shunts (TIPS). Since 2002, it has replaced (CTP score) for allocation of organs in patients awaiting liver transplants in USA. Using MELD for organ allocation has reduce the mortality of waiting list patient for liver transplant.

Model for End-stage Liver Disease is another method of categorizing the patients awaiting liver transplantation. It takes into consideration serum bilirubin, prothrombin time (INR), and serum creatinine. Patient having had hemodialysis

Table 8.26: Child-Turcotte-Pugh Score (CTP)

	1	2	3
Encephalopathy	None	1 and 2	3 and 4
Ascites	Absent/ slight	Moderate	Not controlled by diuretics
Bilirubin mg%	1–2	2–3	>3
Albumin gm%	>3.5	2.8–3.5	<2.8
PT (INR)	<1.7	1.7–2.3	>2.3

Child–Pugh Class A: 5–6, Class B: 7–9, Class C: 10–15

pre-transplant affects the calculation of MELD score. It is a mathematical calculation and is calculated by the formula:

$$\begin{aligned}3.78 &\times \log e\,(\text{bilirubin mg/dL}) + 11.2\\ &\times \log e\,(\text{INR}) + 9.5\\ &\times \log e\,(\text{creatinine mg/dL}) + 6.4\end{aligned}$$

The MELD is modified in case of hepatocellular carcinoma, the minimum score automatically becomes 24 irrespective of other parameters.

Extra MELD points are also given to patients who have developed hepatopulmonary syndrome and their paO_2 values are less than 60 mm Hg, implying the advanced nature of liver dysfunction and priortization of such patients.

There have been further modifications of MELD as well. Among those which have been found useful in categorizing disease severity are Na MELD and Delta MELD. Both these MELD variants do need to be validated on a larger scale.

Pediatric End-stage Liver Disease

For children under the age of 12 years have different criteria for listing them for liver transplantation. Besides age, it takes into consideration serum albumin, prothrombin time (INR), weight and bilirubin. The mathematical calculation is as follows:

PELD Score = 10* (0.480 * (bilirubin) + 1.857 * (INR) - 0.687 * (albumin) + 0.436.

The PELD score calculation takes into account if the child is less than one year and if there is growth failure.

There have been developments in incorporating other parameters for assessing disease severity, the most prominent being serum sodium. Hyponatremia indicates severity of chronic liver disease and is associated with poor prognosis. Serum sodium is incorporated in the recently adopted score in United Kingdom and is called UKELD. The validity of this score in organ allocation or outcome after transplant is yet to be established in prospective studies. The calculation is done as follows:

UKELD – (5.395×INR) + (1.485×S. Creatinine) + (3.13×S. Bilirubin) – (81.565×S. Na) + 435

A score of 49 is required before a patient is listed for transplantation and this signifies 9% one year mortality risk. A score of 60, on the other hand is associated with 50% mortality in one year 5.

FULMINANT HEPATIC FAILURE

The patients with acute liver disease cannot be rated according to CTP or MELD. The most accepted criteria for fulminant hepatic failure is the King`s College Criteria which has separate distinguishing parameters for those having acetaminophen toxicity and others.

Criteria of King's College, London

- Acetaminophen toxicity patients
  - Ph<7.3 or
  - Prothrombin time >6.5 (INR) and serum creatinine level >3.4 mg/dL
- Other patients (Nonacetaminophen)
  - Prothrombin time >6.5 (INR) or
  - Any three of the following variables:
    - Age <10 years or > 40 years
    - Etiology: non, A non, B hepatitis, halothane hepatitis, idiosyncratic drug reaction
    - Duration of jaundice before encephalopathy >7d
    - Prothrombin time >3.5 (INR)
    - Serum bilirubin level >17.6 mg/dL.

Surgery Specific Anesthetic Preparation and Premedication

Preoperative Preparation

Preoperative preparation includes re-evaluation of the patient especially if the patient has been admitted from home. All patients must undergo screening process to rule out any infective issues. Culture of blood, urine and ascitic fluid is done. X-ray chest is done if there was hydrothorax or gross ascites, which can affect lung bases. Arterial blood gases are done to rule out metabolic acidosis, which is seen especially if there is development of portal vein thrombosis. Poor oxygenation is seen hepatopulmonary syndrome for which liver transplant is the answer though these patients have a prolonged intensive care stay. Echocardiography is done to rule out pericardial effusion and any alteration of cardiac function. The need for incentive spirometry is emphasized and patients educated in its use. Premedication with anxiolytics is generally not required except in children or younger patients.

Induction and Intubation

All patients are induced in operating theater and the patient is placed on a gel mattress underneath which is thermostatically controlled with warm water circulating at 39–41°C. Forced air warmer can also be used to keep upper and lower body warm. An ECG monitor, pulseoximeter and automatic blood pressure monitor are attached to the patient before induction. Anesthesia is usually induced with midazolam 1–2 mg, fentanyl 1–1.5 mcg/kg and propofol 1–2 mg/kg.

This may be followed by suxamethonium if the patient has gross ascites or is likely to be full stomach, otherwise a non-depolarizing relaxant can be used to facilitate endotracheal intubation. Anesthesia is maintained with fentanyl 1–2 mcg/kg/hour with air/oxygen/desflurane or isoflurane. Use of nitrous oxide is avoided as it causes distension of intestines on prolonged use, besides there is always possibility of air embolism in liver transplant surgery, which makes presence of nitrous oxide hazardous.

The volatile agent of choice has been isoflurane, which preserves splanchnic blood flow better than other volatile agents.[6] There is evidence that hepatic artery buffer response is better preserved with isoflurane than other inhalational agents. Rocuroniun or vecuronium are the preferred muscle relaxants, rocuronium probably has a slight advantage as this relaxant does not have any active metabolite. In a patient where an early extubation is not planned, either of the agents can be used as none of them has any hepato-toxic effects. Atracurium is metabolized by Hoffman`s elimination which is pH dependent and is unaffected by liver or kidney function. The breakdown product of atracurium is laudanosine which is excreted by the kidney. This becomes relevant in the event of patients with hepatic encephalopathy in presence of pre-existing renal dysfunction as laudanosine has central nervous system effects.

Vascular Access and Various Invasive Monitoring

Vascular Access

Liver transplant surgery is associated with unpredictable blood losses. Losses are expectedly more if there is a history of previous upper abdominal surgery or the patient is highly coagulopathic and has significant portal hypertension. Peripheral venous access may be difficult if the patient has had previous hospital admissions before the transplant.

Large-bore intravenous infusions are set up in the arms if peripheral access is available. After induction of anesthesia is done, central venous cannulation is done. Typically two central venous catheters are inserted, among them one is a large bore for rapid infusion and another triple/four lumen for infusion of drugs and blood products (Fig. 8.25A). In children also two central venous catheters are inserted and the prefer side is right internal jugular vein (Fig. 8.25B). Pulmonary artery catheter (PAC) is floated to monitor pulmonary artery pressures. Internal jugular vein preferably the right side, is the route selected because of the straighter course of the vein. At Medanta, The Medicity Hospital, we use Advance Venous Access catheter 7.5 F which has three lumen and a port for floating pulmonary artery catheter. If veno-venous bypass is

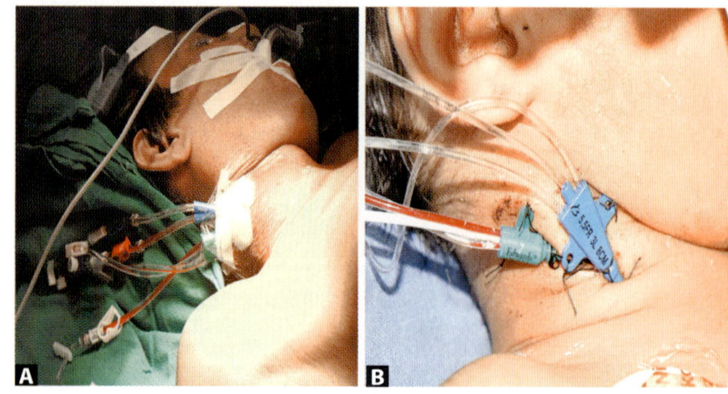

Figs 8.25A and B: (A) Vascular access in adults and children; (B) Preferred site right internal jugular vein

to be used then either 10F catheter is used or axillary vein is used on the left side. If axillary vein is to be used for inflow, open access is usually obtained surgically. Veno-venous bypass has not been used in our institution for the last 300 patients for transplantation.[7]

Intraoperative Monitoring

Special emphasis is made to have comprehensive monitoring of hemodynamic, coagulation, renal and respiratory systems. The hemodynamic changes could be sudden and extreme in nature with cardiac output varying drastically during vena caval clamping and reperfusion. Blood loss could be sudden and massive, besides coagulopathy adding to the continuous blood loss and blood product infusion.

A multifunction patient monitored along with cardiac output monitoring is essential for these patients (Fig. 8.26). Continuous intravascular pressure monitoring is mandatory and there is a case for having two arterial catheters. All patients do have central venous catheters and in selected patients, there is need to have pulmonary artery catheter as well. Pulmonary artery catheter can be used for measuring cardiac output by thermodilution method as well as to monitor pulmonary artery pressures which are increased in patients with portopulmonary hypertension (POPH). Mean pulmonary artery pressure (MPAP) higher than 35 mm Hg have poor prognosis post liver transplant and will require therapeutic measures to keep MPAP well below 35 mm Hg. Mixed venous oxygen saturation can act as a good indicator of graft function at the time of reperfusion.

Another monitoring tool which can be used is trans-esophageal echocardiography (TEE), which is a non-invasive tool. Discretion has to be used in patients with large esophageal varices, which could bleed during insertion and manipulation of the TEE probe. It is useful to assess the volume status as well

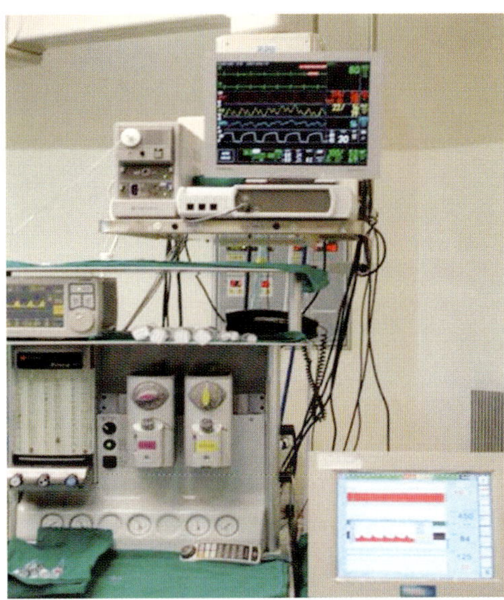

Fig. 8.26: Multifunction patient monitor and lithium dilution cardiac output monitor ring

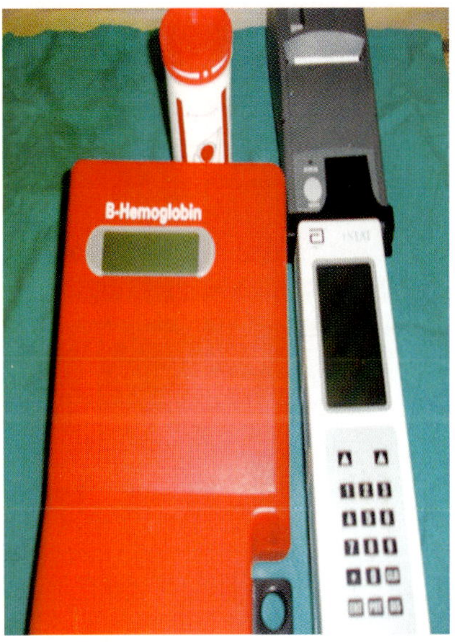

Fig. 8.27: Hemoglobinometer and blood gas analyzer

as contractility of the ventricles. It is also useful in diagnosing air embolism as well as thromboembolism, which is always a possibility in this surgery.

Temperature monitoring is essential as hypothermia affects the activity of clotting factors. The maximum temperature drop occurs in the initial induction stage and early in dissection phase. Patient should not be left exposed, except at the time insertion of lines and during the cleaning and draping procedure. Warming mattress, heating blanket, and fluid warmers are used to keep temperature closer to 37°C.

Arterial blood gases are monitored on a regular basis, starting from induction of anesthesia (Fig. 8.27). This gives an account of blood oxygenation, sodium, potassium, pH, calcium, glucose and hemoglobin. These parameters are subject to change during the surgery and their regular monitoring is essential for safe conduct of anesthesia. The use of blood and blood products could lead to citrate proxicity as it is not metabolized by the liver which is sub-optimal in function. Citrate binds to calcium and will lead to hypocalcemia and would need correction with calcium chloride on a continuous basis if blood or blood products are infused. Equally important is monitoring of sodium as a number of these patients have hyponatremia and rapid correction of sodium can lead to pontine mylinosis, which has a very poor prognosis.

Intraoperative Coagulation

Preoperative coagulation screen and full blood count along with PT/INR should be performed routinely in theater at regular interval. A full coagulation screen, including platelet count, fibrinogen levels and thromboelastography (TEG) are routinely done, to monitor coagulation.[7]

Intraoperatively the coagulation parameters–PT and/or TEG checked and if found abnormal, either FFP and/or platelets are infused. Absolute number of platelets probably do not reflect state of coagulation in these patients of chronic liver disease with portal hypertension and hyperspenism. Thromboelastography is a better modality to ascertain requirement of platelets, prolonged reaction time along with maximum amplitude (mA) less than 40 mm justifies platelet supplementation.

At Medanta, The Medicity, it is a practice to have onsite coagulation monitoring in operating theater and thromboelastography (TEG) is used for assessing coagulation status and administrating blood products (Figs 8.28 and 8.29). TEG is done at the start of the operation, once or twice during dissection phase, anhepatic phase, an hour after reperfusion and at any time there is unexplainable bleeding.

High-risk patients (those with portal hypertension, history of upper abdominal surgery or bacterial peritonitis) may require prophylactic antifibrinolytic therapy. Subclinical fibrinolysis is present in most patients with chronic liver disease and some centers advocate the use of antifibrinolytic therapy in all patients for liver transplant for chronic liver disease as this is known to reduce overall blood and blood product requirement. There are case reports implicating use of antifibrinolytics with thrombotic events in the recipients.

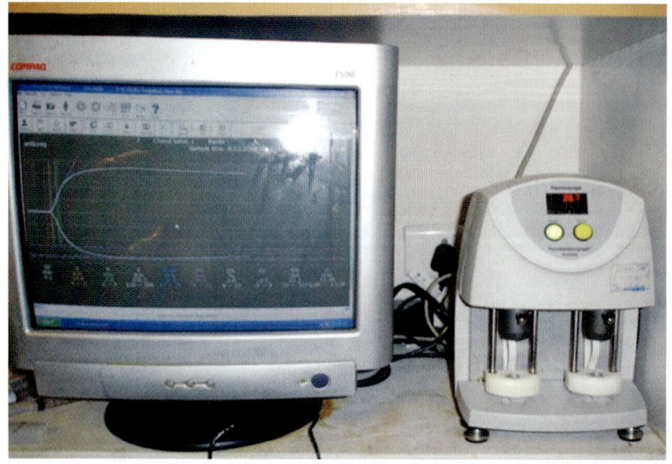

Fig. 8.28: Two channel TEG machine with active monitoring screen

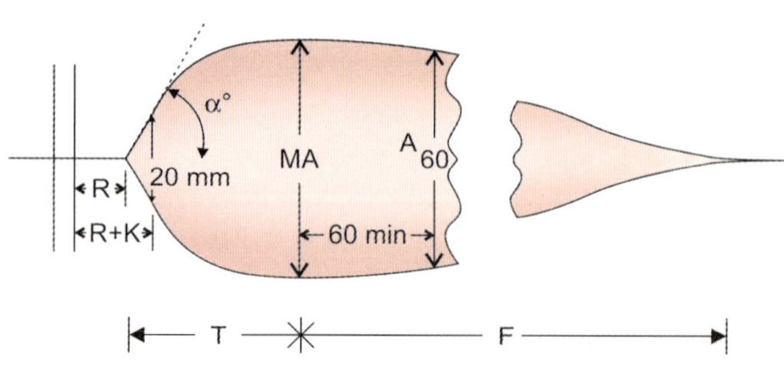

Fig. 8.29: Thromboelastograph showing various components—R, K, R +K time, α angle, MA A 60

Antifibrinolytic therapy is used in the form of Traxemic acid, 1 gm bolus followed by 6 gm over 24 hours. Other option is aprotinin infusion 50,000 unit test dose, and after 15 minutes, 2 million units over 30 minutes, followed by 5,00,000 units per hour till the end of surgery. Patients with Budd-Chiari syndrome, hepatocellular carcinoma or those with a history of deep vein thrombosis or other thrombotic tendency are excluded from prophylactic antifibrinolytic therapy.

Phases of Liver Transplantation

Dissection Phase

The beginning of the surgery itself gives a clue to the likely course of the transplant procedure. Coagulopathy should be corrected promptly and aggressively, as chasing the abnormal numbers leads to more and more blood loss. The major cardiovascular changes associated with this stage are those related to intravascular volume depletion as a result of blood loss, manipulation of liver and handling of the inferior vena cava (IVC). During this period the most important consideration is to maintain intravascular volume by infusion of blood, blood products and colloids, depending on the hematocrit and coagulation status. The blood loss in this phase could be massive especially in those patients with portal hypertension and previous upper abdominal surgery. Calcium chloride/gluconate must be added in adequate dose to avoid hypotension due to continuous blood loss.

Once dissection of the liver is done and all the vessels and bile duct have been isolated, trial clamping of inferior vena cava is performed to see how well this maneuver will be tolerated when new liver is being revascularized. The trial clamping is done for at least one minute to see the hemodynamic effects. There is an expected drop in cardiac output and it is to be assessed whether this period of inferior vena cava clamping can be managed with vasopressors and volume adjustments. Adequacy of the patient's ability to withstand caval clamping is thereby assessed. If the systolic pressure falls to less than 70% of its previous value, (or SAP <80–90 mm Hg, or MAP < 60 mm Hg), in the presence of adequate blood replacement, or if ECG changes occur, bypass support may be needed. In our center at SGRH we rarely resort to veno-venous bypass during inferior vena cava clamping. One reason for that is the patients who are accepted for transplants normally do not have significant heart disease.

Anhepatic Phase

Clamping of portal vein marks the beginning of anhepatic phase and this causes congestion of the bowel.[8,9] If anhepatic phase is likely to be prolonged, portocaval shunt can be established, which will prevent bowel congestion. These can also be obviated by using veno venous bypass, but it has its own inherent side effects of air embolism, etc. which requires monitoring.[10]

Hemodynamic changes during this period are related to IVC cross-clamping and to physiological changes caused by the removal of the liver. Some patients, who were unstable during dissection phase start stabilizing during anhepatic phase because the liver which was producing various vasoactive substances is now out of circulation. On the other hand with liver out, some patient would start showing signs of fibrinolysis as tissue plasminogen activator is not being removed from the circulation. IVC cross-clamping results in a decrease in cardiac

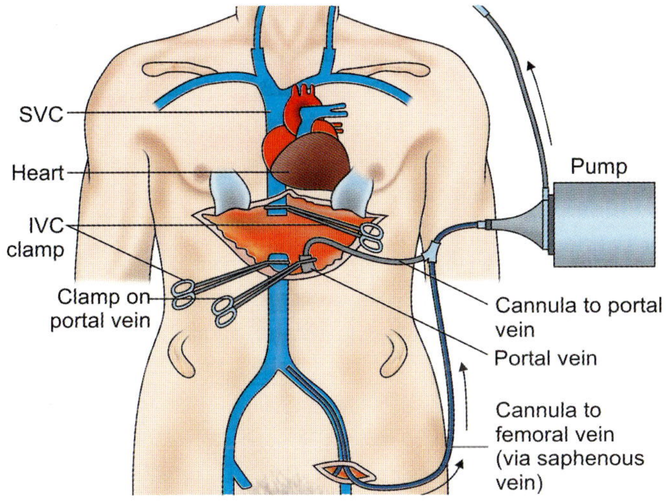

Fig. 8.30: Veno venous bypass

output which is more marked in the absence of extensive collaterals as seen in patients with hepatocellular carcinoma. IVC side clamping is done if the patient does not tolerate cross clamping or if there is preoperative renal dysfunction. Removal of the native liver results in reduction in oxygen consumption, which also contributes to the fall in cardiac output. Absence of liver function results in inability to metabolize citrate; citrate intoxication presents with decreased ionized calcium and myocardial depression. Hypocalcemia must be corrected before reperfusion.

Attempts to increase filling pressures by blood and fluid replacement must be cautious at this stage, because of the danger of fluid overload at the time of liver revascularization, when normal venous return and central blood volume are restored. Piggyback technique decreases the need for VVB.[11]

Veno venous Bypass

Veno venous bypass involves cannulating inferior vena cava and portal vein and the blood from these two sides being pumped back into the upper body circulation via axillary vein or internal jugular vein (Fig. 8.30). Venovenous bypass during liver transplantation started as a routine in cadaveric liver transplant where liver along with vena cava are dissected out and replaced with anatomizing two caval ends with liver attached to it. Other advantages of VVB during liver transplant are it maintains hemodynamic stability, preserves cardiac, pulmonary, cerebral, renal and intestinal flow and function and reduces blood loss. Besides it gives more time for surgical procedure to be carried out. Veroli et al advised the use of VVB in patients with 30% drop in mean arterial pressure and 50% decrease in cardiac index during a 5 min test-clamping of inferior vena cava.[12] However, several studies have failed to show any effect on morbidity or mortality in patients with or without the use of VVB.[13,14]

Administration of vasopressors and strict volume adjustment can help to maintain preload and hemodynamic stability without an increased risk of volume overload and pulmonary edema following reperfusion of the liver.[15] In living donor liver transplant, there is preservation of recipient vena cava and therefore one can even do partial caval clamping and carry out the venous anastomosis.

Reperfusion Phase

Reperfusion of the new liver is accompanied with changes due to ischemia reperfusion injury. The extent of this injury can be minimized by giving prednisolone before reperfusion in the dose of 10 mg/kg. Still reperfusion can cause dramatic cardiovascular changes, which may or may not last for a long time.[16] There is a sudden increase in serum potassium levels, which may used to be offset by giving calcium bolus. There could be sudden decrease in heart rate, mean arterial pressure and systemic vascular resistance due to release of vasoactive substances from ischemic liver graft and from static blood from the gut. It is important to ensure that ionized calcium levels are greater than 1.1 mmol/lt before reperfusion. Treat hypotension with phenylephrine, or noradrenaline, which should be connected through a syringe pump connected to a running infusion. It is common practice to use one of these prophylactically, along with calcium chloride, on unclamping of the portal vein. Normally there is no more blood loss after this stage but at times anestemotic vascular bleed and fibrinolysis continues and may require continued antifibrinolytic therapy and blood product.

Maintenance of Renal Function and Fluid Balance: Kidneys are prone to get affected during the transplant with the rapidly altering cardiac output. Effort must be made to maintain urine output during the procedure, although oliguria is usual and even anuria may occur during the period when inferior vena cava is clamped. Crystalloid infusion in the form of 5% dextrose is started from the beginning to prevent hypoglycemia. Other crystalloid used is Plasmalyte A which is pH corrected solution having pH of 7.4. Hartman`s solution contains lactate which is normally metabolized in the liver and therefore may not be good choice if large volume of fluids are required. Intravascular volume is maintained with Albumin, 6% Hydroxyethyl starch (HES), blood and blood products as indicated by measurements of hematocrit and thromboelastography (TEG). Mannitol is given as free radical scavenger and as osmotic diuretic in a dose of 0.5 to 1.0 g/kg before inferior vena cava clamping, when an abrupt fall or temporary cessation of urine output is usual. Vena cava clamping is done while the venous anastomosis and portal venous system is being established for the new liver and this period of vena cava clamping lasts for less than one hour. Vasopressors may be required at this stage, nor adrenaline, adrenaline, phenylephrine have all been used. There may be need to give intravenous fluids if there is inadequate response to vasopressors. Dopamine 200 mg in 50 mL 5% glucose can be used at 0.5–2 mL hr^{-1} if there is still inadequate urine output with the measures outlined above. The maintenance of urine output is desirable although the use of low-dose dopamine for this reason is unproven.[18]

If there is evidence renal dysfunction preoperatively, one should consider use of veno venous bypass which maintains renal blood flow during periods of portal vein and vena cava clamping which otherwise produces low flow states.

Option to consider in patients with renal dysfunction is to avoid complete venous clamping and instead use a side clamp whereby a partial vena cava clamp is applied and venous return is not hampered.

Chronic liver disease is often associated with hyponatremia and rapid correction of sodium is accompanied with dire consequences. Sodium level should be maintained closer to the preoperative levels and certainly not increase by more than 12 mmols/L in 24 hours which can lead to cerebropontine mylinosis.

Usage of Blood and Blood Products and Blood Conservation Strategies

Blood Conservation Strategies

Liver transplantation is at times associated with large blood losses and various conservation strategies are adopted to minimize blood/blood product requirement. Correction of coagulation defects with plasma transfusion does not necessarily decrease blood loss during liver transplantation, it can even lead to a hypervolemic state which can even increase blood loss during surgery.

Low Central Venous Pressure

To reduce blood losses during liver dissection before the anhepatic phase, various measures can be employed. One of them is lowering of central venous pressure. Central venous pressure can be lowered by fluid restriction, phlebotomy, and by avoiding plasma transfusion in order and hence diminish the transfusion of blood products. This practice of reducing central venous pressure does not result in any deleterious results.[19]

Cell Saver (Fig. 8.31)

The use of intraoperative cell saver shows a reduction of blood and components transfusion. In a prospective study published recently, the use of cell saver was shown not only to reduce transfusion but also could be cost effective.[20] Cell saver use has the potential to reduce the need for hetorologous transfusion, thereby reducing the risks of disease transmission and allied to this the cost is also reduced. One aspect that needs to be kept in mind is that with cell saver, one is using blood which has come out of the abdominal cavity, gone into collection bags, washed, collected into other bags and then reinfused. During this travel from the abdominal cavity to reinfusion, there is possibility of contamination and infection.

Thromboelastography

Routine use of thromboelastography in the surgical theater is another means to reduce transfusion of blood components, especially fresh frozen plasma and platelets. Another means of blood loss reduction is the use of recombinant activated factor VII (rFVIIa). Two recent retrospective studies obtained favorable results with reduced transfusion of packed red blood cells and fresh frozen plasma in the patients treated with rFVIIa.[21,22]

Antifibrinolytic

Use of antifibrinolytic can also reduce intraoperative bleeding, as there is some amount of fibrinolysis going on in most patients

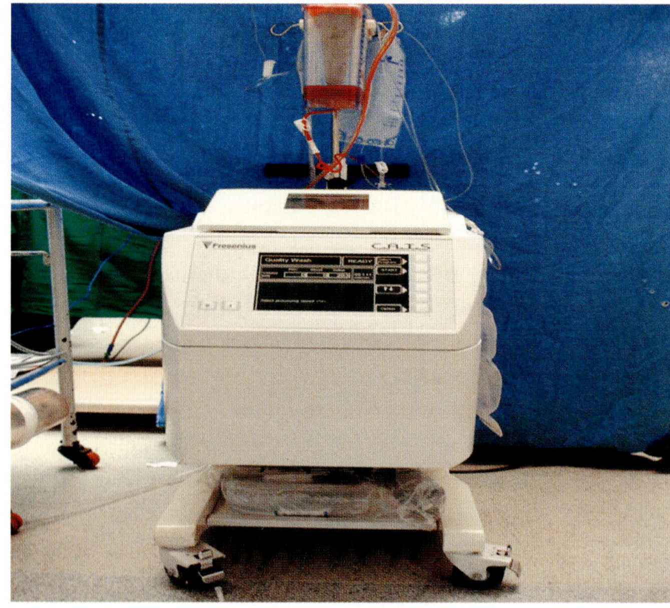

Fig. 8.31: Cell saver

with chronic liver disease. This is due to presence of circulating t-PA during the anhepatic phase and the burst release of t-PA associated with the reperfusion of the liver graft. Aprotinin has been shown to reduce transfusion requirements in surgeries with significant blood loss.[23]

Specific Complications

Major Bleeding

This procedure has a potential to have rapid and sudden blood loss and it is essential to transfuse at a rate sufficient to maintain hemodynamic parameters in the near normal range. Some form of rapid infusion device should be available to correct the changing hemodynamic status. It should be remembered that concentrated and washed cells must be supplemented with colloids. Rapid blood replacement causes citrate intoxication leading to hypocalcemia, and even hyperkalemia.

Air Thrombolism

This is likely to occur during dissection as well as when the graft gets back into circulation. Air embolism is seen at the time of dissection in the area of inferior vena cava. Any hole in the vena cava during dissection, entrain air as vena cava is a fixed structure. This is more likely to happen if the venous pressures are low. Thromboembolism happens during re-perfusion, as micro-thrombi in hepatic circulation or from the venovenous bypass circuit (if used) get back into the circulation.

Metabolic Acidosis

There is likelihood of developing metabolic acidosis during dissection and anhepatic phase. Metabolic acidosis develops due to tissue hypoperfusion resulting from shunting of blood from intestines to systemic circulation. Treatment should be aimed at correcting the volume status and by mild hyperventilation. Sodium bicarbonate should be used cautiously as this adds to sodium load. After reperfusion of the liver, metabolic acidosis typically worsens as a result of sudden release into the circulation of acidotic material from the ischemic liver and obstructed splanchnic bed. This is generally self-limiting and resolves over a few hours without specific treatment. It could lead to what is described as post-reperfusion syndrome which is defined as a 30% or more drop in blood pressure from baseline that lasts for at least 1 minute. This syndrome is seen more in cadaveric donor liver transplant and is rare in LDLT patients.

Hypocalcemia

Ionized calcium measurements are made at regular intervals during the operation. Levels tend to be low even in the early part of the operation in patients with poor liver function, as a result of the citrate in blood products. In spite of calcium administration, these may fall further during anhepatic phase, when citrate metabolism ceases completely. If blood loss is not substantial, values return to normal after reperfusion without the need for further treatment. The aim should be to keep serum calcium within the normal range (1.1–1.3 mmol 1L) at all times, especially during the period preceding reperfusion.

Hyperkalemia

This occurs on release of the clamps on portal and hepatic vein but the effect is short lasting and no specific treatment apart from prophylactic calcium chloride is indicated. When hyperkalemia is present or is likely to occur before reperfusion measures to prevent a further marked increase are essential to reduce the risk of hyperkalemic arrest at reperfusion. These include washing of bank blood (if using cell saver), glucose/insulin infusion and calcium. Other measures used include bleed out of some portal blood and/or bleeding out a predetermined amount of blood from the hepatic veins before establishing reperfusion.

Initial Poor Graft Function

Persistence of metabolic acidosis after reperfusion and continued hemodynamic instability should sound warning bells for poor graft functioning. Congested or grayish appearance of the liver, coagulopathy, poor urine output, and hypotension are signs of poor graft function. Poor graft function is seen in poor quality of liver grafts mainly from cadaver donors. These marginal donors are being accepted for transplantation due to shortages of donor organs and increasing waiting lists. These are more prone for ischemia reperfusion injury compared to normal grafts. This issue is almost non-existent in live donor liver transplants. Management includes continued use of N-acetylcysteine 5–10 mg/Kg/hr, vasopressors and control of metabolic acidosis. It could take 24 hours or longer before the liver functions start improving. There is continuous requirement for supporting coagulation-fresh frozen plasma, cryoprecipitates as well as antifibrinolytics.

Postoperative Care and Management

Monitoring continues in the postoperative period from where it was left in the operating theater. Pulmonary artery pressure

(PAP) monitoring may be discontinued in the intensive care unit, if the pressures are near normal and remain stable. The pulmonary artery catheter should be removed after having seen position on chest X-ray. Most patients post-transplant are ventilated for a variable period depending on their preoperative status and the intraoperative course. Selected patients can be extubated early in the immediate postoperative period on transfer to the intensive care unit. Postoperative routine investigations include hemoglobin, PT, APTT, platelet count, SGOT, SGPT, sodium, potassium, calcium and creatinine.

There has been an interest to fast track some of these patients from the intensive care unit. To successfully fast track it is important to use short-acting drugs and appropriate use of narcotics and benzodiazepine to allow early return of spontaneous breathing and awakening at the end of surgery. Patients with encephalopathy, large blood and blood product requirement, obesity, high Child's Pugh Score are not good candidates for fast tracking. Similarly obesity and preoperative encephalopathy are likely to result in failed attempts at immediate extubation. Therefore one must be very careful in selecting patients for fast tracking. It is not true that endotracheal extubation at the end of surgery will result in shorter intensive-care-unit stay or in significant savings in cost. All patients postoperatively still require close monitoring.

Keeping a low venous pressure enables a better venous drainage from the newly grafted liver. So if PEEP (Positive end expiratory pressure) and intermittent positive pressure ventilation (IPPV) can be avoided or minimized in the perioperative period, it may be beneficial for the new liver. Aggressive chest physiotherapy is done postextubation and incentive spirometry. All patients are counseled pre-operatively about the need to do incentive spirometry in postoperative phase in the intensive care unit, this is though is not possible in patients with encephalopathy.

Vascular Doppler is carried out once a day to know the blood flow in portal vein, hepatic vein and hepatic artery. In children, the Doppler studies are conducted twice a day. The re-exploration rate is much higher in children due to hepatic artery thrombosis or other vascular flows. Some of the children may require heparin infusion postoperatively to prevent thrombotic complications.

Abdominal drain is monitored for the quantity of drainage produced every hour, if required, drain hemoglobin is measured. If drain hemoglobin is close to patient's hemoglobin, intra-abdominal bleed or coagulopathy should be strongly suspected. Thromboelastography (TEG) at this stage may help in differentiating medical bleed from surgical bleed. In surgical bleed the TEG will be near normal.

Postoperative infection is a major hazard in these patients. Over 80% mortality in liver transplant is related to infective issues. Barrier nursing, hand hygiene and appropriate antibiotic therapy should be used in these immunocompromised patients. Immunosuppression in liver transplants can be introduced upto 72 hours posttransplant as liver is much less immunogenic compared to other organs like kidney.

Liver transplantation is at a threshold in this country and is ready to take off and become a routine procedure. The number of liver transplant centers in India has grown significantly in the last five years. It requires dedicated multidisciplinary approach with commitment from surgery, anesthesiology, hepatology, blood transfusion services, intensivists, physiotherapist and intensive care nursing staff.

CLINICAL PEARLS

- Live related and deceased donor liver transplant
- Preoperative evaluation plan, necessary investigation and risk stratification
- Surgery specific anesthetic preparation and pre-medication
- Vascular access and various invasive monitoring
- Phases of liver transplantation
- Usage of blood and blood products and blood conservation strategies
- Complications
- Postoperative care and management

REFERENCES

1. Kamath PS, Wiesner RH, Malinchoc M, et al. A model to predict survival in patients with end-stage liver disease. Hepatology, 2001;33:464-70.
2. United Network for Organ Sharing Liver Disease Severity Score Committee Wiesner R, Edwards E, et al. Model for end stage liver disease (MELD) and allocation of donor livers. Gastroenterology, 2003;124:91-96.
3. Pham PT, Pham PC, Wilkinson AH. The kidney in liver transplantation. Clin Liver Dis, 2000;3:567-90.
4. Samiullah, et al. Evaluation of Creatinine modified Child Pugh score.for predicting short term prognosis in patients with decompensated cirrhosis of liver as compared to original Child Pugh score. J Ayub Med Coll Abbottabad, 2009;21(2):64-67.
5. Asrani SK, Kim WR (May 2010). "Organ allocation for chronic liver disease: model for end-stage liver disease and beyond". Curr. Opin. Gastroenterol, 26(3):209-13.
6. O'Riordan J, O'Beirne HA, Young Y, Bellamy MC. Effects of desflurane and isoflurane on splanchnic microcirculation during major surgery. Br J Anaesth, 1997;78:95-6.

7. Ozier Y, Pessione F, Samain E, Courtois F. Institutional variability in transfusion practice for liver transplantation. Anesth Analg, 2003;97:671-9.
8. Haagsma EB, Gips CH, Wesenhagen H, Van Imhoff GW, Krom RA. Liver disease and its effect on haemostasis during liver transplantation. Liver, 1985;5:123-8.
9. BechsteinWO, Neuhaus P. Bleeding problems in liver surgery and liver transplantation. Chirurg, 2000;71:363-8.
10. Budd JM, Isaac JL, Bennett J, et al. Morbidity and mortality associated with large-bore percutaneous venovenous bypass cannulation for 312 orthotopic liver transplantations. Liver Transplant, 2001:7:359-62.
11. Tzakis A, Todo S, Starzl TE. Orthotopic liver transplantation with preservation of the inferior vena cava. Ann Surg, 1989;210:649-52.
12. Veroli P, el Hage C, Ecoffey C. Does adult liver transplantation without venovenous bypass result in renal failure? Anesth Analg, 1992;75:489-94.
13. Schwarz B, Pomaroli A, Hoermann C, Margreiter R, Mair P. Liver transplantation without venovenous bypass: morbidity and mortality in patients with greater than 50% reduction in cardiac output after vena cava clamping. J Cardiothorac Vasc Anesth, 2001;15:460-2.
14. Wall WJ, Grant DR, Duff JH, Kutt JL, Ghent CN, Bloch MS. Liver transplantation without venous bypass. Transplantation, 1987;43:56-61.
15. Wu Y, Oyos TL, Chenhsu RY, Katz DA, Brian JE, Rayhill SC. Vasopressor agents without volume expansion as a safe alternative to venovenous bypass during cavaplasty liver transplantation. Transplantation, 2003;76:1724-8.
16. Blanot S, Gillon MC, Ecoffey C. Circulating endotoxins during orthotopic liver transplantation and post-reperfusion syndrome [letter]. Lancet, 1993;342:859-60.
17. Estrin JA, Beiani KG, Ascher ML, Lura D, Payne W, Najarian JS. Haemodynamic changes on dumping and unclamping of major vessels during liver transplantation. Transplant Proc, 1989;21:3500-5.
18. Swygert T. Effect of intraoperative low-dose dopamine on renal function in liver transplant recipients. Anesthesiology, 1991; 75:571-6.
19. Luc Massicotte. 1 Serge Lenis Liver Transplantation, 2006;12:117-23.
20. Phillips SD, Deshpande R, Muiesan P, Bowles MJ, Rela M, Heaton ND. A prospective study investigating the cost effectiveness of intraoperative blood salvage during liver transplantation. Transplantation, 2006;81:536-40.
21. Kalicinski P, Markiewicz M, Kaminski A, Laniewski P, Ismail H, Drewniak T, et al. Single pretransplant bolus of recombinant activated factor VII ameliorates influence of risk factors for blood loss during orthotopic liver transplantation. Ped Transpl, 2005;9:299-304.
22. Niemann CU, Behrends M, Quan D, Eilers H, Gropper MA, Roberts JP, et al. Recombinant factor VIIa reduces transfusion requirements in liver transplant patients with high MELD scores. Transf Med, 2006;16:93-100.
23. Lentschener C, Roche K, Ozier Y. A review of aprotinin in orthotopic liver transplantation: can its harmful effects offset its beneficial effects? Anesth Analg, 2005;100:1248-55.

Anesthetic Management of Pediatric Liver Transplantation

Archna Koul, Deepanjali Pant

INTRODUCTION

Pediatric liver transplantation is one of the most successful solid organ transplants. The United Network for Organ Sharing (UNOS) has reported one year graft survival of 81% in 6–10 years old recipients compared to 68%, a decade ago.[1] From 1988 to 2010, a total of 11958 pediatric liver transplantations have been performed in the United States of which 10% have been living related.

In just two decades pediatric liver transplant has matured as a clinical therapy from one performed in only a few countries in the United States and Western Europe to one that is practiced in innumerable medical institutions. Improvement in immunosuppression therapy, surgical techniques and organ preservation have been of key importance in improving survival after transplant. Split liver and living donor liver transplantation have contributed in decreasing waiting list and mortality in pediatric patients.

Pediatric liver transplantation is a high-risk procedure, carrying a significant risk of mortality with a potential for chronic disability and requirement for long-term drug administration. Long-term follow-up, prevention of immunosuppression related complications and aiming at "as normal growth as possible" are the main issues of interest in the present day practice of liver transplant.

Indications for Liver Transplantation

1. Progressive subacute or chronic primary liver disease such as biliary atresia and sclerosing cholangitis.
2. Metabolic diseases of liver such as Wilson's disease, α1 antitrypsin deficiency, oxaluria, tyrosinemia, urea cycle enzyme deficiencies and glycogen storage disorders. Metabolic disorders such as oxalosis or primary hyper-oxaluria and urea cycle enzyme deficiencies manifest solely with extrahepatic manifestations.
3. Hepatic tumors.
4. Fulminant hepatic failure.
5. Secondary liver disease, e.g. biliary cirrhosis secondary to cystic fibrosis and sclerosing cholangitis secondary to Langerhans cell histiocytosis.

In approximately 75% of children with acute liver failure the etiology is unknown.[2]

The most common indications for transplant in children are biliary atresia followed by metabolic disease and acute hepatic necrosis.

Growth is a sensitive measure of liver function in childhood. The point of growth arrest is therefore the ideal time to transplant an infant with biliary atresia and cirrhosis after removing any correctable cause of growth failure.[3]

Cirrhosis is an indication of liver transplant only if there is evidence of functional hepatic decompensation such as coagulopathy, frequent massive GI bleed, malnutrition, growth failure or severe bacterial infection.

Cholestatic disease comprises 54.4% of the total population and is the most common disease among both, registered and transplanted patients. Biliary atresia is by far the most common cholestatic disease in children accounting for 50–75% of liver transplants performed.[4] After undergoing a Kasai's procedure approximately 1/3 of patients have long term success, 1/3 will require urgent transplantation and remaining 1/3rd require non urgent transplantation.[5]

Metabolic causes are the second most common indication for liver transplant. Liver transplant can correct hyperammonemia related to metabolic errors involving urea cycles but it cannot correct CNS injury. Early diagnosis, aggressive support and early liver transplantation before neurological damage occurs, is essential.

Hepatic Tumors: Hepatoblastoma is the most common primary hepatic tumor in childhood accounting for 0.8–2.0% of all pediatric tumors but more than 50% of these patients are unsuitable for radical surgery at diagnosis because of huge intrahepatic extension of tumor and or presence of extra-hepatic disease.[6]

Absolute Contraindications to Liver Transplant

1. Extrahepatic malignancy which is non resectable
2. Uncontrolled systemic or locally invasive infection
3. Irreversible massive brain injury
4. Uncorrectable congenital anomalies affecting major organs
5. Multisystem organ failure.

Relative Contraindications to Liver Transplant

- Malignancy that is considered cured or curable by standard oncological criteria
- Treatable infection
- HIV infection
- Extrahepatic disease
  a. Progressive extrahepatic disease
  b. Substance abuse.

Evaluation of the Transplant Candidate

The primary goal of the evaluation process is to identify appropriate candidates for liver transplantation and to establish a pre-transplantation plan.

The following steps are usually considered

1. Confirm the indication for transplantation
2. Determine the severity of disease
3. Consider alternative treatment to transplantation
4. Exclude contraindications to transplantation
5. Identify active infections and assess immunological status of child
6. Rule out cardiac malformations that might need to be corrected before transplantation
7. Establish a pre-treatment therapeutic plan: immunizations when possible, nutritional support to optimize growth, dental care, prevention or treatment of drug induced side effects (e.g. osteopenia secondary to prolonged steroid intake).

Pediatric End-stage Liver Disease (PELD) Scoring

In 2002, the pediatric end stage liver disease (PELD) score was implemented to allocate decreased donor livers based on the severity of liver disease. PELD numerical scale is currently used for liver allocation in children less than 12 years of age. At the same time 'model for end stage liver disease' (MELD) score was implemented for adults.

The PELD score seeks to accurately predict death or transfer to ICU within 3 months of testing.[8]

A patient with acute liver failure (ALF) (status I) is given priority for liver donors, then patients with highest MELD/PELD score and appropriate blood group are next.

PELD score depends on:

- Total bilirubin
- INR
- Serum-albumin
- Age <1 year
- Height <2 standard deviation from mean

PELD Score
$10 \times [0.480 \times \log e$ (total bilirubin mg/dL)]
$+ 1.857 \times \log e$ (INR)
$- 0.687 \times \log e$ (alb g/dL)
$+ 0.436$ (if pt <1 year of age)
$+ 0.667$ (if pt has growth failure).

Drawbacks of the Scoring System

Extrahepatic manifestations of liver disease such as renal failure, pulmonary hypertension and hepatopulmonary syndrome are not taken into account by the score. Similarly, liver tumors such as hepatocellular carcinoma are potentially greatly disadvantaged. The greatest concern in programs offering both pediatric and adult transplantation are the comparative status of adults and children competing for the same organ as calculated by different scoring systems.

Preoperative Consideration Relevant to Pediatric Patients

The general medical condition of the patient should be assessed, beginning with overall health and nutritional status.

Growth is an important feature of childhood that reflects the functional status of liver. When it becomes evident that no further growth is possible despite maximal nutritional support, transplantation should be performed as soon as possible.

Preoperative evaluation also depends on the indication of transplantation, e.g. patients with Alagille syndrome may have underlying structural heart disease while patients with cystic fibrosis have varying degrees of underlying lung disease.

A thorough assessment of these underlying end-organ complications must be performed before placing the patient on the transplant list (Table 8.27).

The candidate must be evaluated with regard to potential for development of infections after transplantation. The serological CMV status determines the risk for serious infection after transplantation. Ebstein Barr virus is also important because of its association with post transplant lymphoproliferative disease. Varicella serological status should be known so that proper care can be provided in case of exposure. Potential recipients should be immunized before transplantation, if at all possible. This should include vaccines for Rubella, Mumps, Hepatitis B virus, Hepatitis A virus, polio, Varicella, DPT, and *Haemophilus influenzae* B.

Patients with biliary atresia usually have had prior abdominal surgery, increasing the risk of operative blood loss and inadvertant enterotomies during surgical dissection at the

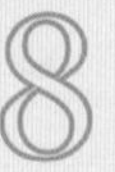

Table 8.27: Preoperative evaluation and investigations[7]

Organ System	*Common findings*	*Implications*	*Investigations*
Pulmonary system	▪ Restrictive function secondary to ascites and pleural effusion ▪ Hypoxemia due to VQ mismatch ▪ Impaired hypoxic pulmonary vasoconstriction ▪ Intrapulmonary shunting ▪ Hepatopulmonary syndrome 7 (HPS)	▪ Propensity to hypoxia ▪ ↓ FRC ▪ Need for supplemental oxygen and adequate preoxygenation ▪ Quick intubation and PEEP ▪ Possibility of systemic air emboli ▪ Pulmonary vasodilator therapy for pulmonary HT ▪ Increased incidence of prolonged postoperative ventilatory requirement	▪ Chest X-ray or Echo ▪ Contrast Echo (Bubble Echo) ▪ Body scanning with technetium labelled albumin to diagnose HPS
Cardiovascular system (CVS)	▪ Hyperdynamic circulation ▪ Increase cardiac output ▪ Decrease SVR ▪ Increase stroke volume and ejection fraction ▪ Pulmonary hypertension or emboli ▪ Pericardial effusion ▪ CAD is very rare in pediatric patients	▪ Decrease sensitivity to catecholamines ▪ Increase mixed venous O_2 saturation ▪ Decreased AV O_2 difference ▪ Severe vasodilatation may compound hypotension due to anesthesia	▪ ABG ▪ Echo
Central nervous system (CNS)	▪ Encephalopathy ▪ Cerebral edema with fulminant hepatic failure	▪ Avoid preoperative sedation ▪ ICP monitoring (avoid in patients with deranged clotting and thrombocytopenia) ▪ Intraoperative measures for ICP reduction	▪ Ammonia levels
Gastrointestinal system	▪ Hepatic dysfunction (loss of synthetic, metabolic and excretory functions) ▪ Portal HT (esophageal varices gastropathy) ▪ Delayed gastric emptying	▪ Decrease plasma oncotic pressure, so decreased dose of anesthetic drugs ▪ Rapid sequence induction of GA with cricoid pressure ▪ Poor nutritional status ▪ Shunt insertion (TIPS) might be required before surgery ▪ Propensity to spontaneous bacterial peritonitis	▪ LFT ▪ Serum proteins ▪ Serum albumin ▪ Total bilirubin ▪ Conjugated bilirubin ▪ Hepatic enzymes ▪ Doppler U/S for hepatic arteries ▪ Liver biopsy
Renal system	▪ Renal dysfunction from prerenal azotemia secondary to diuretics ▪ Hepatorenal syndrome is less common in children than in adults	▪ Perioperative renal failure ▪ Renal replacement therapy might be needed preoperatively	▪ RFT–BUN, serum creatinine, and 24 hours creatinine clearance ▪ Urinary sodium
Immunological	▪ Hypogammaglobulinemia	▪ Increased risk of infections	▪ TLC
Hematological system	Anemia ▪ Thrombocytopenia ▪ Elevated prothrombin time ▪ Hypofibrinogenemia ▪ Dysfibrinogenemia ▪ Fibrinolysis ▪ DIC	▪ Very careful insertion of vascular catheters and NG tubes ▪ Adequate supplies of packed red blood cells, FFP and platelets	▪ CBC ▪ DLC ▪ PT/INR/APTT ▪ Fibrinogen level ▪ FDP levels ▪ Blood typing and antibody screening
Fluid, electrolyte and acid base status	▪ Intravascular volume depletion (secondary to diuretics) ▪ Hypokalemia ▪ Hyponatremia ▪ Metabolic acidosis or alkalosis ▪ Hypoglycemia ▪ Hyperammonemia	▪ Regular monitoring of ABG + electrolytes ▪ Prolonged starvation can cause hypoglycemia ▪ Some cases might require preoperative hemodialysis	▪ ABG ▪ Electrolytes ▪ Blood glucose, fasting and postprandial

time of liver transplant. They may also have other associated anomalies such as cardiac disease and gastrointestinal malrotation.[9]

Some syndromic cholestatic disorders are associated with pulmonary hypertension and preoperative optimization is essential.

Following identification of a potential candidate for liver transplantation, a stepped up evaluation is initiated. In the first phase blood typing, blood chemistries, liver and renal function tests, coagulation profile and viral serologies are done (Table 8.28). Anatomic assessment of liver may include abdominal ultrasound and/or angiography. A liver biopsy may be indicated to confirm the diagnosis or severity of liver disease. Further testing including echocardiography, chest X-ray and ECG are performed. Following acceptance of a patient for transplant by selection committee, steps for optimization of medical condition are initiated.

- Medical therapy to control ascites, infection and encephalopathy
- Nutritional assessment and diet modification, endoscopy and sclerotherapy to treat GI bleeding
- Additional studies—ABG, response to inhaled O_2 and cardiac catheterization
- Vitamin K administration
- Prophylactic dental work, tonsillectomy or adenoidectomy, if required, are performed before transplantation.

Preoperative Visit

At our center when the child is posted for transplantation, the anesthesiologist again visits the patient a night before the surgery to review the history and physical examination, to seek evidence of new changes and complications. All routine investigations are repeated the night before and on the morning of surgery to reassess the hematological and biochemical profile of the patient.

Table 8.28: Additional investigations required

Serological investigations	
Hepatitis B [Surface Ag, Surface Ab, Core Ab and antigen]	
Hepatitis C [HCV Ab, PCR if antibody is positive]	
Hepatitis A [Ig G]	Blood culture
CMV – IgG + 1g M	Urine culture
EBV – IgG + 1g M	Ascitic fluid cell count
HIV	
HSV Ig G	
Measles IgG	
Varicella IgG	
Rubella IgG	

We do not routinely advise any premedication to these children. However very anxious, older children may be prescribed IV midazolam 0.025–0.1 mg/kg or orally 0.5 mg/kg. We do not give an intramuscular injection to these children.

A peripheral intravenous access is usually obtained in the ward and maintenance fluid contaning dextrose [0.45% NS with 5% dextrose] is started. The child is made NPO as per the guidelines. We encourage clear sugar containing oral fluids upto 2 hours before induction of anesthesia.

Infusions of Drugs are Prepared and Kept Ready for use Before Induction of Anesthesia

1. N acetylcysteine (NAC) 120 mg/mL given in all patients, 1.5 mg/kg/hr for 24 hours throughout the surgery for its antioxidant effects
2. Fentanyl 5–10 µg/mL; given at 1–2 µg/kg/hr
3. Atracurium 0.5 mg/kg/hr
4. Norepinephrine 40–80 µg/mL; given at 5–15 µg/kg/min
5. Solumedrol 15 mg/kg given before reperfusion
6. Epinephrine 1: 10,000
7. Lasix 1 mg/kg
8. $NaHCO_3$–1 mEq/kg
9. Ca gluconate 10%, 30–40 mg/kg–if required
10. Heparin 100 U/kg–after arterial anastomosis, if required
11. Antibiotics prepared.

Equipment setup: apart from normal requirements
1. Noninvasive cardiac output monitors
2. Fluid warming device
3. Convective warming device
4. Humidifiers
5. Syringe pumps
6. Fluid pressurizing devices
7. Stat Lab
   a. TEG Monitor
   b. Hemoglobin estimation device
   c. ABG Machine.

Preparation of Patient for Surgery

1. Induction of anesthesia
2. Orotracheal intubation
3. Placement of orogastric tube, urinary catheter and temperature probe

4. Placement of intravascular catheters
   a. IJV/subclavian venous catheter
   b. Intravenous catheter
   c. Intra-arterial catheter
5. Placement of warming devices
6. Attachment of infusions
7. Pressure points padded.

Anesthetic Management

The operation room is prewarmed with forced air warming device. On arrival to operation theater, ECG electrodes, pulse oximetry probe and blood pressure cuff are connected. Since the child already has an intravenous access, intravenous induction is performed with IV thiopentone Na 3–5 mg/kg, fentanyl 2 μg/kg and intubation is facilitated by atracurium and 0.5 mg/kg after adequate preoxygenation. We do not routinely employ a rapid sequence induction and avoid the use of succinylcholine. An endotracheal tube of suitable size is then placed with only allowable leak and pressure controlled ventilation is initiated. After induction and intubation, a nasogastric tube of appropriate size in place, the child is covered with a blanket as much as possible.

Our protocol is to ventilate the lungs with air/oxygen and isoflurane supplemented by fentanyl infusion 2 ug/kg/hr and atracurium 0.5 mg/kg/hr. Invasive monitoring usually includes a Foley's catheter, an arterial line and central venous pressure monitoring. We usually use IJV for inserting a triple lumen catheter size 5.5 F, one lumen of which is used for CVP monitoring and the other two lumens are utilized for giving infusions, drugs and fluids.

During placement of lines and catheters the children are placed on a pressure relieving warming mattress and before draping a convective warming system (Bair Hugger) is placed around them. The children are also draped such that ascites and blood can flow away rather than pool on their bodies. Other useful adjuncts used for temperature maintenance are heat and moisture exchangers in breathing circuit. All fluids and blood products are warmed using a high flow fluid warming device. We do not use pneumatic pressure devices in pediatric patients. In order to monitor cardiac output we use noninvasive cardiac output monitor, which relies upon the arterial waveform contour to derive cardiac output with lithium dilution calibration.

All intravenous lines are placed in the upper limbs because of manipulation of inferior vena cava during surgery. We do not use pulmonary artery catheters because of risk of complications and non availability of appropriate size.

For intravenous maintenance fluid we use with 5% dextrose or 4% dextrose in 0.18% saline initially. The type of maintenance fluid is changed according to serial measurement of blood glucose and electrolytes.

In the liver transplant theatre we have a blood gas analyzer for monitoring ABG and electrolytes, hemoglobin estimation device for measuring Hb and thromboelastogram to monitor coagulation profile. For monitoring temperature we use esophageal temperature probe, though rectal probe can also be used. End tidal CO_2 is also monitored to assist in recognizing the occurrence of air embolism. Ample padding of extremities and all pressure points, including head, concludes the preparation prior to incision.

Anesthesia is maintained with a combination of isoflurane, fentanyl and atracurium.

Blood products (packed cells, fresh frozen plasma platelets and cryoprecipitate) should be kept ready in operation theater.

PHASES OF LIVER TRANSPLANTATION (TABLE 8.29)

Stage 1 or Prehepatic stage or Dissection phase: This stage begins with surgical incision and ends with removal of liver from the circulation. Suprahepatic vena cava, infrahepatic vena cava and structures in portahepatis (Portal vein, hepatic artery, common bile duct) are identified and mobilized.

Stage 1 includes dissection of the liver from the surrounding structures, dissection of hilum and dissection of inferior vena cava. In pediatric patients, piggyback hepatectomy is performed instead of standard complete hepatectomy. Piggyback hepatectomy involves careful dissection of the liver from retrohepatic vena cava with preservation of patient's vena cava.

Problems Commonly Encountered

1. Massive blood loss because of
   - Adhesions or scar tissue from previous surgery
   - Large collateral vessels
   - Coagulopathies
   - Portal HT
2. Ongoing loss of ascitic fluid

   Goal: is to maintain high preload just before stage II, since cross clamping of vena cava will result in an acute decreased preload and cardiac output.
   - Transfusion to be guided by close attention to Hematocrit, PT and TEG with reference to filling pressure and urine output

- Ideal hematocrit is probably between 26–30%[10]
- Ideal INR is around 1.5
- Platelets are transfused only when there is evidence of thrombocytopenia on TEG along with clinical evidence of bleeding. We also use human albumin solution for intravascular volume expansion. Concurrent fluid resuscitation results in a gradual decline in coagulation factors and platelets.[11]

3. ***Surgical factors***: Retractor blades under hemidiaphragm may lead to movement of small patients during transplant and thus position of patient and pressure points should be reassessed regularly.
   Dissection around porta hepatis may necessitate lifting and manipulation of liver and thus interfere with venous return and result in hypotension.
4. Serum glucose and electrolytes should be monitored closely. Ionised calcium may fall precipitously with infusion of FFP and packed cells.

We routinely assess ABG, Hb, blood sugar and TEG after every 2 hours, however in an unstable patient we do it more frequently.

Table 8.29: Phases of liver transplantation

Intraoperative steps	*Problems*
Subcostal incision	**Preanhepatic stage**
↓	▪ Bleeding
Liver mobilization	▪ Coagulopathy
↓	▪ Hypotension due to bleeding and drainage of ascitic fluid
Exposure of vena cava	
↓	
Hilar dissection	
↓	
Arteries clamped high in the hilum to preserve all options for retransplantation	
↓	
Mobilize hepatic artery proximal to gastroduodenal artery	
↓	
Skeletonize portal vein	
↓	
Small hepatic veins from vena cava to the liver are individually ligated and over sewn prior to cross clamp	
↓	
Clamp portal vein	
↓	
Partial side biting clamp of IVC	***Anhepatic stage***
↓	Decreased venous return—hypotension
Recipient liver excised	Decreased urine output
↓	Bowel edema
Graft hepatic vein to host vena cava anastomosis	Accumulation of the products of anerobic metabolism due to mesenteric and caval stasis
Graft portal vein to host portal vein anastomosis	
↓	
Reperfusion	***Reperfusion syndrome***
↓	Pulmonary edema
Arterial anastomosis	Neohepatic stage
↓	
Biliary reconstruction	

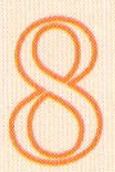

Stage II or Anhepatic phase: The anhepatic stage begins with cross clamping the suprahepatic vena cava, infrahepatic vena cava, portal vein and hepatic artery. In some situations the surgeons may avoid cross clamping the vena cava by isolating the hepatic vein from the recipient vena cava and using a partial side biting clamp on this portion of vena cava. During the an-hepatic phase, the native liver is completely excised, bleeding is controlled in the retrohepatic area and donor liver is sutured in place. In general, vessels are anastomosed in the following order, hepatic veins with vana cara portal rein to portal vein.

The infrahepatic vena caval anastomosis is not completed at this time. The donor liver is flushed with 200–300 mL of gelofusine through portal vein which is drained out from the incomplete infrahepatic vena caval anastomosis. 25–30% of the initial blood entering the liver from portal vein is allowed to exit from infrahepatic vena cava as the suprahepatic vena cava is still clamped to remove perfusate which is rich in potassium and also to clear liver vasculature of entrained air. About 1/3 to 1/4 of the blood volume of the patient is lost via this route and this blood loss is replaced rapidly. The portal vein clamp should be released slowly because this method decreases the bolus effects and lessens the likehood of severe reperfusion syndrome. The suprahepatic vena cava is then opened and infrahepatic vena caval anastomosis is completed. This technique of nonsystemic reperfusion of the transplanted liver reduces the incidence of reperfusion syndrome significantly. The an hepatic phase ends with restoration of blood flow to new liver.

The anesthesiologist must take care after reperfusion not to cause volume overload as congestion of liver graft can seriously impair graft function.

The cross clamp time should be tried to be limited to less than 30 minutes to avoid prolonged stasis in the mesenteric and caval circulation thereby avoiding the accumulation of products of anerobic metabolism and proximal thrombosis.

Problems Encountered

1. Decreased venous return to heart either due to total or partial cross clamping of vena cava, produces a precipitous decrease in preload to the heart. Collateral circulation secondary to portal hypertension modulates the decrease from infradiaphragmatic portion of the body. Children tend to cope up with this situation well by developing tachycardia.

   Cautious administration of fluids and inotropes is necessary to treat hypotension due to decreased venous return.

   We avoid excessive fluid administration as it may lead to high right atrial pressures at reperfusion which can congest the newly transplanted liver and cause bleeding. Avoiding excessive fluid administration and hypervolemia and maintaining low CVP is one of our intraoperative goals during liver transplantation. We have gradually modified our intraoperative techniques so that transfusion of blood and blood products during transplantation is limited to situations where clinical bleeding and or anemia is present. Mounting evidence also supports maintaining a low CVP via intravenous volume restriction because a lower CVP can improve O_2 delivery to the donor graft.[12] It creates a venous gradient between portal and central venous circulation that draws blood through the donor graft. [13]

   Because of the increased portal venous pressure there is tendency towards fluid translocation and bowel edema.

   Though urine output falls during this stage due to decreased renal blood flow, infants and children usually have normal urine output during this period, apparently because there are other pathways by which venous blood can return to central circulation, e.g. via Batson's plexus.

   We use mannitol 0.25–0.5 g/kg infusion during the anhepatic period for its antioxidant effects and for increasing urine output. Osmotic activity of mannitol can aid in removing free water within the congested abdominal organs and thus prevents hepatic distension once the transplanted liver is reperfused. It may also provide renal protection during the anhepatic stage and has free radical scavenging and antioxidant properties.[11]

2. Progressive metabolic changes are decreased pH, increased serum potassium and decreased core temperature. Correction of acid base abnormalities, electrolyte levels and maintenance of hemostasis is aimed at during this stage.

   In preparation for the new graft entering the circulation, methyl prednisolone 10 mg/kg is given. Steroids prevent macrophages from releasing interleukin I thereby initiating immunosuppression.

3. Alterations in hemostasis: Platelet and coagulation factors continue to decline and in absence of hepatic clearance, accumulation of tissue thromboplastin compounds the dysfunction.

Stage III or Reperfusion (Post-anhepatic or Neohepatic Period)

Postreperfusion syndrome is defined as a 30% or more drop in blood pressure from baseline that lasts for a minute or more and occurs within 5 minutes of reperfusion.[14] Pediatric patients have 9% incidence of postreperfusion syndrome as compared to 42% incidence in adult patients.[15] Surgical goals during this period include.

1. Restoration of blood flow into the new liver
2. Completion of hepatic arterial anastomosis
3. Establishment of biliary drainage.

During revascularization of the liver, the clamp on portal vein is opened first, followed by the infrahepatic IVC clamp and the intravascular bed enlarges to include the donor liver. Volume preloading with crystalloids or colloids is done which prevents fall in systolic arterial pressure. Next the suprahepatic vena cava clamp is released. A transient decrease in systolic and diastolic blood pressure occurs at this time despite volume preloading due to return of acidotic blood from lower extremities and bowel which can also suppress myocardial contractility. A transient increase in serum K^+ may lead to systemic vasodilatation. Hypotension may be observed even though pH and serum potassium levels are normal, probably due to kallikrenin like substances. A bolus of calcium gluconate 30–60 mg/kg to maintain ionized calcium 1.1–1.2 mmol/L, an infusion of 0.25–0.5g/kg of glucose followed by intravenous insulin 0.1 U/kg infusion can be administrated to reduce serum potassium concentration; noradrenaline 10–15 ug/kg/min and $NaHCO_3$ 1 mEq/Kg are required at this stage. This reperfusion syndrome usually manifests by fall in mean BP, relative bradycardia and raised pulmonary vascular resistance. Postreperfusion syndrome is provoked by rapid infusion of effluent from the transplanted liver, which is high in potassium and low in pH and temperature. In addition, infusion of air and or microthrombi into heart may precipitate acute pulmonary hypertension. Before reperfusion, ABG and electrolytes should be normalized, body temperature should be increased to 36–37°C if possible, rigorous flushing of liver with colloids and retrograde flushing with patient's blood should be done. In addition FiO_2 should be increased to 1.0 and inhalational anesthesia agents should be discontinued 3–5 mins prior to reperfusion.

In infants and children reconstruction of hepatic arterial inflow may be more difficult and includes reconstruction via a patch graft from recipient aorta to the donor celiac trunk, hepatic artery or aorta.

- Biliary drainage may occur via duct to duct anastomosis in patients with normal extrahepatic ductal system or via Roux-en-Y choledochojejunostomy in children with abnormal extrahepatic bile ducts.

  After revascularization of the graft

  - Acidosis tends to correct spontaneously
  - Serum K+ level tends to fall
  - Blood glucose level often rises
  - Urine output increases.

At this time the drains are inserted and surgical closure is started. Small infants or those with large grafts may be at risk for tight abdominal closure and there may be risk of displacement or compression of the graft. If this seems to be the case, a staged abdominal closure with prosthesis may be employed.

In general trachea of most children undergoing an elective transplant with good postoperative graft function are extubated within 24 hours of surgery.

PROBLEMS ENCOUNTERED DURING LIVER TRANSPLANT

Progressive Metabolic Changes

a. Glucose: Intraoperative hypoglycemia is rarely encountered except in patents of fulminant hepatic failure (FHF) or severe chronic liver disease. Hyperglycemia is frequently encountered which increases progressively from dissection to postoperative phase. Causes of hyperglycemia include
   a. Baseline insulin resistance
   b. Methylprednisolone administration
   c. Stress response due to stress hormones
   d. Therapeutic infusion of catecholamines
   e. Direct infusion of glucose in transfused blood products

   Portal vein unclamping is followed by increase in plasma glucose concentration due to glucose release by the graft liver.

   Small infants may have markedly decreased glycogen stores and are frequently at risk for developing hypoglycemia. For hypoglycemic children, dextrose (0.5–1g/kg) is administered and for hyperglycemia (>250 mg/dL) insulin is administered, 0.1U/kg.
b. Lactate: Throughout the dissection phase there is an increase in plasma lactic acid level which accelerates during anhepatic stage due to impairment of lactate clearance when liver is excluded from the circulation. If the graft is functioning properly, plasma lactate levels decrease on the first postoperative day.
c. Acid base balance: There is biphasic acid base disturbance characterized by initial metabolic acidosis and then protracted metabolic alkalosis. Causes of metabolic acidosis are—tissue hypoperfusion, decreased or absent

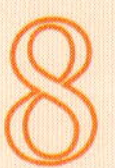

metabolism of lactate, citrate and other metabolic acids by liver, rapid administration of acidic blood products, associated renal impairment and acidic effluent from liver allograft. In general when base deficit > 8–20 mEq/L or pH ≤ 7.25 ($PaCO_2$ < 40 mm Hg), bicarbonate is administrated prior to reperfusion of the graft.

Treatment of metabolic acidosis prior to reperfusion is indicated when there is concomitant myocardial depression and/or there are signs of persistent hyperkalemia.

Metabolic alkalosis in postoperative period is due to clearance of H^+ along with conversion of citrate and lactate to bicarbonate by graft liver.

d. Hyponatremia: is common in these patients due to free water retention that exceeds sodium retention. We have to be very careful as rapid correction of serum sodium associated with intraoperative administration of crystalloid and colloid solutions, blood products and sodium bicarbonate may lead to central nervous system injury.

e. Potassium: Severe hypokalemia may be present initially because of preoperative use of diuretics, gastrointestinal fluid losses and hyperaldosteronism. Intraoperatively, the principle concern is hyperkalemia with may be related to blood products, preservative solution or cellular K^+ efflux in exchange for H^+ due to metabolic acidosis.

Abrupt increase in serum potassium concentration is anticipated with liver reperfusion. ECG changes, especially T wave changes may not be present in infants and small children. Following reperfusion, K^+ tends to decrease due to urinary losses, uptake by muscle cell and allograft liver. K^+ administration is indicated if serum K^+ decreases and the urine output is adequate in post reperfusion phase.

f. Calcium: Ionised hypocalcemia is the most frequently encountered problem due to citrate containing blood products. Profound hypocalcemia during anhepatic phase may cause myocardial depression and hypotension. Calcium replacement therapy is achieved with calcium infusion. Ca^+ requirements decrease following reperfusion. Intraoperative changes in serum ionized Mg^{++} concentration are same as with those of calcium concentration. Cardiac irritability and clotting dysfunction are improved by Mg^{++} replacement.

Hemostasis

Thromboelastography, a specific type of whole blood viscoelastic coagulation monitoring which uses kaolin specific reference values, has been used successfully at our center during liver transplantation to assess the requirement of FFP, platelet, cryoprecipitate and antifibrinolytic agent.

The pediatric patient may be at a particular risk for thrombotic events in immediate postoperative period due to the small size of their vessels. Hepatic arterial thrombosis may cause the graft to be lost in 12 to 24 hours and occurs with greater frequency in infants and children. Because of the potential for graft loss with vessel thrombosis, a slightly anticoagulated state is maintained in infants and small children following liver transplant. This includes avoiding full correction of heparin effects in the operating room, maintaining a slightly higher PT and early administration of aspirin or prophylactic administration of intravenous heparin.

Thrombocytopenia is a common finding in these patients. Intraoperative thrombocytopenia may develop or worsen due to replacement of blood loss during the dissection phase with non-platelet containing solutions. Platelet count decreases slightly during the anhepatic period and decreases significantly upon reperfusion of the graft.

Platelet transfusion is indicated if there is evidence of thrombocytopenia on TEG along with clinical impression of abnormal hemostatic function. Following reperfusion, multiple coagulation defects can appear due to raw surfaces and multiple suture lines.

Oliguria

Despite adequate IV volume, administration of furosemide or mannitol and elevated serum glucose levels, oliguria is very common.

Oliguria during dissection phase is probably due to preexisting hepatorenal syndrome and during anhepatic phase it is due to decreased arteriovenous gradient across kidneys as inferior vena cava is clamped. After revascularization and decompression of vena cava, urine output usually increases markedly.

Hypotension

Hypotension occurs because of several factors

1. Inadequate fluid replacement in response to massive and rapid blood loss
2. Cardiac dysfunction secondary to decreased concentration of ionized calcium as a result of increased citrate concentration
3. Preexisting myocardial disease
4. Surgical manipulation
5. Arrhythmias[16]

Hypothermia

Severe factors contribute to hypothermia. Temperature maintenance is difficult because of long intraabdominal operation, and massive fluid and blood products transfusion. Hypothermia develops more gradually during dissection phase, temperature decreases more rapidly during anhepatic period and immediately upon reperfusion. Implantation of graft that has temperature nearing zero, contributes to hypothermia. There is 1–2°C decrease in body temperature when cold graft is placed in abdomen. There is also an abrupt decrease in core temperature with reperfusion when cold flush solution is infused into systemic circulation.

Surgical Techniques

Reduced size liver transplantation (RSLT): To solve the size mismatch, reduced size liver transplantation was undertaken by procurement of the whole liver from adult cadaver donors, which is reduced in its size on the back table to tailor the size of the graft to that of a single recipient. The remaining resected liver is discarded. In pediatric patient RSLT, either the left lateral segment or the full left lobe is usually retained.[17]

Split liver transplant (SLT): This technique allows the preparation of two split grafts by dividing all vascular and biliary structures and parenchyma for the benefit of two recipients, usually the right lobe is transplanted into adult and the left lobe or left lateral segment into a child.

Living donor liver transplantation (LDLT): This accounts for a substantial number of pediatric cases performed in our center. Left lobectomy is performed during which segments 2 and 3 are separated from the remaining liver. After parenchymal dissection, the left branch of portal vein, the left hepatic artery and the left suprahepatic vein are quickly clamped and dissected.

An adult left lateral lobe produces a graft of approximately 250 gms which is adequate for a recipient up to 20 kg. The full left lobe is usually between 250–500 gms and has been used for medium sized children.

Small size of infants younger than 3 months makes graft selection difficult. All neonatal liver transplants are now performed with technical variant grafts, either from deceased or liver donors. The use of over sized allografts should be avoided because it commonly results in delayed abdominal closure and increased intra-abdominal pressure with subsequent impairment of respiratory function and decreased graft perfusion.

LDLT has Several Advantages for the Child and Transplant Population as Whole

1. It increases the number of organs directly available for pediatric population
2. Most recipients receive their transplant on an elective basis and thus should incur lower morbidity and mortality values and decrease overall cost
3. Minimal cold ischemia time and use of healthy donors may contribute to the absence of primary nonfunction.

Pedatric LDLT is now an accepted therapy for children throughout the world and frequently accounts for 50% or more of pediatric liver transplants performed at regional centers.[18]

Among children < 3 years of age, LDLT graft provides superior graft survival compared with RSLT and SLT. In older children it appears that cadaveric organs may offer better outcome.[19]

Fulminant hepatic failure (FHF): is present when encephalopathy develops within 8 weeks of the onset of symptoms related to liver disease in patients with previously normal hepatic function. In pediatric patients this interval may be extremely short, often less than 2 weeks. More recently it has been divided into 2 subgroups (1) FHF or acute liver failure with hepatic encephalopathy that occurs within 2 weeks from the onset of jaundice. (2) Subfulminant hepatic failure (SFHF), in which hepatic encephalopathy occurs 2 weeks to 3 months after the onset of jaundice. The most common cause of FHF in children is viral hepatitis.[20]

Patients with Grade III or IV coma require intubation and ventilation to protect the airway, otherwise all patients with milder grades of encephalopathy require careful monitoring and review.

Patients in this group are at a specific risk of severe encephalopathy, intracranial hypertension and life threatening cerebral edema.

- The perioperative management of these patients often necessitates the placement of an intracranial pressure monitoring device depending on the coagulation status of the patients
- Volume control with mannitol and hypertonic saline, hyperventilation, osmotic diuretics, barbiturates and rapid correction of coagulopathy with activated factor VII is tried.
- There is increased risk of coagulopathy and GI bleed, sepsis, hypoglycemia, severe acidosis and kidney failure in these patients.

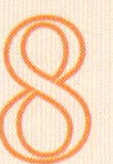

- Elevation of patient's head 25° and maintenance of cerebral perfusion pressure by supporting systemic arterial blood pressure, reducing central venous pressure and avoiding agitation are essential.

MOLECULAR ABSORBENT RECIRCULATING SYSTEM

The MARS is a modified hemofiltration system that can be used as a bridge to transplantation or spontaneous recovery. There have been reports that its application leads to improved hemodynamics, reduced inotropic requirements and improved grades of encephalopathy.[21]

There are 3 compartments—The blood, albumin solution (20%) and conventional filter against a standard dialysis solution. The tubules through which blood passes are lined with albumin impregnated high flux polysulfone dialysis membrane. Highly protein bound toxins can be removed from the binding proteins in the patient's plasma. There is evidence of improved survival in rather small trials; it is quite invasive and expensive. With newer trials it will become clearer what benefits can be expected.

Future

Good intraoperative and postoperative care has led to decrease in mortality of the pediatric patients coming for liver transplant.

The main areas where progress is needed are immunology, chronic rejection and post-transplantation lymphoproliferative disease and provision of sufficient donors.[22]

Experiments with MARS or derivatives from it, e.g. promethus (a plasma fractionation and albumin dialysis) could avoid transplantation altogether. Infusions of human or animal hepatocytes derived from cloning or other genetic manipulation do hold promise in some conditions where liver architecture is preserved, e.g. inborn errors of metabolism.[23]

CLINICAL PEARLS

- Clinical assessment is more important than laboratory values
- Proper vascular access is essential.
- Tight control of sugar and electrolytes of patient is important
- Avoid graft congestion.
- TEG is the key monitor for the coagulation status.
- Slight hypocoagulation is preferred to hypercoagulation status.

REFERENCES

1. United Network for Organ Sharing at www.unos.org assessed 2009.
2. Cox KL, Berquist WE, Castillo RO. Paediatric liver transplantation: indications, timing and medical complications. J Gastroenterol Hepatol, 1999;14:S61-6.
3. Busuttil and Klintmalm. General criteria for paediatric transplantation–Transplantation of liver. 2nd edn. (Elsevier Saunders Publication). 2009;287-300.
4. Busuttil RW, Seu P, Millis JM, Olthoff KM, Hiatt JR, Milewicz A, et al. Liver Transplantion in children. Ann Surg, 1991;213: 48-57.
5. Engelskirchen R, Holschneider AM, Gharib M, Vente C. Biliary atresia a 25-year survey. Eur J Pediatr Surg, 1991;1(3):154-60.
6. Exelby PR, Filler RM, Grosfeld JL. Liver tumors in children in particular reference to hepatoblastoma and hepatocellular carcinoma: American Academy of Pediatrics Surgical Section Survey-1974. J Pediatr Surg, 1975;10:329-337.
7. Victor L, Scott II, Kerri M, Wahi, Kyle, et al. Smiths Anaesthesia for infants and children. 8th edn. 2011;905-928.
8. McDiarmid SV, Merion RM, Dykstra DM, Harper AM. Selection of pediatric candidates under PELD system. Liver transpl, 2004; 10;S23-30.
9. Carmi R, Magee CA, Neill CA, Karrer FM. Extrahepatic biliary atresia and associated anomalies: etiologic heterogeneity suggested by distinctive patterns of associations. Am J Med Genet, 1993;45:683-93.
10. James B, Peter B. Perioperative Issues in Pediatric Liver Transplantation. International Anaesthesiology Clinics. Summer 2006;44:125-147.
11. Hannaman MJ, Hevesi ZG. Anaesthesia care for liver transplantation. Transplant Rev (Orlando), 2011;25:36-43.
12. de Boer MT, Molenaar IQ, Hendriks HG, Slooff MJ, Porte RJ. Minimizing blood loss in liver transplantation: progress through research and evolution of techniques. Minimiziung blood loss in liver transplantation: progress through research and techniques. Dig Surg, 2005;22:265-75.
13. Mandell MS, Tsou MY. The development of perioperative practices for liver transplantation: advances and current trends. J Chin Med Assoc, 2008;71(9):435-41.
14. Aggarwal S, Kang Y, Freeman JA, Fortunato FL, Pinsky MR. Postreperfusion syndrome: cardiovascular collapse following hepatic reperfusion during liver transplantation. Transplant Proc, 1987; 19:54-5.
15. Estrin JA, Belani KG, Ascher NL, Lura D, Payne W, Najarian JS. Hemodynamic changes on clamping and unclamping of major vessels during liver transplantation. Transplant Proc, 1989; 21:3500-5.
16. Borland LM, Roule M, Cook DR. Anaesthesia for paediatric orthotropic liver transplantation. Anaesth Analg, 1985;64: 117-24.
17. Spada M, Riva S, Maggiore G, Cintorino D, Gridelli B. Paediatric liver transplantaion. World J Gastroentrol, 2009;15(6): 648-74.
18. Kim M, Ottohoff, Deirdre A Kelly and William E Harmon. Paediatric solid organ transplantation; 2nd edn. Richard N Fine, Stevenson A Webber, IPTA (Black Well Publishing) 2007.
19. Emond JC. Living donor liver transplantation in children: what to recommend? Am J Transplant, 2004;4:293-4.

20. Hammer GB, Kane EJ. Anaesthesia for liver transplantation in children. Paedriatric anaesthesia, 2001;11:3-18.
21. Schmidt LE, Wang LP, Hansen BA, Larsen FS. Systemic hemodynamic effects of treatment with the molecular adsorbents recirculating system in patients with hyperacute liver failure: a prospective controlled trial. Liver transpl, 2003;9:290-7.
22. McDiarmid SV. Current status of liver transplantation in children. Pediatr Clin North Am, 2003;50:1335-74.
23. Baccarani U, Adani GL, Sainz M, Donini A, Risaliti A, Bresadola F. Human hepatocyte transplantation for acute liver failure: state of the art and analysis of cell sources. Transplant Proc, 2005;37:2702-04.

Pain Management in Liver Transplantation

Nitin Sethi, Pradeep Jain

INTRODUCTION

Organ transplantation is one of the most fascinating medical advance in the last 50 years. There is a wide gap in the supply of the cadaveric organ and the need for the living organs in the current world. Successful adult to adult and adult to child live donor transplantations have helped partially to relieve the refractory shortage of deceased donor grafts. Liver donor surgery involves a large "roof-top" incision and provision of good postoperative pain relief is an important component of perioperative care.[1]

POSTOPERATIVE PAIN RELIEF IN LIVER DONOR

There are inherent challanges associated with postoperative analgesia in the donor group. Optimum pain relief provided by the dedicated pain team in the postoperative period holds a crucial rule. Poor postoperative pain control can have a significant negative impact on the quality of life of an otherwise healthy individual. Studies have shown that the pain in the right lobe donor hepatectomy supersedes the pain of hepatic carcinoma resection.[2]

Liver is a vital organ that controls coagulation. A major liver resection can disturb the balance of thrombosis and bleeding leading to a marked prolongation of the prothrombin time in the postoperative period. A direct correlation between the extent of the liver resection and the maximum postoperative prothrombin time has been demonstrated.[3-6] Hence incorporation of an optimal postoperative pain management regimen that is both effective and safe for living donors can be a great challenge for clinicians.

The epidural infusion of a local anesthetic with an opiate is a well-established analgesia regimen after various surgeries, including living donor hepatectomy, and provides better pain control than IV-PCA; however, increased possibility for trauma secondary to the epidural catheter raises an important safety issue in donors undergoing major liver resection.[5-7] The various modalities of the analgesia for donor hepatectomy.

Epidural Analgesia

Continuous epidural analgesia provides the best form of relief during the first three to four postoperative days. Mid thoracic epidural catheter insertion has been studied by various groups for providing adequate analgesia. The skill in performing the technique, inserting the epidural catheter and the timing of removal of the catheter imparts safety to the analgesia program.

Two schools of thoughts have emerged *'for and against'* the use of epidural analgesia postoperatively in the donor group. The proponents advocate it is relatively safe and effective means of pain control and that the incidence of hematoma, abscess formation or post dural puncture headache is practically very low.[3-6] Some studies have however shown that because of an anticipated postoperative derangement of the coagulation profile and various possible complications including PDPH, infection, nausea, vomiting and neurological complications its use should be discouraged.[7-10]

Numerous case reports have described incidences of epidural hematoma after various surgeries and few of these cases were presumed to have received intraoperative heparin. However in our series we have found epidural analgesia to be exceedingly safe and effective. PT/INR are altered in the immediate postoperative period but is usually followed by a steady trend towards normalization in the following days. The need for fresh frozen plasma (FFP) administration to achieve a safety INR of less than 1.5 for removal of catheter is almost rare.[1]

The patient controlled epidural analgesia (PCEA) settings used are basal rate of 6 mL/hr, demand dosage of 2–6 mL and lock out interval of 20–30 minutes. The combination of bupivacaine with opioid or bupivacaine alone is used. The opioid preferred is fentanyl in the dosage of 2.5–5 µg/mL. Bupivacaine is used in dose ranging from 0.0625% to 0.125%. Morphine when used is in dosage of 0.05 mg/mL. Superiority of any of the combination PCEA has not been shown over others and all have shown to be equally efficacious.[2]

Thoracic Paravertebral Block (TPVB)

The role of thoracic paravertebral block for postoperative analgesia in patients undergoing major abdominal and thoracic surgeries is well established. TPVB is the technique of injecting local anesthetic adjacent to the thoracic vertebra. The idea is to block the somatic and the sympathetic nerve in multiple adjacent thoracic dermatomes above and below the site of injection.

Right thoracic paraverterbral analgesia for hepatectomy has been shown to be safe and does not entail the risk of spinal hematoma seen with the epidural catheters even in presence of moderate hemostatic deficiencies.[11]

In a study by Ashraf et al[12] 24 adult patients aged 18–50 years, of both sexes scheduled for right lobe donor hepatic resection were enrolled. Patients were randomly allocated into two equal groups of 12 patients each. Before induction of general anesthesia all patients received bilateral single site thoracic paravertebral injection at the level of T7–8 in the sitting position. One group received 25 mL of bupivacaine with 0.25% epinephrine while the other was given 25 mL of 0.9% normal saline. Bilateral single site thoracic paravertebral block significantly decreased the pain visual analogue score. Total morphine consumption in the first 24 hours was reduced by more than 50% in paravertebral block group as compared to the placebo group.

Bleeding into the non compressible thoracic paravertebral space is of concern and infection can be devastating. If use of the paravertebral analgesia is prolonged, accumulation of local anesthetic can occur, hence continuing it beyond two days is not propounded.

Intravenous Patient-Controlled Analgesia (IV-PCA) with or without Intrathecal Morphine

The use of intravenous analgesics and systemic opioids in the immediate postoperative period has to be done with caution, since the kinetics of drug distribution and metabolism is not completely investigated after liver resection. Slow metabolism is presumed due to the small remnant liver mass.

Intrathecal opioid either morphine or fentanyl or both combined with IV-PCA morphine has been shown to have good analgesia and less consumption of morphine in the postoperative period. Intrathecal opioid was shown to produce lowered pain scores upto first 18 hours to 30 hours postoperatively without an increase of side effects.[13,14]

At our center we use a continuous infusion of epidural bupivacaine 0.125% till the first postoperative day. From second postoperative day onwards a patient controlled epidural analgesia with a combination of fentanyl (5μg/mL) and bupivacaine 0.125% is administered to the patient.

POSTOPERATIVE PAIN RELIEF IN LIVER RECIPIENT

There are no studies or clinical trials available assessing severity of postoperative pain and its management. In our experience recipients experience minimal postoperative pain and only a few percentage of patients may have moderate to severe pain. Postoperative pain is these patients is well managed with 0.5 μg to 1ug/kg boluses of fentanyl.

CLINICAL PEARLS

- Epidural analgesia provides effective postoperative analgesia in liver donors
- Estimation of coagulation profile is essential prior to removal of epiduxal catheter liver donors.

REFERENCES

1. Feltracco P, Ori C. Anesthetic management of living transplantation. Minerva Anestesiol, 2010;76:525-33.
2. Cywinski JB, Parker BM, Xu M, Irefin SA. A comparison of postoperative pain control in patients after right lobe donor hepatectomy and major hepatic resection for tumor. Anesth Analg, 2004;99:1747-52.
3. Borromeo CJ, Stix MS, Lally A, Pomfret EA. Epidural catheter and increased prothrombin time after right lobe hepatectomy for living donor transplantation. Anesth Analg, 2000;91:1139-41.
4. Choi SJ, Gwak MS, Kim MH, Yang M, Ko JS, Hahm TS, et al. Differences of perioperative liver function, transfusion, and complications according to the type of hepatectomy in living donors. Transpl Int, 2005;18:548-55.
5. Matot I, Scheinin O, Eid A, Jurim O. Epidural anesthesia and analgesia in liver resection. Anesth Analg, 2002;95:1179-81.
6. Wheatley RG, Schug SA, Watson D. Safety and efficacy of postoperative epidural analgesia. Br J Anaesth, 2001;87:47-61.
7. Christie IW, McCabe S. Major complications of epidural analgesia after surgery: results of a six-year survey. Anaesthesia, 2007;62: 335-41.
8. Akpek EA, Arslan G, Erkaya C, Torgay A, Donmez A, Kayhan Z, et al. Anesthetic risks for donors in living related liver transplantation: analysis of 30 cases. Transplant, 2003;16:486-90.
9. Cammu G, Troisi R, Cuomo O, de Hemptinne B, Di Florio E, Mortier E. Anaesthetic management and outcome in right-lobe living liver-donor surgery. Eur J Anaesthesiol, 2002;19:93-8.
10. Salame E, Goldstein MJ, Kinkhabwala M, Kapur S, Finn R, Lobritto S, et al. Analysis of donor risk in living-donor hepatectomy: the impact of resection type on clinical outcome. Am J Transplant, 2002;2:780-8.
11. HO AMH, Karamkar MK, Cheung M, Lam GCS. Right thoracic paraverterbral analgesia for hepatectomy. Br J Anesth, 2004;93(3): 458-61.
12. Ashraf M. Opiod saving strategy; bilateral single site thoracic paravertebral block in right lobe donor hepatectomy. MEJ Anesth, 2008;789-802.
13. Justin et al. Intrathcal morphine combined with intravenous patient controlled analgesia is an effective and safe method for immediate post operative pain control in live liver donors. Liver Transp, 2009;15:381 9.
14. Roy JD, Massicotte L, Sassaine MP, et al: A comparison of intrathecal morphine/fentanyl and patient controlled analgesia with patient controlled analgesia alone after liver resection. Anesth Analg, 2006:103:990-4.

9 CHAPTER

Anesthetic Management of a Transplanted (Renal and Cardiac) Patient for Non-transplant Surgery

Jayashree Sood

INTRODUCTION

Advances in immunosuppressive therapy, surgical techniques, anesthesia, postoperative and intensive care have led to the popularity of organ transplantation.

The organ procurement transplant network data, 2008 has shown the 5 years survival rate for kidney 85.9%, liver 73.1%, heart 69%, pancreas 80% and lung 47.3%.[1]

There are certain principles which need to be followed for any transplanted patient undergoing non-transplant surgery. The patient should undergo a thorough preoperative evaluation especially regarding the functional status of the transplanted organ. Optimization of the transplanted organ is of prime importance. The anesthetic technique chosen should ensure minimal injury to the transplanted organ. Meticulous sterile anesthetic techniques are essential. A balance between immunosuppression and prevention of infection should be maintained. Immunosuppressive drugs and antibiotics should be continued. The postoperative strategy should be planned in advance.

RENAL TRANSPLANTED PATIENT FOR NON-TRANSPLANT SURGERY

The patient survival after 1 year of renal transplantation is 95% with a graft survival of 85%. The 3 year patient survival after renal transplant from United Network of Organ Sharing (UNOS) data is 90%.[2] An increased incidence and duration of survival after renal transplantation, implies that many of these individuals may require surgery either for management of complications, related to the transplant surgery or may encounter an illness, which may necessitate an incidental surgery.[3,4] Since renal transplant is now the most commonly encountered transplanted organ, it is essential that every anesthesiologist should understand the specific problems associated with a transplanted individual, since the patient may come to a hospital where transplant procedures are not performed.[5]

Common surgical procedures for which renal transplanted patients may present are:[6]

a. Procedures related to post renal transplant complications

Early

- Re-exploration required due to bleeding or a sudden decrease in urine output after an initial good urine output. An ultrasound examination often reveals decreased blood flow through the arterial anastomosis. Occasionally it is a kinked ureter which is the cause of decreased urine output.

Delayed

- Exploration of surgical site due to wound infection (Fig. 9.1)
- Graft nephrectomy (removal of the transplanted kidney) (Fig. 9.2) due to "rejection" or "infection" resulting in thrombosis of the renal graft
- Lymphocele
- Incisional hernia at site of surgery (Fig. 9.3)
- New arteriovenous (AV) fistula to be made in case the transplant is unsuccessful
- CAPD insertion after removal of the transplanted kidney (Fig. 9.4)

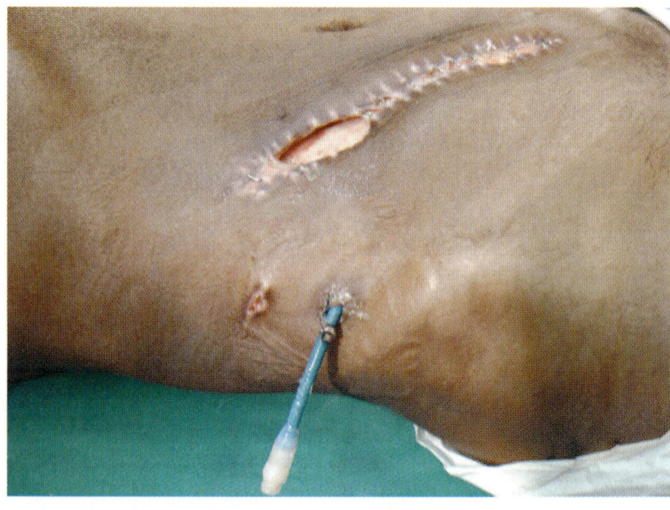

Fig. 9.1: PostKTP collection—perigraft drain

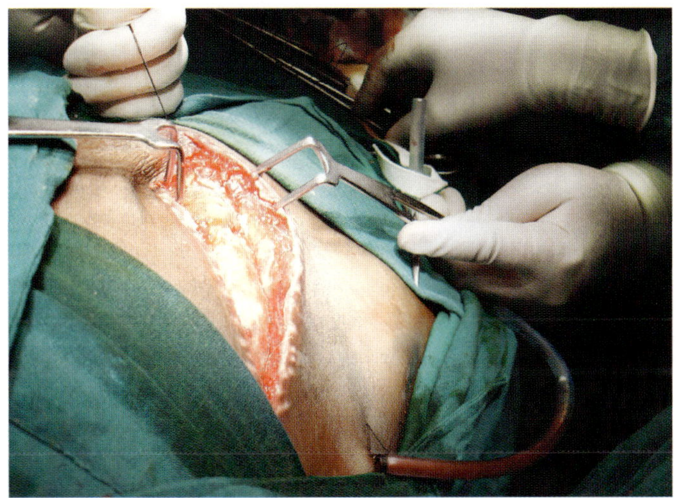

Fig. 9.2: PostKTP—resuturing

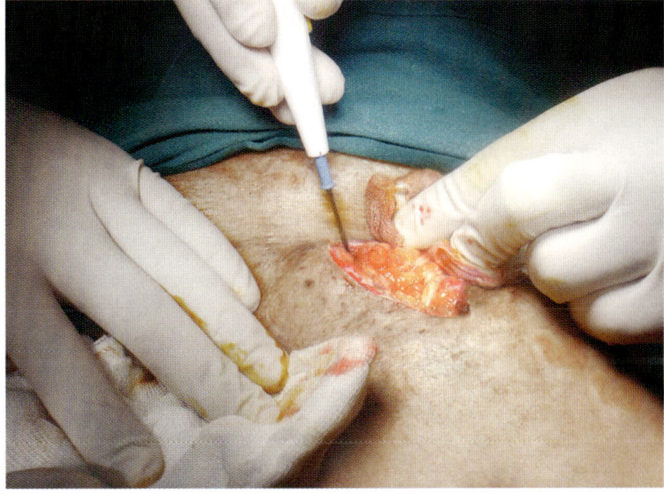

Fig. 9.3: Incisional hernia

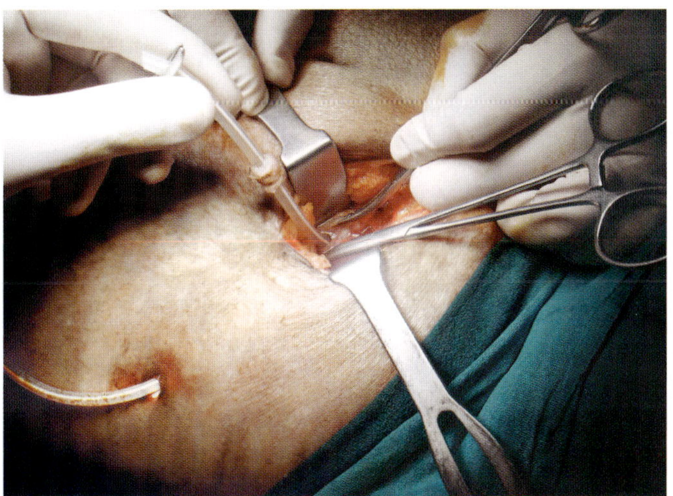

Fig. 9.4: CAPD insertion

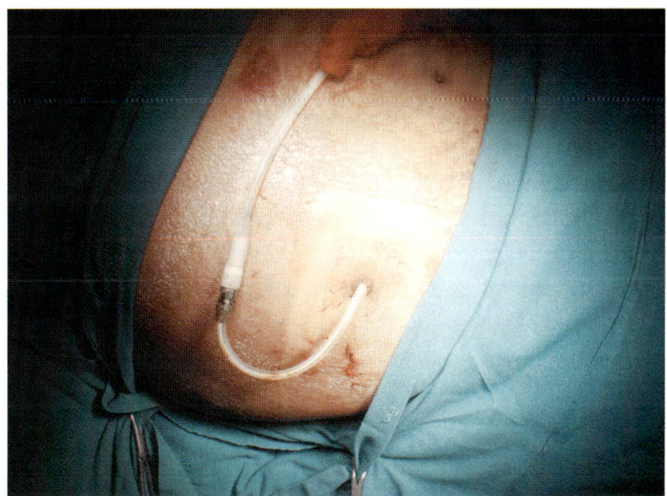

Fig. 9.5: Peritoneal dialysis

b. Procedures unrelated to renal transplant surgery
   - Appendicitis or any other emergency procedure
   - Continuous ambulatory peritoneal dialysis (Fig. 9.5)
   - Cataract

A postrenal transplant patient has several problems. Like all other transplanted patients they are on life long immunosuppressive therapy. The function of the transplanted kidneys is variable. These patients usually have a multisystem involvement with anemia, hypertension and diabetes mellitus. The effect of chronic renal disease on other organs is of great importance and leads to significant co-morbidity.[7] If the patient is on hemodialysis, there may be hypokalemia, hypovolemia and cardiovascular instability.

Compared with other transplant recipients, renal transplant recipients are older with associated co-morbidities which impact anesthesia care.[8]

Principles of Management[2,6]

- Preoperative assessment and optimization of renal function
- Preoperative control of hypertension, diabetes and other co-morbidities
- Immunosuppressive drugs to be continued
- Ascpsis is of vital importance
- Meticulous anesthetic technique to prevent injury to the transplanted kidney
- Aseptic techniques

- Drug excretion may be prolonged, therefore choose drugs that do not rely on the kidneys for excretion. Although the serum creatinine may be normal, the GFR and effective renal plasma flow may be lower than in a normal individual.[2]
- Avoid hypoperfusion of the kidneys due to intravascular volume depletion
- Use diuretics judiciously, only after evaluation of the patient's volume status
- Plan meticulous postoperative care.

Preoperative Assessment[2,6]

- Detailed history of immunosuppression
- Focus on graft rejection and infection
- Assessment of renal function (graft function)
- Assessment of functions of other organs.

Immunosuppressive Therapy[6]

All patients undergoing transplant surgery are started on immunosuppressants which are continued throughout life and therefore, these patients are always susceptible to infection and malignancy. If these recipients require nontransplant surgery there may be alteration of immune competence due to acute illness, stress of surgery and alteration of the immunosuppressive drug regime.[6] This immune instability can result in graft rejection or infection and sometimes both. Various immunosuppressive drugs include calcineurin inhibitors, e.g. cyclosporine and tacrolimus, cytokine receptor signal transduction inhibitors, e.g. sirolimus, nucleoside synthesis inhibitors, e.g. azathioprine, mycophenolate, steroids, monoclonal antibodies and anti-lymphocyte globulin.

Immunosuppressant drugs are associated with side effects which may affect the anesthetic management, e.g. cyclosporine, tacrolimus and steroids result in diabetes, hypertension, renal insufficiency and neurotoxicity often associated with generalized major motor seizures. These patients have very often received several of these drugs and so may have some organ dysfunction. Since immunosuppressive therapy with cyclosporine and tacrolimus is known to be associated with compromise of renal function, like a decrease in renal blood flow and GFR, it is important to estimate renal function preoperatively.

Cyclosporine and tacrolimus are metabolized in the liver through the cytochrome P-450 system and so drugs which are metabolized by the same enzyme (e.g. cimetidine, diltiazem, metoclopramide, nicardipine and verapamil) will result in increased levels of these immunosuppressants. Cimetidine, ranitidine and NSAIDs may produce further renal dysfunction in patients who are on cyclosporine or tacrolimus. Decreased blood levels of cyclosporine and tacrolimus are seen in patients on ticlopidine, carbamazepine and phenytoin.

Azathioprine and mycophenolate cause anemia, leucopenia and thrombocytopenia. Anti-thymocyte globulin and monoclonal antibodies may produce fever and anaphylaxis due to the release of cytokines.

Focus on Graft Rejection and Infection

A balance between risk of rejection due to inadequate immunosuppression and risk of infection due to immunosuppression has to be maintained during the perioperative period.

Immunosuppressed patients are at an increased risk of bacterial, fungal and viral infections; however reducing the dose of immunosuppressants perioperatively may increase the chances of rejection in the perioperative period.

Rejection and infection of the transplanted kidney are important causes of morbidity and mortality and should always be ruled out before incidental surgery. Elective surgery should be postponed, if either acute rejection or infection is suspected. Hypertension, proteinuria and azotemia indicate graft rejection.[2]

If the renal function tests of the transplanted kidney are abnormal, rejection of the organ should be suspected and elective surgery postponed. Renal function should be optimized and only then should surgery proceed.

It is important to rule out the presence of infection in the grafted kidney. Infection in the transplanted kidney predisposes to graft rejection. Fever of unknown origin may be due to infection. It is also important to note that an immunocompromised patient does not show the typical signs of infection like fever and leucocytosis.

Assessment of Renal Function

Assessment of renal function is important because the immunosuppression therapy may compromise renal function. The renal graft could be functioning or the patient may be on maintenance hemodialysis. If the renal transplanted patient has a functioning kidney graft, the serum creatinine levels may be normal.

But patients with renal graft dysfunction and on maintenance hemodialysis may be hypovolemic and hypokalemic producing hemodynamic instability and susceptibility to muscle relaxants respectively.[9]

Assessment of Functions of Other Organs and Optimization of Co-morbidities[10]

A patient who has undergone renal transplant continues to have comorbidities like hypertension, diabetes, congestive heart failure and coronary heart disease. Hypertension may persist due to the side effects of immunosuppressant drugs.[11] Comorbidities should be optimized before surgery.

Investigations

Standard preoperative investigations include a complete blood count, BUN, serum creatinine, serum sodium, potassium, chloride and calcium.

Serum creatinine may be normal or almost normal if the renal allograft is functioning normally.

An electrocardiogram to reveal coronary ischemia or chamber hypertrophy is advised.

If the patient has allograft dysfunction and is on maintenance hemodialysis, signs of end stage renal disease may be evident-like anemia, electrolyte disturbances, platelet dysfunction and metabolic acidosis. A complete blood count, serum electrolytes, platelet count and ABG will reveal these abnormalities.

If the surgery contemplated warrants other investigations they should be done as well.

Preoperative Management

Patients should be fasting overnight. A high risk informed consent should be taken. All investigations should be reviewed on the morning of surgery.

If required, PT, aPTT and platelet count should be repeated on the morning of surgery.

Premedication

All patients should receive oral alprazolam to allay anxiety. The dose of immunosuppressive therapy should not be altered unless the route of administration needs to be changed, for example from oral to parenteral route.

The usual dose of antihypertensive, antianginal and antibiotic drug should be given on morning of surgery. Proton pump inhibitors like pantaprazole and omeprazole may be given as well.

Anesthetic Technique

General, regional and monitored anesthesia care (MAC) have all been used with success if the principles of management are adhered to.[6]

Whichever the method of anesthesia, a strict aseptic technique should be practised including the use of sterile anesthetic circuit, laryngoscopes and bacterial filters. A supplemental stress dose of steroid should be given. A meticulous anesthetic technique is essential for a successful outcome. The anesthetic technique is chosen according to the type of surgery contemplated. Many procedures like AV fistula formation, cataract extraction and lymphocele correction can be done successfully under monitored anesthesia care. Intravenous midazolam and fentanyl, provide, sedation and analgesia respectively. Regional anesthesia including spinal and epidural may be administered if the coagulation profile – PT, aPTT, INR and platelet function are within normal limits. It is contraindicated if the patient is hypovolemic, has platelet dysfunction or uremic/ diabetic neuropathy. Peripheral nerve blocks and local infiltration are other options, however continuous catheter techniques are not advisable due to the potential risk of infection. Anesthesia personnel should wear protective gear to prevent transmission of infection. General anesthesia may be indicated in several surgical conditions. Occasionally GA may be required for marsupialization of a lymphocele in an obese individual. Induction of anesthesia may be done with sleep dose of thiopentone or propofol. Neuromuscular relaxation is obtained with cisatracurium or atracurium, 0.4–0.5 mg/kg[10] and an LMA may be preferred over an endotracheal tube for positive pressure ventilation. Propofol infusion does not modify the cyclosporine levels in humans. Blood levels of cyclosporine are not altered by isoflurane/ nitrous oxide anesthesia. Cyclosporine enhances the effect of muscle relaxants, therefore patients receiving cyclosporine require a smaller dose of non-depolarizing muscle relaxant.[5] Rapid sequence intubation should be considered if there is gastroparesis due to diabetes mellitus. Suxamethonium is safe if serum K^+ is <5.5 mEq/L. Intubation may be difficult if the patient has posttransplant lymphoproliferative disease. Isoflurane, sevoflurane and desflurane are safe, while enflurane is potentially nephrotoxic. Isoflurane is the inhalation agent of choice. Hyperventilation should be avoided since the seizure threshold of patients receiving cyclosporine or tacrolimus is lowered. Monitoring should be appropriate for the nature of the surgical procedure.[6] Minimum intraoperative monitoring includes standard ASA monitoring – SpO_2, NIBP, ECG and $EtCO_2$. CVP monitoring may be helpful to assess fluid status of the patient. Immunosuppressive therapy should be continued. Since cyclosporine and tacrolimus levels must be kept within the therapeutic range, the blood levels should be monitored daily during the perioperative period.

Avoid intravascular volume depletion since it will lead to renal hypoperfusion.[11]

A patient who has been dialyzed preoperatively is more likely to be hypovolemic and hypokalemic and therefore diuretics should be used very judiciously in such circumstances.

Hypokalemia may produce arrhythmias and also prolong the action of muscle relaxants.

All patients should receive deep vein thrombosis (DVT) prophylaxis. Postoperative pain relief may be provided by wound infiltration, IV patient-controlled analgesia (PCA) and patient-controlled epidural analgesia (PCEA). NSAIDs should be avoided.

Opioid tolerance may develop in transplant recipients undergoing repeated surgeries. Although morphine excretion is not affected, it is the accumulation of metabolites, morphine-3-glucoronide which may produce prolonged sedation postoperatively.[12]

Laparoscopic Surgical Procedures in a Transplanted Patient

Many of the surgical procedures being done on renal transplanted patients are being performed successfully by the laparoscopic route. Some examples are lymphoceles and cholecystectomy. The advantages of the laparoscopic approach are a shorter hospital stay and immunosuppressive therapy can be continued by the oral route. The perioperative care should follow all the principles as for any other surgical transplanted patient.

Postoperative Care

The patient should be shifted to a high dependency unit where monitoring should continue. The immediate postoperative care could include dialysis, hemodynamic support or any metabolic correction. A close liaison between the anesthesiologist, nephrologist and nursing staff is necessary for a successful outcome.

HEART TRANSPLANTED PATIENT FOR NON-TRANSPLANT SURGERY

Heart transplantation is now an accepted treatment for a variety of end stage cardiac diseases. Some of the indications for heart transplant include hemodynamic compromise due to severe heart failure-refractory cardiogenic shock and documented dependence on intravenous inotropic support to maintain adequate organ perfusion, pulmonary hypertension, congenital heart disease, severe symptoms of ischemia which are not amenable to coronary artery bypass graft (CABG) surgery or percutaneous interventions and recurrent symptomatic ventricular arrhythmias refractory to all therapeutic interventions.

These transplanted patients may return to the operation theatre for a procedure which may or may not be related to the transplant.

Procedures related to the heart transplant

a. Procedures related to post heart transplant complications

   Early
   - Bleeding
   - Cardiac tamponade
   - Removal of a ventricular assist device

   Delayed
   - I and D of an abscess
   - Sternal wound infections requiring plastic reconstructive surgery

b. Procedures unrelated to the heart transplant surgery, but related to the chronic debilitated medical illness
   - Intra-abdominal emergencies (hypoperfusion of gut), intestinal perforation
   - Malignancy (immunosuppressant induced)
   - Surgery for associated peripheral vascular disease
   - Repair of aortic aneurysms.

Physiological Changes in Heart Transplanted Recipients

The transplanted heart has no sympathetic, parasympathetic or sensory innervation. There is loss of vagal activity which results in a higher resting heart rate, approximately 90–100 beats per minute, but there may be some reinnervation after the transplant. If the cuff of the native atria are left behind to allow surgical anastomosis of the grafted heart then the native pacemaker remains intact and therefore there are 2 P waves in a transplanted heart, but since the native P wave cannot cross the suture line, it has no role in the chronotropic activity of the transplanted heart.

There are several implications due to denervation of the heart. Valsalva maneuver and carotid sinus massage have no effect on the heart rate[13] and there is loss of cardiac baroreflexes. During period of stress (hemodynamic or exercise induced) the denervated heart relies on circulating catecholamines and Frank Starling law to maintain cardiac output by increasing stroke volume.[14] It is preload dependent since it cannot produce tachycardia during hypovolemia. However several years after transplant, reinnervation does take place.[15]

Anesthetic Implications of the Physiological Changes after Heart Transplant

Because of the various physiological changes that take place due to the denervation of the transplanted heart it is important to understand these changes so that modification can be made in the anesthetic technique.

A higher pulse rate is present, as described earlier. There is a blunted heart rate response to inadequate depth of anesthesia or analgesia.[16] There is also absence of sympathetic response to laryngoscopy and intubation of trachea.[17]

Pharmacological Changes in Transplanted Heart

Drugs like anticholinergics (atropine, glycopyrollate), anti-cholinesterases (neostigmine, edrophonium), muscle relaxants producing tachycardia including pancuronium, gallamine; nifedipine and sodium nitroprusside act via the autonomic nervous system and thus do not have significant effect on the transplanted heart. Therefore other positive chronotropic drugs like ephedrine, dobutamine and isoproterenol should be available. Dobutamine and isoproterenol have similar effects on both normal and denervated hearts.

Dopamine acts mainly by the release of norepinephrine and is therefore a less effective inotropic drug in the denervated heart recipient.

Neostigmine may produce bradycardia by direct activation of the cholinergic receptors on the myocardial ganglionic cells, but usually has no effect since it acts indirectly on the myocardium.[18]

Since intact sympathetic nerves are required for the normal uptake and metabolism of catecholamines, the catecholamine response in a denervated heart is different from that of a normal heart. However, the transplanted heart can respond to direct acting sympathomimetic drugs since the receptor density is intact. Both epinephrine and norepinephrine have an augmented inotropic effect in the heart transplanted patients.[1] Both have a higher inotropic to vasoconstrictive ratio (β;α).

Preanesthetic Examination

A thorough preoperative check up should focus on graft infection, rejection and graft function. Rejection usually occurs within the first three months. A patient with graft rejection may have persistent coronary artery disease. They may present with severe myocardial ischemia without any chest pain. Other features of rejection include fatigue, CCF, ventricular and atrial arrhythmias and silent myocardial infarction diagnosed only on ECG. Patient with mild rejection may continue to have a normal myocardial function but severe rejection is associated with severe diastolic and systolic dysfunction.[19]

An endomyocardial biopsy confirms rejection. A pre-operative check up must rule out the above dysfunction.

Arrhythmias including first degree AV block are common in the transplanted heart. Ventricular ectopics are seen in the first few weeks after transplantation, however lignocaine should be used cautiously because of its negative inotropic effects.

A detaled history regarding immunosuppressive and cardiac drugs should be obtained. Preoperative evaluation should include routine tests like complete blood count, serum electrolytes, chest X-ray, ECG and echocardiography. Majority of patients develop hypertension after 5 years of heart transplant due to the cyclosporine therapy. They may have concomitant renal dysfunction as well.

If the patient has an indwelling pacemaker, it should be tested for its proper functioning. Diaphragmatic dysfunction is usually present. All medications should be contined throughout the perioperative period.

Monitoring

The intensity of monitoring will depend on the invasiveness of the surgical procedure. Minor non cardiac procedures may be done with standard monitoring. Multilead ECG and ST trend analysis are recommended. However invasive monitoring including central venous pressure (CVP) and pulmonary capillary wedge pressure (PCWP) should be done in major surgical procedures since the transplanted heart is preload dependent and may be prone to myocardial dysfunction and ischemia. For CVP monitoring, the right internal jugular vein should be avoided because this route is usually used for endomyocardial biopsies.

Hypotensive episodes are often treated with rapid fluid administration in these patients, and PCWP may be a helpful guide to prevent pulmonary edema. Transoesophageal echo-cardiography helps assess preload and diagnose ischemia.

Anesthesia Technique

The choice of anesthesia will depend on the surgical procedure. A judicious, meticulous anesthetic technique with full asepsis is mandatory. Minor surgical procedures may be done under monitored anesthesia care. If there is no renal or liver dysfunction these patients have normal anesthetic agent requirements.

General anesthesia is usually preferred since there may be an impaired response to hypotension after spinal or epidural anesthesia. If regional anesthesia is administered, the aim is to avoid significant vasodilatation and fall in preload.[20]

All induction agents have been used safely when used judiciously. Inspite of the vasodilating properties of propofol it has been used safely. Inhalation agents are well tolerated unless there is decompensated heart failure.[21]

For the treatment of bradycardia, epinephrine and isoproteranol should be available.

CONCLUSION

Transplant recipients are increasing in number and therefore are likely to be encountered by non-transplant anesthesiologists since they may present for a non transplant procedure. It is essential to know the physiology of the transplanted organ, the pharmacology of the immunosuppressive drugs and the surgical condition for which they have presented to ensure a safe anesthetic technique and a good perioperative outcome.

CLINICAL PEARLS

- Transplant surgery is now a common surgical procedure, of which renal transplant is the most common.
- The main areas of concern are immunosuppression, infection and rejection.
- Proper understanding of the physiological changes of transplanted organ with altered pharmacology of drugs is essential.
- Pharmacology of immunosuppressive drugs should be studied.

REFERENCES

1. Organ procurement transplant network Data 2008.
2. Kostopanagiotou G, Smyrniotis V, Arkadopoulos N, Theodoraki K, Papadimitriou L, Papadimitriou J. Review article: anesthetic and perioperative management of adult transplant recipients in nontransplant surgery. Anesth Analg, 1999;89:613.
3. First MR. Cadaveric organ procurement: an overview of two aspects-donor and hospital networks, and minority donation. Transplant Proc, 1997;29:70-2.
4. Barone GW, Sailors DM, Hudec WA, Ketel BL. Trauma management in solid organ transplant recipients. J Emerg Med, 1997;15:169-76.
5. Suthanthiran M, Strom TB. Renal transplantation. N Engl J Med, 1994;331:365-76.
6. Keegan MT, Plevak DJ. The transplant for non-transplant surgery. Anesthesiology Clin N Am, 2004;22:827-61.
7. Zhang R, Leslie B, Boudreaux JP, Frey D, Reisin E. Hypertension after kidney transplantation: impact, pathogenesis and therapy. Am J Med Sci, 2003;325:202-8.
8. Vautour LM, Melton LJ, Clarke BL, Achenbach SJ, Oberg AL, McCarthy JT. Long-term fracture risk following renal transplantation: a population-based study. Osteoporos Int, 2004;15: 160-7.
9. Sharpe MD, Gelb AW. Anesthetic considerations for the previously transplanted patient. Anesthesiol Clin North America, 1994;12:827-43.
10. Sakamoto H, Takita K, Kemmotsu O, Morimoto Y, Mayumi T. Increased sensitivity to vecuronium and prolonged duration of its action in patients with end-stage renal failure. J Clin Anesth, 2001;13:193-7.
11. Lemmens HJM. Kidney transplantation: recent developments and recommendations for anesthetic management. Anesthesiol Clin North America, 2004;22:651-62.
12. Armstrong PJ, Dersten A. Normeperidine toxicity. Anesth Analg, 1986;65:536-8.
13. Shaw IH, Kirk AJ, Conacher ID. Anaesthesia for patients with transplanted hearts and lungs undergoing non-cardiac surgery. Br J Anaesth, 1991;67:772-8.
14. Kavanagh T, Yacoub MH, Mertens DJ, Kennedy J, Campbell RB, Sawyer P. Cardiorespiratory responses to exercise training after orthotopic cardiac transplantation. Circulation, 1988;77:162-71.
15. Huang MH, Ewy GA. Sympathetic reinnervation of the transplanted heart. N Engl J Med, 2001;345:1914-5.
16. Gammie JS, Keenan RJ, Pham SM, McGrath MF, Hattler BG, Khoshbin E, et al. Single- versus double-lung transplantation for pulmonary hypertension. J Thorac Cardiovasc Surg, 1998;115:397-402.
17. Plotkin JS, Johnson LB, Rustgi V, Kuo PC. Coronary artery disease and liver transplantation: the state of the art. Liver Transpl, 2000;6:S53-6.
18. Backman SB, Fox GS, Ralley FE. Pharmacological properties of the denervated heart. Can J Anaesth, 1997;44:900-1.
19. Park DW, Park SW, Park KH, et al. Frequency of and risk factors for stent thrombosis after drug-eluting stent implantation during long-term follow-up. Am J Cardiol, 2006;98:352-6.
20. McFalls EO, Ward HB, Moritz TE, et al. Coronary-artery revascularization before elective major vascular surgery. N Engl J Med, 2004;351:2795-804.
21. Nordmann AJ, Briel M, Bucher HC. Mortality in randomized controlled trials comparing drug-eluting vs. bare metal stents in coronary artery disease: a meta-analysis. Eur Heart J, 2006;27:2784-814.

10 CHAPTER

Anesthetic Considerations for Non-transplant Surgery in the Post-liver Transplant Patients

Vijay Vohra

INTRODUCTION

The success of liver transplant is improving with time and therefore increasing number of patients will present for surgery after having under gone transplantation. This trend is likely to continue in future as more centers are now coming up and the transplant activity is increasing. All this is because of the improved outcome of liver transplant surgery. The long-term survival of liver transplant has improved greatly over the years. Five years survival rate was around 72% in 2002 that improved to 86% in 2008.[1] The reason for this improved survival is multifactorial which includes good selection of patients, improved immuno-suppression, technical skills and perioperative care of the transplanted organ and the patient. These patients will now come to the hospital for both elective and emergency procedures with added responsibility of caring for the transplanted organ and the ongoing immuno-suppression.

In spite of transplantation procedure being highly successful, transplant recipients often present with very complex problems. The functional reserve of the liver could be impaired along with biochemical changes and the primary disease may also affect other organs. Split liver graft and living donor transplant would take between 3 to 12 months to reach the recipient standard liver volume. The immuno-suppressive therapy itself may produce certain side effects like hyperglycemia, hypertension and hyperlipidemia and these in turn lead to coronary artery disease. All patients of organ transplantation should be considered as immuno-compromised and thus, making them more prone to infection and malignancy.

In the early period, after transplantation, infection is the most common cause of mortality.[2] There will be some patients who would show signs of rejection as well and may need modifying Immunosuppressive medication. When these transplanted recipients require nontransplant surgery, immunity level can be altered because of the stress of surgery, alteration in the drug regime or by the acute illness itself. At this time, immunosuppressive medication needs to be adjusted to provide the immune imbalance brought on by severe stress. The possibility of infection and rejection both exists at this stage. These patients could also be emotionally unwell because of chronic medication and repeated hospital visits and therefore need to be handled with due care.

The patient with transplanted liver is therefore could pose many complex problems besides the surgical indication for hospital admission.

Early Postoperative Period Following Transplant

Up to 30% of transplanted patients may require some surgical interventions sooner or later.[3] The reason could be technical whereby the crucial anastomosis of the vessels is less than perfect and/or persistent coagulopathy which may lead to excessive bleeding necessitating exploration in the early postoperative period. Over enthusiastic correction of coagulopathy predisposes to vascular thrombosis, which can be catastrophic in comparison to some blood loss in slightly under corrected coagulation status.

The first few hours after the transplant are critical for the recipients. After multiple vascular anastomosis in the presence of impaired coagulation, there is possibility of bleeding. A constant vigil must be kept on the amount of collection seen in the drainage bags. The color of the drainage fluid should be noted and high drain hemoglobin would indicate the possibility of the derangement of coagulation or surgical bleed. This complication is rare with a kidney transplant where as it is much more common with heart transplant. Hyper acute rejection is an emergency and effort should be made to arrange a new donor organ immediately. When this occurs in kidney transplant, urgent transplant nephrectomy may be required even before a donor organ is available. In the interim period patient can be sustained on hemodialysis. In liver transplant, retransplantation could also be required if there is hepatic artery thrombosis in the early postoperative period. One can also attempt to do revascularization by

Table 10.1: Checklist for postoperative bleeding

1.	Amount of drainage per hour
2.	Color of the drain fluid
3.	Drain hemoglobin, drain/blood Hb ratio
4.	PT INR
5.	Platelet count
6.	Thromboelastography

intervention radiological means but that is possible if thrombosis has developed 5–7 days post liver transplant. For first 2–3 days, if there is hepatic artery thrombosis, the treatment option is re exploration, attempting thrombectomy, and even retransplantation. If thrombectomy has been done, there would be need to continue with thrombolytic therapy in the postoperative period. This increases the chances of bleeding from other cut surfaces especially in the live donor liver transplant where right/left lobe is transplanted.

Early Indications for Surgery

- Bleeding (Table 10.1), vascular thrombosis, biliary stenosis, biliary leak.
- Acute/hyperacute rejection can occur requiring removal of the grafted organ and retransplantation at the earliest subject to the availability of the organ.
- Wound dehiscence requiring resuturing

Checklist for postoperative bleeding: Critical monitoring of the following parameters is done besides hemodynamic monitoring and other parameters relating to intravascular volume status.

Infections in Post-transplant Patients

After transplantation, infection is the main cause of death postoperatively especially in first year.[4] At the time of intense immunosuppression, which is generally in the first few months after transplant, the infections could be life threatening. At the beginning of post-transplant phase, there is a susceptibility to nosocomial bacterial infections, but later on viral infections especially cytomegalovirus and fungal infections are the more predominant infections. It may not be easy to identify the causative organism and there may be need to do more invasive procedures like-open Biopsy requiring general anesthesia. In the transplant patients there is inherent risk of infections because of compromised immune-system. Immune-system can be further affected or altered due to acute illness or the stress of surgery. The immunosuppressive medications will need to be adjusted to offset the severe stress brought about by the surgical stress.

Late Indications for Surgery

- Infections—Opportunistic
- Intraabdominal perforation, collection or obstruction
- Biliary and vascular stenosis
- Lymphoproliferative diseases—Carcinoma
- Coronary artery disease
- Hernia repair

Majority of the complications can fit into one of the two main categories—either due to immunesuppression or technical complications of the transplant procedure.

General Surgical Issues in Transplanted Recipients

Transplanted recipient are at increased risk of requiring surgical interventions compared to normal person of similar demographics. Corticosteroids along with cyclosporine which forms a part of immunosuppression regime, results in increased in risk of developing gall stones and therefore requiring surgery.[5] Renal transplant recipients are at increased risk of pancreatitis, peptic ulcer disease, pseudomembranous colitis and spontaneous bowel perforation.[6]

The detection of peritonitis may be late as the typical signs may be absent in patients taking immunosuppressive medications. The contributing factors associated with perforation of the bowel include corticosteroid therapy, CMV infection and lymphoproliferative disorder.

Wound healing: Immunosuppresive therapy does inhibit wound healing after organ transplantation, the relative contribution of each agent is difficult to ascertain. Comparing azothiaprine with mycophenolate, there is increased incidence of wound problems with the former. These patients could present with wound dehiscence and would require resuturing. Steriods along with obesity have long being recognized as strong inhibitors of wound healing.[7] This patient's of chronic liver diseases, who have undergone liver transplantation, have underline malnutrition, which affects the ability to counter act infection. Serolimus is known to impair fibroblast and angiogenesis.[8] As the wound healing is impaired, there is a higher incidence of incisional hernia. Reported incidence of incisional hernia in liver transplantation is up to 17%.[9] The likely reason for high incidence of hernia is because of combination of factors-immunesuppression as well as persistent malnutrition.

Gastrointestinal complications: Over 30% patients of solid organ transplantation have gastrointestinal complaints and in 10% of these patients, the complaints could be of serious nature requiring intervention.[10,11] The bulk of surgical procedures required would be peptic ulcer disease, colonic perforation, biliary disease and malignancy. Cyclosporine use is associated with increased incidence of cholelithiasis due to cholestasis induced by the drug. Rejection episodes after the transplantation are commonly treated with large dose of steroids, which may also contribute to development of peptic perforation.

Orthopedic issues: Accompanying the increased survival after organ transplantation is the increased incidence of bone fractures due to pretransplant loss of bone, which gets substantiated by immunotherapy after the transplant. An additional factor responsible for fractures is the relative lack of activity in these patients. The reported risk of fractures is highest after liver transplant (13%–53%) whereas after heart transplant the reported risk is 6% to 21%.[12,13] A vascular necrosis as well as osteoporosis is seen in the recipients of organ transplantation. The shifting of organ transplant recipient should be done gently for the fear of fracturing the fragile bony structure.

PREGNANCY

Chronic liver disease is known to cause amenorrhea in women of childbearing age but pregnancy has been reported following successful liver transplantation.

After liver transplant pregnancy proceeds normally but is not completely without complications. Most centers advocate avoiding pregnancy during first 1–2 years of transplant, as it takes time to stabilize immunosuppression regime. There is risk of low birth weight baby's and prematurity. Upto 30% of the mothers developed pre-eclampsia and may need treatment for that. In a series by Jain A et al reported hyperkalemia in 5 out the 7 babies at birth from liver transplant recipient mothers. These mothers were on immunosuppressive therapy with tacrolimus.[14] Up to 50% mothers with liver transplant will require operative delivery in the form of cesarean section. The choice of anesthetic of these mothers will depend on the general condition of the mother and coagulation profile. The aim is to prevent development of hypotension and hypoxia, which could compromise liver blood flow and oxygenation. Regional anesthesia would be the choice in the absence of coagulation and platelet abnormality.

Malignancy

Besides infection, malignancy is the next major cause of morbidity in patients who survive the early course of transplant procedure. Lymphoproliferative disorders are generally seeing in 3 to 6 months after transplant and has been reported in Upto 8% of all transplant recipients.[15] The incidence of lymphoproliferative disorders varies with the intensity of immunosuppression. OKT3 has increased the risk of this disorder by nearly 9 fords.[16] Reduction of immunosuppression and treatment with Anti-viral agents along with surgical removal may be curative for lymphoproliferative disorder. Malignancy in this setting is usually not responsive to chemotherapy and the mortality at this stage approach is high and may reach upto 70%. Other malignant conditions seen in posttransplant patients are—colorectal carcinoma, skin malignancy and lymphoma.

Immunomodulatory Therapy: Implications for Anesthesia

Immunomodulatory therapy has allowed liver transplantation to become an acceptable procedure for end stage liver disease. Besides their effect on immune system, there are other side effects of this therapy. Each of the immunesuppressive agents have their side effects as well as toxic effects. One has to watch out for the side effect and monitor the dose of the drug to have optimum immunomodulatory effect. These drugs are used in combination and most patients will start their immunosuppression with up to 3 drugs.

Hyperglycemia

Corticosteroids are well known to increase the incidence of diabetes in normal population. Hyperglycemia is also seen to be associated with the use of immunosuppressant cyclosporine. Cyclosporine directly decreases the release of insulin from Islet Cells of Langerhans in the pancreas. This drug has been reported to double the incidence of diabetes in transplant recipients.[17] Steroids increase the insulin resistance and thus the transplanted patient may require higher doses of insulin to control blood sugar. The reported incidence of steroids related diabetes after transplantation ranges from 3.4% to 46%.[18] A Large number of patients develop metabolic Syndrome while on immunosuppressive drugs and require control of blood sugar and hypertension. Steroids are generally included in all the regimes but tapered of slowly over a period of months to years.

Hypertension

Almost half of the patients after solid transplant develop hypertension. The responsible drugs are corticosteroids, cyclosporine and tacrolimus. The other contributing factors could be recurrent renal disease like diabetic nephropathy and rejection.

Hypertension is often is not easy to treat and may require multidrug therapy. Calcium channel blockers and angiotensin converting enzyme (ACE) inhibitors have a favorable effect of transplanted kidney but do not offer any distinct advantage in liver transplant recipients. ACE inhibitors delay the progress of diabetic nephropathy and thereby reduce the proteinuria. Calcium channel blockers reduce the arterial vasoconstriction thereby controlling the blood pressure. Some calcium channel blockers like verapamil, nicardepine and diltiazem interfere with drug metabolism through inhibition of cytochrome P–450 and affect the levels of cyclosporine.

Hyperlipidemia

Cholesterol both total and low-density cholesterol are increased in renal and heart transplant patients. There is also increase in triglycerides level, which predisposed of pancreatitis. Hyperlipidemia produced in conjunction with cyclosporine does not respond to dietary measures and statins are required to lower the high cholesterol levels.[19] Statins are not totally benign drugs and must be given cautiously in patients receiving cyclosporine as this combination is known to cause rhabdomyolysis and acute renal failure. Low dose statin may be required in such circumstances after the transplant surgery to prolong patient survival.[20]

Coronary Artery Disease

The risk factor of coronary artery disease gets aggravated following transplantation and start of Immunosuppressive Drugs. There could be acceleration of coronary artery disease if present before the transplant procedure. The risk of ischemic heart disease postrenal transplant is upto 3 times of that expected from the similar age group patients. Similarly both peripheral and cerebral vascular disease incidence rises. The reason for developing coronary artery disease is increased incidence of diabetes, hypertension and hyperlipidemia. Other risk factor that could contribute in the coronary artery disease includes the history of smoking, diabetes of more than 25 years duration an age more than 45 years. All patients with a presence of risk factor must be investigated for coronary artery disease at regular interval. Coronary angiography should be reserved for patients who do not have significant renal dysfunction as the contrast used can cause renal damage. Keeping this in mind, dobutamine echocardiography or CT Angiography may a choice in this patient for detection coronary artery disease.[23]

Renal Dysfunction

Both cyclosporine and tacrolimus, which are used in transplant recipients, are known to cause renal dysfunction. Hypertension induced by these agents may also contribute the development of kidney injury. Both serum creatinine and creatinine clearance will be altered after prolonged use of these immunosuppressive agents.[21] It is estimated that 32% of heart transplant, 20% of lung transplant and 18% liver transplant recipients will have renal insufficiency at five years and 29% of these patients will eventually require renal replacement therapy.[22]

Adrenal Insufficiency

Methyl prednisolone is the most commonly used drug as a part of immunosuppressive regime for transplant patients. Varying amount of dose—up to 1000 mg is given before the new organ is perfused with the patient's blood. Steroids are continued in the postoperative period but there is now tendency to use smaller maintenance dosages. A dose of prednisolone 20 mg/day for three weeks is known to cause functional suppression of hypothalamic/pituitary/adrenal axis.[24] A patient with adrenal insufficiency will develop persistent hypotension with no obvious signs of hypovolemia. Response to vasopressors is obtunded in adrenal insufficiency. Traditionally a dose of hydrocortisone 50 mg given 8 hourly is given for the stress period and then quick return to the pre-surgical dosages. The dose of steroids can be tapered quickly over 3 days whereas a prolonged high dose will require a slower return of the steroid dose to maintenance levels.

Platelet Dysfunction

First 24 hours after the transplant is the crucial period during which there is an increased risk of vascular thrombosis, which could lead to loss of graft. This is more common in renal transplant patients who may have acquired coagulation defects, raised homocysteine levels and antiphospholipid antibodies are some of the abnormalities that are detected. This makes a case for prothrombotic screening including clotting factor deficiency, factor V Leiden gene mutation, and prothrombin gene mutation. Suspicion of thrombotic tendencies must arise if there is history of deep vein thrombosis, frequent thrombus formation in the arterio-venous fistula and clotting of dialysis filter. If the transplanted patients are at an increased risk of developing thrombosis, anticoagulation is generally continued in the postoperative phase for a variable period lasting upto six months.

This prothrombotic scenario is commoner in kidney transplant recipients and is not seen in liver transplant recipients, where thrombocytopenia is more likely seen due to hypersplenism. Patients with significant hypersplenism may take upto 6 weeks after liver transplant before their platelet count improve significantly. Surgical procedures if required at this stage may necessitate giving platelet transfusion to prevent excessive bleeding. Thrombocytopenia is also caused by the immunosuppressant drugs mycophenolate and azothiaprine.

Immunosuppressive agents do have side effects as described in the Tables 10.2 and 10.3 and could be a strong factor in the development of metabolic syndrome in the post-transplant period. Post-transplant hypertension and renal dysfunction are major morbid issues with these drugs. There use is monitored is very closely in the initial period after the transplant to provide optimal immunosuppression. Thereby preventing rejection of the transplanted liver. The long-term aim is always to have minimal immunosuppression and thereby limit the hazards of these drugs.

Table 10.2: Side effects and toxicity of commonly used immunosuppressive agents

Drug	Side effect or toxicity
Corticosteroids	1. Hyperglycemia
	2. Peptic ulcers
	3. Pancreatitis
	4. Cushing's syndrome
	5. Osteoporosis
	6. Myopathy
	7. Glaucoma, cataract, avascular necrosis
Cyclosporine	1. Hypertension
	2. Hepatoxicity
	3. Neprotoxicity
	4. Hypomagnesemia
	5. Increased cancer risk
Azathiaoprine	1. Pancreatitis
	2. Cholestatic jaundice
	3. Gastrointestinal upset
	4. Hepatitis
Mycophenolate	1. Thrombocytopenia
	2. Pancytopenia
	3. Gastrointestinal upset
	4. Anemia
Tacrolimus	1. Nephrotoxicity
	2. Hypertension
	3. Glucose intolerance
	4. Possible cardiomyopathy (high dosage)
	5. Neurological: headache, tremors, hyperesthesia
OKT3	1. Hypotension
	2. Pulmonary edema
	3. Neurological: headache, confusion, seizures

Table 10.3: Drug interactions of immunomodulatory drugs

Drug	Interactions
Cyclosporine	Calcium channel blockers increase cyclosporine blood levels
Mycophenolate mofetil	Proton pump inhibitors (PPI)
Tacrolimus	Cyclosporine, fluconazole, metoclopramide, erythromycin, verapamil, methylprednisolone-enhance effect. Phenytoin, nifedapine, carbimazapine, rifampicin decrease blood concentration
Sirolimus	Diltiazem, erythromycin, ketoconazole, bromocriptine and verapamil increased blood levels. Rifampacin decreased blood concentration
Corticosteroids	Anticoagulants, bronchodilators effect enhaced, antidiabetic and anticonvulsant effect could be decreased

Preoperative Evaluation

Any transplanted patient coming for surgery, some of the issues that must be kept in considerations are:

- Common complications of immunosuppressants and if any one of them are present in the patient
- Status of the transplanted organ
- Presence of the opportunistic infections.

With these aspects in the mind, the preoperative evaluation process can commence. All basic issues have to be taken care of as for any surgery. These should be incorporated with additional recommendations for transplanted patient. All basic issues have to be taken care of as for nay surgery Table 10.4. It is good to involve the transplant hepatology team as well or the perioperative care of these patients.

1. The basic assessment should be performed as per any other patients coming for surgery.
2. The anesthetic record of the previous transplant procedure should be reviewed. Review the postoperative course and examine if there were any factors, which could contribute to readmission. History of intraabdominal collection requiring drainage or exploration at the time of transplant could raise suspicion of intraoperative pathology. The status of the graft function and the relevant laboratory investigations and biopsy results should be assessed.
3. Laboratory tests documenting the graft function are essential and are helpful in assessing any deterioration of function postoperatively.
4. Identify any incriminating factors during last transplant
5. Duration of time elapsed since the transplant

Table 10.4: Preoperative evaluation: Core issues to be emphasized during preoperative evaluation

- State of the transplanted liver–functional status
- Immunosuppression drugs–dosages and dose modification
- Immunosuppression side effects
- Corticosteroids dose adjustments
- Infection issues (due to immune suppression)
- Viral hepatitis status–C, B–? reactivation post-transplant

6. Find out the details of immunosuppressive agents. Immunosuppressant drugs should be re-evaluated in the context of the surgery. If there is infection, there may be need to downgrade the immunosuppressive regime.
7. Look for the presence of any infection. May need to do cultures of urine, blood and other cultures even if there are no apparent symptoms.
8. Assess function of the transplanted liver
9. Function of other organs—may be compromised due to immunosuppressive therapy or dysfunction of the transplanted organ.

The basic investigation should include serum electrolytes, creatinine, complete blood count including platelets, chest X-ray, electrocardiogram, blood culture and culture from other site of infection.

Blood should be cross-matched as antibodies could be present in the recipient. The blood product obtained should be CMV negative as the risk of transmitting infection is high. CMV infection is a potential source of morbidity in immunocompromise patients. Additional doses of antibiotics may be required in the presence of infection and the dose of corticosteroids and as well as Immunosuppressant may need to be modified. Immunosuppressant must be continued although over all absorption in the perioperative period may be altered. Parental steroids can safely substitute oral steroids by equivalent doses and there could be need to give an additional dose to overcome this period of additional stress.

Preoperative Investigations

Complete blood count	TLC, DLC, platelet count
LFT's	Bilirubin, SGOT/SGPT, Alk phosphatase
Renal function tests	Serum creatinine, Na, K, Ca, BUN
X-ray chest	P/A for lung parenchyma, heart size
Eletrocardiogram	12 lead for ischemia, arrhythmias
Echocardiography	LV function, pericardial effusion

Anesthetic Technique

Up to 10% of patient return to the operating theater within 24 to 48 hour after transplantation reason for re operation in these patient is generally hemorrhage. Patient may have developed decreased urine output and even intraabdominal compartment syndrome due to collection of fluid/blood in the peritoneal cavity. Most of these patients will have invasive monitoring and additional large bore vesicular excess in place. Some of them may even be intubated and on the ventilator but may have difficulty in ventilation and maintaining oxygenation. These patients may have cardiovascular collapse once the abdomen is opened and the tamponade effect on the bleeding vessels is released. There should be arrangement for the some kind of rapid infusion system (Level 1) or something similar. Surgical source of bleeding is looked for, the common sites being the raw surface of the liver, abdominal wall, liver laceration and the vascular anastomosis.

After the first 1 or 2 days, the other possibility of transplanted patient coming to operation theater is vascular thrombosis. Hepatic artery thrombosis is seen more commonly in children and may present with elevated enzymes and hemodynamic instability. This is an emergency and needs active surgical interventions, as this can eventually lead to graft failure.

Patient could be admitted due to immunosuppression related complications, like pneumonia requiring bronchoscopy. There could be development of intraabdominal collections, which may require surgical evacuation if ultrasound guided drainage is unsuccessful. Biliary complications are common in living donor liver transplantation (LDLT) compared to diseased donor liver transplantation (DDLT).

Most surgical procedures would require general anesthesia, as residual coagulopathy may persist for a few weeks after transplant. The recipients of liver transplants have a very low analgesic requirements and the best option of providing them analgesia is through patient control analgesia devices without any background infusion.[25]

After a successful liver transplant, majority of the multisystem dysfunction as seen in end stage liver disease, start returning towards normal in two to three weeks. Platelet count may take up to six weeks before it starts improving. Metabolic functions are first to correct and are monitored with gradual lowering of serum lactate levels followed by slower recovery of synthetic functions observed by improving serum albumin levels among other parameters. Albumin levels may take weeks to months before returning back to normal after successful liver transplant. Induction agents—barbiturates and propofol are largely bound to albumin in the blood and would have an enhanced effect in the presence of low serum albumin due to increased free fraction of the drug.

Renal function improves in most patients with hepatorenal syndrome after transplant but if the kidney does take a hit during the liver transplant surgery, there could be worsening of renal functions. If the patient was suffering from intrinsic renal disease, this could worsen inspite of taking adequate renal protective measures.[26]

Hypoxemia seen in the preoperative period in patients with hepatopulmonary syndrome (HPS), will take weeks to corrects itself and sometimes take even longer to resolve completely. These recipients may require long-term oxygen therapy for a variable period of time. Supplemental oxygen may still be required if there is persistence of basal atelectasis due the presence of preoperative ascites, upper abdominal surgery. Portopulmonary hypertension (POPH) is an even more entity to resolve post-liver transplant. The treatment for POPH must continue postoperatively with nitric oxide, epoprostanol, or sildenafil. POPH persisting post-operatively can affect the outcome of liver transplantation surgery hence the need to monitor these patients more closely.

The clinical condition is the guide to the choice of anesthesia like in any other situation. Meticulous hygiene technique should be used to minimize the risk of the patient developing infections. Critically ill transplant recipients must be handled with all percautions. The choice of anesthetic technique— general anesthesia, intravenous sedation, regional anesthesia or local infiltration should be according to the type of surgery planned, patient wish and the experience of the anesthetist. Care should be taken not to cause undue hypotension during regional anesthesia as this can compromise portal blood flow and compromise liver function. Epidural space is known to accumulate fat due to steroid therapy in these patients. This may cause technical difficulty in performing epidural block, which could be challenging. Monitoring again depends on the clinical condition and emergent nature of the procedure. A patient who is well, standard monitoring of arterial blood pressure, oxygen saturation and electrocardiogram may be all that is required. When invasive monitoring is used, intra vascular catheter should be removed as soon as possible to avoid developing infection.

Avoiding hypoxia during anesthesia is a good practice but is more relevant in present context as it can aggravate POPH. Hypoxemia could be persisting because of HPS, which could take months to recover after the transplant. Inhalational agents can be used butt all of them can affect splanchnic blood flow and thus portal blood flow. The hepatic artery buffer response is altered with the use of volatile agents but is better maintained with isoflurane. Propranol and other drugs known to decrease the hepatic blood flow should be avoided.

Regional anesthesia should be considered if the coagulation profile has returned to normal and platelet count is more than 100,000/mm^3. Post liver transplant it would take upto six weeks before there is improvement in platelet count and normal platelet will not be seen for 3–6 months. Weight gain and metabolic syndrome is a feature in many of the post liver transplant patients. There could be increased fat content in the epidural space, which may hinder identification of space as well as higher spread of the epidural drug.

Transmission of infectious disease must be kept in mind and institutional protocols including universal precautions must be strictly followed as a large percentage of the patients are suffering from hepatitis B or hepatitis C.

Risk of Disease Transmission to Attending Personnel

The indication for liver transplantation over the years has seen many fold increase in hepatitis C. The transplanted patient may be a carrier of infective viral hepatitis B or C. Health workers likely to be involved in the looking after transplant patients should all be immunized for hepatitis B and must ensure that the serum antibody titers have reached above 100 units/L.

Hepatitis B is seen in large number of patients in kidney and liver transplant. Besides, these transplant patient are more vulnerable to developing Hepatitis B and C And HIV because of multiple blood infusions.[27] It is best to adopt universal precautions, which prevents transmission of disease and must be followed in all patients. There is a window period when viral markers do not show up but the patient may be in infective state.

Recurrence hepatitis C after having undergone liver transplantation is not uncommon. Even if the patients are not symptomatic, viremia may still be persisting with distinct possibility of viral transmission.

Needle stick injury must be guarded against besides using protecting eye covers and mask. There should be clear institutional guidelines to follow in the disposal of waste from operating theater should be handled carefully as per the hospital policy.

Postoperative Care

Chronic liver disease leading to end stage liver disease and culminating in liver transplant can be a very traumatic journey for the patient. The transplanted patient would have gone through a lot of agony and could be either become a very positive and disciplined person or could be an emotional wreck. They need to be handled with compassion and caring attitude. Undergoing another surgery after having got liver transplant done might sound trivial by all standards but could pull the patient down morally. Effort should be made to be very compassionate and provide all support needed for this group of patients.

For someone who has undergone major surgical procedure, must be looked after in high dependency unit with close monitoring. The stakes here are higher whereby the current surgical procedure demands postoperative care and the effect of this surgical procedure may affect the function of the transplanted liver. Post-operative period is crucial because from maximal monitoring in operating theater, the patient now moves to an area where there may not be clear understanding as to what went on while in the operating theater. So for a variable period in the postoperative course the monitoring should be continuation of what was being done in the operating room. The level of monitoring can be gradually modified as the time progresses.

Pain relief in the postoperative period can be effectively achieved by both parenteral analgesia or by regional analgesic techniques. For instituting regional anesthetic techniques, platelet counts should be > $100,000/mm^3$ and prothrombin time (P T) International Normalized Ratio (INR) should be less than 1.5 Postoperative pain control should be discussed before the surgical procedure itself and must be instituted early in the postoperative period. Most patients will be using systemic medications—narcotics like morphine, the dose varying depending on physical status and the type of surgery. Patient control analgesia is the best method of providing pain control in patients who are being managed in the wards. In intensive care unit, the nursing staff and the doctors can monitor the analgesia, as the requirement in these patients could be highly variable.

Right diaphragmatic dysfunction persists for a variable length of time post liver transplant and a period of up to 6 months has been reported before return of normal diaphragmatic activity. A raised diaphragm in the postoperative phase may therefore be quite normal and not a sign of basal lung collapse.

The number of transplanted patients is steadily increasing and they will present to the hospitals for various elective and emergency procedures. It is important to recognize changes due to organ transplantation and the effect of immuno-suppressive agents. In a normally functioning graft, there may not be many problems. But it does become a challenging issue if the graft function is less than perfect and surgery is of emergent nature.

CLINICAL PEARLS

- Assessment of liver function-liver enzymes SGOT/ SGPT for any acute episodes. Prothrombin time and serum albumin for synthetic function. This will be an indicator of graft function, rejection or acute insult to liver
- Critical look at immunosuppressive regime as it may need to e modified due to increased stress of the surgery or if there is evidence of infection.
- Look for side effects and toxicity of immunosuppressive agents as the dose requirement keeps varying with immune status at a particular time.
- Extraprecautions in exercising asepsis in handling of the recipient due to their immune compromised status.
- Universal precautions to prevent transmission of infections/ viral hepatitis to theatre personnel.
- Review of the previous anesthetic notes and postoperative course to assist in formulating anesthetic plan for the surgery.

REFERENCES

1. Source; OPTN/SRTR Data as of October 1,2010.
2. Forton J, et al. Percutaneous radiofrequency thermal ablation of hepatocellular carcinoma: a safe and effective bridge to liver transplantation. Liver Transplantation, 2002;8:1065-70.
3. Cheng DCH, Anaesthesia for non-cardiac surgery in heart-transplanted patient. Can J Anaesth, 1993;40:981-6.
4. FORTUN J liver transpl, 2002;8:1065-70.
5. Boline GB, et al. Cholecystectomy in the potential heart transplant patients. J Heart Lung Transplant, 1991;10:269-74.
6. Lao A, Bach D. The UGI series in renal transplant candidates. J Can Assoc Radiol, 1988;39:195-7.
7. Anstead GM. Steriods, Retiniods and wound heeling. ADV Wound Care, 1998;11:277-8.
8. Gregory CR, et al. Treatment with Rapamycin and Mycophenolic acid reduces arterial intimal thickening produced by mechanical injury and allows endothelial replacement. Transplantation, 1995; 59:655-61.
9. Gomez R, et al. Incidence and predisposing factors for incisional hernia in patients with liver transplantation. Hernia, 2001;5:172-6.
10. Goldberg HJ, et al. Colon and rectal complications after heart and lung transplant. J Am Coll Surg, 2006;202:55-61.
11. Sariko S, et al. Severe gastrointestinal complications after 1515 adult kidney transplantation. Transplant Int, 2004;17: 505-10.
12. Leidig-Bruckner G, et al. Frequency and predictors of osteoporotic fractures after cardiac or liver transplantation: a follow up study. Lancet, 2001;357(9253:342-7).
13. Poayko MD, et al. Bone disease in liver transplantation recipients: incidence, timing and risk factors. Transplant Proc, 1991;23(1Pt 2): 1462-5.
14. Jain A, et al. FK506 and pregnancy in liver transplantation. Trans-plantation, 1993;56:1588-1589.
15. Penn I, Why do immunosuppressed patients develop cancer? Crit Rev Oncolog, 1989;1;27-52.
16. Petri WA. Junior, Infections in heart transplant patients. Clin Infect Dis, 1994;18:141-6.

17. Nilsen JH, et al. Direct effect of cyclosporine A on human pancreatic B cells. Diabetes, 1986;35:1049-52.
18. Friedman EA, et al. Post transplant diabetes in kidney transplant recipients. AM J Nephrol, 1985;5:196-202.
19. Moor RA, et al. The effect of American Heart Association Step One Diet on hyperlipidemia following renal transplantation. Transplantation, 1990;49:60-2.
20. Kobashigawa JA, et al. Low dose lovastatin safely lowers cholesterol after cardiac transplantation. Circulation, 1990;82 Supplement IV; 281-3.
21. Olson LJ, et al. Mayo Clinic Proc, 1992;67:775-84.
22. Ojo AO, Held PJ, et al. Chronic renal failure after transplantation of non-renal organ. N Engl J Med, 2003;349(10);931-40.
23. Braun WE, et al. Coronary artery diseases in transplant recipients. Cleveland Clinic J medicine, 1994;61:370-85.
24. Bromberg JS, et al. Stress steroids are not required for patient receiving a renal allograft and undergoing operation. J Am Coll Surg, 1995;180(5);532-6.
25. Eisenach JC, et al. Comparison of analgesic requirement after liver transplantation and cholecystectomy. Mayo Clin Proc, 1989; 64:356-9.
26. Gines P, et al. Hepatorenal Syndrome. Lancet, 2003;362:1819-27.
27. Jeffers LJ, et al. Prevalence of antibodies to hepatitis C virus among patients with cryptogenic chronic hepatitis and cirrhosis. Hepatolgy, 1992;15:187-90.

11 CHAPTER

Pregnancy in a Transplanted Patient

Jayashree Sood

INTRODUCTION

The first successful pregnancy after kidney and liver transplant surgery was reported in 1963[1] and 1978[2] respectively. One year survival reported is more than 80–90% for most transplant recipients. Improved surgical techniques and better immunosuppressive therapies have allowed women in the reproductive age group to become pregnant after transplant procedures. Therefore, anesthesiologists may be required to manage these patients in hospitals not involved in transplantation procedures.

For many years, the data regarding pregnancy outcomes was provided by case reports and case series. A voluntary National Transplantation Pregnancy Registry (NTPR) was established in 1991 at the Thomas Jefferson University in North America, to study the safety of pregnancy and its outcomes.[3] As of August 2012, more than 2,000 recipients have reported more than 3,000 pregnancies in female recipients or fathered by male transplant recipients. Later other smaller registries, e.g. European Dialysis Transplant Association Registry and United Kingdom Transplant Pregnancy Registry were established.[4,5]

Anesthesiologists are faced with a number of challenges when a pregnant woman who has previously undergone transplantation procedure presents for instrumental delivery or cesarean section. One has to consider the physiological and pharmacological changes related to pregnancy, effect of pregnancy on graft function, physiological and pharmacological problems of allograft denervation, interaction of immunosuppressants with anesthetic drugs and their side effects, increased risk of infection, the potential for rejection of transplanted organ, status of the transplanted organ and status of other organs which may have been affected by immunosuppression or dysfunction of the transplanted organ.

Effect of Pregnancy on Graft Function

Pregnancy has no effect on graft function if the graft has been previously stable.[6,7] However, an increase in serum creatinine level with a failure to return to pre-pregnancy level may be seen in parturients with pre-existing renal dysfunction.[4] There are biopsy proven incidences of acute rejection in 2–4% of pregnancies depending on calcineurin inhibitor exposure.[8] A lower incidence of adverse events and fewer graft losses have been seen in parturients post liver transplant[3,8] and post heart transplantation,[4,9] while poor graft survival following pregnancy has been documented in pancreas and lung transplants.[3]

Problems of Allograft Denervation

Heart transplant recipients have denervated hearts, as a result of which there is an increased incidence of cardiac arrhythmias during pregnancy. Furthermore, there is an increased sensitivity to sympathomimetic agents.[10] There may be absence of typical chest pain that occurs during myocardial infarction. Allograft vasculopathy is also common post cardiac transplant.[10]

Delivery

Delivery should be a planned procedure in post-transplant recipients. Close collaboration among obstetrician, transplant physician and anesthesiologist is essential.

Preoperative Assessment

The basic aim is to rule out the presence of rejection. Rejection results in progressive deterioration of organ function. One may have decreased the dose of immunosuppressants during pregnancy to avoid the effect on fetus but this may precipitate rejection. Surgery during rejection is a major factor which increases morbidity.[11]

Presence of infection should also be ruled out preoperatively. Immunosuppressed patients may not present with the typical signs and symptoms of intra-abdominal sepsis, i.e. fever, leucocytosis and physical signs of peritonitis. Elective surgery should be postponed in presence of infection.[12]

In patients on warfarin, sudden withdrawal of azathioprine causes bleeding because its metabolite 6-mercaptopurine induces microenzymes which metabolize warfarin.[13]

Transplant organ function should be evaluated thoroughly. Renal function should be assessed as it could be compromised by therapy with tacrolimus and cyclosporine. Hepatobiliary and pancreatic diseases should be evaluated. Upper gastrointestinal bleeding secondary to peptic ulcer disease, gastritis or cytomegalovirus gastroenteritis should be ruled out.

The functional adequacy of other organ systems should be determined.

A detailed airway assessment should be done as there could be severe perioperative airway obstruction by post-transplant lymphoproliferative disease.[14]

Investigations

A complete blood count, liver and renal function studies, routine blood sugar, serum amylase and lipase, viral serology and ECG should be undertaken. There may be evidence of thrombocytopenia in a parturient taking azathioprine and antithymocyte globulin, so a coagulation profile is necessary.

Daily blood levels of immunosuppressants should be monitored, especially cyclosporine and tacrolimus and maintained within the desired limits (cyclosporine 50–150 gm/L, tacrolimus 4–8 pg/dL).

Post lung transplant parturients should be assessed by pulmonary function tests and arterial blood gas analysis. An echocardiogram should be considered in post cardiac transplant pregnancy.

ANESTHETIC CONSIDERATIONS

Interactions of Immunosuppressants with Anesthetic Drugs

It is recommended that patients should be given oral cyclosporine 4–7 hours prior to anesthesia to achieve optimal blood levels because of prolonged gastric emptying and delayed absorption associated with the pre-existing liver disease.[15] Exposure to isoflurane also results in delayed gastric emptying and absorption of cyclosporine from proximal small bowel in rats.[16] An enhanced effect of phenobarbital and muscle relaxants with immunosuppressants has been observed in animal studies. However, clinically relevant doses of azathioprine do not show this effect in humans. But, a reduced dosage of these drugs should be administered and a prolonged recovery time should be expected.[17] Propofol[18] and epidural bupivacaine[19] are considered safe. In clinical doses, toxic effects of bupivacaine with compromised renal function have not been demonstrated.

A wide variety of anesthetic techniques (general, regional, neuroleptic) have been adopted in a post-transplant parturient.

These patients may be on low dose aspirin. Its use prior to surgery should be withheld. Blood pressure should be controlled and infection treated aggressively. Meticulous fetal surveillance by the obstetrician is mandatory.

If the patient has been stable on a particular regime of immunosuppressants then it should be continued throughout the pregnancy at the pre pregnancy dosages. Therapeutic levels of these drugs should be maintained and monitoring should be continued till at least 1 month post partum. Fluid shifts, restoration of pregravid renal blood flow and reactivation of autoimmune diseases can result in significant changes in blood levels of immunosuppressants. Subtherapeutic levels of immunosuppressants may precipitate rejection. Oral and intravenous doses of prednisolone and azathioprine are approximately equivalent.[20]

Stress coverage by steroids is not indicated, although with repeated surgeries some transplant recipients may develop tolerance to steroids.[21] The regimen is titrated to clinical effect and potential of side effects anticipated. Metabolites of morphine (morphine 3-glucoronide and morphine 6-glucoronide) may accumulate and result in prolonged sedation postoperatively.[22] There may be an overt diagnosis of preeclampsia in this subset of patients, due to hypertension and proteinuria secondary to immunosuppressants. Presence of preeclampsia and associated edema may compromise the airway.

Standard premedication should be given prior to cesarean section. Antacid prophylaxis should be considered in patients on chronic steroid therapy secondary to peptic ulcerative disease. Ranitidine should be used cautiously in a parturient receiving cyclosporine or tacrolimus as it is associated with increased chances of renal dysfunction.[23]

Routine prophylactic antibiotic to prevent subacute bacterial endocarditis is not recommended in heart transplanted parturients.[24] The parturient on chronic steroid therapy should be handled gently to avoid skin damage and bone fractures. An aseptic technique should be used during the procedure with regard to securing intravascular access, intubation, using of disposable anesthetic accessories and regional anesthesia. Standard monitoring is recommended. Continuous ECG monitoring should be done in all patients. Invasive monitoring should be established after weighing the risk benefit ratio. DVT prophylaxis is mandatory. Watch for cardiac arrhythmias in post cardiac transplant parturients.

Anesthesia Technique

The choice of anesthesia technique depends on the functional status of the transplanted graft, cardiovascular and hematological status of the parturient and the indication for cesarean section. Anesthetic management is similar to that of a normal parturient except for a few changes specific to the transplanted graft. Central neuraxial block is not contraindicated in these patients, rather it decreases the chances of pulmonary aspiration, avoids dealing with a difficult airway, causes less fetal depression and provides superior postoperative pain relief. During labor, an epidural provides the advantages of reducing pain induced sympathetic responses and decreases acute blood pressure fluctuations. Parturients on cyclosporine A have an increased chance of neurotoxicity. A careful neurological examination and documentation of paresthesias should be done prior to a regional block.[25]

A parturient with a normal cardiovascular status may be offered regional anesthesia. Spinal anesthesia has the advantage of faster onset of action and less dose requirement as opposed to epidural anesthesia. An epidural has the advantage of achieving a desired level of block by small incremental doses with a gradual fall in blood pressure. Regional anesthesia warrants normal coagulation status and platelet count of the parturient, although in cases of marginal derangement of coagulation profile, spinal anesthesia with a narrow gauge needle, i.e. 27G can be given.[26]

General anesthesia should be considered when there are contraindications to regional anesthesia, for example patient refusal, local anesthesia toxicity, altered coagulation profile, compromised cardiac function or an obstetric indication. A rapid sequence induction is recommended to avoid risk of pulmonary aspiration. Suxamethonium is safe to use if serum potassium levels are below 5.5 mEq/L. There exists a higher risk of aspiration post lung transplant because of the absence of cough reflex, so these parturients should be monitored closely in the postoperative period.[27] Careful attention to serum sodium and magnesium levels should be given in patients taking cyclosporine or tacrolimus.

Pregnancy in Renal Transplanted Patients

Advances in renal transplantation medicine and techniques have made post-transplant pregnancy a viable option for women of child bearing age. Post kidney transplant pregnancies are high risk, but can progress successfully without adversely affecting the survival and function of the allograft.

The currently available immunosuppressant drugs are not teratogenic, however in the 2nd and 3rd trimester they affect the immune system of the fetus such that they are immunocompromised for a short period resulting in prematurity and low birth weight babies with adverse effects on the liver, pancreas and lymphocytes.[28-32] Other risks are anemia, arterial hypertension, proteinuria, infections and acute graft rejection. Bacterial infections include urinary tract infection and acute pyelonephritis of the graft.

The incidence of preeclampsia and premature labor in the transplanted parturient is higher than in normal pregnancy. The incidence of hypertension during pregnancy after transplant appears to be dependent on the type of immunosuppressive agents used. It is estimated to be 22–29% with corticosteroids, 68–73% with cyclosporine and 47–54% with tacrolimus.[33]

Perioperative Management of a Parturient After Renal Transplant

The most frequent indications for elective caesarian section in these parturients are hypertension and preeclampsia. In case a caesarian section (CS) is planned, the principles of anesthetic management would include those for a CS and also those for patients undergoing any surgery after a renal transplant. Meticulous asepsis should be maintained.

Signs of rejection, i.e. azotemia, proteinuria and hypertension should be looked for. Adequate intravascular volume should be maintained and renal hypoperfusion, diuretics and nephrotoxic drugs, i.e. nonsteroidal anti-inflammatory drugs should be avoided. In a parturient on cyclosporine or tacrolimus therapy avoid cimetidine, ranitidine, cotrimoxazole, vancomycin and gentamycin. These drugs increase chances of renal dysfunction.[17,34] Pregnancy leads to a substained decrease in cyclosporine levels, so these should be monitored during pregnancy. The patients may be undergoing dialysis in the event of graft dysfunction. Dialysis may result in hypovolemia and hypokalemia leading to cardiovascular instability, arrhythmias and increased susceptibility to muscle relaxants.

If general anesthesia is given, hyperventilation should be avoided in these patients as they have a lower seizure threshold secondary to cyclosporine therapy.[35] The choice of non-depolarizing muscle relaxant depends on the renal status of the parturient. Cyclosporine augments the action of neuromuscular blocking drugs due to cremaphor, the solvent of a cyclosporine.[36] Use of peripheral nerve stimulator is recommended. Atracurium has least renal elimination and is the drug of choice in these patients. Extubation is done when the patient is fully awake. Meticulous intraoperative fluid and electrolyte management should be done. Hypotension secondary to denervated kidney increases the susceptibility to acute tubular necrosis which is further potentiated by the nephrotoxicity of cyclosporine. Adequate hydration and a urine output of more than 1 mL/kg/hr should be maintained.

Postoperative pain relief should be supplemented by a narcotic intravenously or by epidural route. Avoid non steroidal anti-inflammatory drugs which increase gastrointestinal bleeding and exacerbate cyclosporine toxicity by decreasing renal blood flow through prostaglandin inhibition.[37]

Parturients on azathioprine may have thrombocytopenia, and uremia may result in platelet dysfunction so caution should be exercised with regional anesthesia.[33]

Bupivacaine has been used in these patients without any adverse effects.[2]

Parturient with Liver Transplantation

Denervation of the liver does not affect its hemodynamics. The liver's synthetic ability usually normalizes within 2 weeks of transplant and the coagulation profile returns to normal by the third postoperative week. The anesthetic technique is quite similar to that of a normal parturient. The inhaled anesthetics are considered safe with no added risk of hepatitis. The liver is a storage organ of blood and during shock states it helps in resuscitation by its vasoconstrictive response.[38] However, liver transplantation impairs this response, so aggressive fluid resucitation and early blood replacement is recommended during shock. One must also avoid over transfusion of blood products and maintain blood viscosity with the hematocrit around 25%. Hemoconcentration results in hepatic arterial thrombosis with increased mortality.[39]

Parturient with Heart Transplantation

Most recipients after heart transplant return to NYHA class 1 functional capacity. They have a higher resting heart rate (91–101 bpm) due to absent sympathetic, parasympathetic or sensory innervation and loss of vagal influence. The ECG demonstrates two P waves. The native pacemaker remains intact when the cuff of the atria is saved to permit surgical anastomosis to the grafted heart. Since this pacemaker signal does not traverse the graft suture line it has no influence on chronotropic activity of the transplanted heart. The intrinsic mechanism and coronary autoregulation remain intact.[40]

Graft rejection should be ruled out. It presents as accelerated coronary artery disease with fatigue, ventricular arrhythmia, congestive heart failure and silent myocardial infarction on ECG. Mild rejection does not compromise cardiac contractility but severe rejection results in significant systolic and diastolic dysfunction.

Carotid sinus massage and the Valsalva maneuver have no effect on the heart rate.[17,40] Denervation results in the loss of baroreceptor reflexes, loss of sympathetic responses to laryngoscopy and tracheal intubation, and blunted heart rate response to an inadequate depth of anesthesia or analgesia.

Since, the receptor density of catecholamines is unchanged, the transplanted heart responds to direct acting drugs. An augmented inotropic effect is seen with sympathomimetics (epinephrine or norepinephrine) as opposed to a vasoconstrictor effect.[10]

Dopamine acts by release of norepinephrine. It is a less effective inotrope in the denervated heart with primary dopaminergic and alpha effects. Ephedrine has a blunted response on blood pressure and heart rate, so direct acting drugs like isoproterenol and dobutamine are preferred which have the same effect in transplanted and normal hearts. Atropine is ineffective in increasing heart rate so isoproterenol and ephedrine should be readily available. Neostigmine can be used safely as it has no effect on heart rate in the denervated heart.[10]

All preoperative drug therapy should be continued. Proper functioning of pacemaker should be confirmed. Invasive monitoring (CVP and PA catheter) is generally not required. General anesthesia is preferred. Inhaled anesthetics are well tolerated unless significant heart failure sets in. Regional anesthesia is associated with impaired response to hypotension. Avoid significant vasodilatation and acute decrease in preload.[40]

Parturient with Lung Transplant

Rejection should be ruled out, as evidenced by a decrease in total leucocyte count, pulmonary function tests (↓FEV and VC) and arterial blood gas analysis (↑$AaDO_2$ gradient). Denervation does not affect the pattern of breathing. Bronchial hyperresponsiveness causes bronchoconstriction, so preoperative nebulization with bronchodilators should be done. Chronic rejection mimics upper respiratory tract infection with fever, leucopenia, hypoxemia, fatigue and shortness of breath. Chest X-ray demonstrates perihilar infiltration or opacification of graft and pulmonary function tests demonstrate obstructive defect with decreased FEV and VC.[41]

In addition, below the level of tracheal anastomosis there is loss of afferent sensation resulting in loss of cough reflex with retention of secretions and increased chances of silent aspiration. Therefore, regional anesthesia is preferred. It avoids tracheal intubation and its effect on the hyperresponsive tracheobronchial tree, potential for chest infection and the increased risk of aspiration.[42]

Diuretics should be used and crystalloid infusion should be restricted because of disruption of lymphatic drainage in the transplanted lung. Fluid causes interstitial fluid accumulation.[27,40,42] Chest physiotherapy, postural drainage and incentive spirometry in the postoperative period is recommended.

Parturient with Pancreatic Transplant

Pregnancy is associated with a good metabolic control and therefore worsening glucose control indicates likelihood of rejection.[43]

Perioperative management of the parturient is similar to that of the diabetic parturient. Monitor urinary amylase level for pancreatic graft function.[44] Pancreatic ductal cells secrete significant amounts of bicarbonate and water. Loss of bicarbonate in urine results in dehydration and metabolic acidosis.[45] Bicarbonate levels should be monitored in urinary bladder drainage of pancreatic secretions. These patients do not require insulin to compensate for the stress response to surgery.

Parturient with Intestinal Transplant

Denervation and lymphatic innervations affect intestinal permeability and absorption. The intestinal mucosal damage secondary to rejection, ischemia or enteritis results in infections into the bloodstream.[46] Full aseptic technique should be used. Difficult venous access due to chronic use of parenteral nutrition should be expected.

CLINICAL PEARLS

- Successful pregnancies are now possible after solid organ transplantation.
- The National Transplantation Pregnancy Registry (NTPR) helps in raise awareness of the successful pregnancy after transplant surgery.[47]
- It is important to understand the physiological changes secondary to transplantation and the changes brought about by pregnancy on the transplanted parturient.
- A multidisciplinary team is essential for optimizing maternal and fetal outcomes.

REFERENCES

1. Murray JE, Reid DE, Harrison JH, Merrill JP. Successful pregnancies after human renal transplantation. N Engl J Med, 1963;269:341-3.
2. Walcott WO, Derick DE, Jolley JJ, Snyder DL. Successful pregnancy in a liver transplant patient. Am J Obstet Gynecol, 1978; 132(3):340-1.
3. Armenti VT, Daller JA, Constantinescu S, Silva P, Radomski JS, Moritz MJ, et al. Report from the National Transplantation Pregnancy Registry: outcomes of pregnancy after transplantation. Clin Transpl, 2006;57-70.
4. Sibanda N, Briggs JD, Davison JM, Johnson RJ, Rudge CJ. Pregnancy after organ transplantation: a report from the UK Transplant Pregnancy Registry. Transplantation, 2007;83:1301-7.
5. McKay DB, Josephson MA, Armenti VT, August P, Coscia LA, Davis CL, et al. Reproduction and transplantation: report on the AST consensus conference on reproductive issues and Transplantation. Am J Transplant, 2005;5:1592-9.
6. Naqvi R, Noor H, Ambareen S, Khan H, Haider A, Jafri N, et al. Outcome of pregnancy in renal allograft recipients: SIUT experience. Transplant Proc, 2006;38:2001-2.
7. Oliveira LG, Sass N, Sato JL, Ozaki KS, Medina Pestana JO. Pregnancy after renal transplantation: a five-yr single-center experience. Clin Transplant, 2007;21:301-4.
8. Armenti VT, Radomski JS, Moritz MJ, Gaughan WJ, Gulati R, McGrory CH, et al. Report from the National Transplantation Pregnancy Registry (NTPR): outcomes of pregnancy after transplantation. Clin Transpl, 2005;69-83.
9. Branch KR, Wagoner LE, McGrory CH, Mannion JD, Radomski JS, Moritz MJ, et al. Risk of subsequent pregnancies on mother and newborn in female heart transplant recipients. J Heart Lung Transplant, 1998;17:698-702.
10. Taylor DO, Edwards LB, Boucek MM, Trulock EP, Aurora P, Christie J, et al. Registry of the International Society for Heart and Lung Transplantation: twenty-fourth official adult heart transplant report 2007. J Heart Lung Transplant, 2007;26:769-81.
11. Howard TK. Postoperative intensive care management of the adult. In: Busuttil RW, Klintmalm GB, eds. Transplantation of the liver. Philadelphia:WB Saunders, 1996:551-63.
12. Fishman JA, Rubin RH. Infection in organ-transplant recipients. N Engl J Med, 1998;338(24):1741-51.
13. Singleton JD, Conyers L. Warfarin and azathioprine: an important drug interaction [letter]. Am J Med, 1992;2:217.
14. Hammer GB, Cao S, Boltz MG, Messner A. Post-transplant lymphoproliferative disease may present with severe airway obstruction. Anesthesiology, 1998;89:263-5.
15. Brown MR, Brajtbord D, Johnson DW, et al. Efficacy of oral cyclosporine given prior to liver transplantation. Anesth Analg, 1989;69:773-5.
16. Gelb AW, Freeman D, Robertson KM, et al. Isoflurane alters the kinetics of oral cyclosporine. Anesth Analg, 1991;72:801-4.
17. Csete M, Sipher MJ. Management of the transplant patient for nontransplant procedures. Adv Anesth, 1994;11:407-31.
18. Pertek JP, Chaoui K, Junke E, et al. Effects of propofol on blood concentration of cyclosporine. Ann Fr Anesth Reanim, 1996;15: 589-94.
19. Hammouda GE, Yahya R, Atallah MM. Plasma bupivacaine concentrations following epidural administration in kidney transplant recipients. Reg Anesth, 1996;21:308-11.
20. Klintmalm GBG, Husberg BS, Starzl TE. The organ transplanted patient: immunological concepts and immunosuppression. In: Makowka L, (ed). The Handbook of Transplantation Management. Austin, TX: Landes, 1995:72-108.
21. Bromberg JS, Alfrey EJ, Barker CF, et al. Adrenal suppression and steroid supplementation in renal transplant recipients. Transplantation, 1991;51:385-90.
22. Hanna MH, D'Costa F, Peat SJ, et al. Morphine-6-glucuronide disposition in renal impairment. Br J Anaesth, 1993;70:511-4.

23. Killenberg PG, Cotton PK. Drug interactions with commonly used immunosuppressive agents. In: Killenberg PG, Clavien P-A, eds. Medical Care of the Liver Transplant Patient. Malden, MA: Blackwell Science, 1997:341-58.
24. Wilson W, Taubert KA, Gewitz M, Lockhart PB, Baddour LM, Levison M, et al. Prevention of infective endocarditis: guidelines from the American Heart Association: a guideline from the American Heart Association Rheumatic Fever, Endocarditis, and Kawasaki Disease Committee, Council on Cardiovascular Disease in the Young, and the Council on Clinical Cardiology, Council on Cardiovascular Surgery and Anesthesia, and the Quality of Care and Outcomes Research Interdisciplinary Working Group [published erratum appears in Circulation. 2007;116:e376-7]. Circulation, 2007;116:1736-54.
25. Wijdicks EF. Neurotoxicity of immunosuppressive drugs. Liver Transpl, 2001;7(11):937-42.
26. Parikh BK, Shah VR, Bhosale GP, Praveen CS. Anesthesia for parturient with renal transplantation. Transplantation India, 2005; 4(2):14-18.
27. McCarthy PM. Immediate postoperative care after thoracic organ transplantation. In: Shumway SJ, Shumway NE, eds. Thoracic transplantation. Oxford: Blackwell Science, 1995;205-18.
28. Berg UB, Bohlin AB. Renal function following kidney transplantation in children treated with cyclosporine. Pediatr Nephrol, 1992;6:339-44.
29. Fischer T, Neumayer HH, Fischer R, Barenbrock M, Schobel HP, Lattrell BC, et al. Effect of pregnancy on long-term kidney function in renal transplant recipients treated with cyclosporine and with azathioprine. Am J Transplant, 2005;5:2732-9.
30. Vennarecci G, Pisani F, Tisone G, et al. Kidney transplantation and pregnancy. Transplant Proc, 1997;29:2797-8.
31. Bayle F, Favier M, Ayoubi JM, et al. Pregnancy outcome in kidney allograft recipients. Transplant Proc, 1997;29:2458.
32. Esplin MS, Branch DW. Immunosuppressive drugs and pregnancy. Obstet Gynecol Clin North Am, 1997;24:601-16.
33. Little BB. Immunosuppressant therapy during gestation. Semin Perinatol, 1997;21:143-8.
34. Sharpe MD, Gelb AW. Anaesthetic considerations for the previously transplanted patient. Anesth Clin N Am, 1994;12:827-43.
35. Berden JH, Hoitsma AJ, Merx JL, et al. Severe central nervous system toxicity associated with cyclosporine. Lancet, 1985;1:219-20.
36. Gramstad L, Gjerlow JA, Hysing ES, Rugstad HE. Interaction of cyclosporine and its solvent, cremophor, with atracurium and vecuronium: studies in the cat. Br J Anaesth, 1986;58:1149-55.
37. Mueller EA, Kovarik JM, Koelle EU, et al. Pharmacokinetics of cyclosporine and multiple dose diclofenac during co-administration. J Clin Pharmacol, 1993;33:936-43.
38. Henderson JM, Millikan WJ, Hooks M, et al. Increased galactose clearance after liver transplantation: a measure of increased blood flow through the denervated liver? Hepatology, 1989;10:288-91.
39. Tisone G, Gunson BK, Buckels JA, Mc Master P. Raised hematocrit: a contributing factor to hepatic artery thrombosis following liver transplantation. Transplantation, 1988;46:162-3.
40. Gelb AW, Sharpe MD. Organ transplantation: anesthetic considerations for the previously transplanted patient. In: Benumof JL, (ed). Anesthesiology Clinics of North America. Philadelphia: WB Saunders, 1994;827-43.
41. Takao M, Higenbottam TW. Lung transplantation. In: Bone RC, (ed). Pulmonary and critical care medicine. Update 1. St. Louis: Mosby-Year Book, 1994;1-12.
42. Faberowski LW, Mahla ME, Gravenstein N. Spinal anesthesia for nonpulmonary surgery in a lung transplant recipient. J Neurosurg Anesthesiol, 1999;11:46-8.
43. Barrou BM, Gruessner AC, Sutherland DE, Gruessner RW. Pregnancy after pancreas transplantation in the cyclosporine era: report from the International Pancreas Transplant Registry. Transplantation, 1998;65:524-7.
44. Sutherland DER, Gruessner R, Gillingham K, et al. A single institution's experience with solitary pancreatic transplantation: a multivariate analysis of factors leading to improved outcome. Clin Transplant, 1991;141-2.
45. Case RM, Charlton M, Smith PA, et al. Biology of normal and cancerous pancreatic exocrine cells. Amsterdam: Elsevier, 1980;41-54.
46. Furukawa H, Reyes J, Abu-Elmagd K, et al. Intestinal transplantation at the University of Pittsburgh: six years experience. Transplant Proc, 1997;29:688-9.
47. Coscia LA, Constantinescu S, Moritz MJ, Frank AM, Ramirez CB, Doria C, et al. Report from the National Transplantation Pregnancy Registry (NTPR): outcomes of pregnancy after transplantation. Clin Transpl, 2008;89-105.

12 CHAPTER Anesthesia for Bone Marrow (Stem Cell) Transplantation

Naresh Dua

INTRODUCTION

Stem cell or bone marrow transplantations are a type of intervention strategies that introduce new cells into damaged tissue in order to treat disease or injury. Many medical researchers believe that stem cell treatment has the potential to change the face of human disease and alleviate suffering.[1] The ability of stem cells to self-renew and give rise to subsequent generations with variable degrees of differentiation capacities, offers significant potential for generation of tissues that can potentially replace diseased and damaged areas in the body, with minimal risk of rejection and side effects.[2] Medical researchers anticipate that adult and embryonic stem cells transplantation also called hematopoietic cell transplant will soon be able to treat cancer, Type 1 diabetes mellitus, Parkinson's disease, Huntington's disease, celiac disease, cardiac failure, muscle damage, neurological disorders and many others.[3]

Bone marrow is the soft spongy area in the center of some of the larger bones of the body. The bone marrow produces all the different cells that constitute blood; such as red blood cells, white blood cells and platelets. All of them develop from a type of precursor cell found in the bone marrow, called a hematopoietic stem cell (Fig. 12.1). The body at any given moment is able to direct hematopoietic stem cells to develop into the required blood components. This is a very active process. The bone marrow produces millions of different cells every hour. Most of the stem cells stay in the marrow until they are transformed into the various blood components, which are than released into the bloodstream. A small number of stem cells can be found in the circulating blood.[4] Some of the most effective treatments for cancer, such as chemotherapy and radiation, are toxic to the bone marrow. In general, the higher the dose, the more toxic are the effects on the bone marrow.

Patients have usually received very high doses of chemotherapy or radiation therapy, which kills cancer cells and destroys all the normal cells developing in the bone marrow, including the critical stem cells. After the chemo or radiotherapy the patients require a healthy supply of stem cells to be reintroduced, or transplanted. These transplanted stem cells then reestablish the blood cell production process in the bone marrow.

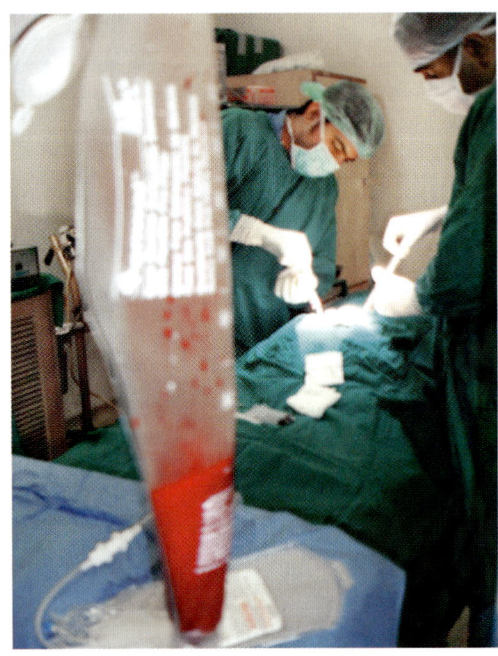

Fig. 12.1: Bone marrow transplantation (BMT)

The cells that are to be transplanted can be taken from the bone marrow (called a 'bone marrow transplant (BMT)'), from the bloodstream (called a 'peripheral blood stem cell transplant'), or occasionally from blood obtained from the umbilical cord at the time of birth of a normal newborn (called an 'umbilical cord stem cell transplant').

TYPES OF BONE MARROW TRANSPLANTATION

There are two main types of bone marrow transplantation: autologous and allogeneic.

Autologous Transplant

In autologous transplantation, patient's hematopoietic stem cells are removed before the high dose chemotherapy or radiation is given and are then frozen for storage and later use. After patient's chemotherapy or radiation is complete, the harvested cells are thawed and returned to the patient.[5]

Allogeneic Transplant

In allogeneic transplantation, the hematopoietic stem cells come from a donor, ideally a brother or sister with a similar genetic makeup. If the patient does not have a suitably matched sibling, an unrelated person with a similar genetic makeup may be used.

Non-myeloablative Transplant

A non-myeloablative transplant, sometimes referred to as a "mini" or reduced intensity transplant, allows patient to have less intensive chemotherapy before transplantation with allogeneic hematopoietic stem cells. This approach may be recommended if the patient cannot undergo standard bone marrow transplantation because of patient's age or other illnesses.

The physician determines whether allogeneic or autologous transplantation is indicated, based on several factors including the type of cancer, patient's age and overall health, and the availability of a suitable donor. As a general rule, autologous transplantation is associated with fewer serious side effects, since the patient receives cells from his/her own body. However, an autologous transplant may be less effective than an allogeneic transplant in treating certain kinds of cancer.

In an allogeneic transplant, the donor's immune system, which is generated from hematopoietic stem cells, recognizes donor cells, including the tumor cells, as foreign and rejects them. This beneficial reaction is called the *graft versus tumor* effect. In many cancers, the immune response caused by the transplanted cells improves the overall effectiveness of the treatment. This immune response helps to kill any residual cancer cells remaining in patient's body.

Indications

Bone marrow transplantation is indicated in various types of cancer and leukemias, aplastic anemias, peripheral vascular disease, Type I diabetes mellitus (DM), Parkinson's disease, Huntington's disease, celiac disease, cardiac failure, muscle damage, neurological disorders and many others.

Cancer

The development of gene therapy strategies for treatment of intra-cranial tumors offers much promise, and has shown to be successful in the treatment of some dogs;[6] although research in this area is still at an early stage. Using conventional techniques, brain cancer is difficult to treat because it spreads so rapidly. Researchers at the Harvard Medical School transplanted human neural stem cells into the brain of rodents who had intracranial tumors. Within days, the cells migrated into the cancerous area and produced cytosine deaminase, an enzyme that converts a non-toxic pro-drug into a chemotheraputic agent. As a result, the injected substance was able to reduce the tumor mass by 81 percent. The stem cells neither differentiated nor turned tumorigenic.[7]

Brain Damage

Stroke and traumatic brain injury lead to cell death, characterized by loss of neurons and oligodendrocytes within the brain. Healthy adult brains contain neural stem cells which divide to maintain general stem cell numbers, or become progenitor cells. In healthy adult animals, progenitor cells migrate within the brain and function primarily to maintain neuron population for olfaction (the sense of smell). Stem cells may also be used to treat brain degeneration, such as in Parkinson's and Alzheimer's disease.[8,9]

Heart Damage

Several clinical trials targeting heart disease have shown that adult stem cell therapy is safe, effective, and equally efficient in treating old and recent infarcts.[10] Adult stem cell therapy for treating heart disease was commercially available in at least five continents at the last count (2007).

Possible mechanisms of recovery include:[6]

- Generation of heart muscle cells
- Stimulation of growth of new blood vessels to repopulate damaged heart tissue
- Secretion of growth factors
- Assistance via some other mechanism—it may be possible to have adult bone marrow cells differentiate into heart muscle cells.

Diabetes

Diabetic patients lose the function of insulin-producing beta cells within the pancreas. Human embryonic stem cells may be grown in cell culture and stimulated to form insulin-producing cells that can be transplanted into the patient.

However, clinical success is highly dependent on factors that transplanted cells should[8]

- Proliferate
- Differentiate in a site-specific manner
- Survive in the recipient (prevention of transplant rejection)
- Integrate within the targeted tissue
- Integrate into the host circuitry and restore function.

Wound Healing

In an adult, wounded tissue is most often replaced by scar tissue, which is characterized in the skin by disorganized collagen structure, loss of hair follicles and irregular vascular structure. Stem cells can also be used to stimulate the growth of human tissues.

Baldness

Hair follicles also contain stem cells, and some researchers predict research on these follicle stem cells may lead to successes in treating baldness through an activation of the stem cells progenitor cells. This treatment is expected to work by activating the already existing stem cells on the scalp.

Teeth Formation

In theory, stem cells taken from the patient could be coaxed in the laboratory into turning into a tooth bud which, when implanted in the gums, will give rise to a new tooth, and would be expected to grow within two months. It will fuse with the jawbone and release chemicals that encourage nerves and blood vessels to connect with it. The process is similar to what happens when humans grow their original adult teeth. Many challenges remain, however, before stem cells could be a choice for the replacement of missing teeth in the future.[11]

Preanesthetic Evaluation for BMT/Stem Cell Transfusion

a. **Donor selection:** There are many possible choices for a hematopoietic stem cell donor. These are described below.

   Matched donor—To help minimize the problems that can be caused by the expected immune response, a donor who has similar genetic makeup as the patient is preferred so that the patient's cells seem "less foreign" to the transplanted donor cells. Siblings (i.e. brothers and sisters who share the same parents as the patient) are typically the only members of patient's family that are tested for being a donor because they have a one in four chance of sharing genetic characteristics with the patient; these characteristics are critical for the patient's body to accept the graft. In general, parents and relatives are not suitable donors since they do not share the same parents, and therefore do not have the same genetic material.

   An exception is called a haploidentical transplant, which may be considered under certain circumstances.

   Matched unrelated donor—If no siblings are available, or if testing the blood of the siblings does not reveal a match, a matched unrelated donor may be used. The search for an appropriate donor can be accomplished using transplant registries throughout the world.

   Mismatched related or unrelated donor—Some patients are offered treatment with cells from a partially matched family member (called mismatched related donor). The hematopoietic stem cell product may be specially prepared to minimize the immune response in the patient. Another alternative is to use umbilical cord blood, collected from a healthy newborn infant at the time of delivery; this blood is a rich source of hematopoietic stem cells.

b. **Physical examination:** Physical examination of the donor must be thoroughly done along with history of previous surgeries, chemotherapy and radiotherapy in context to diagnosis. The patient may already have a line in situ for chemotherapy such as chemoport or Hickmann's line. In patients who have received radiotherapy in oropharyngeal cancers, detailed airway examination for a difficult airway should be done. The pediatric age group donor should be treated with tender care as they are already undergoing mental stress due to their sibling's disease and financial burden on family. Thorough preoperative psychosocial analysis and support should be given to these patients. Preoperative fasting should strictly be done according to operative time.

c. **Biochemical investigations:** The American Society of Anaesthesiologists (ASA) I donors should have basic investigations before undergoing general or regional anesthesia which include complete blood count (CBC) and blood coagulation profile along with required investigations as according to their age, while the autologous BMT donor patients must have detailed workup with all investigations such as complete blood count, liver function tests, renal function tests, blood coagulation profile, serum ferritin, and serum electrolytes along with trace metals (Mg^{++}, $PO4^{++}$) estimations.

Anesthetic Considerations

Overnight fasting of approximately 6 hours is recommended for ASA I adult donors. Pediatric age group donors require fasting of 4 hours for semi solids and two hours for clear fluids.

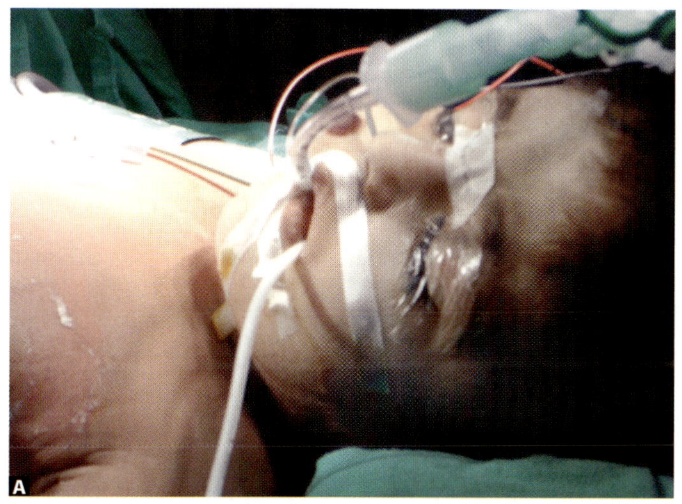
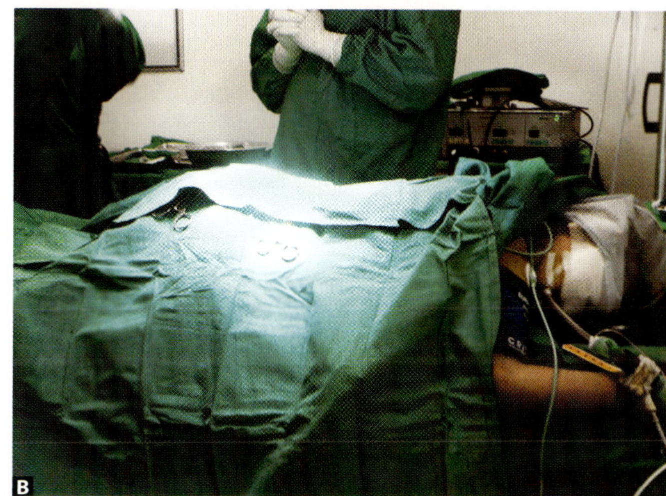

Fig. 12.2A and B BMT donor under general anesthesia

Standard monitors are applied. Induction is achieved with oxygen and sevoflurane followed by intravenous cannulation. Maintenance of general anesthesia should be preferably done with O_2, air and inhalation anesthetic agents along with opioids and muscle relaxants (Fig. 12.2A and B). Since there is a controversial role of N_2O in depressing the bone marrow, it is avoided. Patients should receive an antiemetic drug (ondansetron, granisetron) for postoperative nausea and vomiting. Perioperative analgesia should be adequate to prevent sympathetic stimulation leading to tachycardia. A caudal epidural analgesia may be given to the child preoperatively to minimize the anesthetic drug requirements. As per an adult donor patient and hematologist request, either regional or general anaesthesia may be employed. Before induction, pre-instituted central venous cannulae (Hickman's line, chemoport, intravenous jugular line, femoral line) should be checked for forward and backward flow.

For regional anesthesia, preoperative coagulation profile must be within normal range. Local anesthetic instillation, intravenous paracetamol and diclofenac must be given for good postoperative pain relief.

Postoperative Care

In the post-anesthesia care unit (PACU), the patient should be observed for bleeding from puncture site, postoperative nausea and vomiting, pain and respiratory depression.

Postoperative Complications and its Management

The postoperative care of patients who undergo BMT, either under regional or general anesthesia, remains the same as any other surgical patient.

The patients have to be observed in PACU till the discharge criteria are met.

Common problems noted are:

1. **Pain** at the bone marrow aspiration puncture sites. Multimodal analgesia with short acting opioids, NSAIDs and local anesthetic infiltration (2% xylocaine or 0.125%–0.25% bupivacaine) should be given.
2. **Nausea and vomiting:** Preoperative use of $5HT_3$ receptor antagonists with steroids can prevent postoperative nausea and vomiting.
3. **Respiratory depression/hypoxemia:** The constitutionally weak allergenic BMT patients who already have received chemotherapy or radiotherapy may have episodes of desaturation after reversal of general anesthesia. Supportive management with oxygen through ventimask or venturi mask should be provided.
4. **Bleeding from donor bone marrow site:** Occlusive pressure bandage is often required to prevent bleeding for puncture sites at iliac crest.

CLINICAL PEARLS

- Stem cell or bone marrow transplantations are a type of intervention strategies that introduce new cells into damaged tissue in order to treat disease or injury.
- The bone marrow produces all the different cells that constitute blood; such as red blood cells, white blood cells and platelets. A small number of stem cells can be found in the circulating blood.
- Preoperative bone marrow patients have usually received very high doses of chemotherapy or radiation therapy, which

kills cancer cells and destroys all the normal cells developing in the bone marrow, including the critical stem cells.

- There are two main types of bone marrow transplantation: autologous and allogeneic.
- Bone marrow transplantation is indicated in various types of cancer and leukemias, aplastic anemias, peripheral vascular disease, Type I diabetes mellitus (DM), Parkinson's disease, Huntington's disease, celiac disease, cardiac failure, muscle damage, neurological disorders and many others.
- There are many possible choices for a hematopoietic stem cell donor: matched, matched unrelated and mismatched related or unrelated.

REFERENCES

1. Lindvall O, Kokaia Z. Stem cells for the treatment of neurological disorders. Nature, 2006;441:1094-6.
2. Weissman IL. Stem cells: units of development, units of regeneration, and units in evolution. Cell, 2000;100:157-68.
3. Singec I, Jandial R, Crain A, Nikkhah G, Snyder EY. The leading edge of stem cell therapeutics. Annu Rev Med, 2007;58:313-28.
4. Léger CS, Nevill TJ. Hematopoietic stem cell transplantation: a primer for the primary care physician. CMAJ, 2004;170:1569.
5. Socié G, Mary JY, Esperou H, et al. Health and functional status of adult recipients 1 year after allogeneic haematopoietic stem cell transplantation. Br J Haematol, 2001;113:194.
6. LeCouteur RA. Current concepts in the diagnosis and treatment of brain tumours in dogs and cats. J Small Animal Pract, 2008;40: 411-416.
7. Stem Cells Tapped to Replenish Organs thescientist.com, Nov 2000. By Douglas Steinberg.
8. Cell Basics: What are the potential uses of human stem cells and the obstacles that must be overcome before these potential uses will be realized?. In Stem Cell Information World Wide Website. Bethesda, MD: National Institutes of Health, US Department of Health and Human Services, 2009.
9. http://www.sciencedaily.com/releases/2009/07/090720190726.htm
10. Strauer BE, Schannwell CM, Brehm M. "Therapeutic potentials of stem cells in cardiac diseases". Minerva Cardioangiol, 2009;57: 249-67.
11. Yen AH, Sharpe PT. "Stem cells and tooth tissue engineering". Cell Tissue Res, 2008;331:359-72.

13 CHAPTER

Corneal Transplantation

Savitar Malhotra

INTRODUCTION

Keratoplasty is the replacement of diseased cornea by a homologous tissue graft. Cornea was the first solid tissue that was successfully transplanted in 1886 by von Hippel. Initially, lamellar keratoplasty was the procedure of choice but with improvements in techniques and the realization of the importance of the endothelium, penetrating keratoplasty has become more common.[1] Thus, in this chapter a corneal transplant would refer mainly to *Penetrating Keratoplasty*.

INDICATIONS FOR PENETRATING KERATOPLASTY (TABLE 13.1)

The indications may be broadly divided into four categories. All indications fall under one or more of these categories.

1. Gross distortion of corneal surface from spherical to irregular
2. Irregularity of corneal surface
3. Increased thickness of the stroma
4. Opacity of the stroma.

The indications for corneal transplant may also be classified as *tectonic* (to improve corneal integrity) and *visual* (to restore the vision).[1]

Table 13.1: Common indications for penetrating keratoplasty

- Keratoconus
- Ectasias/thinnings
- Pseudophakic corneal edema
- Fuchs endothelial dystrophy and primary endotheliopathies
- Noninfectious ulcerative keratitis
- Mechanical and chemical injuries
- Corneal degenerations
- Aphakic corneal edema
- Stromal corneal dystrophies
- Congenital opacity
- Viral/postviral keratitis
- Microbial/postmicrobial keratitis

Eye Banking

For a successful penetrating keratoplasty, endothelial viability is paramount.[1] The donor corneoscleral button can be preserved in different media and by different methods (Figs 13.1 and 13.2). Some of the commonly used methods are:

- Storage in tissue media
  - McCarey-Kaufman tissue transport medium: It contains dextran, antibiotics, chondroitin sulfate and antioxidants. The tissue can be stored upto 4 days at 4°C in this medium.[2]
  - Optisol GS: It contains vitamins, amino acids, antioxidants and ATP precursors. The tissue can be safely stored for upto 2 weeks in this solution.
- Cryopreservation: It involves freezing the whole globe at –70 to –80°C. It requires complicated freezing and thawing techniques, but has the advantage of enabling storage for more than 1 year.
- Organ culture: Here the corneal tissue is maintained at 34°C and allows for active cellular metabolism. Both the procedure and equipment is complex and microbial contamination is also higher. The tissue can be preserved for over a month in organ culture.

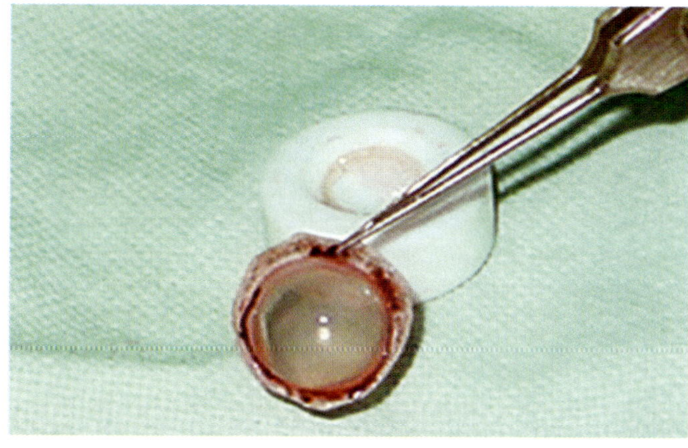

Fig. 13.1: Donor cornea

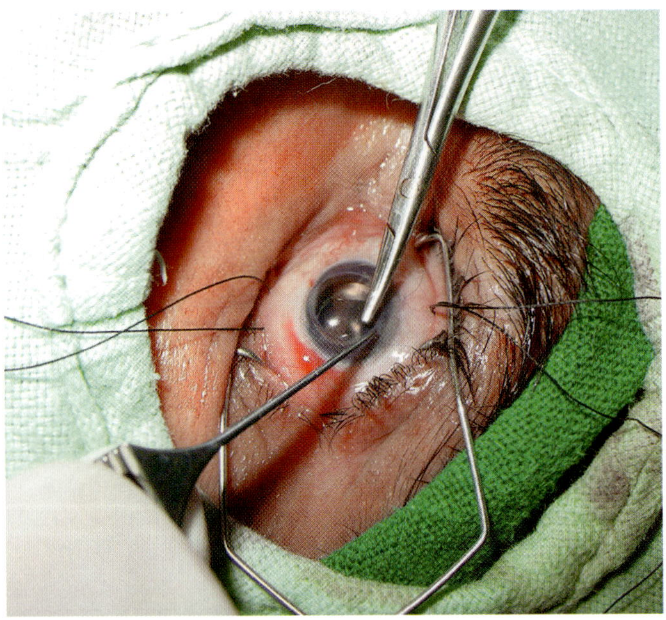

Fig. 13.2: Donor cornea sutured in place postoperatively

Donor Selection

The outcome of a corneal transplant depends to a large extent on donor selection. Proper donor selection is important both for patient safety as well for successful grafting.

Contraindications for donor cornea use:

Criteria by Eye Bank Association of America (EBAA)[3]

- Death of unknown cause
- Unknown CNS disease or certain infectious diseases of the CNS (e.g. Subacute sclerosing panencephalitis, creutzfeldt-Jakob disease, progressive multifocal leukoencephalopathy, Reye syndrome, congenital rubella, rabies, active viral encephalitis, encephalitis of unknown origin).
- HIV infection, syphilis, or active viral hepatitis
- Active septicemia
- Bacterial or fungal endocarditis
- Leukemias, or active disseminated lymphomas
- Ocular or intraocular inflammation (iritis, scleritis, conjunctivitis, viritis, retinitis, choroiditis)
- Hepatitis B, Hepatitis C, or HIV infection
- Malignant anterior segment tumors, adenocarcinoma eye (primary or metastatic) and retinoblastoma
- Prior refractive corneal surgery.
- Congenital or acquired eye disorders: any central donor corneal scar or pterygia involving the central 8 mm clear zone (optical area of the donor button), keratoconus, keratoglobus, fuchs dystrophy.

Preoperative Evaluation

A corneal transplant surgery can be performed on an ambulatory basis. Nevertheless, a complete ophthalmic and medical examination of the patient is of prime importance. The patients are usually on a 'waiting list' for a prospective donor, but it is advisable to repeat the eye and physical examination prior to surgery so that any recent changes in the eye or physical status may not preclude safe conduct of the surgery.

A detailed pre-anesthesia evaluation should be aimed to determine fitness of the patient. Any comorbid illness should be recognized and controlled prior to the procedure. Cardiac, pulmonary, and endocrinological disease may require specific anesthesia precautions. The patient's systemic medications may influence blood coagulation, wound healing, and tear production. Medications, to which there is a prior history of allergy, should be carefully avoided. Preoperative investigations are usually done according to any associated comorbidity. In a clinically fit patient no investigations may be needed.

A complete eye examination is done by the surgeon. Surface problems like dry eye, trichiasis, exposure blepharitis, and rosacea must be recognized and treated prior to penetrating keratoplasty. Issues that could compromise the final vision should be taken care of, e.g. neurologic factors (optic nerve damage), intraocular factors (media opacity, uncontrolled glaucoma, amblyopia, macular abnormalities, retinal disease, and ocular inflammation).

Factors associated with poor prognosis are deep corneal vascularization, ocular surface disease, active anterior segment inflammation, peripheral corneal thinning, previous graft failures, poor compliance, and increased intraocular pressure.

A detailed social history helps in predicting the compliance of the patient with the treatment regimen and whether the patient will report immediately on any untoward happening.

Anesthesia Management

Most of the graft procedures can be performed under an orbital regional anesthesia. General anesthesia may be used if the patient is aphakic, or if the vitreous may be exposed or involved during the procedure. Other indications for general anesthesia are pediatric patients, an uncooperative patient, and patients with movement disorders, etc.

Investigations Required

Routine tests are not indicated for patients undergoing keratoplasty under a regional block. Tests may be done only when thought necessary in patients with significant comorbidity to improve the general health of the patient rather than the surgical outcome.

Fasting Requirement

As for other eye surgeries done under a regional block, fasting of the patient is not essential. But if for some reason, the procedure is planned under general anesthesia, preoperative fasting for at least six hours for solids is recommended.[4]

Premedication

Appropriate premedication can help in allaying any anxiety that the patient may have towards the procedure. The need of a premedication should be assessed during the preoperative visit or evaluation. Premedication is useful before both general and regional anesthesia.

Preparation

Prior to giving an ophthalmic block or general anesthesia, monitors for blood pressure, pulse oximetry and electrocardiogram should be placed. Vitals of the patient should be carefully noted and any abnormal value should be carefully managed. The surgeon or the anesthesiologist giving the block should note the *relation of the eye in the orbit*. This helps to decide the angle of the block needle during the block and to avoid penetrating the sclera.[5]

Sedation Analgesia for Orbital Regional Anesthesia

An ophthalmic block is a painful procedure. Use of sedation and analgesia decreases anxiety and pain associated with the block and thus makes the experience less traumatic for the patient.[6] Sedatives and analgesics can be chosen from different classes of agents including benzodiazepines, opioids, intravenous induction agents, and alpha-2 agonists. Some practitioners prefer deep sedation or brief general anesthesia to coincide with the placement of the block. This provides a painless procedure to the patient, but it is not without risks. Some of the possible complications are apnea, loss of airway and hypoxia, vomiting, and aspiration.[5]

Some practitioners are of the view that sedation should be just adequate to keep the patient calm and cooperative so that he/she can report the pain of injection. More than usual pain may suggest and warn against injection into an inappropriate location like a nerve, extraocular muscle, subperiosteal or the globe.

Two types of blocks are commonly used

- Retrobulbar (intraconal)
- Peribulbar (extraconal)

Retrobulbar (intraconal): A neutral gaze is maintained with the patient in the supine position. A wheal is made with a local anesthetic solution (e.g. lignocaine 0.5%) at the inferotemporal corner of the orbit. Through this wheal a 25G, 31mm needle is inserted tangentially to the globe so that its tip lies in a space behind the globe. A volume of 4–5 mL is injected in this space.

Peribulbar (extraconal): The patient position and the puncture site is the same as in the retrobulbar block. In this block, instead of going tangentially behind the globe, the needle is inserted parallel to it, so that the tip stays outside the cone. A volume of 6–8 mL is required for a successful block.

Complications associated with anesthesia for keratoplasty.

- Complications of monitored anesthesia care
  - Postoperative nausea vomiting
  - Oversedation or undersedation
  - Inadvertent local anesthetic injection.
- Complications of general anesthesia
  - Airway and respiratory complications
  - Awareness
  - Delayed awakening
  - Inadequate muscle relaxation which may result in coughing or movement leading to retinal detachment, corneal laceration, lens subluxation or expulsion of intraocular contents. This can be prevented by monitoring the neuromuscular block and depth of anesthesia.
- Complications of anesthesia and surgery
  - Oculocardiac reflex
  - Corneal abrasions of the nonoperative eye.

CLINICAL PEARLS

- Keratoplasty is now a common surgical procedure.
- Proper donor selection is important.
- Meticulous perioperative care results in a successful outcome.

REFERENCES

1. S Arthur Boruchoff, John P Frangie. Penetrating keratoplasty. In: Albert, Jakobiec Azar Gragoudas, eds. Principles and Practice of Ophthalmology. WB Saunders Company; 2000. p 1027-1039.
2. H Kaz Soong. In: George L Spaeth, editor. Ophthalmic Surgery-Principles and Practice. WB Saunders; 2003. p 139-160.
3. O'Day DM. Donor selection. In: Brightbill FS, (ed). Corneal surgery, theory, technique and tissue, St Louis: Mosby- Year Book; 1993. p 549-562.
4. Steeds C, Mather SJ. Fasting regimens for regional ophthalmic anaesthesia. A survey of members of the British Ophthalmic Anaesthesia Society. Anaesthesia, 2001;56:638-42.
5. Fanning GL. Orbital Regional Anesthesia. Ophthalmol Clin N Am, 2006;19:221-32.
6. Woo JH, Au Eong KG, Kumar CM. Conscious sedation during ophthalmic surgery during local anesthesia. Minerva Anestesiol, 2009;75:211-9.

14 CHAPTER

Perioperative Management of Heart Transplantation

Arun Maheshwari, Monish S Raut

INTRODUCTION

Cardiac transplantation has become the treatment of choice for many symptomatic cardiac failure patients, despite maximal medical management. Post cardiac transplantation, survival has improved due to advances in immunosuppressive and anti-infective treatment (Fig. 14.1).

Though the number of potential recipients is increasing, the number of heart donors available is not able to meet the demand. Worldwide upto approximately 50,000 patients are waiting for cardiac transplantation, but only 5,000 transplantations are occurring annually.[1] In India, the first heart transplantation was done on 3rd August 1994 at All India Institute of Medical Sciences, but only 104 heart transplantations have been done so far in the country till 2011 (data collected from various hospitals).

Up to 10% of patients with cardiac failure have advanced heart disease, this in itself is a risk factor for high mortality and morbidity.[2] In the most advanced phase of cardiac failure, cardiac transplantation has been the only means of improving the quality of life and survival in these patients. With the advances in immunosuppression therapy, 1-year survival after cardiac transplantation reaches 90%, and 50% of patients surviving >11 years.[3] Advanced knowledge of immunological mechanisms, immunosuppressive therapies and the advent of endomyocardial biopsy, have all contributed to improved survival of heart transplantation surgeries (Fig. 14.2).[4-6] Heart transplantation is now an established treatment for a variety of end-stage cardiac diseases.

In 1989, the US United Network of Organ Sharing (UNOS) introduced a high priority UNOS status 1 listing, to give preference to candidates who are the least likely to survive without transplantation. This was reclassified as UNOS status 1A and 1B in 1999, with the intention of making shorter the waiting time and betterment in survival in waiting list candidates.[7,8] The majority of these candidates are extremely ill sick cardiac failure patients who are dependent on inotropes or mechanical circulatory support (MCS) devices as a bridge to transplantation (BTT).[9]

Pathophysiology of Heart Failure

Better knowledge of the pathophysiology of failing heart has influenced the pharmacological management of heart failure (Table 14.1). Rather than focusing on inotropic agents to improve systolic function, the main aim of treatment is now breaking the pathways of neurohormonal and immunologic systems which are triggered in heart failure.[12,13]

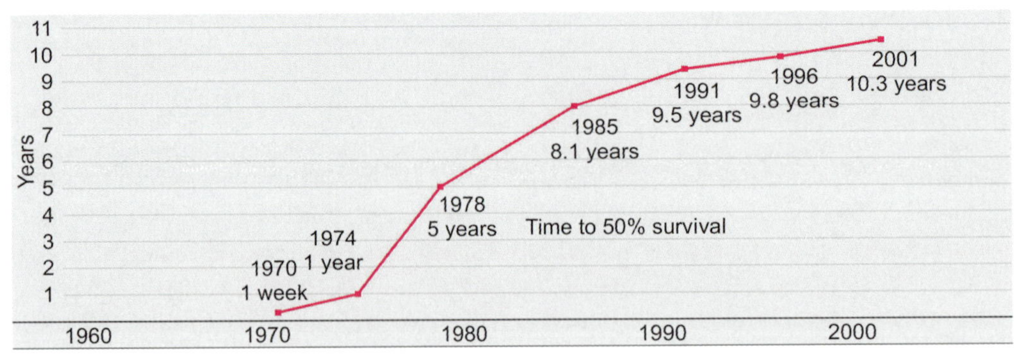

Fig. 14.1: History of heart transplantation associated with progressive improvement in survival. (Adapted from J Am Coll Cardiol 2008;52: 587–98.)

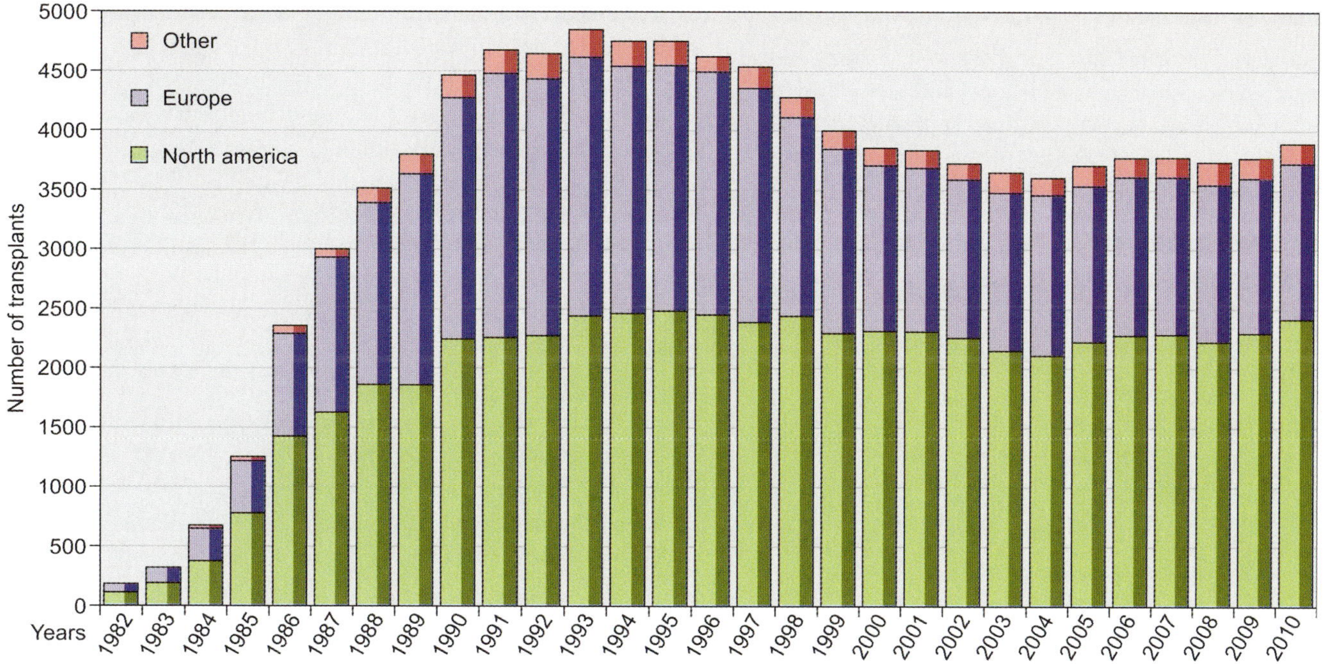

Fig. 14.2: Cardiac transplantations performed worldwide. (From the registry of the International Society of Heart and Lung Transplantation: J Heart Lung Transplant. Oct 2011)

Table 14.1: Pathophysiology of failing failure

- Failure of the left ventricle leads to an increase in the left ventricular end-diastolic volume and pressure
- Enhancement of resting myocardial fiber length for optimising effective contraction
- Stroke volume is maintained at the expense of increasing the left atrial pressure, increased diastolic pressure and increased pulmonary venous congestion
- CO is maintained by elevation in catecholamines and renin production

The main effect of this triggering is the increase in vasoconstriction.[10,11] Chronically elevated circulating catecholamines lead to down-regulation of expression and function of β-adrenoceptor and α_2-adrenergic receptors.[13] As a result, the responsiveness to β-adrenergic receptor agonists is decreased and myocardial catecholamines are depleted.[14,15] There is profound evidence that the immune system plays a role in the progression of heart failure. Several cytokines, namely plasma tumor necrosis factor-α, soluble tumor necrosis factor-receptor II, and interleukins-1, -2 and -6, are elevated in patients with heart failure.[10,18] Immunomodulatory therapy can be a promising tool in the management of such patients.[19]

A few months of maximal medical therapy is given to assess the therapeutic response. If no reversible causes are present and the presence of class III/IV symptoms persist despite optimal therapy, than the transplant evaluation process begins. However, if the patient is in cardiogenic shock or on intravenous inotropic agents and which cannot be reduced because of hypotension, end-organ dysfunction, or symptoms, then the options for this patient are limited to cardiac transplantation, mechanical device support, or palliative care (Fig. 14.3).

BRIDGE TO TRANSPLANTATION (BTT)

The therapeutic focus is on restoration of hemodynamic stability, end-organ perfusion, and symptomatic relief as a bridge to transplantation. The various methods by which this can be done are:

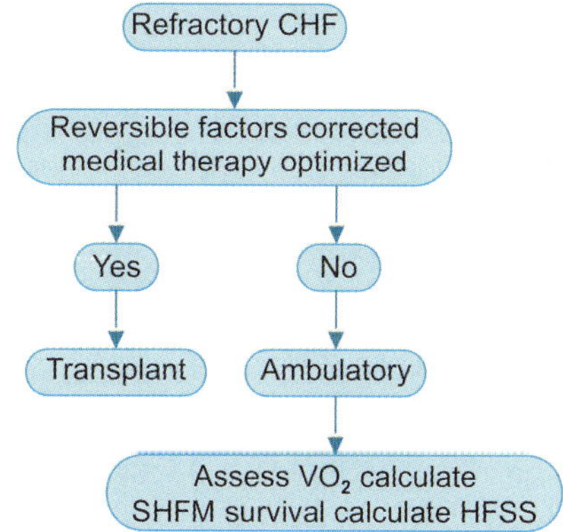

Fig. 14.3: VO_2 oxygen consumption
SHFM Seattle Heart Failure Model; HFSS Heart Failure Survival Score

Medical Management

The aims of treatment are to decrease circulating catecholamines, reduce ventricular afterload, and relieve pulmonary venous congestion. As survival has improved with medical therapy even for patients with progressive heart failure, the role of cardiac transplantation has been reassessed.[9]

Surgical Management

Though heart transplantation has become the established surgical treatment for heart failure patients, but the scarcity of donor hearts has made investigators think of alternative surgical strategies.

I. Coronary revascularization
II. Repair of regurgitant valves
III. Dynamic cardiomyoplasty
IV. Partial left ventriculectomy
V. Resection of akinetic anterior wall

INDICATIONS FOR HEART TRANSPLANT

The ACC/AHA guidelines state the following as indications for heart transplant (Table 14.2).[20]

CRITERIA FOR HEART TRANSPLANTATION

Though heart transplantation is aimed to improve survival, but evaluation of prognostic factors in cardiac failure patients should be considered during the selection process (Table 14.2). Some important predictors implying poor prognosis are hyponatremia, NYHA class III/IV and low LV systolic function.

Peak VO_2

In general, the peak VO_2 (VO_2 max) appears to give the most objective assessment of functional capacity in patients with HF and may be the best predictor to list an individual patient for cardiac transplantation. The 2002 Task force of the ACC/AHA recommended the use of exercise testing with ventilatory gas analysis for this purpose (Table 14.3)[21] and the 2005 ACC/AHA heart failure guidelines (with 2009 update) include peak VO_2 criteria for cardiac transplantation.[22] Guidelines also include the recommendations for associated comorbidities and their implications for heart transplantation[22] (Tables 14.4 to 14.6).

Peak VO_2 has been the major factor used to guide the selection of heart transplant candidates, but no single variable can stratify the risk profile of the patient optimally. Hence, many risk models have been developed that use factors identified in multivariable survival analysis to establish a risk score for prognosis in these patients.[23-27] These include the **Heart Failure Survival Score (HFSS)** and the **Seattle Heart Failure Model (SHFM).**

These scores are helpful when other predictors are inconclusive to decide listing of patients for heart transplantation.[9]

Table 14.2: Indications of heart transplantation

Absolute indications
- Hemodynamic compromise due to HF
  - Refractory cardiogenic shock
  - Peak VO_2 < 10 mL/kg/min
  - Parenteral inotropic support dependent, to maintain cardiac output and perfusion
- Intractable and recurrent symptomatic ventricular arrhythmia
- Ischemic symptoms limiting daily activities and not amenable to CABG or PCI

Relative indications
- Peak VO_2 of 11 to 14 mL/kg per minute (or 55 percent predicted) and major limitation of the patient's daily activities
- Recurrent fluid imbalance despite on medical management
- Recurrent unstable ischemia not treatable by other interventions

Table 14.3: Recommendations of cardiopulmonary testing for heart transplantation

Class I:
1. A maximal cardiopulmonary exercise (CPX) test is defined as one with a respiratory exchange ratio (RER) >1.05 and achievement of an anerobic threshold on optimal pharmacologic therapy (level of evidence: B)
2. In patients intolerant of a β-blocker, a cutoff for peak VO_2 of ≤14 mL/kg/min should be used to guide listing (level of evidence: B)
3. In the presence of a β-blocker, a cutoff for peak VO_2 of ≤12 mL/kg/min should be used to guide listing (level of evidence: B)

Class IIa:
1. In young patients (<50 years) and women, it is reasonable to consider using alternate standards in conjunction with peak VO_2 to guide listing, including percent of predicted (≤50%) peak VO_2 (level of evidence: B)

Class IIb:
1. In the presence of a sub-maximal CPX test (RER <1.05), use of ventilation equivalent of carbon dioxide (Ve/Vco_2) slope of >35 as a determinant in listing for transplantation may be considered (level of evidence: C)
2. In obese (body mass index [BMI] >30 kg/m^2) patients, adjusting peak VO_2 to lean body mass may be considered. A lean body mass–adjusted peak VO_2 of <19 mL/kg/min can serve as an optimal threshold to guide prognosis (level of evidence: B)

Class III:
1. Listing patients based solely on the criterion of a peak oxygen consumption (VO_2) measurement should not be performed (level of evidence: C)

Table 14.4: Recommendation for co-morbidities (age, obesity and cancer) and their implications for heart transplantation

Class I:

1. Patients should be considered for cardiac transplantation if they are ≤70 years of age (level of evidence: C).
2. Pre-existing neoplasms are diverse and many are treatable with excision, radiotherapy or chemotherapy to induce cure or remission. In these patients needing cardiac transplantation, collaboration with oncology specialists should occur to stratify each patient as to their risk of tumor recurrence. Cardiac transplantation should be considered when tumor recurrence is low based on tumor type, response to therapy and negative metastatic work-up. The specific amount of time to wait to transplant after neoplasm remission will depend on the aforementioned factors and no arbitrary time period for observation should be used (level of evidence: C).

Class II a:

1. Overall, pre-transplant BMI >30 kg/m^2 or percent ideal body weight (PIBW) >140% are associated with poor outcome after cardiac transplantation. For obese patients, it is reasonable to recommend weight loss to achieve a BMI of <30 kg/m^2 or percent BMI of <140% of target before listing for cardiac transplantation (level of evidence: C)

Class II b:

1. Carefully selected patients >70 years of age may be considered for cardiac transplantation. For centers considering these patients, the use of an alternate-type program (i.e. use of older donors) may be pursued (level of evidence: C)

Heart Failure Survival Score

One model that has been validated prospectively is the Heart Failure Survival Score (HFSS).[23] The Heart Failure Survival Score (HFSS) is calculated by taking the absolute value of the sums of the products of each component variable's value and its model coefficient. Survival predictors in HFSS are

1. Serum Na^+ level
2. HR at resting state
3. Peak VO_2
4. LVEF
5. Interventricular conduction delay on ECG
6. MAP
7. CAD

Pulmonary artery occlusion pressure can be considered as the eighth variable in an invasive version of HFSS.

The HFSS classifies patients into low, medium, and high risk categories, based upon a sum of the variables mentioned above multiplied by defined coefficients.

Table 14.5: Recommendations for diabetes, renal dysfunction and peripheral vascular disease

Class II a:

1. Diabetes with end-organ damage other than non-proliferative retinopathy or poor glycemic control (glycosylated hemoglobin [HbA1C] >7.5) despite optimal effort is a relative contraindication for transplant (level of evidence: C).
2. Renal function should be assessed using estimated glomerular filtration rate (eGFR) or creatinine clearance under optimal medical therapy. Evidence of abnormal renal function should prompt further investigation, including renal ultrasonography, estimation for proteinuria, and evaluation for renal arterial disease, to exclude intrinsic renal disease. It is reasonable to consider the presence of irreversible renal dysfunction (eGFR <40 mL/min) as a relative contraindication for heart transplantation alone (level of evidence: C).

Class II b:

1. Clinically severe symptomatic cerebrovascular disease, which is not amenable to re-vascularization, may be considered a contraindication to transplantation. Peripheral vascular disease may be considered as a relative contraindication for transplantation when its presence limits rehabilitation and re-vascularization is not a viable option (level of evidence: C)

Table 14.6: Recommendation for psychosocial evaluation

Class I :

1. Psychosocial assessment should be performed before listing for transplantation. Evaluation should include an assessment of the patient's ability to give informed consent and comply with instruction including drug therapy, as well as assessment of the support systems in place at home or in the community (level of evidence: C).

Class II a:

1. Mental retardation or dementia may be regarded as a relative contraindication to transplantation (level of evidence: C).

Class II b:

1. Poor compliance with drug regimens is a risk factor for graft rejection and mortality. Patients who have demonstrated an inability to comply with drug therapy on multiple occasions should not receive transplantation (level of evidence: C).

The Seattle Heart Failure Model

The Seattle Heart Failure Model has included the impact of newer heart failure therapies on survival, including ICDs and CRT.

CARDIAC TRANSPLANTATION CONTRAINDICATIONS

There has been a gradual relaxation in the conventional cardiac transplantation exclusion criteria as experience with increasingly complex cases has grown. Exclusion criteria include severe, irreversible, end-organ disease and conditions incompatible with immunosuppression (Table 14.7). In particular, evaluation of pulmonary vascular resistance (PVR) and its reversibility is critical in the preoperative evaluation of cardiac transplant candidates, as pulmonary hypertension is a predictor of postoperative right ventricular (RV) failure and mortality.[28]

THE CARDIAC TRANSPLANT DONOR

Most deceased donor organs are recovered from donors who meet criteria for brain death and have ongoing cardiac function. Brain death is irreversible, and the ability to recover organs for transplantation exists only because the technology of the intensive care unit can maintain physiologic homeostasis, including circulation and respiration. Without this support, "brain death" occurs almost simultaneously with "cardiac death."

Table 14.7: Contraindications to HT

Absolute
- Systemic illness with a life expectancy <2 y despite HT, including
  - Active or recent solid organ or blood malignancy within 5 y (eg. leukemia, low-grade neoplasms of the prostate with persistently elevated prostate-specific antigen)
  - AIDS with frequent opportunistic infections
  - Systemic lupus erythematosus, sarcoid, or amyloidosis that has multisystem involvement and is still active
  - Irreversible renal or hepatic dysfunction
  - Significant obstructive pulmonary disease (FEV1 <1 L/min).
- Fixed pulmonary hypertension
  - Pulmonary artery systolic pressure >60 mm Hg
  - Mean transpulmonary gradient >15 mm Hg
  - Pulmonary vascular resistance >6 Wood units

Relative
- Age >72 years
- Morbid obesity (body mass index >35 kg/m2) or cachexia (body mass index <18 kg/m^2)
- S. creatinine >2.5 mg/dL or creatinine clearance <25 mL/min*
- S. bilirubin >2.5 mg/dL, serum transaminases >3X, INR >1.5 off warfarin
- Any active infection (with the exception of device-related infection in VAD recipients)
- Severe pulmonary dysfunction with FEV1 < 40% normal
- Active peptic ulcer disease
- Severe diabetes mellitus with end-organ damage (neuropathy, nephropathy, or retinopathy)
- Severe peripheral vascular or cerebrovascular disease
  Peripheral vascular disease not amenable to surgical or percutaneous therapy
  Symptomatic carotid stenosis
  Ankle brachial index <0.7

Uncorrected abdominal aortic aneurysm >6 cm
- Recent pulmonary infarction within 6 to 8 week
- Irreversible neurological or neuromuscular disorder
- Active mental illness or psychosocial instability
- Heparin-induced thrombocytopenia within 100 days

Donor Selection and Contraindications

The primary factor limiting cardiac transplantation is the shortage of donors. Over the past decade, the median waiting time for cardiac transplantation has increased in all age groups, with approximately 30% of patients dying before cardiac transplantation.[29] Therefore, in an attempt to increase donor numbers, the criteria for cardiac organ donation have been relaxed in recent years with an increased acceptance of older donors with and without evidence of CAD (Table 14. 8).

However, the risk of failed transplantation increases with donor age and the presence of concomitant disease.[30] Absolute and relative contraindications for heart donation are listed in Table 14.9.

Perioperative Management of the Cardiac Transplant Donor

Post transplant cardiac function is directly dependent on donor care before organ harvesting. Thus, the goal of medical management after brain death is to ensure optimal myocardial and end-organ perfusion. The basic management goals are to achieve hemodynamic stability and optimal function of all organs that may be transplanted (Table 14.10).

Organ Harvest Technique

After heparinisation, perfusion sensitive organs—kidney and liver are removed before heart removal. Median sternotomy

Table 14.8: Extended-donor criteria

- Donor age >55 years
- Cocaine use
- Long-term alcohol abuse
- Significant pressor or inotrope requirement (>10 mcg/kg/min. dopamine or dobutamine)
- ECG abnormalities (left ventricular hypertrophy, regional wall abnormality)
- Long-standing diabetes mellitus
- Death by poisoning (carbon monoxide, cyanide)
- Prolonged ischemic time (>4 h)
- Malignant brain tumors
- Single-vessel coronary artery disease
- Undersized organ (mismatch >30%), especially in patients with pulmonary hypertension.

Table 14.9: Contraindications to heart donation

Absolute
- Positive serology for syphilis, HTLV-4, and HIV
- Presence of malignancy with extracranial metastatic potential left ventricular ejection fraction <40%
- Significant valvular abnormality
- Significant coronary artery disease

Relative
- Sepsis
- Hepatitis B surface antigen positive
- Hepatitis C antibody positive
- Repeated need for cardiopulmonary resuscitation
- High-dose inotropic support exceeding 24 hours

Table 14.10: Goals of perioperative management
- Maintenance of optimal tissue and organ perfusion
- Maintenance of fluid and electrolyte balance
- Maintenance of adequate blood gases
- Prevention of secondary infection
- Maintenance of normal temperature

is performed and donor heart is removed en bloc. SVC and IVC ligations are done to allow exsanguinations. Cold crystalloid cardioplegia is administered after aortic cross clamp. The aorta and pulmonary arteries are transected but keeping the native donor arterial segments as long as possible. Pulmonary veins are individually divided finally after lifting the donor organ out of the thoracic cavity. Hypothermia is the major method of donor heart preservation. Thus, the donor heart is kept in a plastic bag containing ice-cold saline and transported in an ice-filled cooler. Donor heart ischemic time should be less than 4 hours to get optimal myocardial function after transplantation.

SURGICAL TECHNIQUES FOR CARDIAC TRANSPLANTATION

Orthotopic Implantation

Orthotopic cardiac transplantation, the surgical technique of choice, involves the replacement of part (or occasionally all) of the recipient's heart with a healthy donor allograft. More than 98% of cardiac transplants currently performed are orthotopic.[31]

Types of orthotopic implantation are

a. Biatrial anastomosis (Fig. 14.4A): The biatrial implantation technique preserves portions of the recipient's native atria to create two atrial anastomoses. Biatrial implantation was the original technique described for cardiac transplantation and has been performed successfully for more than 3 decades.[32] It is most common because the ischemic time is shorter. Complications include atrial dysfunction due to size mismatch of atrial remnants and arrhythmias (sinus node dysfunction, bradyarrhythmias, and AV conduction disturbances) that necessitate pacemaker implantation in 10–20% of patients.
b. Bicaval anastomosis (Fig. 14.4B): The bicaval implantation technique is a modification of the classic biatrial technique.[33] In this technique, only a single, small, left atrial cuff containing the pulmonary veins is preserved in the recipient, and bicaval and left atrial anastomoses

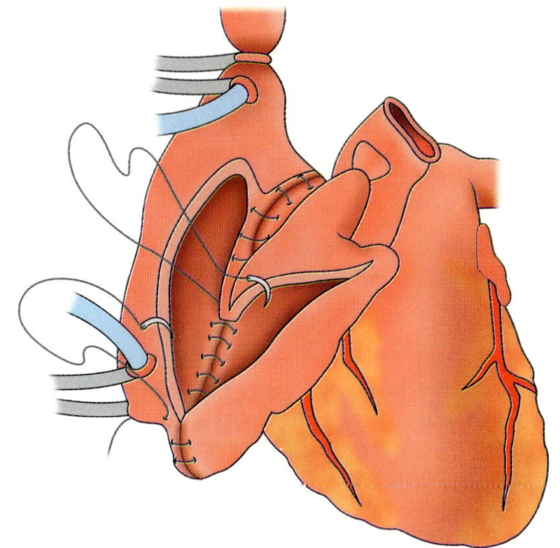

Fig. 14.4A: Biatrial technique

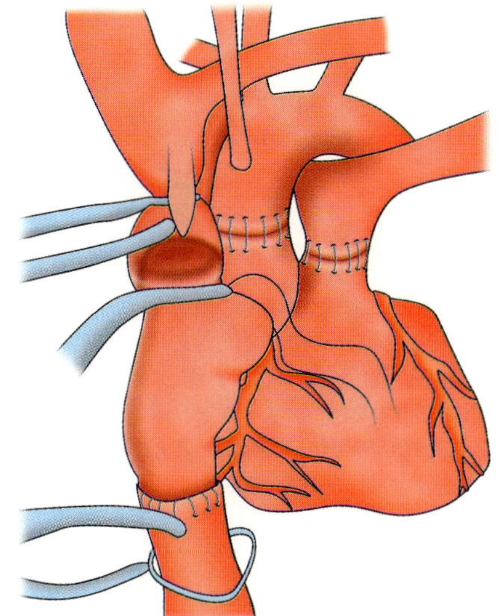

Fig. 14.4B Bicaval technique

are performed. It decreases incidence of arrhythmias, the need for a pacemaker, and risk for mitral or tricuspid regurgitation. However narrowing of the SVC and IVC make biopsy surveillance difficult and ischemic time can be prolonged.

Heterotopic Cardiac Transplantation

Heterotopic transplantation accounts for less than 1% to 2% of cardiac transplantation procedures performed each year.[31] In this technique, the recipient's heart is not excised. Instead, the donor heart is placed within the right anterior thorax and anastomosed to the recipient's native heart such that a parallel circulation is established (Fig. 14.5). It is rarely performed today. It may be indicated if orthotopic transplantation is not possible because of elevated pulmonary vascular resistance or when a donor heart is too small to sustain the recipient. Even in these selected cases, results are not equivalent to orthotopic transplant.

PREOPERATIVE ASSESSMENT OF THE PATIENT UNDERGOING HEART TRANSPLANT

The **preoperative anesthetic evaluation** include battery of tests as enumerated (Table 14.11)

- History
- Physical examination
- Review of the past medical record.
- Matching Donor and Recipient-Since ischemic time during cardiac transplantation is crucial, donor recipient matching is based primarily not only on HLA typing but also on severity of illness, ABO blood type (match or compatible), response to PRA, donor weight to recipient ratio (must be 75% to 125%), geographic location to donor, and length of time at current status.

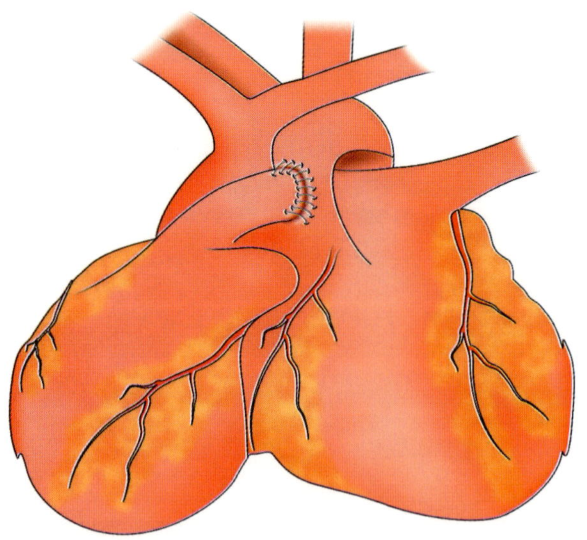

Fig. 14. 5: Heterotopic heart transplant

The PRA is a rapid measurement of preformed reactive anti-HLA antibodies in the transplant recipient. In general if PRA< 10 to 20% then no crossmatch is necessary. If PRA is > 20% then a T and B cell crossmatch should be performed.

Patients with elevated PRA will need plasmapheresis, immunoglobulins, or immunosuppressive agents to lower PRA.

Table 14.11: Preoperative work up

I. Clinical Laboratory Studies:
  A. Blood type and antibody screen
  B. Complete blood count with differential
  C. Urinalysis
  D. Random chemistry profile with T4
  E. Coagulation Profile.
  F. Percent reactive antibody (send 1 cc in a red top tube to Histocompatibility)
  G. Eletrolytes, Kidney Function Tests, Liver Functions Tests
  H. HLA typing and crossmatching (completed when donor is identified)
  I. Prostatic Specific Antigen (as indicated)
  J. Stool for occult blood (as indicated)

II. Other Tests:
  A. Echocardiogram
  B. Right heart catheterization
  C. Chest radiograph
  D. Coronary angiography (if indicated)
  E. Pulmonary function tests (if indicated)

III. Consults:
  A. A Infectious Diseases
  B. Dentistry
  C. Social Services
  D. Psychiatry (as indicated)
  E. Neurology (as indicated)
  F. Nephrology (as indicated)
  G. Gastroenterology (as indicated)

IV. Pre transplantation Infectious Diseases Screening:
  A. RPR or VDRL
  B. Hepatitis B surface antigen
  C. Hepatitis C antibody
  D. HIV screen
  E. Coccidioidomycosis titer
  F. PPD skin test

Perioperative Management

A. Induction

Anesthetic induction should be planned to minimize prolonged donor heart ischaemic time, ideally less than 4 hours (Table 14.12). Commence CPB immediately upon donor arrival.

Routine invasive and non invasive hemodynamic monitoring should be applied namely standard five-lead ECG, noninvasive BP measurement, pulse oximetry, capnography, nasopharyngeal temperature, urinary output, systemic arterial and central venous and/or PA pressure monitoring.

A PA catheter is helpful in post CPB period permitting monitoring cardiac output, ventricular pressure, and calculation of SVR and PVR. These indices are helpful for assessment and treatment of post CPB pulmonary hypertension and RV dysfunction. Use of TEE (Trans Esophageal Echocardiogram) is helpful and can be substituted in place of PA catheter.

Aim to maintain HR and contractility, avoid acute changes in preload and afterload, and prevent increases in PVR. A rapid or modified rapid sequence anesthetic induction with maintenance of cricoid pressure during positive-pressure ventilation should be considered as all patients should be considered full stomach.

Midazolam, in boluses, is commonly used for sedation and to produce amnesia. It should be used cautiously as a small dose may produce severe hypotension. Various drugs can be used for induction like – etomidate (0.2 to 0.3 mg/kg) in combination with fentanyl (5 to 10 mcg/kg) or sufentanil (5 to 8 mcg/kg).

Table 14.12: Anesthetic induction

- Timing of induction is crucial as soon as donor heart arrives (communication with transplant team)
- Minimize pre-operative sedation
- Patient in OR and induction begun on arrival of donor heart to OR
- Surgical team, CPB & perfusionist ready
- Monitors: Standard CAS monitors: 5 lead ECG, NIBP, pulse oximeter, awake arterial line, large bore IV canula, BIS
- Vascular access (left IJ), +/- PA catheter, nasal temp probe
- Continue existing inotropes, vasopressors, and assist devices
- TEE probe
- Rapid Sequence Induction
- Minimize cardiac depressants (propofol)
- Etomidate 0.3 mg/kg
- High doses of opioids (fentanyl 5–10 mcg/kg)
- Rocuronium 1mg/kg

Routinely a high-dose narcotic regimen is used. Bradycardia occurring in response to high-dose narcotics should be treated promptly, as CO in patients with end-stage heart disease is heart rate dependent.

Muscle relaxants are used according to the critical comorbid nature of the patient. Atracurium may be preferred as it has minimal cardiac and extra cardiac interactions. Pancuronium can be helpful in narcotic induced bradycardia. Vecuronium and rocuronium are other options.

Various drug interactions should be anticipated as these patients are on multi drug therapy. Patients receiving digitalis–diuretic combinations have an increased risk of dysrhythmias in the presence of hypokalemia.

The cardiac transplant recipient is at increased risk for infection due to ongoing immunosuppressive therapy. Broad spectrum antibiotic coverage is routinely administered

The Role of Intraoperative Transesophageal Echocardiography (TEE)

Intraoperative TEE is an invaluable tool for the management of the cardiac transplant recipient. Various roles of TEE are:

- Monitor chamber functions, valve abnormalities
- Identify intracavitary size and thrombus
- Estimate PA and chamber pressures
- Evaluate cannulation and cross clamp sites
- Evaluate efficacy of de-airing procedures and surgical anastomosis

In the post CPB period, TEE may reveal acute mitral and tricuspid regurgitation, low diastolic compliance and reduced ventricular contractility. Right ventricular (RV) enlargement and tricuspid valve regurgitation secondary to pulmonary hypertension may be seen in up to 66% of patients.[34]

B. Maintenance

Narcotic based maintenance anesthesia is preferred. Supplemental inhalational agents and benzodiazepines are administered as required. In spite of negative inotropic effects, most inhalational agents are well tolerated and decrease the risk of awareness. Sympathetic response to light planes of anesthesia is often blunted in these patients so all measures should be taken to prevent awareness.

C. CPB

Moderate hypothermia (28° to 30°C) commonly is used during CPB to improve myocardial protection. Hemofiltration and/or mannitol administration can be helpful during CPB in patients with congestive heart failure with large intravascular blood volume and coexistent renal impairment. Femoral venous and arterial cannulation sites frequently are chosen in patients undergoing repeat sternotomy because of the risk of injury to the heart and great vessels. Although immunosuppressive regimens vary among transplantation centers, high-dose intravenous methylprednisolone is frequently preferred before aortic cross-clamp release to reduce the incidence of hyperacute rejection.

CPB termination requires the patient to be normothermic and with electrolyte/acid–base abnormalities corrected. De-airing of the heart before aortic cross-clamp removal is essentially done under the guidance of TEE (Table 14.13). Inotropic agents should be started during rewarming. In the post CPB period, the following parameters are preferable–

- MAP > 65 mm Hg
- HR 90–110/min
- CVP 12–16 mm Hg
- PCWP 14–18 mm Hg

Postoperative Pain Management

Attaining high quality postoperative analgesia is important. Intravenous systemic opioids form the cornerstone of post cardiac transplantation analgesia. While NSAIDs (specifically COX-2 inhibitors) have received much recent attention, very important clinical issues regarding their safety (gastrointestinal effects, renal effects, hemostatic effects, immunologic effects) need to be resolved. While PCA techniques are commonly used, their clinical superiority over traditional nurse controlled analgesic techniques remain unproven. As a general rule, it is probably best to avoid intense, single modality therapy for the treatment of acute postoperative pain. Multimodal analgesia, with drugs acting at different site, of actions are used.

Chest Pain Late after Cardiac Transplantation

Sympathetic re-innervation of the transplanted heart can occur[35-39] and therefore angina pectoris should be considered in the differential diagnosis of chest pain which develops some years after cardiac transplantation. Chest pain in the presence of coronary allograft vasculopathy (CAV) can be managed medically. CAV is generally diffuse and so may not be treatable by percutaneous or surgical intervention and the option of re-transplantation may not be feasible due to the scarcity of donor organs. Refractory angina pectoris may lead to a significant deterioration in the quality of life and necessitates recurrent hospital admissions.

The use of spinal cord stimulation in the management of chronic refractory angina pectoris in other clinical settings is now well established.[40-42] There has been one previous report of the successful management of refractory post-transplant angina by spinal cord stimulation.[43]

Table 14.13: Weaning from CPB

- Evacuation of air from heart
- IV methylprednisolone before reperfusion
- Assessment of myocardial and valvular function
- Assessment of rate and rhythm
- Temperature, Hemoglobin, electrolytes, ventilation, oxygenation
- Look for denervated heart, dysrhythmias , right heart failure

IMMEDIATE POST-OPERATIVE CONSIDERATIONS

a. A denervated transplanted heart

The newly transplanted heart is denervated and does not respond to direct autonomic nervous system stimulation or to drugs that act indirectly through the autonomic nervous system (e.g. atropine). Instead, the denervated transplanted heart only responds to direct-acting agents such as catecholamines. Since transient, slow nodal rhythms are common after aortic cross-clamp release, a direct-acting β-adrenergic receptor agonist commonly is commenced before CPB termination to achieve a HR of 90 to 110 beats/min. Many centers use isoproterenol. dopamine, dobutamine, or epinephrine also are effective (Table 14.14). Newly transplanted hearts unresponsive to pharmacologic stimulation may require temporary epicardial pacing.

b. Right ventricular dysfunction

RV failure is a significant cause of early morbidity and mortality. RV dysfunction should be treated aggressively after bypass (Table 14.15). After heart transplantation, causes of acute RV failure can be transient pulmonary

Table 14.14: The denervated heart

- Denervated donor atrium but source of electrophysiologic response
- Absence of sympathetic and parasympathetic innervation to donor heart
- ECG shows 2 P waves
- Electrical activity may not cross suture line
- Absence of vagal effect on sinus and AV nodes
- Presence of recipient atrial activity but not conducted
- Absence of reflex tachycardia due to hypovolemia, hypotension
- Indirectly acting sympathomimetic agents may not have preferable effect (anticholinergics, anticholinesterases, pancuronium, ephedrine)
- Directly acting sympathomimetics produce desired effects (isoproterenol, norepinephrine, epinephrine, phenylephrine, dopamine)

Table 14.15: Management of right heart failure

- Optimize preload-avoid over distension and under filling
- Inotropic and chronotropic support-milrinone, dobutamine
- Maintain coronary perfusion-vasopressors
- Lower PVR-nitrates, prostaglandins, nitric oxide (NO)
- Mechanical support-IABP, RV assist device

vasospasm, pre-existing pulmonary HTN in the recipient, tricuspid or pulmonic valve insufficiency secondary to early postoperative RV dilation, and donor–recipient size mismatch. Inadequate myocardial protection, prolonged donor heart ischemic time and surgical manipulation of the heart can also contribute to postoperative RV dysfunction. Direct observation of the surgical field and TEE can reveal RV distension and hypokinesis.

The goal of therapy for RV dysfunction is a PVR < 6 Woods units or a transpulmonary gradient < 5–10 mm Hg. Pulmonary vascular resistance can be reduced by increasing FiO_2, correction of acid–base abnormalities, and hyperventilation ($PaCO_2$ of 25 to 30 mm Hg) . Inotropic support and pulmonary vasodilation can improve RV function. Pharmacologic agents commonly used for pulmonary vasodilators commonly used are nitrates, prostacyclin [prostaglandin I_2 (PGI_2)], prostaglandin E_1 (PGE_1), phosphodiesterase-III inhibitors, and inhaled NO.

c. Left ventricular dysfunction

Inadequate myocardial perfusion, prolonged donor heart ischemic time, intracoronary embolization of intracavitary air or surgical manipulation can contribute to post-CPB LV dysfunction . Prolonged, high-dose inotropic support before organ harvest is a risk factor. Continued postoperative inotropic support with dobutamine, norepinephrine or epinephrine may be needed to maintain adequate cardiac output.

d. Coagulation abnormalities

Coagulation abnormalities may be due to preoperative anticoagulation, CPB-induced platelet dysfunction, chronic hepatic venous congestion, hemodilution of clotting factors and hypothermia. Blood products can be administered (guided by frequent measurements of platelet count and clotting factors) after exclusion of surgical bleeding. All blood products should be cytomegalovirus (CMV) negative, and leukocyte depleted because of the potential risk of infection and graft-versus-host disease. Platelets and RBCs should be given through leukocyte filters.

e. Renal dysfunction

Increased serum creatinine and oliguria, is common in the immediate postoperative period. Cyclosporine-associated renal toxicity, pre-existing renal dysfunction, CPB and perioperative hypotension are risk factors for renal impairment. Diuretics and optimization of CO and systemic BP can improve most cases. Significant renal dysfunction may require dose adjustment or substitution of nephrotoxic drugs, such as cyclosporine.

f. Pulmonary dysfunction

Postoperative lung complications, such as pneumonia, pleural effusion and atelectasis are common and may be decreased by regular endobronchial suctioning, PEEP ventilation, and chest physiotherapy. Bronchoscopy to clear pulmonary secretions often is useful. Pulmonary infection in the immunosuppressed recipient should be treated early and aggressively.

g. Hyperacute allograft rejection

Cardiac allograft hyperacute rejection is caused by preformed anti-human leukocyte antigen (HLA) antibodies present in the recipient. Although extremely rare, hyperacute rejection results in severe cardiac dysfunction and death within hours of transplantation. Assisted mechanical circulatory support until cardiac retransplantation is the only therapeutic option.

CARDIAC TRANSPLANTATION COMPLICATIONS

a. Infection

Immunosuppression can predispose to raised incidence and spectrum of opportunistic infections.[44-46] Important causes of infection in the first month post transplant : infection derived from either the donor or recipient and infectious complications of the transplant surgery and hospitalisation. In the period one to six months post-transplant, the nature of common infections changes. Major infections due to opportunistic pathogens[47-79] include: pneumocystis carinii pneumonia (PCP), protozoal, fungal infections, viral pathogens- HBV, TB and non-tuberculous mycobacteria (NTM), herpes group, HCV.

More than six months post transplant, many patients are on low levels of immunosuppression. These patients are prone to community-acquired pneumonias due to respiratory viruses, pneumococcus, legionella, or other common pathogens.

b. Acute allograft rejection

Acute heart allograft rejection remains an important clinical problem. The high incidence of cellular rejection is at 1 month after transplant, then declines rapidly over the next 5 months, reaching a low constant rate by the end of the first year.[50-52] Newer immunosuppressive strategies have resulted in significant delays in the time that acute cellular rejection occurs.[53] Endomyocardial biopsy can establish the diagnosis of acute cellular rejection. Biopsy is performed as part of routine surveillance or, when symptoms are suggestive of or echocardiographic evidence of new left ventricular dysfunction.[54-56]

c. Systemic hypertension

After heart transplantation, cardiac denervation and immunosuppressive therapy commonly cause increased sympathetic nervous system activity, renal impairment and neuroendocrine activation. Cyclosporine raises thromboxane production and renal vascular resistance, and its chronic administration can lead to the development of hypertension.

d. Allograft coronary artery vasculopathy

Beyond the first year, transplant vasculopathy (also called transplant coronary artery disease or cardiac allograft vasculopathy) is the second most common cause of death, after malignancy.

Transplantation results in cardiac denervation and reinnervation is incomplete. Hence vasculopathy generally advances silently . Affected patients rarely present with classic symptoms of angina due to afferent denervation . Common presentations are silent MI, sudden death, and progressive heart failure.

The most common screening approach is yearly coronary angiography. Given the poor outcome in patients with established transplant vasculopathy, effective prevention is needed. Retransplantation is the only definitive therapeutic option.

CARDIAC TRANSPLANTATION SURVIVAL AND PROGNOSIS

Patient survival has steadily improved since the early days of heart transplantation.

- There is appreciable mortality in the first six months followed by a mortality rate of about 3.4 percent per year thereafter.
- The half-life of patient survival has progressively improved from 8.9 years in 1982 to 1991 to 10.3 years in 1992 to 2001 to a projected half-life of approximately 11 years in 2002 to 2005.

1. Future directions

Newly developing therapeutic strategies for end stage heart failure will have great impact on selection and management of future cardiac transplant recipients. Development of noninvasive methods to diagnose myocardial rejection and new immunosuppressive agents will improve cardiac transplant recipient survival. Surgical modalities such as total artificial heart currently are being considered as promising and can reduce the current donor heart shortage problem. Recent advances in myocardial gene therapy eventually may eventually abolish the requirement for heart transplantation eventually.

The Sir Ganga Ram Hospital Experience of Cardiac Transplantation

SGRH has done successful heart transplantation and organ harvesting of brain dead patients. Anesthetic management of the donor during organ harvesting was tailored to maintain optimal organ perfusion and cellular oxygenation with fluid, electrolytes and acid -base balance. The harvested heart was immediately brought to the cardiac operation room for transplantation.

Preoperative premedication protocol included the immunosuppressant drug mycophenolate mofetil and oral midazolam. After induction, a Swan-Ganz catheter was inserted and the pulmonary artery (PA) pressure was recorded. Moderate hypothermia (28°–30°C) was used during cardiopulmonary bypass. Hemofiltration and mannitol administration were used during cardiopulmonary bypass (CPB). Mean arterial pressure was maintained between 50–60 mm Hg. Orthotopic cardiac transplantation was done using bicaval anastomosis. Methyl prednisolone 1 gm was given before cross-clamp removal. Cardiac ischemic time was less than 3 hours. Inotropic and vasopressor support by adrenaline, noradrenaline, vasopressin, milrinone, and isoprenaline infusion was continued. Transesophageal echocardiography was used to assess cardiac function (Figs 14.6A and B). Inhaled nitric oxide in the doses 10–20 ppm was administered. Nitrogen dioxide and methemoglobin levels were monitored. Cardiac index was maintained at 2.5–3 $l/min/m^2$ and PVR was maintained at 100–140 $dynes.sec.cm^{-5}$.

Postoperatively, the immunosuppressant drug protocol included thymoglobulin, methyl prednisolone, tacrolimus and mycophenolate mofetil. Tacrolimus dose was adjusted to keep serum level at 5–15 mcg/lit. Postoperatively, analgesia was maintained with inj tramadol 10–20 mg/hr infusion and inj paracetamol 500 mg TDS. Endomyocardial biopsy done 2 weeks after surgery and repeated after 1 week, did not reveal any rejection changes. Histopathological examination of the patient's native heart showed granulomatous changes suggestive of myocardial tuberculosis, so anti-tubercular treatment was started.

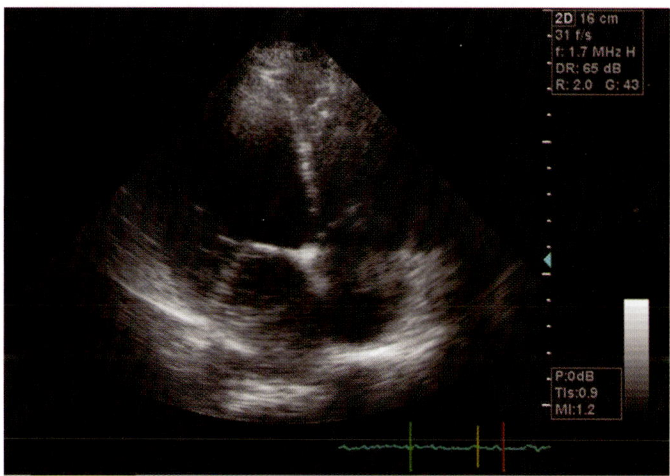

Fig. 14.6A: Preoperative native heart echocardiogram

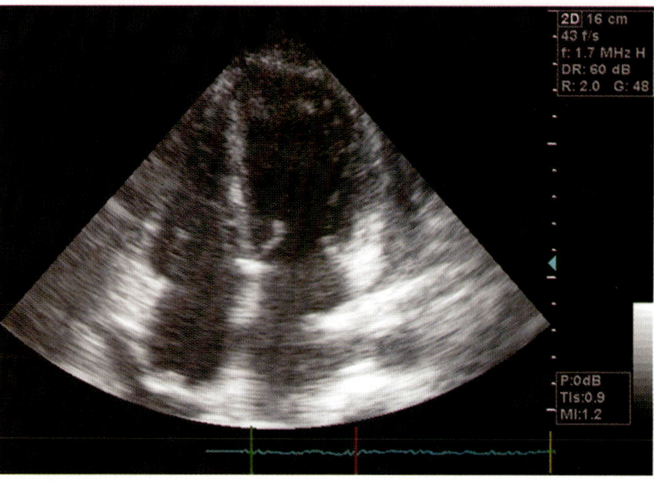

Fig. 14.6B: Transplant heart echocardiogram

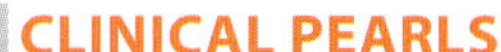

CLINICAL PEARLS

- The key factor limiting the number of cardiac transplants is a shortage of donors.
- Potential recipients have end stage heart disease, New York Heart Association class IV symptoms, ejection fraction less than 20% and physiological age less than 60 years.
- Transesophageal echocardiography and pulmonary artery catheterization play a major role in assessing cardiac function and as hemodynamic monitoring tools.
- After transplantation, the patient has a denervated heart, and heart rate increases only gradually with stress due to circulating catecholamines.
- Denervation means direct acting cardiovascular drugs must be used to obtain a response
- Allograft coronary vasculopathy is a frequent long term complication.
- The 1 year survival is 79% with a subsequent mortality of about 4% per year.

REFERENCES

1. Taylor DO, Edwards LB, Boucek MM, et al. Registry of the International Society for Heart and Lung Transplantation: twenty-fourth official adult heart transplant report--2007. J Heart Lung Transplant, 2007;26:769.
2. American Heart Association. Heart Disease and Stroke Statistics: 2008 Update. Dallas, Tex: American Heart Association, 2008.
3. Aurora P, Edwards L, Christie J, Dobbels F, Kirk R, Kucheryavaya A, et al. Registry of the International Society for Heart and Lung Transplantation: eleventh official pediatric lung and heart/lung transplantation report: 2008. J Heart Lung Transplant, 2008;27:978-983.
4. Caves PK, Stinson EB, Billingham ME, et al. Percutaneous endomyocardial biopsy in human heart recipients.Ann Thorac Surg, 1973;16:325.
5. Oyer PE, Stinson EB, Jamieson SA, et al. Cycolsporin A in cardiac allografting: a preliminary experience Transplant Proc. 1983;15:1247.
6. Hosenpud JD, Bennett LE, Keck BM, et al. The registry of the international society of heart and lung transplantation: fifteenth official report—1998. J Heart Lung Transplant, 1998;17:656.
7. Renlund DG, Taylor DO, Kfoury AG, Shaddy RS. New UNOS rules: historical background and implications for transplantation management: United Network for Organ Sharing. J Heart Lung Transplant, 1999;18:1065-70.
8. Current US waiting list for heart transplant candidates: based on OPTN data as of January 1, 2007. 9. Mehra, MR, Kobashigawa, J, Starling, R, et al. Listing criteria for heart transplantation: International Society for Heart and Lung Transplantation guidelines for the care of cardiac transplant candidates--2006. J Heart Lung Transplant, 2006;25:1024.
9. Ferrari R, Ceconi C, Curello S, et al. The neuroendocrine and sympathetic nervous system in congestive heart failure. Eur Heart J, 1998;19:F45.
10. Mann DL. Basic mechanisms of disease progression in the failing heart: the role of excessive adrenergic drive. Prog Cardiovasc Dis, 1998;48:1.
11. Middlekauff HR, Mark AL. The treatment of heart failure: the role of neurohumoral activation. Intern Med, 1998;37:12.
12. Bristow M, Kantrowitz N, Ginsburg R, et al. Beta-adrenergic function in heart muscle disease and heart failure. J Mol Cell Cardiol, 1985;17:41.
13. Chidsey CA, Braunwald E, Morrow AG. Catecholamine excretion and cardiac stores of norepinephrine in congestive heart failure. Am J Med, 1965;39:442.
14. Anker SD. Catecholamine levels and treatment in chronic heart failure. Eur Heart J, 1998;19:F56.
15. Valdemarsson S, Bergdahl A, Edvinsson L. Relationships between plasma levels of catecholamines and neuropeptides and the survival time in patients with congestive heart failure. J Intern Med, 1994;235:595.

16. Kawaguchi A, Gandjbakhch I, Pavie A, et al. Cardiac transplant recipients with preoperative pulmonary hypertension: evolution of pulmonary hemodynamics and surgical options. Circulation, 1989;80:III-90.
17. Lommi J, Pulkki K, Koskinen P, et al. Hemodynamic, neuroendocrine and metabolic correlates of circulating cytokine concentrations in congestive heart failure Eur Heart J, 1997;18:1620.
18. Niebauer J, Volk HD, Kemp M, et al. Endotoxin and immune activation in chronic heart failure: a prospective cohort study [see comments]. Lancet, 1999;353:1838.
19. Pagani FD, Miller LW, Russell SD, Aaronson KD, John R, Boyle AJ, For the HeartMate II Investigators. Extended mechanical circulatory support with a continuous-flow rotary left ventricular assist device. J Am Coll Cardiol, 2009;54:312-321.
20. Focused update incorporated into the ACC/AHA 2005 Guidelines for the Diagnosis and Management of Heart Failure in Adults: Circulation, 2009;119(14):391.
21. Hunt SA, Abraham WT, Chin MH, et al. 2009 focused update incorporated into the ACC/AHA 2005 Guidelines for the Diagnosis and Management of Heart Failure in Adults: a report of the American College of Cardiology Foundation/American Heart Association Task Force on Practice Guidelines: developed in collaboration with the International Society for Heart and Lung Transplantation. Circulation, 2009;119:e391.
22. Aaronson KD, Schwartz JS, Chen TM, et al. Development and prospective validation of a clinical index to predict survival in ambulatory patients referred for cardiac transplant evaluation. Circulation, 1997;95:2660.
23. Alla F, Briancon S, Juilliere Y, et al. Differential clinical prognostic classifications in dilated and ischemic advanced heart failure: The EPICAL study. Am Heart J, 2000;139:895.
24. Hansen A, Haass M, Zugck C, et al. Prognostic value of Doppler echocardiographic mitral inflow patterns: Implications for risk stratification in patients with chronic congestive heart failure. J Am Coll Cardiol, 2001;37:1049.
25. Lee DS, Austin PC, Rouleau JL, et al. Predicting mortality among patients hospitalized for heart failure: derivation and validation of a clinical model. JAMA, 2003;290:2581.
26. Levy WC, Mozaffarian D, Linker DT, et al. The Seattle Heart Failure Model: prediction of survival in heart failure. Circulation, 2006;113:1424.
27. Gardner RS, McDonagh TA, Macdonald M, et al. Who needs a heart transplant?. Eur Heart J, 2006;27:770.
28. Dabol R, Edwards NM. Cardiac transplantation and other therapeutic options in the treatment of end-stage heart disease. Compr Ther, 2000;26:109-113.
29. Nisco SJ, Reitz BA. Developments in cardiac transplantation. Curr Opin Cardiol, 1994;9:237-246.
30. Practice parameters for determining brain death in adults (summary statement). The Quality Standards Subcommittee of the American Academy of Neurology. Neurology, 1995;45:1012.
31. Nisco SJ, Reitz BA. Developments in cardiac transplantation. Curr Opin Cardiol, 1994;9:237-246.
32. Aziz TM, Burgess MI, El-Gamel A, et al. Orthotopic cardiac transplantation technique: a survey of current practice. Ann Thorac Surg, 1999;68:1242-46.
33. Taylor AJ, Bergin JD. Cardiac transplantation for the cardiologist not trained in transplantation. Am Heart J, 1995;129:578-592.
34. Schmid ER, Burki C, Engel MH, et al. Inhaled nitric oxide versus intravenous vasodilators in severe pulmonary hypertension after cardiac surgery. Anesth Analg, 1999;89:1108-1115.
35. Wilson RE, Christensen BV, Olivari MT, Simon A, White CW, Laxson DD. Evidence for structural sympathetic reinnervation after orthotopic cardiac transplantation in humans. Circulation, 1991;83:1210-1220.
36. Schwaiger M, Hutchins GD, Kalff V, Rosenspire K, Haka MS, Mallette S, et al. Evidence of regional catecholamine uptake and storage sites in the transplanted human heart by positron emission tomography. J Clin Invest, 1991;87:1681-90.
37. Bengel FM, Ueberfuhr P, Ziegler SI, Nekolla S, Reichart B, Schwaiger M. Serial assessment of sympathetic reinnervation after orthotopic heart transplantation. A longitudinal study using PET and C-11 hydroxyephedrine. Circulation, 1999;99: 1866-71.
38. Kaye DM, Esler M, Kingwell B, McPherson G, Esmore D, Jennings G. Functional and neurochemical evidence for partial cardiac sympathetic reinnervation after cardiac transplantation in humans. Circulation, 1993;88:1110-18.
39. De Marco T, Dae M, Yuen-Green MS, Kumar S, Sudhir K, Keith F, et al. Iodine-123 metaiodobenzylguanidine scintigraphic assessment of the transplanted human heart: evidence for late reinnervation. J Am Coll Cardiol, 1995;25:927-31.
40. Mannheimer C, Eliasson T, Augustinsson LE, Blomstrand C Emanuelsson H, Larsson S, et al. Electrical stimulation versus coronary artery bypass surgery in severe angina pectoris: the ESBY study. Circulation, 1998;97:1157-63.
41. Ekre O, Eliasson T, Norrsell H, Wahrborg P, Mannheimer C; Electrical Stimulation versus Coronary Artery Bypass Surgery in Severe Angina Pectoris. Long-term effects of spinal cord stimulation and coronary artery bypass grafting on quality of life and survival in the ESBY study. Eur Heart J, 2002;23: 1938-45.
42. Mannheimer C, Eliasson T, Andersson B, Bergh CH, Augustinsson LE, Emanuelsson H, et al. Effects of spinal cord stimulation in angina pectoris induced by pacing and possible mechanisms of action. BMJ, 1993;307:477-480.
43. Maritano M, Centofanti P, La Torre M, Barbato L, De Luca A, Fiore G, et al. New therapeutic option for cardiac ischemia in transplant vasculopathy: spinal cord stimulation. J Heart Lung Transplant, 2004;23:368-370.
44. Winston DJ, Emmanouilides C, Busuttil RW. Infections in liver transplant recipients. Clin Infect Dis, 1995;21:1077.
45. The AST Infectious Disease Community of Practice, Amercian Society of Transplantation, Infectious Disease Guidelines for Transplantation. Am J Transpl, 2009;9(Suppl 4):S1.
46. Hadley S, Karchmer AW. Fungal infections in solid organ transplant recipients. Infect Dis Clin North Am, 1995;9:1045.
47. Fishman JA. Vancomycin-resistant Enterococcus in liver transplantation: what have we left behind? Transpl Infect Dis, 2003;5:109.
48. Talbot TR, Hatcher J, Davis SF, et al. Scedosporium apiospermum pneumonia and sternal wound infection in a heart transplant recipient. Transplantation, 2002;74:1645.
49. Fishman JA. Pneumocystis carinii and parasitic infections in transplantation. Infect Dis Clin North Am, 1995;9:1005.
50. John R, Rajasinghe HA, Chen JM, et al. Long-term outcomes after cardiac transplantation: an experience based on different eras of immunosuppressive therapy. Ann Thorac Surg, 2001;72:440.
51. Kubo SH, Naftel DC, Mills RM Jr, et al. Risk factors for late recurrent rejection after heart transplantation: a multiinstitutional, multivariable analysis. Cardiac Transplant Research Database Group. J Heart Lung Transplant, 1995;14:409.

52. Hershberger RE, Starling RC, Eisen HJ, et al. Daclizumab to prevent rejection after cardiac transplantation. N Engl J Med, 2005;352:2705.
53. Winters GL, Marboe CC, Billingham ME. The International Society for Heart and Lung Transplantation grading system for heart transplant biopsy specimens: clarification and commentary. J Heart Lung Transplant, 1998;17:754.
54. Billingham ME, Cary NRB, Hammond ME, et al. A working formulation for the standardization of nomenclature in the diagnosis of heart and lung rejection: Heart Rejection Study Group. J Heart Transplant, 1990;9:587.
55. Stewart S, Winters GL, Fishbein MC, et al. Revision of the 1990 working formulation for the standardization of nomenclature in the diagnosis of heart rejection. J Heart Lung Transplant, 2005; 24:1710.
56. Dengler TJ, Zimmermann R, Braun K, et al. Elevated serum concentrations of cardiac troponin T in acute allograft rejection after human heart transplantation. J Am Coll Cardiol, 1998; 32:405.

15 CHAPTER

Heart Transplant: Overview

Sumir Dubey

Cardiac surgery is a relatively young specialty; the history of cardiac surgery spans just over 100 years. The developments in the specialty are a result of vision, dynamism and persistent efforts of pioneering surgeons coupled with developments in technology. Until the late 19th century it was believed that heart was the inscrutable and throbbing seat of human soul, an organ too delicate to allow intervention. The advances and research during the world war and in the post war era allowed surgeons to make rapid strides in the development of heart surgery. The invention of heart lung machine and cross circulation laid the foundation for modern cardiac surgery.

Historical Aspects

Alex Carrel is widely regarded as the father of vascular and transplant surgery. In the early 20th century, he along with Charles Guthrie, performed the first animal heterotopic heart transplant.[1]

In 1964, a team of surgeons at Jackson, Mississippi in USA performed the first human heart transplant when they transplanted a chimpanzee heart into a dying man's chest. This heart worked for 90 minutes before it stopped, but heralded the beginning of heart transplantation in humans.[2]

The first successful human to human heart transplant was performed by Dr Christian Barnard on 3rd December 1967, at Cape Town, South Africa.[3] He implanted a young woman's heart killed in a car crash into the chest of a South African grocer. The gentleman survived for eighteen days, but succumbed to pneumonia following immunosuppressants. The success of Barnard inspired surgeons across the world and a series of heart transplants were performed in different parts of the world. However, the results were consistently poor with more than 80% mortality in the first year. This discouraged surgeons and thus after a small period of excitement the transplant numbers dropped to insignificant levels in 1970's.

The modern heart transplant program owes it to persistent efforts of some pioneering surgeons, notable among them was the Stanford University team led by Norman Shumway. The other significant developments were understanding of transplant immunology, the discovery of cyclosporine A and percutaneous endomyocardial biopsy, all of which changed the scenario and brought about a resurgence of heart transplantation in the 1980's. Thereafter heart transplant was standardized and became a standard treatment for end-stage heart failure. In the present era the numbers of cardiac transplants world wide are limited only by the availability of donors.

INDICATIONS FOR HEART TRANSPLANT

Heart transplant is indicated for a patient with severe symptoms of heart failure, intractable angina or rhythm disturbances where there exists no other alternative form of remedial pharmacological and/or non-pharmacological therapy and the patient carries a poor prognosis.

The major goal of transplant is to improve survival and quality of life. According to the *International Society for Heart and Lung Transplantation Registry,* the most common indications for heart transplantation are cardiomyopathies (50%), ischemic heart disease not amenable to surgical or percutaneous intervention on maximal medical therapy (41%), congenital heart disease (3%), re-cardiac transplant (3%) and valvular heart disease (2%).[4]

In the current era, medical and device therapies have dramatically improved the prognosis of heart failure patients. Since, the donor is a scarce resource, it is emphasized that all heart failure patients should be on maximal medical therapy, including devices prior to accepting a patient as a heart transplant candidate.

It is difficult to determine the prognosis and survival odds of a heart failure patient. Many predictors of poor prognosis have been identified including functional class, low ejection fraction, hyponatremia and maximal oxygen comsumption (VO_2). A peak VO_2 value of < 14 mL/kg/min identifies a patient with poor prognosis and an optimal candidate for listing for transplantation. However, VO_2 has its limitation as it is a continuous variable and is affected by age, gender, medical therapy and physical conditioning.

Limitations in using individual parameters for prognostication led to use of clusters of factors together in formulation of various risk models like *Heart Failure Survival Score* (HFSS) and *Seattle Heart Failure Model*. These models are useful for guiding decision making in heart failure patients where individual predictors may be equivocal.

The HFSS model includes predictors of survival namely presence of coronary artery disease, resting heart rate, LV ejection fraction, mean arterial blood pressure, IVCD, serum Na^+ and peak VO_2. Some include PCWP as the eighth variable. The HFSS classifies patients in low, medium and high-risk categories. The HFSS model does not include the impact of medical management.

The *Seattle Heart Failure Model* was developed to incorporate the impact of optimal medical therapy and devices and provide a more valid estimate of survival in modern era. Various such models provide prognostic information for heart failure patients but each has its limitations and therefore recommendation for cardiac transplant cannot be based solely on such models only. It is important that the patient is evaluated by a team of doctors; with it is mandatory that the patient besides eligibility based on his heart failure has emotional, psychological and intellectual stability to comply with the complex and long management post-transplant.

CONTRAINDICATIONS FOR HEART TRANSPLANT

Pulmonary hypertension is an incremental risk factor for right heart failure and mortality after transplant. Severe and irreversible pulmonary hypertension is a contraindication for transplantation. Though there are no clearly defined values, a pulmonary vascular resistance of greater than 4–6 Woods or a trans-pulmonary gradient of more than 15 mm Hg serve as guidelines for exclusion of patients from transplantation. Pulmonary hypertension may result from pulmonary vasoconstriction due to neurohumoral factors; therefore the need for use of pulmonary vasodilators during assessment with right heart catheterization and evaluation on maximal optimal medical therapy.

All patients following transplant need immunosuppressants, hence any active systemic infection is a contraindication for surgery. Certain chronic infections like HIV are a challenge as immunosuppressive regimes in the immunocompromized population lead to increased morbidity and even mortality. There are a few reports of transplants in HIV positive cases but long-term data are lacking. It also poses a moral and ethical question on the use of a scarce societal resource.

Any active malignancy, other than skin, which limits survival span, is an absolute contraindication to heart transplant. Patients who have a history of malignancy in the past may be accepted for transplant, if the risk of tumor recurrence is low. In addition a reasonable period of remission, tumor type and response to therapy and metabolic workup is considered in accepting for a transplant.

Peripheral vascular disease, cerebrovascular disease or any irreversible dysfunction of a major organ are contraindications to transplant, as they can impact survival and quality of life following transplant. Diabetes and obesity are other significant comorbidities which can significantly impair post-transplant survival but these are not contraindications in present era.

Emotional and psychological stability with ability to comply with an intensive, long and uncertain pre and post-operative medical course is crucial in ensuring good outcome after transplant. History of substance abuse like alcohol, tobacco and drugs are also taken into consideration in eligibility for heart transplant.

CARDIAC DONOR

The availability of donor heart remains the major limiting factor in heart transplantation. The number of heart transplants have plateaued since the last decade due to non-availability of donor hearts.

A brain-dead patient is a potential donor. Once brain-death has been certified and consent for organ donation obtained, the prospective donor is screened for transplant.

The suggested criteria for donor selection for heart transplant are[5]:

- Age less than 55 years.
- No history of previous MI/cardiac disease, extra-cerebral malignancy or ongoing sepsis.
- No history of severe chest trauma, prolonged hypotension, shock or cardiac arrest and resuscitation.
- Patient should be hemodynamically stable or need minimal inotropes.

Once the donor is identified and qualifies the criteria for heart donation, the patient is screened for ABO blood group, size, weight and serology for HIV/HBV/HCV. Hereafter the donor is assessed by a cardiologist. Routinely an ECG and echocardiogram are done to evaluate for heart function, valve or structural abnormalities. Coronary angiography is advised if the age is more than 45 years for male and 50 years for female donor.

In an effort to expand the donor pool, some centers float a pulmonary artery catheter (PAC) if the initial echocardiogram reveals LV dysfunction. After aggressive hemodynamic management the donor is reassessed. It has been observed that 10–30% of patients have LV dysfunction following brain death; these hearts, after optimization, may be deemed fit for transplant.[6]

The final screening for the donor heart is done by the surgeon at the time of organ harvest. The surgeon inspects the organ for left ventricular function, scars, trauma, congenital anomalies, and palpable plaques in coronary arteries.

Donor management is an essential part of organ preservation. Brain death is usually followed by hemodynamic instability. It is common to observe vasodilatation (neurogenic shock), hypothermia, and diabetes insipidus following brain death. Donor management involves aggressive fluid management to maintain adequate filling pressures, usually a CVP of 6–10 mm of Hg. Metabolic perturbations like electrolyte disturbances, metabolic acidosis, hypercarbia, and hypoxia are addressed. Inotropes and vasoconstrictors may be needed to maintain a mean blood pressure > 60 mm Hg. Central diabetes insipidus, consequence of pituitary dysfunction, requires fluid replacement and vasopressin infusion. Several studies have demonstrated the benefits of hormonal resuscitation-bolus of methylprednisolone, triiodothyronine infusion and vasopressin. Insulin is required to maintain optimal blood sugar values and maintain serum osmolarity. Hypothermia is prevented by active external warming, warm fluid and warm inspired air. Antibiotics are administered prophylactically.

Donor and Recipient Matching

The prospective recipient and donor must be ABO blood type compatible. ABO incompatibility may result in fatal hyperacute sensitization. They should be size matched, the weight difference not exceeding 20%. In case of a recipient with high PVR, the donor size should be at least equal to that of recipient to decrease the possibility of acute right heart failure in the early postoperative period. All recipients undergo Panel Reactive Antibody test (PRA). If the value exceeds 10%, it indicates recipient sensitization. In such a scenario the incidence of rejection is significant and it becomes mandatory to have negative cross match between recipient and donor, prior to transplantation.

It has been observed that matching at the HLA-DR locus is associated with lower incidence of rejection. However, at the present time, prospective HLA-DR matching is logistically not feasible.

Donor Cardiectomy

Donor Heart retrieval is a part of the multiorgan procurement from the donor. Initially, the cardiac harvesting starts with a median sternotomy and longitudinal pericardiotomy. The heart is inspected by the surgeon for any damage or anomalies. The superior vena cava, azygous and inferior vena cava are dissected, mobilized and taped. The aorta is separated from the pulmonary artery. Hereafter, the abdominal team starts dissection and preparation for explantation of the liver, kidneys and pancreas.

Once the abdominal team is ready with the preparations, heparin is administered intravenously. The SVC is doubly ligated and divided. An aortic cross clamp is applied and single dose of antegrade cold cardioplegia is administered. The IVC is divided/incised for efflux of the cardioplegia. The left heart is vented through a nick on the right superior pulmonary vein or left atrial appendage. The heart is cooled rapidly with ice-cold slush. Once the cardioplegia is administered, the team proceeds with cardiectomy. The SVC and IVC are transected taking long segments. The apex is retracted and the pulmonary veins are divided. If the lungs are also being harvested, a cuff of atrial tissue is left behind with the pulmonary veins on either side. The aorta is transected just proximal to the innominate artery and pulmonary artery beyond the bifurcation. The procured heart is placed in ice-cold saline, bagged and placed in a box for transportation.

Organ Preservation

Optimal organ preservation is mandatory for allograft function post-transplant. Suboptimal donor management, hypothermia, and ischemic reperfusion injury are associated with myocardial dysfunction post-transplant.

At present ischemia time upto 4 hours is considered safe with current methods. A single dose of cold cardioplegia during cardiectomy followed by storage at 4–10°C in cold saline is the most widely practiced technique of graft storage and transplantation.

The harvested donor heart is most often transported in cold saline or a preservative solution in accordance with the individual center protocol. Preservative solutions are either intracellular type solutions characterized by low Na^+ and calcium and moderate to high K^+(University of Winsconsin, Eurocollins, Bretschnieder) or extracellular type solutions which have higher Na^+ Mg^{++}, Ca^{++} content and moderate to low K^+ (St. Thomas, Hopkins, Krebs). Comparisons between various solutions have shown variable results.[7] Additives like colloids, impermeants to maintain osmolality, antioxidants and nutritional substrates may be added; there are no standard recommendations. Continuous hypothermic perfusion of the graft has also been tried to provide uniform myocardial cooling, substrate supplementation and metabolic washout.

This technique is limited by increase in interstitial edema of the allograft and difficulties associated with a complicated perfusion apparatus.[8]

Myocardial preservation and extension of safe ischemic time is an area of active research. An organ care system which involves perfusion of the harvested donor heart with warm oxygenated, substrate enriched blood which allows the heart to be in a beating and functional state during transportation has been developed.[9] This system was evaluated for safety and preservation of myocardial function in the proceed trial in USA.[10]

CARDIAC RECIPIENT

Orthotopic heart transplant is the most commonly used technique for transplantation. Heterotopic heart transplantation is uncommon and reserved for special situations like recipients with pulmonary hypertension and size mismatch.

The communication between donor and recipient team is important to optimize *ischaemia time* and recipient *bypass time*. The recipient is prepared for cardiectomy. The cardiopulmonary bypass is established in a standard manner; a high ascending aortic cannulation for arterial return and bicaval cannulation for venous return. The patient is heparinized and cardiopulmonary bypass initiated.

There are three major techniques for orthotopic heart transplant (i) Standard biatrial technique (ii) Bicaval and (iii) Total heart transplantation.

The **biatrial technique** was originally described by Shumway[11] and Lower[12] from the Stanford group. This is still widely practiced with some modifications. In the standard biatrial technique, the recipient cardiectomy involves excision of the heart at mediastinal level and division of aorta and pulmonary artery (Fig. 15.1).

The donor heart is prepared by joining all four pulmonary veins and creating a matching left atrial cuff, and separating the proximal portion of aorta and pulmonary artery (Fig. 15.2).

The transplantation starts with left atrial anastomosis at the far side starting at the left superior pulmonary vein (Fig. 15.3).

After the left atrial anastomosis, the right atrium is anastomosed followed by pulmonary artery and the aorta (Figs 15.4 and 15.5). After thorough deairing of the chambers, the cross clamp is released and the donor heart is reperfused.

The biatrial technique results in figure of '8' configuration of the atria. This creates large atrial cavities and abnormal geometry. There is also dyssynchrony of the donor and recipient atrial innervations. These have been correlated to the higher incidence of tricuspid and mitral regurgitation, atrial thrombus and tachyarrhythmias, post transplant.[13]

The **bicaval technique** was initially reported in clinical practice by Sievers and colleagues in 1991.[14] Sarsam and associates subsequently described the bicaval Wythenshawe technique in 1993.[15] In the bicaval technique, recipient cardiectomy is modified to leave behind a left atrial cuff, SVC and IVC stumps (Fig. 15.6); the RA is excised (cf biatrial technique). The technique involves left atrial cuff anastomosis

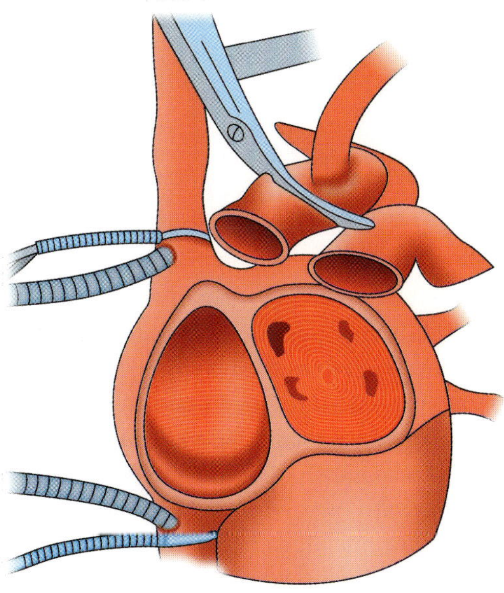

Fig. 15.1: Biatrial technique—recipient cardiectomy

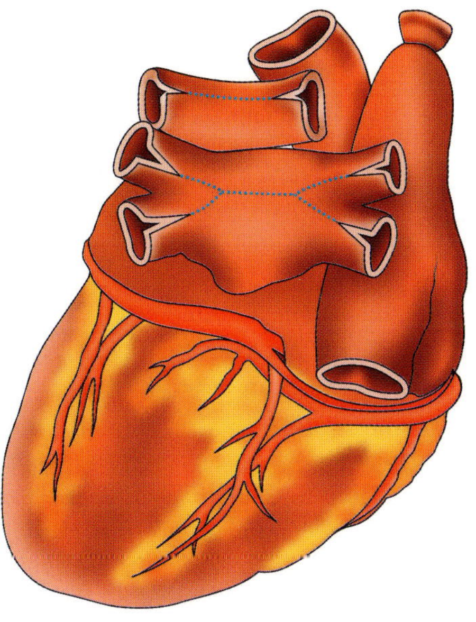

Fig. 15.2: Biatrial technique—donor heart

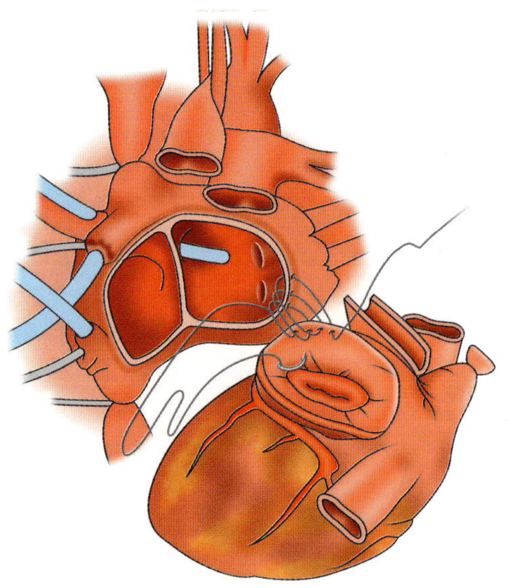

Fig. 15.3: Biatrial technique—left atrial anastomosis

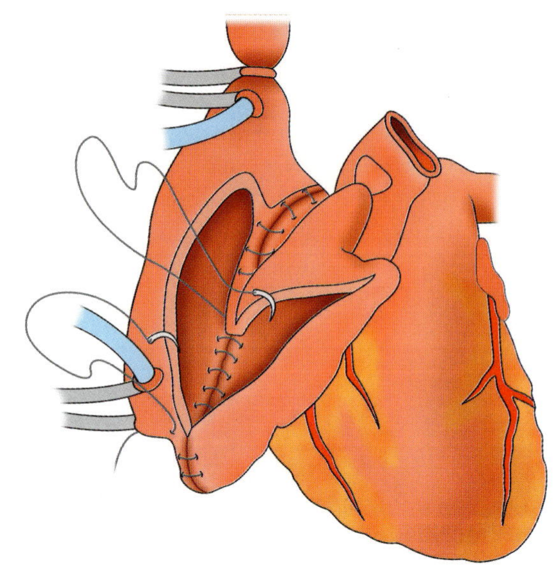

Fig. 15.4: Biatrial technique—right atrial anastomosis

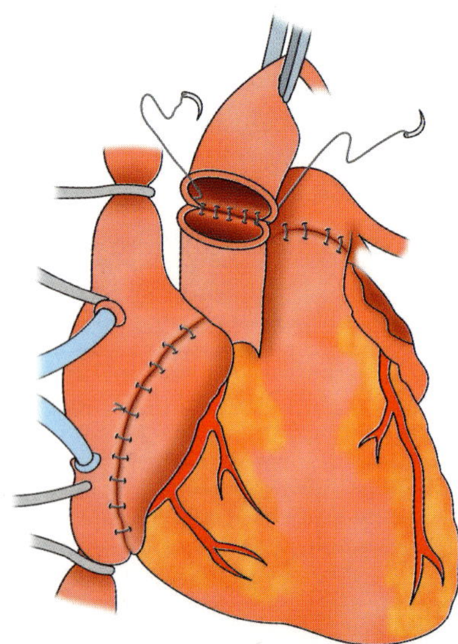

Fig. 15.5: Biatrial anastomosis—completed right atrial anastomosis

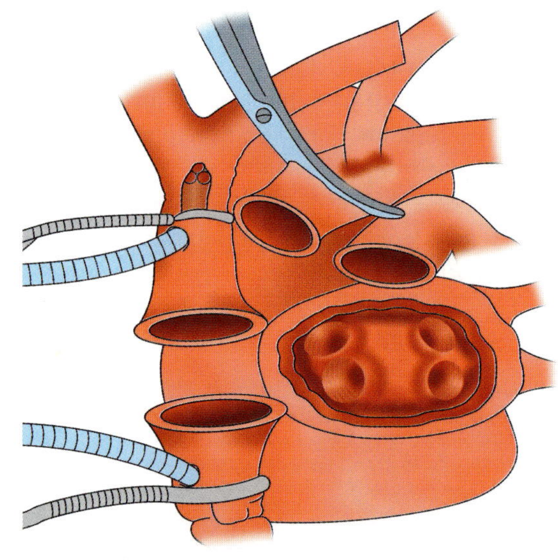

Fig. 15.6: Bicaval technique—recipient cardiectomy

and individual SVC and IVC anastomosis to the corresponding structures on the donor heart (Fig. 15.7). This is followed by the anastomosis of the pulmonary artery and aorta.

The bicaval technique prevents atrial distortion and enlargement. This technique is believed to result in improved atrial function, reduced atrial tachyarrhythmias and better preservation of sinus node function,[13, 16] however it is prone to SVC/IVC anastomotic stenosis, thrombosis and SVC syndrome.

The bicaval technique retains the right atrial morphology. The presumed theoretical advantages of maintained tricuspid competence, node function and synchronous atrial activity result in improvement in hemodynamics, lower RA pressure, chamber sizes, exercise capacity, lower incidence of tricuspid incompetence and decreased early and late arrhythmias.[16]

The **total technique** (complete atrioventricular cardiac transplantation with separate caval and pulmonary vein anastomoses) was introduced into clinical practice by the Harefield group[17] before it was reported by Carpentier's group in 1989.[18] The total heart transplant involves removal of the entire recipient heart including both the atria, leaving

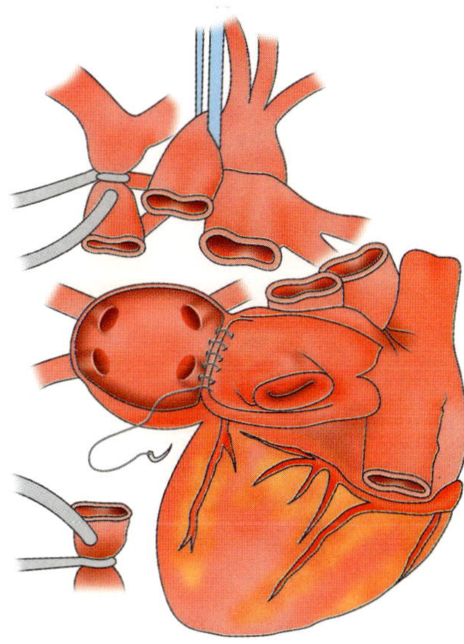

Fig. 15.7: Bicaval technique—atrial anastomosis

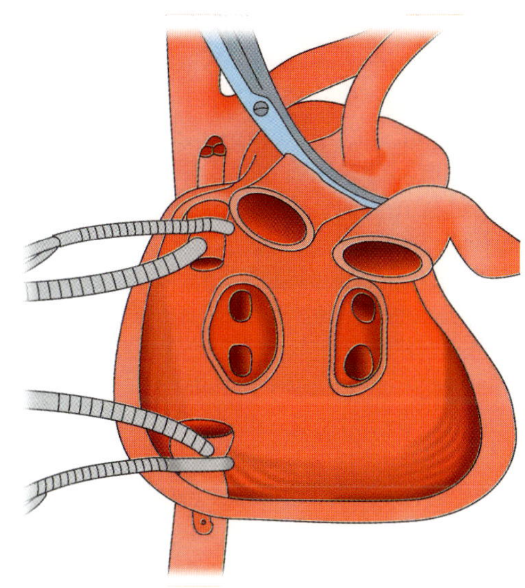

Fig. 15.8: Total heart transplant—recipient cardiectomy

behind a cuff of right and left pulmonary veins, the vena cava (SVC and IVC), aorta and pulmonary artery (Fig. 15.8). The suturing involves individual anastomosis of the left and right pulmonary venous cuffs to the corresponding openings in the donor left atria, separate SVC and IVC anastomosis followed by pulmonary artery and aortic anastomosis. The total heart transplant is technically more challenging and takes longer time. There is a risk of bleeding from the inaccessible posterior suture lines of pulmonary veins. It may also lead to narrowing, twisting, distortion and reduced patency of pulmonary veins. Total heart transplant has all the advantages of bicaval technique. Besides there is intact left atrium and thus the morphology of the left atrium is preserved which is associated with lower incidence of mitral regurgitation and LA thrombus.[13,19]

Heterotopic Heart Transplant

Heterotopic heart transplant is rarely performed today. It is usually reserved for recipients with significant pulmonary hypertension with raised pulmonary vascular resistance where the possibility of post transplant right heart failure is extremely likely. Another indication, though uncommon now, would be when the donor size is significantly smaller compared to the recipient size.

In this technique, the recipient's heart is not excised. Instead, the donor heart is placed within the right anterior thorax and anastomosed to the recipient's native heart such that a parallel circulation is established. The opening in donor's left atrium is sutured to the recipient's left atrial-right superior pulmonary vein junction. A side-to-side right atrial anastomosis and end to side aortic and pulmonary artery anastomosis are constructed (Fig. 15.9). Disadvantages of heterotopic cardiac transplantation include high operative mortality, requirement for continued medical treatment of the failing native heart, potential of native heart to be a source for thromboembolism and compromised pulmonary function due to placement of donor heart in the right chest.

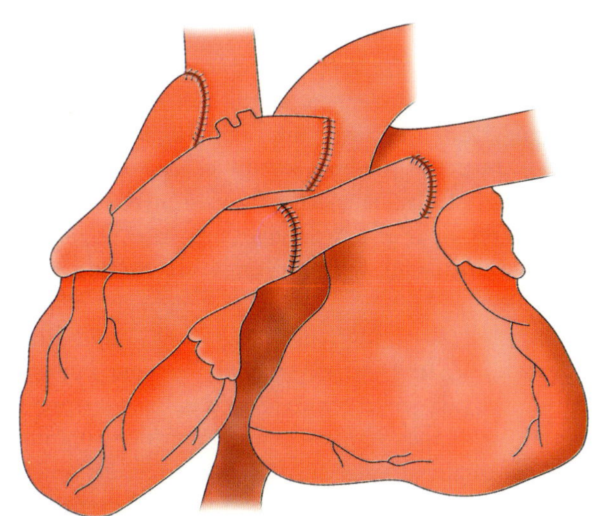

Fig. 15.9: Heterotropic heart transplant

Postoperative Management

The postoperative course following heart transplant is eventful and requires intensive monitoring and anticipation. There are issues related to hemodynamics, renal, and hematological dysfunction, immune response and susceptibility to infections.

The management of post-operative heart transplant is similar to care following open heart surgery. Routine monitoring of ECG, invasive blood pressure, filling pressures, cardiac output and saturation are mandatory.

The transplanted heart has some differences from the native heart. It is denervated and does not respond to direct autonomic nervous system stimulation or to drugs that act indirectly through the autonomic nervous system (e.g. atropine); there is also a delayed response to stress (hypovolemia, hypoxia) as the allograft depends on circulating catecholamines for its response.

Transient, slow nodal rhythms are common after aortic cross-clamp release and early in the postoperative period. Bradyarrhythmias due to sinus node dysfunction are probably caused by surgical trauma to the sinoatrial node or its blood supply. Isoprotenol, a direct-acting β-adrenergic receptor agonist, is suggested to achieve an optimal heart rate. Newly transplanted hearts unresponsive to pharmacologic stimulation may require temporary epicardial pacing.

Sustained atrial flutter and fibrillation in the later post-operative period are commonly associated with allograft rejection. Thus, the presence of these arrhythmias should prompt a search for acute rejection by endomyocardial biopsy. Complex ventricular ectopy or atrioventricular block may be caused by either acute rejection or severe cardiac allograft vasculopathy.

The most common mechanism of early allograft failure is right heart failure secondary to the inability of the unprepared RV of the allograft to overcome elevated pulmonary pressures and afterload. It may also result from transient pulmonary vasospasm, tricuspid valve insufficiency secondary to early postoperative RV dilation and donor–recipient size mismatch. Additional factors that may contribute to postoperative RV dysfunction include a prolonged donor heart ischemic time, inadequate myocardial protection, and surgical manipulation of the heart. RV distension and hypokinesis may be diagnosed by TEE or direct observation of the surgical field. Other findings suggesting RV failure include elevations in CVP, PA pressure, and transpulmonary gradient (greater than 15 mm Hg). Increased FiO_2, correction of acid–base abnormalities, and hyperventilation ($PaCO_2$ of 25 to 30 mm Hg) may reduce PVR. RV function may be improved by inotropic support and pulmonary vasodilation. Pulmonary vasodilators as nitroglycerine, nitroprusside, prostacyclin, prostaglandin I_2 (PGI_2), prostaglandin E_1 (PGE_1), phosphodiesterase-III inhibitors, and inhaled NO may be used. Uncommonly refractory right heart failure may require right ventricle assist device.

Early LV dysfunction occurring in the operative and immediate postoperative period is often due to ischemic injury due to inadequate preservation (due to donor ischemia, donor hemodynamic instability, insult from hypothermia and surgical handling) or due to the use of a suboptimal donor heart. It is associated with a need for increased use of inotropic agents or other circulatory support (such as intraaortic balloon pumping). Hyperacute rejection also can occur at this time but is now rare.

The most important causes of late LV dysfunction are allograft rejection and allograft vasculopathy. Prompt treatment of allograft rejection can result in dramatic improvement and empiric therapy may be indicated if the clinical suspicion is high, even in the absence of biopsy-proven rejection. Other uncommon causes of delayed LV dysfunction include typical coronary atherosclerosis, opportunistic myocardial infections, and rarely recurrent myocardial disease.

Coagulation defects may result from hepatic dysfunction secondary to chronic hepatic venous congestion, preoperative anticoagulation, CPB-induced platelet dysfunction, hypothermia, and hemodilution of clotting factors. This is corrected by administration of blood products guided by repeated measurements of clotting factors and clinical judgement.

Renal function needs optimization in the immediate postoperative period. Preoperative renal dysfunction from heart failure, nephrotoxic effect of cyclosporine and other immunosuppressants, perioperative hypotension, and CPB put the kidneys at risk. Significant renal dysfunction may require dose adjustment or substitution of nephrotoxic drugs, such as cyclosporine.

Postoperative pulmonary complications, such as atelectasis, pleural effusion, and pneumonia, are common. Management includes PEEP, regular endobronchial suctioning and chest physiotherapy. Pulmonary infection should be treated early and aggressively as these are immunosuppressed patients.

Immunosuppressant Therapy

The Human Leukocyte Antigen (HLA) on the allograft elicits a host defense response. The principle of immunosuppressive therapy is to modulate the host's immune response to prevent rejection while sparing immunity against infection and malignancy. Immune reactivity and rejection episodes are highest early in the first three to six months, and decrease over time. Therefore, immunosuppressive therapy is the most intense early after surgery and gradually decreased in intensity over a year and eventually maintained on minimum maintenance dose. All immunosuppressive protocols employ multidrug regimes to achieve comprehensive and sequential immunosuppression and also reduce toxicity by reduction in doses of individual agents.

Immunosuppressive regimes may be classified as induction, maintenance or anti rejection. Induction regimes provide intense early postoperative immune suppression when the risk of graft failure is highest. Approximately half of the transplant centers employ induction or augmented immunosuppression in the early posttransplant period.[20] Besides providing intense immunosuppression early, a major advantage of induction therapy is that it delays the initiation of nephrotoxic immunosuppressive drugs in patients with compromised renal function. Though induction therapy is associated with decreased early rejection, there are concerns regarding increased late rejection after therapy completion and increased probability of infection and malignancy.[21-23] The induction therapy is most beneficial for younger patients, Afro-American race, high panel-reactive antibody (PRA) values, and patients on ventricular assist device (VAD) with high levels of preformed antibodies, where the risk for rejection is highest.[24]

The induction therapy is employed in a quarter of heart transplant recipients at present and protocols vary across different centers. The most commonly employed agents are polyclonal anti thymocyte antibodies, monoclonal antibodies and interleukin-2 inhibitors.

Polyclonal anti thymocyte antibodies are derived from immunization of animals after injecting them with human thymocytes. These preparations cause rapid depletion of T lymphocytes by causing complement mediated cytolysis and cell mediated opsonization in liver and spleen. The major side effects are serum sickness reaction, leucopenia, thrombocytopenia, predisposition to opportunistic infections and possible increased incidence and aggressiveness of post-transplant malignancies.

The most commonly used monoclonal antibody was Muromonab (OKT3) which binds to cell receptor-CD3 complex on circulating lymphocytes.[25] It is associated with significant short and long-term adverse reactions like cytokine release syndrome, opportunistic infections, lymphoproliferative disorders and increased risk of acute antibody mediated rejection (AMR) after long-term use. The use of OKT3 has declined at present due to its adverse effects and availability of other agents. Alemtuzumab, a humanized rat monoclonal antibody is being investigated in heart transplantation. It is a powerful cytolytic agent and has prolonged effect lasting for approximately 6 months and even more. It targets the CD52 antigen on the 'T' and 'B' cell lymphocytes.[26]

The use of interleukin-2 receptor antagonist is increasing in induction therapy for patients undergoing heart transplantation. These agents act by inhibiting IL-2 mediated T-lymphocyte proliferation. The commonly employed agents are basiliximab and daclizumab. These are not combined with cell lymphocytolytic therapy. The use of IL-2 as an induction agent in the background of standard triple drug maintenance immunosuppression regime is associated with decreases in the incidence of biopsy proven rejection, hemodynamically significant graft dysfunction, death and retransplantation.[27]

Maintenance immunosuppression is the cornerstone of post-transplant management and survival. Cyclosporine, following its introduction made a major impact on heart transplant results in the mid 1980's and was responsible for the resurgence of heart transplantation. This was a significant move from broad and nonspecific immunosuppression to more targeted immunosuppression with selective inhibition of lymphocyte activation and proliferation. Majority of maintenance immunosuppression regimes employ three drugs regime which includes a calcineurine inhibitor, an antiproliferative agent and glucocorticoids.

Calcineurine Inhibitors (CNI): This group of drugs inhibits the calcium-calcineurine pathway, a type of signal transduction pathway. The end result is blunting of lymphocyte activation and proliferation in response to an antigen. The two available CNI agents are cyclosporine and tacrolimus both of which are derived from a fungus. These drugs differ with respect to efficacy and side effect profile. Various trials have shown similar survival but more favorable adverse effect profile with tacrolimus when compared to cyclosporine. Tacrolimus is associated with lower incidence of biopsy proven acute cellular rejection.[29] These are continued indefinitely but higher blood levels are targeted in the first 6 or 12 months and then continued at lower intensity. The major limitations of cyclosporine are nephrotoxicity, hypertension and hyperlipidemia. Tacrolimus is associated with less hypertension and dyslipidemia but possibly a higher incidence of new onset diabetes.[28]

Antiproliferative agents or antimetabolite group of drugs interfere with nucleic acid synthesis and prevent both T and B lymphocyte proliferation. The two commonly used agents are azathioprine and mycophenolate mofetil (MMF). MMF is the most commonly used agent in this group as it has been shown to be superior to azathioprine in terms of mortality and graft loss.[29] The drug is available both as an oral preparation and powder for injection. The major adverse effects are leucopenia. MMF is not nephrotoxic.

Glucocorticoids: Corticosteroids are an integral part of any immunosuppressive regime. These are non-selective and influence all aspects of immune-response. In the initial period of triple-drug immunosuppressive therapy for heart transplant, methylprednisolone is used immediately after surgery and subsequently followed by oral prednisolone. These are used in high dose doses initially and then tapered to be stopped. The timing of steroid withdrawal varies between different centers from a few months to a year. Steroids are the treatment or choice for acute rejection episodes. Long term use is associated with osteoporosis, myopathy, diabetes, infection, weight gain, hyperlipidemia and severity of cardiac allograft vasculopathy (CAV).

Proliferation Signal Inhibitors (PSI): These agents have been introduced recently into clinical heart transplant and are indicated in patients with renal insufficiency, CAV or malignancy to reverse or slow the progress. These agents are not started de novo following transplant because of frequent side effects and interference with wound healing.[30] The two members of this class, sirolimus and everolimus bind to a protein and inhibit a protein kinase in the cytoplasm called mammalian target of rapamycin (mTOR) causing cell cycle arrest and thus inhibition of lymphocyte proliferation. They have been shown to be superior in preventing rejection compared to azathioprine when combined with CNI. The PSI can potentiate the nephrotoxic effects of CNI, therefore the doses of CNI need to be reduced when the two are used together. The major adverse effects are bone marrow suppression, oral ulcerations, lower limb edema, wound healing complications and pleural and pericardial effusions.[31] Their major advantage is that they may decrease the incidence and progression of CAV.[31]

Complications

Rejection

Acute Cellular Rejection (ACR): Acute cellular rejection is the most common mechanism of rejection in the first 6 months of heart transplantation. Approximately 20–40% of the heart transplant recipients will have at least one episode of ACR in the first year following transplant. This is predominantly 'T' cell mediated in response to direct allorecognition. ACR is characterized by infiltration of myocardium predominantly with lymphocytes, macrophages, plasma cells and myocardial necrosis. These changes are histologically classified in a grading system developed by ISHLT.

Acute Antibody Mediated Rejection (AMR): This is relatively less common occurring approximately in 10% of the patients. This should be suspected in patients with evidence of graft dysfunction which does not show features of ACR (lymphocyte infiltration) on the biopsy specimen. Patients who are allosensitized are at a greater risk of AMR. This form of rejection is mediated by 'B' cells which leads to antibody injury to endothelium, endothelial dysfunction, microvascular coagulation, ischemia and allograft dysfunction. It is noteworthy that AMR and ACR may coexist in a quarter of acute rejection episodes.

Hyperacute Rejection: This is extremely rare and occurs within a few minutes to few hours of transplantation. It is triggered by pre-formed antibodies to ABO antigens, HLA exposed on vascular endothelial cell or non HLA on vascular endothelium. The antibody mediated rejection leads to activation of the complement cascade and thrombosis characterized grossly by marked congestion, edema and hemorrhages. Microscopically it shows swelling, extravasation, thrombosis, interstitial edema, inflammatory infiltrate and tissue necrosis. It carries a grave prognosis. Management includes immunoglobulins, plasmapheresis, assist device and re-transplantation.

Symptoms: Rejection episodes may be asymptomatic or with non-specific symptoms of fatigue, malaise, nausea or fever. As the graft dysfunction progresses, they may manifest with congestive heart failure. Rejection may also manifest with A-V block and bradyarrhythmias. In advanced stage there would be symptoms of low cardiac output or may have sudden cardiac death. Since the signs and symptoms of rejection have low sensitivity and specificity, surveillance for rejection is mandated. The surveillance has to be more intense in the early months and frequency gradually tapered over one year.

Monitoring of Acute Rejection

Invasive

Endomyocardial biopsy (EMB): This is an invasive procedure performed with bioptome which is introduced from the right internal jugular vein and 4–5 biopsy samples are obtained from the right ventricle. The two dreaded complications are cardiac perforation and tricuspid regurgitation from iatrogenic injuries. The frequency of EMB varies between transplant centers. Initially the biopsy is done more frequently (every fortnight) in the first three months and then gradually decreased over one year.

Non-invasive

Electophysiological parameters are simple and inexpensive. QRS amplitude, signal averaged ECG, heart rate variability, QT depression may indicate rejection but have low sensitivity and specificity. Evoked ventricular responses have high negative predictive prognostic value.

Imaging: Echocardiogram and recently magnetic resonance imaging are the most frequently employed. Echocardiography is a standard tool and is routinely used for evaluation of allograft function, diastolic dysfunction, tissue doppler velocities, and presence of pericardial effusion. These may indicate rejection but are non-specific.

Recently MRI has attracted attention and correlation between T2 relaxation times and rejection has evinced interest.

Biochemical Markers: The various biochemical markers used to identify rejection like BNP, troponin levels, CRP, markers of T-cell activation like IL and TNF have yielded inconsistent results and have limited utility.

A new methodology *Gene Expression Profiling* is being evaluated for screening of rejection. The screening involves evaluation of transcription of genes mediating the immune process. Assessment of a single or cluster based scoring system may provide a basis for risk assessment of rejection episodes in future.

Management of Rejection

Acute cellular rejection (ACR) may be asymptomatic and diagnosis made on a routine EMB surveillance or may manifest with signs and symptoms of graft dysfunction (symptomatic). Symptomatic ACR should be hospitalized in intensive care and EMB obtained as soon as possible. High dose intravenous corticosteroids are the first line therapy followed by cytolytic immunosuppressant therapy in case of hemodynamic compromise or failure of response in 12–24 hours. Hemodynamic support with inotropes and vasopressor is instituted and antibiotic prophylaxis against opportunistic infection is administered. Adjustment is made to the maintenance therapy namely increasing the doses of CNI/ MMF or addition of agents (PSI) or conversion to an alternative immunosuppressive regime. Serial echocardiograms are used to follow changes in graft function and EMB done 1–2 weeks later to asses the response.

Asymptomatic severe rejection (grade 3R) is treated similar to symptomatic ACR. However, moderate ACR (Grade 2R) may be treated with IV or oral corticosteroids. Severe and moderate rejection need adjustments in the immunosuppression regime. Asymptomatic mild ACR requires surveillance and monitoring only.

Antibody mediated rejection (AMR): Hyperacute: This is grave and treatment is instituted as soon as the diagnosis is established. Management includes corticosteroids, plasmapharesis, immunoglobulins, polyconal antibodies, IV CNI/MMF and mechanical circulatory support. Urgent re-transplantation should be considered if the above measures do not result in acceptable improvement of graft function.

Acute AMR: Asymptomatic AMR warrants reassessment of adequacy of immunosuppression and close monitoring. The management of symptomatic AMR targets removal of circulating antibodies and reduction in the synthesis of more alloantibodies and monoclonal antibodies. Circulating antibodies can be removed by plasmapharesis, immunopheresis and IV immunoglobulins. Ritiximaban antibody directed against B lymphocyte is being evaluated.

Infections

Infections are frequent after heart transplant and lead to significant morbidity and mortality. The greatest risk occurs in the first six months when infection can be life threatening.

Infection in the early postoperative period (< 1 month) is mainly associated with technical or nosocomial factors. These are generally wound infections, mediastinitis or pneumonias. *Staphylococcus* and gram negative bacilli are the major culprits and management requires prevention, chemoprophylaxis and specific antimicrobial therapy based on culture and sensitivity once the infection is established.

Infection in between 1 to 6 months is generally associated with opportunistic organisms or re-activation of latent infection. Infections beyond 6 months are generally community acquired.

Cytomegalovirus (CMV) infection is probably the most important cause of mortality and morbidity following heart transplant. CMV infections besides causing morbidity from septic complications are also associated with rejection episodes, acceleration of cardiac allograft vasculopathy (CAV) and lymphoproliferative disorders (malignancy). This infection may occur from donor transmission, reactivation of latent disease or new infection. Prophylaxis with anti-viral agents like ganciclovir is recommended and extended prophylaxis along with CMV infection surveillance is recommended for high-risk group (CMV+ve donor, seropositive recipient, etc.).

Fungal infections especially mucocutaneous candidiasis is common and responds to local antifungal treatment. Invasive candidiasis (esophageal, gut) or opportunistic aspergilosis in lung/CNS can be lethal. These are treated with fluconazole/ variconazole or amphoterecin B. Prophylactic fluconazole may be administered in the first 6–12 weeks post-transplant.

The incidence of opportunistic protozoal *P. carnii varies* from 1–10%. Patients are recommended trimethoprim-sulfamethoxazole chemoprophylaxis for *P. carnii* for at least 6 months post-transplant.

Other important protozoal infection is with toxoplasmosis which may be transmitted from donor, reactivation or an acquired new infection. T Gondi usually causes CNS infection.

Cardiac Allograft Vasculopathy (CAV)

This is a unique and challenging problem in patients with long-term success in cardiac transplantation. The incidence of angiography proven CAV varies between 40–50% at 5 years after transplantation. CAV mimics atherosclerosis but has distinctive features. It is characterized by diffuse, concentric intimal hyperplasia which affects both epicardial vessels and micro-vasculature. Calcification is uncommon. It is believed to be initiated as an immune mediated injury. Hypertension, hyperlipidemia, diabetes and donor age predispose to CAV. Besides, repeated episodes of acute rejection and CMV infection are also related to CAV incidence.

The CAV generally begins within several weeks and progresses at a variable rate. CAV presents as myocardial ischaemia which in a denervated heart manifests as ventricular arrhythmia, heart failure or sudden death. Coronary obstruction and thus CAV is picked up on coronary angiography. Intravascular ultrasound (IVUS) is probably more sensitive as it may better define the vessel characteristics and intimal thickening.

Non-invasive surveillance of CAV may be done by dobutamine stress echo, myocardial perfusion scan, fast CT coronary angiography and tissue doppler imaging.

Prevention is the best form of cure for CAV. Control of risk factors like hypertension, diabetes, hyperlipidemia, smoking cessation, exercise and diet are probably helpful but empirical. Statin therapy may influence progress of CAV. Certain immunosuppressants like PSI are known to control and even reverse some changes associated with CAV. The only definitive treatment of advanced CAV is cardiac re-transplantation.

Malignancy

Chronic immunosuppression is associated with increased incidence of malignancy. Malignancy and CAV are the major limiting factors in post-transplant long-term survival. The most common malignancies associated post-transplants are lymphoproliferative disorders and skin malignancy. Besides, the incidence of solid organ malignancy like lung, breast, and prostate is also increased. Malignancy in a post-transplant patient carries a grave prognosis and conventional therapy has limited success.

Hypertension, hyperlipidemia, renal dysfunction are well described and managed with routine protocols.

Results

The cardiac transplantation results have gradually improved in the last 3 decades. The maximal improvement is in the first year survival and has been mainly driven by improvement in immunosuppression, rejection surveillance, prophylaxis and treatment of rejection. There has been no substantial difference in post 1 year transplant survival in last 3 decades.

According to ISHLT 2012 report, the median survival for 96,273 adults and pediatric heart transplants is 10 years. Patients who survive beyond 1 year have a 63% likelihood of survival 10 years post-transplant and 27% survival 20 years post-transplant.[4] The survival after heart transplantation at 1 year was influenced by the underlying etiology for heart transplantation; non-ischemic cardiomyopathy (86%), ischemic cardiomyopathy 84%, re-transplantation 81% and valvular and congenital heart disease 79%.[4]

The leading causes of death after heart transplantation are acute rejection, graft failure, cardiac allograft vasculopathy and malignancy. Graft failure and infections are the major cause of death in the early period after transplant. However beyond 3 years allograft vasculopathy and malignancy are the major contributors to mortality.

According to ISHLT data donor age, allograft ischemic time (>200 mins), very young or very old age of the recipient, renal dysfunction and need for dialysis, and etiology of the heart disease (congenital vs cardiomyopathy) were risk factors for mortality in first post-transplant year. The need for mechanical circulatory support before transplant also conferred increased risk for 1 year mortality; the risk was higher for ECMO and temporary pulsatile support compared to long-term ventricular assist device (VAD) support. Besides the factors described above, the five year mortality is influenced by the number of acute rejection episodes, need for dialysis, treated infection prior to transplant, and immunosuppression regime.

CLINICAL PEARLS

- Heart transplant is the standard of care for patients with advanced heart failure.
- A certified brain dead patient is a potential donor, who is less than 50 years of age, hemodynamically stable with no history of cardiovascular disease, malignancy or ongoing sepsis.
- Recipient and donor for heart transplant should be ABO blood group compatible.
- A cold ischemic time up to 4 hours is considered safe for heart transplantation.
- Bicaval orthotropic heart transplantation is the preferred surgical technique.
- Triple-drug regimen remains the cornerstone for immunosuppressive therapy.
- Episodes of acute rejection and infection are the major risks in early transplant years. Cardiac allograft vasculopathy and malignancy are the major cause of morbidity and mortality in later transplant years.

- Heart transplantation improves survival and quality of life. The mean survival is 80% at 1 year after transplant. The median survival is 10 years.

REFERENCES

1. Carrel A, Guthrie CC. The transplantation of veins and organs. Am. Med, 1905;10:1101.
2. Hardy JD, Chavez CM, Kurrus FD, et al. Heart transplantation in man. JAMA, 1964;188:114.
3. Barnard CN. A human cardiac transplant: An interim report of a successful operation performed at Groote Schuur Hospital, Cape Town. S Afr Med J, 1967;41:1271.
4. Stehik J, Edwards LB, Kucheryavaya AY, et al. The Registry of ISHLT: 29th official Adult Heart Transplant Report-2012, the J Heart & Lung Transplantation, 2012;31:1052-64.
5. Nwakanma LU, Shah AS, Coute JV, Baumgartner WA. Heart Transplantation, Cohn L ed. Cardiac surgery in the Adult. New York; Mc Graw Hill, 2008;1539-78.
6. Wheeldon DR, Polten CD, Oduo A, et al. Transforming the unacceptable donor: outcomes from adoption of standardized donor management technique. J Heart lung transplant, 1995;14:734.
7. Demertzis S, Wipperman J, Schapper J, et al. Univ of Wisconsin versus St. Thomas Hospital Solution for human donor heart preservation.
8. Oshima K, Morishita Y, Yamagishi T, et al. Long term heart hypothermic perfusion apparatus. J Heart Lung Transplant, 1999; 18:852.
9. Yeter R, Hubler M, Pasic M, et al. Organ preservation with organ care system. Applied Cardiopulmonary Pathophysiology, 2011; 15:207-212.
10. Vellota JB, Balram LB, Fischbein MP, et al. Heart Transplantation; Sabiston and Spencer's Surgery of Chest, 8th edn. Frank Settle, Pedro J. del Nido and Scot Swansow, eds. Elsevier Inc. Shumway NE, Lower R, Stofer RC. Transplantation of the heart. Adv. Surgery, 1966;2:265-84.
11. Shumway NE, Lower RR, Stofer RC. Transplantation of the heart. Adv Surg, 1966;2:265-284
12. Lower RR, Stofer RC, Shumway NE. Homovital transplantation of the heart. J Thoracic Cardiovasc Surgery, 1961;41:96-201.
13. Aziz TM, Burgess MI, Gamel AE, et al. Orthotopic heart transplantation technique. A survey of current Practice. Ann Thoracic Surg, 1999;68:1242-6.
14. Sievers HH, Weyend M, Kraatz EG, et al. An alternative technique for orthotopic cardiac transplantation, with preservation of normal anatomy of the right atrium. Thorac Cardiovasc Surg, 1991;39; 70-2.
15. Sarsam MA, Campbell CS, Yonan NA, et al. An alternative technique in orthotopic cardiac transplantation. J Cardiovasc Surg, 1993;8:344-9.
16. Schnoor M, Schafer T, Luhmann D, et al. Bicaval vs standard technique in orthotopic heart transplantation: A systematic review and metanalysis. J Thorac Cardiovasc Surg, 2007;134:1322-31.
17. Yacoub MH, Banner NA. Recent developments in lung and heart lung transplantation. In. Morris PJ, Tilney NE eds. Transplantation reviews, vol 3. Philadelphia: WB Saunders, 1989:1-12.
18. Drefus C, Jebara V, Mihaileaunu S, Carpentier A. Total orthotopic heart transplantation: an alternative to the standard technique. Ann. Thorac Surg, 1991;52:1181-4.
19. Blanche C, Nessim S, Quartel A, Takkenberg JJ, Czer LS, Trento A. Heart Tx with bicaval and pulmonary venous anastomoses. J Cardiovac Surg, 1997;38:561-6.
20. Stehlik J, Edwards LB, Kucheryavaya AY, et al. The Registry of the International Society for Heart and Lung Transplantation: twenty-seventh official adult heart transplant report-2010. J Heart Lung Transplant, 2010;29:1089.
21. Adamson R, Obispo E, Dychter S, et al. Long-term outcome with the use of OKT3 induction therapy in heart transplant patients: a single-center experience. Transplant Proc, 1998;30:1107.
22. Swinnen LJ, Costanzo-Nordin MR, Fisher SG, et al. Increased incidence of lymphoproliferative disorder after immunosuppression with the monoclonal antibody OKT3 in cardiac-transplant recipients. N Engl J Med, 1990;323:1723.
23. Opelz G, Döhler B. Lymphomas after solid organ transplantation: a collaborative transplant study report. Am J Transplant, 2004; 4:222.
24. Higgins R, Kirklin JK, Brown RN, et al. To induce or not to induce: do patients at greatest risk for fatal rejection benefit from cytolytic induction therapy? J Heart Lung Transplant, 2005;24:392.
25. Caillat-Zucman S, Blumenfeld N, Legendre C, et al. The OKT3 immunosuppressive effect. In situ antigenic modulation of human graft-infiltrating T cells. Transplantation, 1990;49:156.
26. Morris PJ, Russell NK. Alemtuzumab (Campath-1H): a systematic review in organ transplantation. Transplantation, 2006;81:1361.
27. Hershberger RE, Starling RC, Eisen HJ, et al. Daclizumab to prevent rejection after cardiac transplantation. N Engl J Med, 2005;352:2705.
28. Grimm M, Rinaldi M, Yonan NA, et al. Superior prevention of acute rejection by tacrolimus vs. cyclosporine in heart transplant recipients-a large European trial. Am J Transplant, 2006;6:1387.
29. Kobashigawa J, Miller L, Renlund D, et al. A randomized active-controlled trial of mycophenolate mofetil in heart transplant recipients. Mycophenolate Mofetil Investigators. Transplantation, 1998;66:507.
30. Kuppahally S, Al-Khaldi A, Weisshaar D, et al. Wound healing complications with de novo sirolimus versus mycophenolate mofetil-based regimen in cardiac transplant recipients. Am J Transplant, 2006;6:986.
31. Keogh A, Richardson M, Ruygrok P, et al. Sirolimus in de novo heart transplant recipients reduces acute rejection and prevents coronary artery disease at 2 years: a randomized clinical trial. Circulation, 2004;110:2694.

16 CHAPTER

Lung Transplantation

Bimla Sharma, Neetu Jain, Pramoj Jindal

INTRODUCTION

Lung transplantation (LT) is the definitive therapy currently available for patients with end-stage pulmonary disease who are refractory to medical treatment.[1] Successful LT dates back to early 1980s, although attempts at human lung transplantation had been made since 1963, when Hardy and co-workers first reported a unilateral lung graft.[2] The recipient lived only for 18 days, but that report provided impetus for the development of LT as a treatment modality. Two decades later, Joel Cooper performed the first lung transplantation with long-term survival. This patient lived for six years before dying of renal failure.[3] However, recent advances in anesthesia, critical care, immunosuppressant therapy, and infection surveillance have made significant contributions in improving the graft function and survival of patients.

The lung transplantation technique has undergone gradual improvement and refinement over the last 30 years. There have been changes in the types of sutures and flush solutions used for the procedures. The major changes in last decade have been the successful living donor and ex-vivo lung transplant programs. The International Society for Heart and Lung Transplantation reported that 3,519 lung transplantation procedures have been performed in 2010, the highest number reported of any year to date.[4] The increased number of procedures has largely been the result of consistent growth in the number of bilateral lung transplants since the mid-1990s, with an unchanged number of single-lung transplants performed annually during this time.

The lung transplantation program has recently been introduced in India.

INDICATIONS

Since LT became technically feasible in 1980s, the spectrum of diseases for which transplantation can be offered has expanded greatly. The indications for lung transplantation include diseases of the pulmonary airways, parenchyma, and vasculature and can be divided into the following groups.

1. Chronic obstructive pulmonary disease (COPD, e.g. emphysema)
2. Suppurative pulmonary disease (e.g. cystic fibrosis)
3. Restrictive pulmonary disease (e.g. pulmonary fibrosis)
4. Pulmonary hypertension (with or without congenital heart disease).

Advanced COPD, idiopathic pulmonary fibrosis (IPF), cystic fibrosis (CF), emphysema due to alpha-1 antitrypsin deficiency, and idiopathic pulmonary arterial hypertension account for approximately 85 percent of all procedures performed worldwide.[4] The remaining 15 percent consist of a variety of diagnoses that span the spectrum of end-stage lung disease from sarcoidosis to lymphangioleiomyomatosis (LAM) to pulmonary Langerhans' cell histiocytosis.[5-10]

CONTRAINDICATIONS

Contraindications for lung transplantation include active malignancy, active sepsis, active tuberculosis, severe neuro-muscular disease, refractory nonadherence to medical care, multiple organ dysfunction, human immunodeficiency virus (HIV) and hepatitis C infection with histologic liver disease. Other contraindications include psychosocial instability, active use of tobacco products during waiting period, obesity or cachexia and history of substance abuse.[11] There is also a list of relative contraindications including issues such as chronic airway infection with multiple resistant organisms, mechanical ventilation, and renal insufficiency.[12] This list varies from center to center and probably will change over time. The age of the recipient may be an important factor in decision for transplantation. The physiological age rather than a strict chronological criterion and the type of transplant procedure also influence the significance of age as a contraindication. Criteria for recipients have been relaxed significantly since the first operations in the 1960s. Presently, the age limit for heart-lung transplant recipients is 55 years, and 60 years for bilateral-lung transplant recipients. It is 65 years for single-lung transplant recipients.[13] The concerns for a potential recipient selected for procedure of lung transplant include long organ waiting time till a suitable organ is procured, maintenance of healthy lifestyle during waiting period, avoiding smoking and improvement of physical condition and rehabilitation.

DONOR CHARACTERISTICS

I. Lung Allocation

There is a great disparity between the number of patients waiting for lung transplantation and the available number of donor organs. This has profound effect on the very sick patients, waiting for lung transplantation. Organ allocation in the USA since May 2005 is based on a Lung Allocation Score (LAS) which replaced the old seniority system by the new priority system with a goal to decrease wait-list mortality.[14] This score is an attempt to balance the urgency for the need of transplant and post transplant chances of survival measure. It has decreased the number of patients on the waiting list by 50%. There was also a decrease in the waiting time from a median of 792 days in 2004 to 200 days or less in each year of 2005–2008.[15]

II. Pulmonary Allograft Procurement and Preservation

Organ Acquisition

Organ availability is the most critical factor in any organ transplantation. Original donor requirements were age less than 40 years, non smokers, and an O_2 index (PaO_2/FiO_2) greater than 350. Many centers are now liberalizing their acceptance criteria.

The lungs and the heart may be used for separate recipients, therefore, the donor lung and cardiac procurement surgery is synchronized.[16] The key goals are aimed to prevent in situ thrombosis and vasospasm and to stabilize the lung for cold storage.

Criteria for selection of brain dead donors for lung transplantation are as follows:

1. No COPD–by history or evaluation of chest X-ray
2. Intubation period < 5 days
3. No fungus on sputum gram stain
4. $PaO_2/FiO_2 > 250$
5. Only small infiltrates on chest X-ray
6. Donor age is center specific

Principles of Management

Medical centers not performing organ transplantations may be involved in optimization of potential organ donors before organ harvest, as proper organ function after transplantation depends significantly on appropriate donor management. Before declaration of brain death, the patient's medical management must be centered on his or her welfare and aimed at recovery. After declaration of brain death, management focus changes from patient's welfare to preservation of organs. Even at this stage, there are some issues that must be considered. Renal transplantation teams prefer liberal fluid administration to provide brisk dilute urine output before harvest but this may worsen the post-transplantation pulmonary edema. From the perspective of the lung harvest team, clearly, lung preservation is the prime focus.

Fluid management is aimed at providing a mean arterial pressure (MAP) of 60 mm Hg by raising central venous pressure (CVP) to 6 to 8 mm Hg and pulmonary capillary wedge pressure (PCWP) to 8 to 12 mm Hg followed by vasoactive drugs, as necessary.[17]

Ongoing medical care after the diagnosis of brain death must be optimal in order to preserve donor organ function. Physiologic derangements in the brain-dead donor include loss of temperature regulation, hypovolemia, hypokalemia, and an acute hormonal deficiency state that commonly includes a reduction in circulating thyroid hormone.[18,19] Up to 40% of donors have systolic dysfunction and ventricular arrhythmias.[20]

Normothermia of the donor should be maintained. Diabetes insipidus should be appropriately treated. FiO_2 should be decreased to maintain PaO_2 at 100 mm Hg (ideally FiO_2 <0.4) and positive end-expiratory pressure (PEEP) 5 cm H_2O should be applied. Minimal and a strict aseptic pulmonary toilet should be done to avoid lung contamination. Newer studies on donor management have focused on organ perfusion as the determining factor in the decision-making process.

Donation After Cardiac Death

Prior to or at the time of declaration of death, the patient is first systemically heparinized 30 minutes before withdrawal of clinical support.[21] After certification of death, the donor is reintubated. A flexible bronchoscopy is performed to rule out aspiration of gastric contents during cardiac arrest and to clear out secretions. A median sternotomy is rapidly performed concurrently; the pericardium is opened and the pulmonary artery cannulated and flushed, before any other dissection is performed. After flushing, the procedure followed is same as that for donation after brain death.

Intraoperative Management

Intraoperative management of the donor is determined by the organs that are being harvested. In the operating room, the multiorgan donor is placed supine and undergoes an extensive midline sternotomy-laparotomy incision from neck to pubis. Commonly administered drugs include a broad-spectrum antibiotic, a nondepolarizing muscle relaxant (to suppress movement associated with spinal reflex activity), and 15 mg/kg methylprednisolone (to moderate inflammatory response). The use of methylprednisolone is associated with improved oxygenation, reduced increases in extravascular lung water, and increased lung yield.[22] During dissection and pulmonary allograft procurement, the donor might require large volumes of fluid resuscitation and is at risk of hypothermia. It is usual for the pulmonary donor to receive a bolus of prostaglandin E1 (PGE1) 500 mcg into the main lung donor artery, followed by cold preservation solution. PGE_1 administration promotes pulmonary vasodilation which in turn helps in uniform spread of the preserving solution.[23] It is recommended that 5 cm H_2O of PEEP be applied during allograft excision and 5 cm H_2O of continuous positive airway pressure (CPAP) applied after excision to maintain partial inflation of the lungs. It is then stored in ice at 0 to 4°C for transfer to its eventual destination.

Role of Inhaled Nitric Oxide (NO)

Administering inhaled NO during excision is helpful probably by attenuating ischemic and oxidant injury during storage and reperfusion.[24] It decreases pulmonary vascular resistance and is reported to mediate several other clinical benefits. It improves oxygenation, decreases inflammatory response to surgery and trauma and impedes microbial growth and the effect is limited only to the pulmonary system.[25] Its use in successful management of lung transplant patients is well documented.[26,27]

Ischemia Time

The shortage of donor organs has led to an extension of the timing criteria to allow for greater transport distances and better donor/recipient matching. Ischemic times up to 8 hours are generally considered acceptable.[28,29] Ueno et al compared early allograft function and outcomes among those who had short (less than 5 hours, n = 20), intermediate (5 to 8 hours, n = 39) and long (more than 8 hours, n = 15) ischemic times.[30] Early allograft function was impaired in those with long ischemic times, but there were no significant differences in other outcomes. This suggests that the acceptable ischemic time in pulmonary transplantation could be longer than previously thought. In spite of advances in lung preservation techniques, it is optimal to limit the donor lung ischemic period to 4 hours.[31]

Preservative Solutions

Balanced (colloid) solutions have been found to be superior to conventional intracellular high potassium, low sodium crystalloid preservative solutions.[32,33] Typically, low-potassium dextran (LPD)-glucose solution (e.g. Perfadex®) is used worldwide for lung transplantation. Preservation with Perfadex is associated with a decreased incidence of primary lung graft dysfunction at 48 hours.[34] Prostaglandin E_1 (PGE_1, alprostadil) and I_2 (PGI_2, prostacyclin, iloprost) are also used for pretreatment or as additives to flush solution to ameliorate ischemia-reperfusion injury.[35,36]

RECIPIENT

Logistical planning and close communication between the surgical and medical team for both donor and recipient is important, detailed discussion and obtaining written informed consent from patient's relatives is mandatory. The donor lungs should be visually inspected and bronchoscopy should be done to identify the bronchial anatomy. The possibility that the donor lungs may be rejected and that the recipient may arrive at the recovery room without a transplant must be explained to the relatives.

Screening, Preoperative Evaluation and Preparation

Donor compatibility is based primarily on ABO compatibility. Major histocompatibility complex (MHC) status is also assessed preoperatively. A detailed physical examination, psychological evaluation and several investigations to assess cardiopulmonary functions are carried out before enrolling the patient into transplant program. Though these parameters are assessed regularly, a review of laboratory and functional data is done immediately before transplantation especially focussing on pulmonary hypertension and cardiac dysfunction. It has been reported that diabetes, atrial fibrillation, elevated systolic pulmonary artery pressure, and low cardiac index before transplantation are associated with a higher risk of death after transplantation.[37]

The recipient is shifted to intensive care unit (ICU) or operating room holding area. Medical records are reviewed and results of recent studies, especially echocardiograms, pulmonary function tests and radionuclide scans are evaluated. Fasting status is determined, adequate blood and products are arranged and anesthetic management and risks are discussed with patient and family.

Premedication with anxiolytics and analgesics is often necessary to allay anxiety as catecholamine release may worsen RV function or pulmonary hypertension. In the operating room, an adequate intravenous access is secured with one or two large bore (14 or 16 gauge) peripheral intravenous catheters. Narcotics should be used cautiously in COPD patients as it may lead to CO_2 retention and hypoxia and exacerbate pulmonary hypertension. Prophylactic antibiotics directed at bacterial, viral and fungal agents are started preoperatively. Immunosuppressants like cyclosporine A and azathioprine are also started preoperatively and high dose steroid therapy-methylprednisolone 1 gm IV is administered along with bronchodilators to protect against airflow obstruction. Aspiration prophylaxis must be given to patients who are not fasting adequately. Supplemental oxygen via nasal cannula with 1–2 L/min must be administered in the holding area and during transfer to operating room.

CHOICE OF PROCEDURE

Four types of transplant procedures are currently available; single lung transplantation (SLT), bilateral lung transplantation (BLT), heart-lung transplantation (HLT) and transplantation of lobes from living related donors.

Single Lung Transplant (SLT)

A single-lung transplant is most commonly chosen for nonseptic end-stage pulmonary disease. An initial decision is required to choose the side of implantation. When the function of the two lungs is equal or when the need for cardiopulmonary bypass (CPB) anticipated, the right side is preferred because of the greater ease of surgical exposure and the institution of CPB via the ascending aorta and right atrium.[38] Single lung transplantation has been used successfully in recipients with pulmonary hypertension.[39] However, it provides less lung function as a buffer for late complications. A standard posterolateral thoracotomy incision is made for SLT, while ventilation is being given to the contralateral lung; the lung to be excised is deflated and mobilized. During dissection the phrenic and vagus nerves and recurrent laryngeal nerve on left side are identified and preserved. The native lung is extracted, and the donor lung is implanted. The three anastomoses to be performed in their posterior-to-anterior anatomic sequence are: bronchus, pulmonary artery, and pulmonary veins to left atrium.

Bilateral Lung Transplant (BLT)

It is indicated primarily for conditions that necessitate removal of both infected lungs, e.g. cystic fibrosis and bronchiectasis. In some centers, double-LT for recipients with pulmonary hypertension is preferred to avoid hyperperfusion and pulmonary edema in the transplanted lung, which is sometimes seen in these patients when a single lung is transplanted. Others recommend the routine use of BLT in young patients with end-stage emphysema because of improved survival and functional status after transplantation.[40,41]

The most commonly used incision for bilateral lung transplant is bilateral, anterolateral thoracotomy with the patient in supine position. The incision can be modified in case the use of CPB is anticipated.

The BLT is performed in 97 percent of pediatric lung transplant cases and in slightly more than 50 percent of adult cases. The original double–lung technique was performed through a median sternotomy with the recipient on cardiopulmonary bypass, and the donor lungs were implanted en bloc with a single tracheal anastomosis.[42]

Complications related to ischemia of the bronchi and trachea around the carina led to the introduction of bilateral sequential lung implantation (BSLT) as the method of choice.[43,44] It was introduced in 1989 and has become a standard approach since then.[45] It is performed through a transverse thoracosternotomy, and the lungs are implanted separately and sequentially.[46] The incision provides excellent exposure of the pleural space, and the bronchial anastomoses are less prone to complications than the tracheal anastomosis. In the majority of cases, CPB can be avoided by supporting the recipient with the contralateral lung.

Heart Lung Transplant (HLT)

End-stage pulmonary disease and concomitant cardiac diseases such as Eisenmenger syndrome with irreparable cardiac defects, IPAH with right ventricular decompensation and advanced lung disease with concurrent severe left ventricular dysfunction or extensive coronary artery disease are some of the indications reserved for HLT.[47]

There is a decline in the number of HLT as most diseases are amenable to isolated lung transplantation. Bilateral sequential lung transplant and improved pharmacologic management of pulmonary hypertension have largely replaced heart-lung transplantation. During the past two decades, the proportion of adult transplants for diagnoses of congenital heart disease and PAH has remained largely unchanged, and the proportion of heart-lung transplant for cystic fibrosis has decreased. Similar to prior reports, there are significant geographic differences in major indications. The reported data between January 2000 and June 2011 show that European and other non-North American centers performed a greater proportion of transplants for cystic fibrosis and that a greater proportion of procedures at North American centers were performed for congenital heart disease.[4] Anesthetic management of these patients is similar to that of isolated heart or lung transplant patients. Since a tracheal anastomosis is performed, a single-lumen endotracheal tube is adequate.

Living Donor Lobar Transplantation

It was introduced in 1993 to overcome the shortage of cadaveric lung donors.[48] Many reports of successful living-donor lobar transplantation have been described.[49-51] It is used as an alternative to cadaveric LT, primarily for cystic fibrosis.[52] Two healthy blood group compatible living donors are selected, one to undergo removal of the right lower lobe and the other for removal of the left lower lobe. These lobes are then implanted in the recipient in place of the whole right and left lungs. This technique has been demonstrated to benefit a small group of patients who would have succumbed to disease while waiting for a cadaveric donor. The main challenges include the size disparity between the donor lobe and recipient pleural thoracic cavity and the abundant blood flow (the entire cardiac output) supplying the two relatively undersized lobes. The overall survival at 1, 3, and 5 years is 67%, 51%, and 48%, respectively for adult recipients.[49-52] Recipient outcomes have been satisfactory and donor morbidity has been minimal.[53]

Retransplantation

Retransplantation is infrequently done. In the International Society for Heart and Lung Transplantation (ISHLT) registry, it was indicated in only 4% of lung and heart-lung procedures.[54] The most common reasons for retransplantation are; early graft failure, intractable airway complications and chronic rejection.[55] Retransplantation should be considered only for carefully selected patients who are ambulatory and who would meet most other general guidelines for a first transplant.

Novel Approaches to Facilitate Lung Transplantation

A. Expansion of Lung Donor Pool

Novel sources of donor lungs and aggressive management of the lung donor can increase the number of donor lungs available.

a. Living related lobar transplantation is routinely performed in Japan in increasingly innovative scenarios. The results are superior or comparable to standard cadaveric lung transplant.[56,57]

b. Cadaveric donors

   Lungs from donors after cardiac death (DCD) are used to increase the donor pool.[58] There are two advantages of DCD lung donation. Firstly, brain death induced neurogenic pulmonary edema is avoided. Secondly, lung injury resulting from systemic inflammation following brain death may also be avoided.

c. Ex-vivo lung perfusion (EVLP) (Fig. 16.1)

   The technique is used to reassess the adequacy of lung function from DCD and high-risk brain death donors prior to transplantation. It can also act as a platform for the delivery of novel therapies to repair injured organs ex-vivo.[59] Normothermic perfusion provides functional and more accurate assessment of the lung function in comparison to in vivo assessment. It allows therapeutic interventions to optimize the donor lung prior to transplantation.

   Renewed interest in ex-vivo lung perfusion has been triggered by the need to develop a method to assess marginal donor lungs which could include those with edema or from non-heart-beating donors.

   Development of ex-vivo lung perfusion could affect several aspects of transplantation in coming years and be one of the most important advances of the past two decades. The extension of preservation time will allow immunological compatibility testing and appropriate assessments of organ function to be done to enable organs to be obtained from distant locations. Additionally, several biomarkers could allow rapid and accurate diagnosis of lung problems during the preservation period and improve the treatment of each individual patient. A pilot study has recently reported about use of a mobile organ care system (OCS)—the integrated and portable OCS Lung—which is a fresh development in ex-vivo lung perfusion.[60]

d. Single lung transplantation in place of bilateral lung transplantation

   Shortage of donor organs has led to more cases of single lung transplantation being performed. Infectious lung disease is the only absolute contraindication to SLT.

B. Extracorporeal Life Support as a Bridge to Lung Transplantation (ECLS)

Patients who are excellent candidates for lung transplantation often die on the waiting list because they are too sick to survive until an organ becomes available. Improvements in

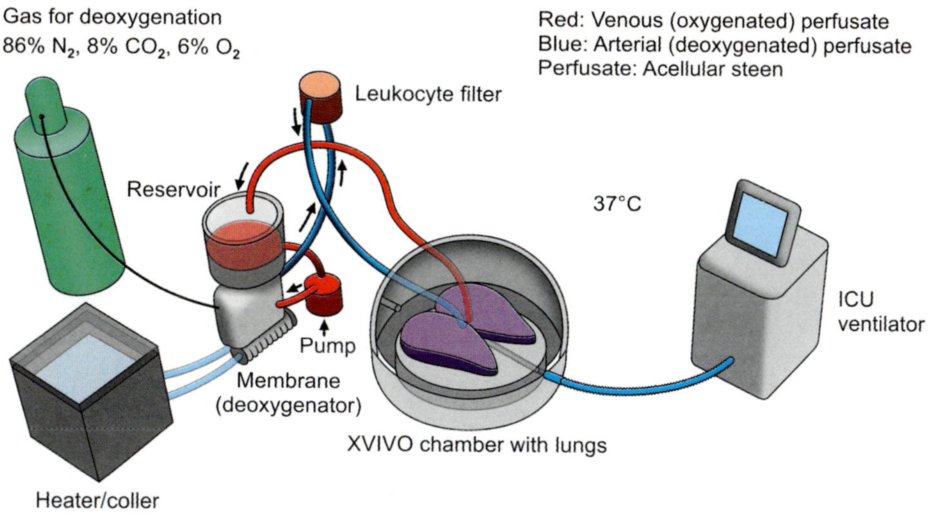

Fig. 16.1: Ex vivo lung perfusion equipment "Reprinted from: Clinics in Chest Medicine; 32(2); Marcelo Cypel, Jonathan C. Yeung, Shaf Keshavjee; Novel Approaches to Expanding the Lung Donor Pool: Donation After Cardiac Death and Ex Vivo Conditioning; 233–244; June 2011; with permission from Elsevier".]

lung transplant outcomes, patient selection, and artificial lung device technologies have made it possible to bridge these patients to successful life-saving transplantation. Extracorporeal life support (ECLS) should be tailored to minimize morbidity and provide the appropriate mode and level of cardiopulmonary support for each patient's physiologic requirements. Novel device refinements and further development of ECLS in an ambulatory and simplified manner will help maintain these patients in better condition until transplantation.[61]

C. Alternatives to Lung Transplantation: Lung Volume Reduction Surgery (LVRS) for COPD

The LVRS or reduction pneumoplasty may be indicated in patients as an alternative treatment for select patients with COPD undergoing consideration for lung transplantation. It is performed either through a median sternotomy or a bilateral thoracoscopy with an aim to remove a part (30%) of the patient's most severely compromised lung. Postoperatively the chest mechanics and the lung functions improve but this may take about 1–2 months. The National Emphysema Treatment Trial (NETT) has demonstrated short-term and long-term effectiveness, and the essential factors that predict the success or failure of lung volume reduction surgery (LVRS).[62,63]

A variety of novel, less invasive bronchoscopic techniques are currently undergoing study and show promise to effectively produce lung reduction in a broader group of patients with advanced emphysema. Additional well-designed prospective studies are needed to determine the optimum role of LVRS versus bronchoscopic LVR in the treatment of severe emphysema.[64]

D. Lungs Repair

Research is also being carried out to achieve lung repair with gene therapy or stem cells. Transtracheal delivery of gene vectors can localize the effect to the lung graft. The introduction of anti-inflammatory cytokines to lung cells is one attractive approach.[65,66]

ANESTHETIC MANAGEMENT

Induction

After arrival of the patient in the operating room, standard monitoring including ECG, NIBP, SpO_2, temperature, BIS and invasive hemodynamic monitoring in form of arterial blood pressure, central venous pressure and pulmonary artery pressure is instituted. Pulmonary artery pressure monitoring is especially important. During surgery, care must be taken to make sure that the pulmonary artery catheter is withdrawn from the pulmonary artery to be stapled and refloated to the nonoperative lung. Capnography, inhalational agent monitoring, transoesophageal echocardiography (TEE) are started after tracheal intubation. Various modifications of pulmonary artery catheter and continuous arterial blood gas monitoring may be instituted depending on case profile and institutional practice. Strict asepsis should be maintained while placing intra arterial, central venous and pulmonary artery catheters. Thoracic epidural catheter (T6–T8) should be considered for postoperative pain relief except in patients in whom CPB may be required in which case the epidural may be placed postoperatively.

During induction, the recipient may need aspiration prophylaxis due to emergent nature of procedure.[22] Preoxygenation should precede induction of anesthesia followed by rapid or modified rapid sequence induction. Prolonged preoxygenation for about 15 minutes is indicated in obstructive lung disease and high residual volumes patients to ensure proper denitrogenation.

Thiopentone, etomidate, propofol, and ketamine have all been used safely. But specific properties of each drug in the setting of the patient's underlying disease should be considered. Thiopentone may be used as an induction agent especially in young patients with normal heart function. Etomidate is also used at various institutions because of its cardiostability. Succinylcholine (1.5 mg/kg) is frequently used for rapid – sequence induction. For modified rapid–sequence induction, slow titration of opiates is used to reduce the effects of rapid withdrawal of sympathetic tone, which may result in cardiovascular collapse.[12] Muscle relaxation may be achieved by a non histamine releasing agent such as vecuronium. Pancuronium may be used to maintain mild tachycardia and cardiac output, especially in patients with right heart failure.

In patients with impaired ventricular function or greater degrees of pulmonary hypertension, most notably, those with primary pulmonary hypertension or cyanotic congenital heart disease, induction of anesthesia needs to be modified further. Such patients should be optimized before induction of anesthesia, which could require commencement of an inotrope infusion, usually in conjunction with a selective pulmonary vasodilator such as inhaled nitric oxide (NO).[67,68] Inhaled nitric oxide represents the first choice for treatment of PH and RV failure associated with systemic hypotension during lung transplantation. Intraoperative situations such as severe hypotension requiring CPB must be identified before development of systemic shock, which represents a late ominous sign of RV failure. Need for emergency CPB or femoral artery cannulation should be anticipated and kept ready in high risk group.

Post induction hypotension may result from decreased cardiac output from hypovolemia, vasodilation and negative inotropic effects from the induction agents, worsening pulmonary hypertension with RV dysfunction or failure. The negative effects of positive pressure ventilation on venous return and epidural local anesthetics may also contribute to hypotension.

Airway Management

Pulmonary isolation is required for patients undergoing SLT and most of those undergoing BSLT. The most commonly used device is a disposable polyvinyl chloride double lumen tube DLT, although the univent tube (Fuji Systems, Japan) or a bronchial blocker is employed occasionally.

Most patients can be managed with a left-sided DLT, with the bronchial cuff positioned just distal to the carina so that it does not impinge on the bronchial anastomosis. Segmental bronchial lavage at induction through a single lumen tube, before placement of the DLT helps in suctioning via the DLT in patients with copious secretions. This should be followed by frequent aspiration through both lumens with 8–12 F suction catheters which are superior to the narrow suction port of the fiberoptic bronchoscope.[31] In addition; the DLT facilitates oxygenation and examination of the bronchial anastomoses. The positioning of DLTs has been assisted by an improvement in DLT designs with shorter endobronchial segments and increased familiarity of anesthesiologists with fiberoscopic lobar anatomy. Bronchial blockers may also be employed for lung isolation but they require repositioning during midsurgery as they get easily dislodged.

Patients undergoing heart lung transplantation, bilateral lung transplantation or those requiring CPB are managed with a single lumen tracheal tube. Patients with known or suspected abnormalities of airway anatomy should be intubated awake after topical anesthesia is applied to the airway.

At times pulmonary ventilation may be impaired or pulmonary isolation compromised; this requires vigilance and manipulation of the endobronchial device. Initially, a FIO_2 of 1.0 is chosen, and this can be reduced after pulmonary allograft implantation. Nitrous oxide is best avoided during pulmonary transplantation, as it can increase PVR, and the recipient is then at risk of air embolism following reperfusion of the allograft.

Maintenance of Anesthesia

Anesthesia can be maintained using a variety of techniques including a balanced technique with low doses of inhaled anesthetics, opiates, muscle relaxants and supplemented by neuraxial blockade through thoracic epidural catheter. A moderate dose of narcotic (5 to 15 ug/kg fentanyl or the equivalent), combined with low doses of a potent inhalation anesthetic, offers the advantages of stable hemodynamics, a high inspired oxygen concentration, a rapidly titratable depth of anesthesia, and the possibility of extubation in the early postoperative period.

Anesthetic maintenance may also be based on intravenous infusions owing to the frequent need for airway access (e.g. suctioning, bronchoscopy), which causes problems in maintaining a stable level of inspired anesthetic vapour. Nitrous oxide is seldom used because of bullous emphysematous disease, pulmonary hypertension, or intraoperative hypoxemia.[69] It is also generally not used because of the requirement for a high inspired oxygen concentration throughout the procedure and its possible deleterious effects if gaseous emboli or an occult pneumothorax is present.[23]

For mild to moderate PAH, fluid restriction, intravenous arterial dilators (nitroglycerine, SNP), direct pulmonary vasodilators (PGE1, prostacyclin) or inhaled NO (20–40 ppm) may be used. In severe cases up to 80 ppm inhaled NO may be required or cardiopulmonary bypass may be instituted. Inotropes such as dobutamine, milrinone may also be required. Inhaled or infused sildenafil has been demonstrated to have an additive effect to inhaled iNO and may be used more often in the future.[70]

Fluid administration should be judicious and excessive fluids should be avoided. The CVP should be maintained at or below 7 cm H_2O with intermittent fluid administration or vasoactive drugs. A study reported that CVP greater than 7 mm Hg correlated with longer intensive care unit stays and higher mortality.[71]

In patients undergoing bilateral LT for cystic fibrosis with significant adhesions or a history of previous intrathoracic surgery, continuous infusion of an antifibrinolytic (€ aminocaproic acid or aprotinin infusion) has been proposed to reduce intraoperative bleeding. Transfusion therapy should be discussed between members of both the anesthesiology and surgical staff and remains a team decision.[72] The anesthesiologist must know whether the patient has antibodies to cytomegalovirus and must closely check blood products to confirm that they coincide with the patient's status. Parameters of end organ perfusion such as urine output must be monitored.

Ventilatory Strategies

After initiation of positive-pressure ventilation it is vital to avoid hyperinflation in patients with increased pulmonary compliance or bullous disease. High airway pressure may cause barotrauma as rupture of bulbous emphysema causes pneumothorax. Acute reductions in SaO_2 accompanied by difficulty in ventilating the lungs and refractory hypotension should generate strong suspicions that a tension pneumothorax has developed. In the event of hemodynamic instability with positive-pressure ventilation, the ventilator should be disconnected from the patient. If hyperinflation is the cause of hypotension, blood pressure will increase within 10 to 30 seconds of the onset of apnea. Ventilation then can be resumed at a tidal volume and/or rate compatible with hemodynamic stability. Disruption of tracheobronchial anastomosis may also occur due to high airway pressure.

Volutrauma may occur due to dynamic hyperinflation of compliant lung and circulatory collapse may ensue due to decreased venous return. The ventilatory strategies which may be used in LT to avoid barotrauma and volutrauma are; low tidal volumes 6–8 mL/kg, reduced respiratory rate (6–10/min), maximal expiratory time (1:E=1:3) , increased inspiratory flow rate, use of pressure control ventilation, high frequency jet ventilation and allowing elevated levels of $PaCO_2$ or permissive hypercapnia.[23,73]

One lung ventilation (OLV) is required in all patients except those who need CPB. It increases intrapulmonary shunt, PVR and further worsens hypoxaemia, hypercarbia and acidosis. To improve oxygenation during OLV, intermittent lung inflation, CPAP to nonventilated lung and or PEEP to ventilated lung may be required. Intermittent suctioning of secretions should be done to prevent regional atelectasis. In cases of refractory hypoxaemia, recruitment manoeuvres are used to recruit atelectatic lung tissue. Hypoxic pulmonary vasoconstriction may be improved by reducing concentrations of inhalational anaesthetics and avoiding vasodilators such as nitroglycerine. In patients with pre-existing or recent onset pulmonary hypertension, OLV may be most challenging. Pulmonary vasodilatiors like NTG, nitroprusside, nitric oxide, prostaglandin I_2 with 100% oxygen may be used to decrease pulmonary vascular resistance.

With restrictive lung disease, higher inflation pressures and positive end-expiratory pressure (PEEP) are often required. In both patients with obstructive disease and patients with restrictive disease, optimal balance of ventilation with hemodynamic stability often necessitates tolerating a degree of hypercapnia. In patients with pulmonary hypertension, mechanical ventilation usually produces less cardiovascular disturbance if caution is exercised not to increase pulmonary vascular resistance (e.g. from hypoxia, hypercarbia, or lung hyperinflation).

Pulmonary Artery Clamping

To anticipate the effects of pulmonary artery clamping, test clamping of PA is done and effects on pulmonary artery pressure (PAP) and right ventricular function are evaluated. It is important to monitor PAP, CVP, and cardiac output. Transoesophageal echocardiography can be used to directly evaluate right ventricular function, distension, new tricuspid regurgitation, and right ventricular cardiac output. It is extremely useful for managing the patient's cardiopulmonary status and recognizing an urgent need for CPB.[68] It also used to examine the sites of pulmonary artery and venous anastomosis. This may aid in the detection of functional complications that may resolve through medical or surgical management.

Role of Cardiopulmonary Bypass and ECMO

The CPB is not routinely required and its use varies with recipient lung disease. Its role is anticipated in adult patients with severe pulmonary arterial hypertension, restrictive lung disease and pediatric recipients. It may also be indicated in patients with unstable hemodynamics or refractory hypoxemia.[46,74] In patients with restrictive disease, bypass is usually indicated if the fall in cardiac index is more than 1.0 to 1.5 L/min/m^2 after clamping the pulmonary artery.[74,75] These patients are anticoagulated with heparin with majority of dissection performed before its administration.

The ECMO has been suggested as an alternative method of CPB during lung transplantation. It offers several advantages over CPB.[76,77] It may improve the outcome by lessening the amount of pulmonary edema, especially in patients who need CPB, it clears the field of bypass cannula making left—sided transplant as unimpeded as the right sided transplant and lung perfusion in the newly transplanted lung can be easily controlled.

Reperfusion

At the time of reperfusion 1 gm methylprednisolone is given intravenously. Mannitol may also be used, both for its diuretic and its free radical superoxides-cavenging activity.[78] Before reperfusion, the anesthesiologist bronchoscopically assesses the bronchial anastomosis and removes secretions and blood. The implanted lung is re-expanded with a slow continuous airway breath to reduce the effect of rapid rexpansion and barotrauma. Peak pressures on ventilator should be aimed to less than 40 mm Hg and plateau pressure should be maintained at less than 35 mm Hg.

The pulmonary venous clamp is removed that allows retrograde blood flow, followed by reperfusion of graft by declamping the pulmonary artery. The time of reperfusion may be critical as pulmoplegia and anerobic metabolites washout may be associated with systemic hypotension and coronary embolization. This may be detected by arrhythmias or new regional wall motion abnormalities on TEE.

Some centers purposely maintain systolic pressure in the range of 80–90 mm Hg to avoid bleeding and reduce PAP. The PAP frequently decreases significantly after reperfusion of the lung. Some patients may develop acute lung injury or transfusion-related lung injury that manifests with pulmonary edema, persistent hypoxemia, elevated PAP, and decreased cardiac output. This may require vasopressor and inotropic support and inhaled NO. Packed red blood cells should be transfused to maintain a hematocrit of 30–35%, especially if mixed venous oxygen saturation is below 65%. In extreme cases, ECMO or high frequency jet ventilation may be required to maintain oxygenation and ventilation. If other modalities are not available, individually ventilating each lung with a DLT and two ventilators is possible.

Pediatric Considerations

Cystic fibrosis, congenital heart disease (CHD), and primary pulmonary hypertension are the main indications for lung transplantation in children.[79] CHD is the most common indication for lung transplantation in infants, while cystic fibrosis is the most common indication in adolescents. Bilateral lung transplantation is the operation of choice due to the underlying pulmonary vascular disease or infectious process in these children, Single-lung transplantation is less commonly performed in this age group. Transplantation is recommended when the life expectancy of the child is 2 years or less. In contrast with the adult population, CPB is frequently utilized during lung transplantation in children.

Postoperative Care and Assessment of Graft Function

All effort is focussed on identification and appropriate management of evolving graft function.[56] Most lung transplant patients are electively ventilated for 6–24 hours. The aim of ventilation is to maintain adequate oxygenation using low airway pressures and low tidal volume to prevent barotrauma, volutrauma and anastomotic dehiscence. Selected patients undergoing SLT may be extubated on the table.

Low-level positive end-expiratory pressure (PEEP) is a standard part of postoperative ventilatory support. Some patients may require ventilation for longer times depending on graft function, function of respiratory muscles, phrenic nerve injury, untreated pain or unstable hemodynamics. Early allograft function should be assessed by arterial blood gas analysis, chest X-ray and if indicated, repeat bronchoscopy or lung biopsy. Early bronchoscopy and judiciously targeted antibiotics minimize deleterious effects of donor derived infections. The presence of infiltrates on chest X-ray is almost universal after LT. The causes include ischemic reperfusion injury associated with alveolar endothelial leakage and impaired interstial fluid clearance due to absence of lymphatic drainage. Other causes include infection and rejection; these usually occur later and may require prolonged ICU stay.

In patients with primary pulmonary hypertension who receive a single LT, there is an increased risk of noncardiogenic reperfusion pulmonary edema due to preferential "luxury" perfusion of the transplanted lung with low PVR as compared to native diseased lung. These patients are more prone to respiratory failure and may required prolonged ventilation and gradual weaning.

Patients with COPD or emphysema, undergoing single LT are at risk of hyperinflation of remaining native lung because of its high compliance. This can lead to mediastinal shift and hemodynamic disturbances and may require DLT and differential lung ventilation. PEEP is not used, or is limited to low pressures (e.g. 5 cm H_2O), because it may overinflate the more compliant native lung.[80]

Postoperatively, most lung transplant patients are on infusion regimens of short acting sedatives such as propofol to facilitate weaning from mechanical ventilation. Adequate ventilation and clearance of secretions are assisted by effective pain relief using epidural infusions of local anesthetics and narcotics. Uncontrolled pain will predispose to atelectasis, sputum retention and infection. Peripheral infusions of intravenous opiates may be used for patients without an epidural catheter. Multimodal analgesic techniques using opioid-sparing agents such as paracetamol and tramadol may be used while nonsteroidal anti-inflammatory drugs (NSAIDs) and cyclooxygenase-2 inhibitors are generally used with caution.

General Management

Patients may require inotropic or vasopressor support to maintain hemodynamic stability while avoiding large fluid volumes to keep the lungs dry. Blood transfusion is kept to a minimum to reduce the risk of transfusion related acute lung injury. Inhaled nitric oxide may be required to lower pulmonary artery pressure and intrapulmonary shunting. Head-up position also helps to reduce preload, improve lung inflation, and lower pulmonary artery pressure.

Renal dysfunction may occur within few days of surgery and may require careful management with pulmonary artery monitoring and judicious use of antibiotic and immunosuppressive therapy.

Physiologic Effects of Lung Transplantation

Successful lung transplantation whether single or bilateral can significantly improve lung function. The innervation, lymphatics, and bronchial circulation are disrupted when the donor pneumonectomy is performed. The principal effect of lung denervation is loss of the cough reflex, which places patients at risk of aspiration and pulmonary infection. Mucociliary clearance is impaired during the early postoperative period. Lymphatic drainage disrupted by transaction of the trachea and bronchi may be re-established during the first 2 to 4 weeks postoperatively. Often a blunted ventilatory response to carbon dioxide persists even though pulmonary function improves. Denervation of the heart is another consideration in patients undergoing heart-lung transplantation.

COMPLICATIONS

The complications can be grouped as early or late. Early graft dysfunction, episodes of rejection, infection and airway complications are the major early complications of lung transplantation. Primary graft dysfunction (PGD), analogous to acute respiratory distress syndrome (ARDS) arises within the first 72 hours following lung transplantation, and is a leading cause of early morbidity and mortality. The severity of PGD has been graded on a scale of 0–3.[81] As per this grading, a study found that recipients who were PGD grade 3 at 48 hours after transplant had 33 percent 90-day mortality.[82]

Management of PGD includes fluid restriction, diuretics, PEEP, inhaled NO and ECMO for severe cases. Immunosuppression is usually initiated before surgery and the induction phase of therapy is continued for 5 to 10 days. The exact regimen varies among antilymphocyte/antithymocyte globulins or interleukin-2 receptor antagonists. Acute rejection episodes are usually treated with intense steroid therapy and optimization of other immunosuppressant dosages. A challenge arises in differentiating acute rejection from infection as a source of shunting and chest radiograph infiltrates. Transbronchial biopsy is often necessary to make the distinction from histologic specimens.

Bacterial pneumonia is the most frequent infection in the first 2 weeks. Although unusual in the first 2 weeks after transplantation, cytomegalovirus in the second most common source of infectious pneumonitis. Broad-spectrum antibiotics are given perioperatively and the regimen is adjusted based on the results of donor and recipient cultures. Antibiotic therapy for patients with cystic fibrosis is challenging and the chosen drug is guided by the patient's cultures and prior history of the organisms colonizing his or her lung. Prophylactic acyclovir appears to be effective in reducing infection caused by herpes simplex and trimethoprim sulfamethoxazole is given to prevent infection from pneumocystis carinii.[83]

Other postoperative complications include hemorrhage, right ventricular failure, neurologic injury (brain, phrenic nerve, and brachial plexus), drug toxicity (immonosuppressants, antibiotics, sedatives) and muscle weakness (myopathy, neuropathy, malnutrition). About 20% patients may develop anastomotic airway complications affecting their survival.[84] It has been reported that endoscopic evaluations within 21 days after transplantation may help predict this problem.[85] Pleural complications such as empyema may also occur.

Late complications include chronic rejection characterized by bronchiolitis obliterans syndrome (BOS), post transplant lymphoproliferative disorders including lymphomas, skin carcinomas, perineal carcinoma, cervical cancer and Kaposi's sarcoma. The incidence of BOS approaches 50% within five years of transplantation.[86] This is followed by a survival of 50% after three years and 30% to 40% after five years.[87]

CLINICAL PEARLS

- Broader donor criteria, use of marginal donors and living lobar lung transplant are being practised so as to reduce the donor supply mismatch. The novel approaches such as EVLP and ECLS have made their way from experimental stage to clinical use in lung transplantation. Research is also taking place on feasibility of pulmonary xenotransplantation. The surgical and technical aspects of lung transplantation have been refined, though slowly, over the least three decades. There is better understanding of the management of complex pathophysiology of PGD. In spite of considerable improvement in the operative survival, the long-term survival of these patients is only around 50%, way behind other transplanted organs.

REFERENCES

1. Rosenberg AL, Rao M, Benedict PE. Anesthetic implications for lung transplantation. Anesthesiol Clin North America, 2004;22:767-88.
2. Hardy JD, Webb WR, Dalton ML Jr, Walker GR Jr. Lung homotransplantation in man. JAMA, 1963;186:1065-74.
3. Cooper JD, Pearson FG, Patterson GA, et al. Technique of successful lung transplantation in humans. J Thorac Cardiovasc Surg, 1987;93:173-81.
4. Christie JD, Edwards LB, Kucheryavaya AY, et al. International Society of Heart and Lung Transplantation. The Registry of the International Society for Heart and Lung Transplantation: 29th Adult Lung and Heart-lung Transplant Report-2012. J Heart Lung Transplant, 2012;31(10):1073-86.
5. Shorr AF, Davies DB, Nathan SD. Outcomes for patients with sarcoidosis awaiting lung transplantation. Chest, 2002;122:233.
6. Shorr AF, Davies DB, Nathan SD. Predicting mortality in patients with sarcoidosis awaiting lung transplantation. Chest, 2003;124:922.
7. Milman N, Burton C, Andersen CB, et al. Lung transplantation for end-stage pulmonary sarcoidosis: outcome in a series of seven consecutive patients. Sarcoidosis Vasc Diffuse Lung Dis, 2005;22:222-28.
8. Kpodonu J, Massad MG, Chaer RA, et al. The US experience with lung transplantation for pulmonary lymphangioleiomyomatosis. J Heart Lung Transplant, 2005;24:1247-53.
9. Pechet TT, Meyers BF, Guthrie TJ, et al. Lung transplantation for lymphangioleiomyomatosis. J Heart Lung Transplant, 2004;23:301-8.
10. Dauriat G, Mal H, Thabut G, et al. Lung transplantation for pulmonary langerhans' cell histiocytosis: a multicenter analysis. Transplantation, 2006;81:746.
11. Orens JB, Estenne M, Arcasoy S, et al. Pulmonary Scientific Council of the International Society for Heart and Lung Transplantation. International guidelines for the selection of lung transplant candidates: 2006 update-a consensus report from the Pulmonary Scientific Council of the International Society for Heart and Lung Transplantation. J Heart Lung Transplant, 2006;25(7):745-55.
12. Faro A, Mallory GB, Visner GA, et al. American Society of Transplantation executive summary on pediatric lung transplantation. Am J Transplant, 2007;7:285-92.
13. DeMeo DL, Ginns LC. Clinical status of lung transplantation. Transplantation, 2001;72:1713-24.
14. Gries CJ, Mulligan MS, Edelman JD, et al. Lung allocation score for lung transplantation: impact on disease severity and survival. Chest, 2007;132:1954-61.
15. Yusen RD, Shearon TH, Qian Y, et al. Lung transplantation in the United States, 1999-2008. Am J Transplant, 2010;10:1047-68.
16. Puri V, Patterson GA. Adult lung transplantation: technical considerations. Semin Thorac Cardiovasc Surg, 2008;20:152-64.
17. SAFE Study Investigators, Australian and New Zealand Intensive Care Society Clinical Trials Group, Australian Red Cross Blood Service, et al. Saline or albumin for fluid resuscitation in patients with traumatic brain injury. N Engl J Med, 2007;357:874.
18. Dujardin KS, McCully RB, Wijdicks EF, et al. Myocardial dysfunction associated with brain death: clinical, echocardiographic, and pathologic features. J Heart Lung Transplant, 2001;20:350-7.
19. Buckley T. Management of the Multiorgan donor. In Oh TE (ed): Intensive Care Manual, 4th edn. Sydney 1997, Butterworth-Heinemann.
20. Daemen JW, Kootstra G, Wijnen RM, et al. Nonheart-beating donors: the Maastricht experience. Clin Transpl, 1994:303-16.
21. Cypel M, Sato M, Yildirim E, et al. Initial experience with lung donation after cardiocirculatory death in Canada. J Heart Lung Transplant, 2009;28:753-8.
22. Venkateswaran RV, Patchell VB, Wilson IC, et al. Early donor management increases the retrieval rate of lung for transplantation. Ann Thorac Surg, 2008;85:278-86.
23. Quinlan JJ, Murray AW, Casta A. Anesthesia for heart, lung, and heart-lung transplantation. In: Kaplan JA(ed): Kaplan's Cardiac Anesthesia. Elsevier Inc; 2011;p742-44.
24. Fujino S, Nagahiro I, Triantafillou AN, et al. Inhaled nitric oxide at the time of harvest improves early lung allograft function. Ann Thorac Surg, 1997;63:1383-9.
25. Trulock EP, Christie JD, Edwards LB, et al. Registry of the International Society for Heart and Lung Transplantation: twenty-fourth official adult lung and heart-lung transplantation report-2007. J Heart Lung Transplant, 2007;26:782-95.
26. Cornfield DN, Milla CE, Haddad IY, et al. Safety of inhaled nitric oxide after lung transplantation. J Heart Lung Transplant, 2003;22:903-7.

27. Hoehn T, Huebner J, Paboura E, et al. Effect of therapeutic concentrations of nitric oxide on bacterial growth in vitro. Crit Care Med, 1998;26:1857.
28. Thabut G, Mal H, Cerrina J, et al. Graft ischemic time and outcome of lung transplantation: a multicenter analysis. Am J Respir Crit Care Med, 2005;171:786-91.
29. Keshavjee S, Davis RD, Zamora MR, et al. A randomized, placebo-controlled trial of complement inhibition in ischemia-reperfusion injury after lung transplantation in human beings. J Thorac Cardiovasc Surg, 2005;129:423-8.
30. Ueno T, Snell GI, Williams TJ, et al. Impact of graft ischemic time on outcomes after bilateral sequential single-lung transplantation. Ann Thorac Surg, 1999;67:1577-82.
31. Slinger PD and Campos JH. Anesthesia for thoracic surgery. In Miller R.D. (ed): Miller's Anesthesia, 7th ed. Philladelphia, Churchill Livingstone, 2010,p1819-1888.
32. Rabanal JM, Ibañez AM, Mons R, et al. Influence of preservation solution on early lung function (Euro-Collins vs Perfadex). Transplant Proc, 2003;35:1938-39.
33. Arnaoutakis GJ, Allen JG, Merlo CA, et al. Low potassium dextran is superior to University of Wisconsin solution in high-risk lung transplant recipients. J Heart Lung Transplant, 2010;29:1380-87.
34. Marasco SF, Bailey M, McGlade D, et al. Effect of donor preservation solution and survival in lung transplantation. J Heart Lung Transplant, 2011;30:414-9.
35. de Perrot M, Fischer S, Liu M, et al. Prostaglandin E1 protects lung transplants from ischemia-reperfusion injury: a shift from pro-to anti-inflammatory cytokines. Transplantation, 2001;72:1505-12.
36. Gohrbandt B, Sommer SP, Fischer S, et al. Iloprost to improve surfactant function in porcine pulmonary grafts stored for twenty-four hours in low-potassium dextran solution. J Thorac Cardiovasc Surg, 2005;129:80-6.
37. Plantier L, Skhiri N, Biondi G, et al. Impact of previous cardiovascular disease on the outcome of lung transplantation. J Heart Lung Transplant, 2010;29:1270-76.
38. Wain JC. Lung Transplantation, in Fishman, AP, ed. Fishman's Pulmonary Diseases and Disorders, 4th edn. New York, McGraw Hill, 2008;pp 1769-98.
39. Gammie JS, Keenan RJ, Pham SM, et al. Single- versus double-lung transplantation for pulmonary hypertension. J Thorac Cardiovasc Surg, 1998;115:397-402.
40. Sundaresan RS, Shiraishi Y, Trulock EP, et al. Single or bilateral lung transplantation for emphysema? J Thorac Cardiovasc Surg, 1996;112:1485-94.
41. Bavaria JE, Kotloff R, Palevsky H, et al. Bilateral versus single lung transplantation for chronic obstructive pulmonary disease. J Thorac Cardiovasc Surg, 1997;113:520-7.
42. Patterson GA, Cooper JD, Goldman B, et al. Technique of successful clinical double-lung transplantation. Ann Thorac Surg, 1988;45:626-33.
43. Griffith BP, Magee MJ, Gonzalez IF, et al. Anastomotic pitfalls in lung transplantation. J Thorac Cardiovasc Surg, 1994;107:743-53.
44. Pasque MK, Kaiser LR, Dresler CM, et al. Single lung transplantation for pulmonary hypertension: technical aspects and immediate hemodynamic results. J Thorac Cardiovasc Surg, 1992; 103:475-82.
45. Pasque MK, Cooper JD, Kaiser LR, et al. Improved technique for bilateral lung transplantation: rationale and initial clinical experience. Ann Thorac Surg, 1990;49:785-91.
46. Egan TM, Detterbeck FC. Technique and results of double lung transplantation Chest Surg Clin N Am, 1993;3:89-111.
47. Aurora P, Boucek MM, Christie J, et al. Registry of the International Society for Heart and Lung Transplantation : Tenth Official Pediatric Lung and Heart/Lung Transplantation Report-2007. J Heart Lung Tansplant, 2007;26:782.
48. Starnes VA, Barr ML, Cohen RG. Lobar transplantation: Indications, technique and outcome, J Thorac Cardiovasc Surg, 1994;108:403-10.
49. Woo MS, MacLaughlin EF, Horn MV, et al. Living donor lobar lung transplantation: the pediatric experience. Pediatr Transplant, 1998;2:185-90.
50. Starnes VA, Woo MS, MacLaughlin EF, et al. Comparison of outcomes between living donor and cadaveric lung transplantation in children. Ann Thorac Surg, 1999;68:2279-83.
51. Barr ML, Schenkel FA, Cohen RG, et al. Recipient and donor outcomes in living related and unrelated lobar transplantation. Transplant Proc, 1998;30:2261-3.
52. Cohen RG, Barr ML, Schenkel FA, et al. Living-related donor lobectomy for bilateral lobar transplantation in patients with cystic fibrosis. Ann Thorac Surg, 1994;57:1423-28.
53. Starnes VA, Barr ML, Cohen RG, et al. Living-donor lobar lung transplantation experience: intermediate results. J Thorac Cardiovasc Surg, 1996;112:1284-90.
54. Hosenpud JD, Novick RJ, Breen TJ, et al. The Registry of the International Society for Heart and Lung Transplantation: twelfth official report--1995. J Heart Lung Transplant, 1995;14:805-15.
55. Novick RJ, Schäfers HJ, Stitt L, et al. Recurrence of obliterative bronchiolitis and determinants of outcome in 139 pulmonary retransplant recipients. J Thorac Cardiovasc Surg, 1995;110: 1402-13.
56. Snell GI, Westall GP. Selection and management of the lung donor. Clin Chest Med, 2011;32:223-32.
57. Bando T, Date H, Minami M, et al. First registy report : lung transplantation in Japan : the Japanese Society of Lung and Heart-Lung Transplantation. Gen Thorac Cardiovasc Surg, 2008;56(1): 17-21.
58. Levvey B. Excellent early results of Australian DCD lung transplantation. J heart Lung Transplant, 2010;31(2):S63-4.
59. Cypel M, Yeung JC, Keshavjee S. Novel approaches to expanding the lung donor pool: donation after cardiac death and ex vivo conditioning. Clin Chest Med, 2011;32:233-44.
60. Warnecke G, Moradiellos J, Tudorache I, et al. Normothermic perfusion of donor lungs for preservation and assessment with the Organ Care System Lung before bilateral transplantation: a pilot study of 12 patients. Lancet, 2012;S0140-6736(12): 61344-50.
61. Cypel M, Keshavjee S. Extracorporeal life support as a bridge to lung transplantation. Clin Chest Med, 2011;32:245-51.
62. Fishman A, Martinez F, Naunheim K, et al. A randomized trial comparing lung volume reduction surgery with medical therapy for severe emphysema. N Engl J Med, 2003;348(21):2059-73.
63. Naunheim KS, Wood DE, Mohsenifar Z, et al. Long-term follow-up of patients receiving lung volume reduction surgery versus medical therapy for severe emphysema by the National Emphysema Treatment Trial Research Group. Ann Thorac Surg, 2006;82(2):431-43.
64. Ernst A, Eberhardt R, Gompelmann D, Herth FJ. Low degree of collateral ventilation measurement in heterogeneous emphysema subject treated by endobronchial lung volume reduction predicts ELVR success. Am J Respir Crit Care Med, 2010;181:A1571.
65. Borro JM. New methods to facilitate lung transplantation. Lancet, 2012;S0140-6736(12):61691-2.

66. Cypel M, Liu M, Rubacha M, et al. Functional repair of human donor lungs by IL-10 gene therapy. Sci Transl Med, 2009;1:49.
67. Pasero D, Martin EL, Davi A, et al. The effects of inhaled nitric oxide after lung transplantation. Minerva Anestesiol, 2010;76:353-61.
68. Della Rocca G, Brondani A, Costa MG. Intraoperative hemodynamic monitoring during organ transplantation: what is new? Curr Opin Organ Transplant, 2009;14:291-6.
69. Csete M, Glas K. Transplant Anesthesia. In Barash PG, Cullen BF, Stoelting RK, Cahalan M, Stock MC (eds). Clinical Anesthesia, 6th edn. Wolter Kluwer/Lipponcott Williams & Wilknis 2009; Section VII, Chapter 54, pg1393-1420.
70. Lepore JJ, Maroo A, Pereira NL, et al. Effect of sildenafil on the acute pulmonary vasodilator response to inhaled nitric oxide in adults with primary pulmonary hypertension. Am J Cardiol, 2002;90:677-80.
71. Pilcher DV, Scheinkestel CD, Snell GI, et al. High central venous pressure is associated with prolonged mechanical ventilation and increased mortality after lung transplantation. J Thorac Cardiovasc Surg, 2005;129:912-18.
72. Wang Y, Kurichi JE, Blumenthal NP, et al. Multiple variables affecting blood usage in lung transplantation. J Heart Lung Transplant, 2006;25(5):533-8.
73. Myles PS. Lessons from lung transplantation for everyday thoracic anesthesia. Anesthesiol Clin North America, 2001;19:581-90vii.
74. de Hoyos A, Demajo W, Snell G, et al. Preoperative prediction for the use of cardiopulmonary bypass in lung transplantation. J Thorac Cardiovasc Surg, 1993;106:787-95.
75. Hirt SW, Axel H, Thorsten W, et al. Predictive criteria for the need of extracorporeal circulation in single-lung transplantation. Ann Thorac Surg, 1992;54:676-80.
76. Ko WJ, Chen YS, Lee YC. Replacing cardiopulmonary bypass with extracorporeal membrane oxygenation in lung transplantation operations, Artif Organs, 2001;25:607-12.
77. Pereszylenyi A, Lang G, Steltzer H, et al. Bilateral lung transplantation with intra and postoperatively prolonged ECMO support in patients with pulmonary hypertension, Eur J Cardiothorac Surg, 2002;21:858-63.
78. Roffey P. Anesthetic concerns in lung transplant. Current opinion in organ transplantation, 2003;8:249-51.
79. Webber SA. The current state of, and future prospects for, cardiac transplantation in children, Cardiol Young, 2003;13:64-83.
80. Yonan NA, el-Gamel A, Egan J, et al. Single lung transplantation for emphysema: predictors for native lung hyperinflation. J Heart Lung Transplant, 1998;17:192-201.
81. Christie JD, Carby M, Bag R, et al. ISHLT Working Group on Primary Lung Graft Dysfunction. Report of the ISHLT Working Group on Primary Lung Graft Dysfunction part II: definition. A consensus statement of the International Society for Heart and Lung Transplantation. J Heart Lung Transplant, 2005;24:1454-9.
82. Miñambres E, González-Castro A, Rabanal JM, et al. Comparative study of two preservation solutions in the initial function after bilateral human lung transplantation. Med Intensiva, 2007;31:1-5.
83. Myles PS. Pulmonary transplantation. In: Kaplan JA, Slinger PD, eds. Thoracic Anesthesia. Philadelphia: Elsevier Science, 2003;295-314.
84. Murthy SC, Blackstone EH, Gildea TR, et al. Impact of anastomotic airway complications after lung transplantation. Ann Thorac Surg, 2007;84:401-9.
85. Fuehner T, Dierich M, Duesberg C, et al. Endoscopic indicators for obstructive airway complications after lung transplantation. Transplantation, 2010;90(11):1210-4.
86. Boehler A, Estenne M. Post-transplant bronchiolitis obliterans. Eur Respir J, 2003;22:1007-18.
87. Valentine VG, Robbins RC, Berry GJ, et al. Actuarial survival of heart-lung and bilateral sequential lung transplant recipients with obliterative bronchiolitis. J Heart Lung Transplant, 1996;15:371-83.

17
CHAPTER

Xenotransplantation

Manish Kohli

INTRODUCTION

Organ transplantation is one of the greatest achievements of modern medicine. Allotransplanation is the transplantation of living organs, tissues or cells from one human to another or between individuals within the same species. It includes either organs, e.g. kidneys, heart, lungs, liver, and pancreas or tissues, e.g. bone marrow, bone, heart valves, eye tissue, and skin. As the demand for organs suitable for transplantation in human beings is increasing day-by-day and with the shortage of human donors there is an increasing interest in alternative therapies.[1, 2] Artificial alternatives are used such as hemodialysis for renal failure and mechanical pumps to assist a failing left ventricle awaiting heart transplantation.[3] Even if efforts to persuade individuals to donate organs are increased, and even if consent to donate should become a legal presumption, there is little prospect of developing a sufficient supply of transplantable human organs to meet the growing demand.[4,5] The United Network for Organ Sharing (UNOS) reported that 560 patients on the UNOS waiting list died while waiting for a liver transplant during calendar year 1993.[6]

Xenotransplantation is the transplantation of living organs, tissues or cells from one species to another (e.g. from nonhuman primates or pigs to humans), and is viewed as a potential solution to the shortage of human organs for transplantation. Xenotransplantation in humans is defined by the United States Public Health Service as any procedure that involves the transplantation, implantation or infusion into a human recipient of either (i) Live cells, tissues, or organs from a nonhuman animal source or (ii) Human body fluids, cells, tissues or organs that have had ex vivo contact with live nonhuman animal cells, tissues, or organs.[7] Xenotransplantation products (Flow chart 17.1) are defined as live cells, tissues, or organs used in xenotransplantation.[6,8]

Animal tissues have been used as grafts to humans for decades. Heart valves from pigs have been used successfully to replace damaged heart valves in humans. Blood vessels

Flow chart 17.1: Xenograft platform

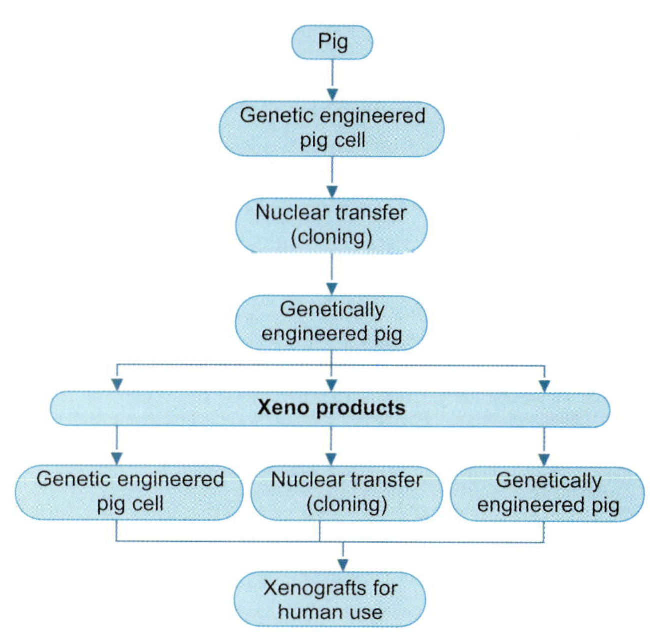

from cows were used to replace damaged blood vessels in humans prior to the development of synthetic materials such as Dacron and Goretex. Most xenotransplantation activity is still in the preclinical stage, involving basic research on technical developments and immunological response and research on infectious risks. Biotechnology is developing fast and hence it is hoped that this form of surgical therapy will soon become a clinical reality.[9,10] Initially, the ideal source animals were thought to be nonhuman primates, since they are close to humans phylogenetically and therefore represent the best immunological match. However, primates are not ideal as donors because of their small litter size, the long latency before pregnancy and the high frequency of viral infection among primates. Thus, most xenotransplant researchers are concentrating on animals like pigs other than primates.[10]

HISTORY

The story of Lord Ganesha and other religious stories signify that the idea of xenografts is not a new concept in Hindu mythology. Nevertheless, the history of previous attempts in modern medicine to implant animal organs into human recipients have all met with failure. Xenotransplantation was attempted early in the twentieth century resulting in early death for all recipients. More sophisticated efforts occurred in the late 1960s and early 1970s during the period when anti-rejection drugs began to make allografts more feasible. Although one recipient of a xenograft survived for 9 months, most patients died within a matter of minutes, hours, or days after engraftment of organs from chimpanzees or baboons.[11]

In 1984, a well-known xenograft involved the transfer of a baboon's heart into 14-day-old "Baby Fae" whose own heart was unable to sustain life for more than a few days, by Dr Leonard Bailey at Loma Linda Hospital, California, USA. Cyclosporin A was used to prevent organ rejection. "Baby Fae" died of progressive graft necrosis 20 days after receiving the baboon heart. This case generated enormous controversy and coverage by news media.[12,13] However, with the advent of the new drug FK506 and other immunosuppressive agents, at least two new xenotransplant efforts were attempted in the 1990s.One technique involved using a donor baboon liver as a "bridging" procedure to sustain patients awaiting human liver transplants. The liver can be removed with relative ease because, although connected to the subject's liver, it remains extracorporeal. Similar experimental techniques were planned involving baboon hearts as bridges for pediatric cardiac patients.

Before new major animal-to-human xenograft research programs are initiated, both the scientific and the ethical aspects of such programs should be carefully considered and debated. Many of the scientific issues were addressed in the *Institute of Laboratory Animal Research Journal (ILAR).*[14] This article addressed ethical aspects of xenotransplantation from animals to humans.

Current State of the Science

New drugs and new combinations of existing immunosuppressive drugs can reduce the likelihood of both short and long-term organ rejection.[15] Improvement in understanding of both human and animal immune systems and their histocompatibility and with development of new agents to control graft-versus-host disease, animal breeding programs for the production of transgenic animals and advancement in surgical techniques have all increased the possibility of successful transfer of organs from animals to humans.

Advantages of Xenotransplantation over Allotransplantation

1. Alternative source to allotransplants
2. Potentially unlimited supply of organs and hence patients will not have to wait endlessly for suitable organ donors
3. Scheduling is not dependent on the unpredictable availability of a donor human organ, allowing for both advance planning and the intentionally timed harvesting of an organ for immediate transplantation as well as immunologic pretreatment of the recipient, if necessary[16]
4. Xenogenic cells are less susceptible to human disease, e.g. human immunodeficiency virus [HIV] and hepatitis B virus
5. Risk of several infections can be reduced by allowing lifelong control of exposure of the source animals to potential infections and extensive prescreening prior to organ harvest
6. Transplantation of pancreatic islet cells can cure diabetes
7. Cellular xenografts could treat Parkinson's and Huntington's disease, multiple sclerosis and the effects of strokes
8. Vehicle for gene delivery
9. Rescue therapy for artificial devices
10. In vivo organogenesis.

OBSTACLES OF XENOTRANSPLANTATION

The science of genetic engineering has been used extensively for xenotransplantation. Since 2000, such efforts have waned because of a moratorium on xenotransplantation resulting from the infectious risk, so clinical application seems remote.[17] The cost and legal liability are severe regulatory hurdles. In addition to it, the technical inputs required in the field collectively pose a daunting barrier.

Other Obstacles of Xenotransplantation

1. Immunologic problems (risks of hyperacute and acute rejection)[18-21]
2. Risk of xenogenic infections, e.g. porcine endogenous retrovirus (PERV)[22]
3. Legal concerns
4. Social concerns
5. Financial concerns versus potential benefits
6. Ethical concerns that animals have the same "rights" as humans do and therefore should not be put to death, even if it saves human lives. The fact is that our society values human life and we have customs and laws to protect humans[4,8]

7. Religious viewpoints: Some oppose xenotransplantation because they regard it as interfering with nature
8. Government viewpoints

The obstacles of xenotransplantation are largely determined by the type of xenograft.[23] The main obstacle is derived from the interaction of the host immune system with the graft. All xenografts elicit a comparable immune response, but the impact of that response depends on how the graft derives its vascular supply. Thus,

1. Cell and tissue xenografts are susceptible mainly to cellular rejection,whereas
2. Organ xenografts suffer severe vascular disease.

Cellular and Tissue Xenografts

Cells are less susceptible to humoral injury because blood is fed to the graft organs through blood vessels of the recipient that naturally grow into the graft and blood vessels of the recipient are obviously not targeted by antibodies and complement.[24] In vivo, cell and tissue xenografts are mainly the target of cell-mediated immunity (cellular rejection) and this process can be controlled with immunosuppressants (Flow chart 17.2). Some examples of tissue xenografts are porcine neural tissue (substantia nigra cells) which have been implanted in pancreatic islets[25] and in patients with Parkinson's disease. Similarly, cellular xenografts like hepatocytes can also be transplanted.

Organ Xenografts

Unlike cellular transplants, organ xenografts have the advantage that their function is not limited by anatomical localization. However, organ xenografts are highly susceptible to vascular disease caused by the immune system of the recipient (Flow chart 17.3).

Flow chart 17.2: Consequences of cellular and organ xenografts

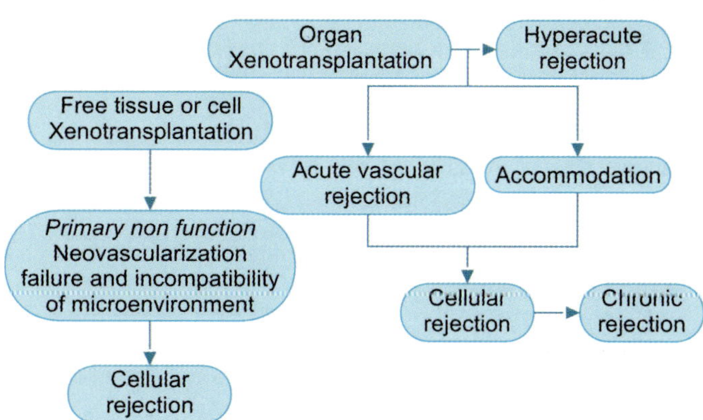

Flow chart 17.3: Vascularization of various grafts

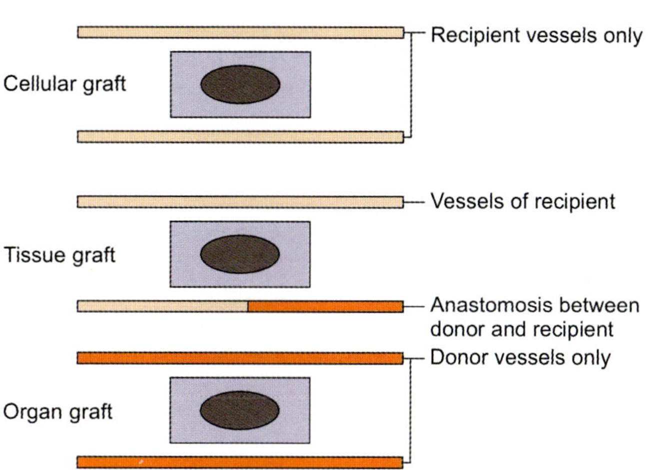

Biological Obstacles for Organ Xenografts and their Management

Immune

Vascularized organs are initially subject to hyperacute rejection, i.e. within a period of minutes to hours. This is an immune-mediated rejection which can be averted by different pretreatments and is no longer considered a hinderance to xenotransplantation.[18,26] By contrast, acute vascular rejection, which arises over days to months, is a severe obstacle.[27] This type of rejection may be triggered by antiswine antibodies that recognize Galα1, 3Gal, a saccharide expressed by pigs and other lower mammals,[28] or by antibodies against swine proteins.[29] By genetic manipulation of pigs the gene for the enzyme α1, 3-galactosyltransferase has been deleted, so that the endothelium of the blood vessels of the pig no longer expresses the important Galα1, 3Gal antigen against which humans have natural preformed antibodies. An immunosuppressive regimen has been developed which controls the rejection response of the graft for periods of two to six months but does not result in high levels of infection or malignancy. Another problem is low-grade endothelial cell activation by anti-non Gal antibodies or cellular constituents of the recipient's blood, due to which thrombotic microangiopathy develops in the grafted organ. This problem has been overcome by genetically introducing a human gene, such as the tissue factor pathway inhibitor, that will maintain the anticoagulant state of the endothelium.[30,31] Among the immune and inflammatory hurdles to transplanting organs between species, the most difficult to manage is that by the complement system which destroys invading bacteria and viruses. Genetic engineering has been used to treat these difficult immune problems. [32]

Accommodation

Some organ grafts survive and function despite the existence of a humoral immune response to the graft by the immune system of the recipient. This condition, first identified in ABO-incompatible kidney allografts, is called "accommodation".[33] Vascular cells of the xenograft express "survival gene" products such as Bcl-2, BclX and A20 that inhibit apoptosis and hemoxygenase (HO)-1. HO-1 may be protective through carbon monoxide generated by the gene product. Expression or up-regulation of just a few of these genes may not induce a state of accommodation because grafts with increased expression of HO-1 or complement regulatory factors may still undergo acute vascular rejection. Accommodation is multifactorial.[34,35]

Physiologic Barriers

Consideration would have to be given to relative drug dose differences between xenografts and the recipients because the xenograft may respond differently to toxic human drug doses, possibly because of differing receptor numbers or sensitivities.[32,36,37] The use of genetic engineering might overcome this problem. For example, adrenergic receptors could be expressed as a strategy to augment cardiac function.[38] Other physiologic defects are incompatibilities of complex systems (complement, coagulation, and metabolic) between the pig and human.

Coagulation Barriers

Endothelial cells of xenografts are activated by the immune system during acute vascular rejection, leading to the formation of a highly procoagulant surface.[39] For example, porcine tissue-factor-pathway inhibitor and thrombomodulin are poorly compatible with human factor Xa and human thrombin, respectively.[40,41]

Metabolic Barriers

Metabolic incompatibilities exist between the recipient and the xenograft. For example, atrial natriuretic factor produced by the porcine heart may not function in the human kidney, hence pharmacotherapy may be needed to help control sodium balance. In the porcine liver, the complex metabolic systems (clotting factors and complement regulatory factors) may differ substantially from homologous systems in the human since extracellular nucleotide metabolism (ecto-ATP-Dases CD39 and CD73) is inherently different across species.[42,43] These enzymes are important for the production of adenosine, a potent platelet inhibitor and natural immunosuppressant in the extracellular compartment. Exogenous administration of precursors of adenosine metabolism with enzyme catabolic inhibitors or the use of genetic engineering to reconstitute enzyme deficiencies across species may be novel methods of overcoming this metabolic barrier. The metabolic function of porcine kidneys has also to be borne in mind when considering kidney xenografts. For example, porcine kidneys produce a higher urine volume, and have differences in pH and excretion of phosphate and uric acid. Porcine erythropoietin seems not to activate the human receptors, so lifelong therapy with recombinant erythropoietin will be needed.[44] Antibodies to porcine erythropoietin produced by the xenograft may cross-react with therapeutic recombinant erythropoietin thus decreasing or eliminating the function of recombinant erythropoietin.[45]

Infections

A recent study suggests that viruses (PERV) could be eradicated from pig herds being bred for xenotransplantation.[7,46,47]

ANESTHETIC AND PERIOPERATIVE CONSIDERATIONS

There are currently few animal models that mimic the sick pretransplant recipient state, thus little information is available about xenograft function in very ill patients. There are multiple factors that have an impact on xenograft survival.

Disease Related

Consideration would have to be given to choosing anesthetic regimens that optimally promote graft function. For example, if hepatic function is abnormal in the recipient, a general anesthetic without the potential for liver toxicity is a rational choice to improve the host environment for the xenograft. Another consideration is coagulation abnormalities such as acute vascular thrombosis leading to neurologic complications and precluding the use of epidural or spinal techniques.[40,41]

Surgery Related

Perioperative procedures, blood loss, hypothermia, sepsis, coagulopathy are various considerations for transplantation.

Patient Related

The pretransplant physiologic milieu of the sick recipient along with different co-morbidities involved and compromised functional reserve of other organs will altogether make the anesthetic management difficult. The patient's state of immunosuppression and its related complications,[48] presence of infection and appropriate perioperative antibiotic regimens and antiretroviral prophylaxis or vaccination before xenotransplantation[49] are some important considerations to be keep in the mind before induction of anesthesia. In addition to it, the pediatric transplant recipients may have associated congenital abnormalities (physiologic or metabolic) that influence the xenograft's environment.[50]

Donor Animal Related

Preoperative management in the xenotransplant setting could be challenging for the anesthesia provider because a number of new areas would have to be mastered: animal physiology, manual skills in animals (intubation, cannulation) and administration and pharmacokinetics of anesthetic drugs in animals. In addition, it is difficult to achieve therapeutic levels of critical immunosuppressive drugs.

FUTURE OF XENOTRANSPLANTATION

Recent developments have brought forward a number of approaches that might be used to replace the function of failing organs such as implantable devices, stem cells and new immunosuppressive agents. Stem cells appear promising for focal defects, but their role in replacing global organ function, as in heart failure, is not yet clear.[51] During the next several years, several advances that may facilitate the application of clinical xenotransplantation are anticipated. Pigs with a targeted disruption of a1, 3-galactosyltransferase, which therefore lacks expression of Gala1 and 3Gal, and porcine organs that resist acute vascular rejection are being studied, thereby improving the potential outcome of xenotransplantation.[52]

Table 17.1: Perioperative considerations

Stage	Considerations
Preoperative	Source (animal) management; impact of drugs and distinct requirement of drug doses for the xenogeneic organs; recipient comorbidities; impaired graft function due to sick patient's (pretransplant) environment; novel immunosuppression techniques (e.g. column adsorption); antibiotics, antiretroviral or vaccine prophylaxis
Operative	Hematological abnormalities; unpredictable response of xenograft to anesthetics in vivo
Postoperative	Hematological and metabolic abnormalities

New methods are being developed to circumvent these complications.

Other new approaches to replacing organ function will be forthcoming, and some of these approaches will be complementary to xenotransplantation. For example, stem cells may be used to generate myocytes to replace infarcted tissue, perhaps using animal hosts (i.e. as a xenograft).[47] As another example, cells harvested from animals genetically engineered to express angiogenic factors on demand could be introduced into ischemic organs to promote revascularization. As still another example, an engineered or xenogenic organ might someday be used to rescue the recipient of a poorly functioning implantable device. Thus, the best options for replacing or augmenting the function of an organ will be achieved by simultaneous advancement of multiple technologies resulting in a multimodal or hybrid approach.[53,54]

A human organ might be grown in an animal as a xenograft. In vitro organogenesis, stem cells that are potentially derived from an individual with organ failure, might be used to grow a new organ, but tissues formed in vitro are very small, cannot support physiologic function and may lack vascularization.[55] A future application of xenotransplantation may be in vivo organogenesis. In vivo organogenesis has the advantage that it might be performed using stem cells from the affected individual but this may be technically challenging and a sick patient may not offer the best environment in which to grow a new organ.[56]

Xenotransplantation is viewed as a potential solution to the existing shortage of human organs for transplantation. The anesthetic management for major surgery is difficult with the multisystem involvement of the diseased patient on organ support systems along with risk of transmitting infections from donor animal, complications of immunotherapy and anesthetic management of donor animal. Cell and tissue xenografts are more susceptible mainly to cellular rejection, whereas organ xenografts suffer severe vascular disease. Genetic engineering finds a possible solution to the problem but things are still at an experimental stage. The best option left with us is a multimodal approach using in vitro organogenesis along with use of stem cells and genetically hybrid animals.

CLINICAL PEARLS

- Xenotransplantation is the transplantation of living organs, tissues or cells from one species to another.
- Most xenotransplantation activity is still in the preclinical stage and researchers are concentrating more on animals like pigs rather than primates.
- Despite its numerous advantages over allotransplantation certain obstacles like legal, financial, ethical and social

issues need to be overcome. The risk of xenogenic infections and immunologic problems pose a major barrier to the ongoing research.

- The development of newer immunosuppressive drugs in various combinations and advances in gene therapy offer a solution to the existing problem.
- The pharmacokinetics and pharmacodynamics of anesthetic and immunosuppressive drugs and manual skills in animals like intubation and cannulation needs to be mastered.
- The choice of anesthesia technique will depend on the physiological milieu of the recipient, multisystem involvement, status of immunosuppression, preexisting infection and surgery related concerns like blood loss, sepsis, coagulopathy and graft rejection.
- A successful xenotransplant provides unlimited supply of organs and hence patients will not have to wait endlessly for suitable organ donors.

REFERENCES

1. Buckley RH. Transplantation immunology: organ and bone marrow. J Allergy Clin Immunol, 2003;111(Suppl 2):S733-44.
2. Evans RW. Coming to terms with reality: Why xenotransplantation is a necessity. In: Platt JL, (Ed). Xenotransplantation. Washinton, DC: ASM Press; 2001:29.
3. Rose EA, Gelijns AC, Moskowitz AJ, Heitjan DF, Dembitsky SLWW, Long JW, et al. Longterm use of a left ventricular assist device for end-stage heart failure. N Engl J Med, 2001;345:1435-43.
4. Cooper D. Ethical aspects of xenotransplantation of current importance. Xenotransplantation, 1996;3:264-74.
5. Cooper D. Clinical xenotransplantation–how close are we? Lancet, 362(9383),557-5.
6. Starzl TE, Fung J, Tzakis A, et al. Xenotransplantation, 1993;1:27-29. 1994 Annual Report of the US Scientific Registry of Transplant Recipients and Organ Procurement and Transplant Network.
7. Boneva RS, Folks TM, Chapman LE. Infectious Disease Issues in Xenotransplantation Clinical Microbiology Reviews, 2001:1-14.
8. Tannsjo T. Ethical aspects of transplantation surgery. Transplant Proc, 2003;35:1210-3.
9. Hammer C. Xenotransplantation: the good, the bad, and the ugly or how far are we to clinical application? Transplant Proc, 2003; 35:1256-7.
10. Cooper D, Ye Y, Rolf L, Zuhdi N. The pig as potential organ donor for man. In Xenotransplantation. D Cooper, E Kemp, K Reemtsma & D White, eds. Springer, Heidelberg,1991;481-500.
11. Millard C, Shumway NE, Starzl TE, et al. Xenografts: Review of the literature and current status. J Am Vet Med Assoc, 1985;254: 3353-56.
12. Annas GJ. Baby Fae: The «anything goes» school of human experimentation. Hastings Center Report, 1985;15:15-17.
13. Platt J. New directions for organ transplantation. Nature, 329(Suppl) 1998:11-17.
14. McCarthy CR. Ethical Aspects of Animal-to-Human Xenografts. ILAR Journal, 1995;V37(1).
15. Makowka L History, Progress, and Future of Transplantation. Paper delivered at Workshop on Transplant Medicine and Surgery, sponsored by The American Society of Laboratory Animal Practitioners (ASLAP) and the Association of Primate Veterinarians (APV), Pittsburgh, Penn., 1994 October 16.
16. Baily LL, Nehlsen-Cannarella SL, Concepcion W, Jolley WB. Baboon-to-human cardiac xenotransplantation in a neonate. JAMA, 1985;254:3321-29.
17. Remuzzi G. Xenotransplantation: a challenge for the future of transplant medicine. Schweizerische Medizinische Wochenschrift, 1998;128:952-60.
18. Platt JL. Hyperacute xenograft rejection. Austin, TX: RG Landes, 1995.
19. Bach FH, Winkler H, Ferran C, Hancock WW, Robson SC. Delayed xenograft rejection. Immunol Today, 1996;17:379-84.
20. Lin SS, Hanaway MJ, Gonzalez-Stawinski GV, Lau CL, Parker W, Davis RD, et al. The role of anti-Gala1–3Gal antibodies in acute vascular rejection and accommodation of xenografts. Transplantation, 2000;70:1667-74.
21. Xu H, Gundry SR, Hancock WW, Matsumiya G, Zuppan CW, Morimoto T, et al. Prolonged discordant xenograft survival and delayed xenograft rejection in a pig-to-baboon orthotopic cardiac xenograft model. J Thorac Cardiovasc Surg, 1998;115:1342-9.
22. Clark DA, Fryer JF, Tucker AW, McArdle PD, Hughes AE, Emery VC, et al. Porcine cytomegalovirus in pigs being bred for xenograft organs: progress towards control. Xenotransplantation, 2003;10:142-8.
23. Khalpey Z, Koch CA, Platt JL. Xenograft transplantation. Anesthesiology Clin N Am, 2004;22:871-85.
24. Saadi S, Platt JL. Humoral rejection and endothelial cell activation. Xenotransplantation, 2002;9:239-41.
25. Bjorklund A. Cell replacement strategies for neurodegenerative disorders. Novartis Foundation Symposium, 2000;231:7-15.
26. Platt JL, Vercellotti GM, Dalmasso AP, Matas AJ, Bolman RM, Najarian JS, et al. Transplantation of discordant xenografts: a review of progress. Immunol Today, 1990;11:450-6.
27. Cascalho M, Platt JL. The immunological barrier to xenotransplantation. Immunity, 2001;14:437-46.
28. Galili U, Clark MR, Shohet SB, Buehler J, Macher BA. Evolutionary relationship between the natural anti-Gal antibody and the Gal a1–3Gal epitope in primates. Proc Natl Acad Sci USA, 1987;84:1369-73.
29. McCurry KR, Kooyman DL, Alvarado CG, Cotterell AH, Martin MJ, Logan JS, et al. Human complement regulatory proteins protect swine-to-primate cardiac xenografts from humoral injury. Nat Med, 1995;1:423.
30. Lai L, Kolber-Simonds D, Park KW, Cheong HT, Greenstein JL, Im GS, et al. Production of a-, 3-galactosyltransferase knockout pigs by nuclear transfer cloning. Science, 2002; 295:1089-92.
31. Phelps CJ, Koike C, Vaught TD, Boone J, Wells KD, Chen SH, et al. Production of alpha 1,3-galactosyltransferase-deficient pigs. Science, 2003;299:411-4.
32. White D, Wallwork J. Xenografting: probability, possibility, or pipe dream? Lancet, 1993;342:879-80.
33. Sato K, Balla J, Otterbein L, Smith RN, Brouard S, Lin Y, et al. Carbon monoxide generated by heme oxygenase-1 suppresses the rejection of mouse-to-rat cardiac transplants. J Immunol, 2001; 166:4185-94.
34. Park WJP, Grande ND, Nath KA, Platt JL, Gloor JM, Stegall MD. Accommodation in ABO incompatible kidney allografts, a novel

mechanism of self-protection against antibody-mediated injury. Am J Transplant, 2003;3:952-60.

35. Holzknecht ZE, Platt JL. Accommodation and the reversibility of biological systems. Transplantation, 2001;71:594-5.
36. Schmoeckel M, Bhatti FNK, Zaidi A, Cozzi E, Waterworth PD, Tolan MJ, et al. Orthotopic heart transplantation in a transgenic pig-to-primate model. Transplantation, 1998;65:1570-7.
37. Sablinski T, Latinne D, Gianello P, Bailin M, Bergen K, Colvin RB, et al. Xenotransplantation of pig kidneys to nonhuman primates: I. development of the model. Xenotransplantation, 1995;2:264-70.
38. Akhter SA, Skaer CA, Kypson AP, McDonald PH, Peppel KC, Glower DD, et al. Restoration of β-adrenergic signaling in failing cardiac ventricular myocytes via adenoviral-mediated gene transfer. Proc Natl Acad Sci USA, 1997;94:12100-5.
39. Buhler L, Basker M, Alwayn IPJ, Goepfert C, Kitamura H, Kawai T, et al. Coagulation and thrombotic disorders associated with pig organ and hematopoietic cell transplantation in nonhuman primates. Transplantation, 2000;70:1323-31.
40. Buhler L, Goepfert C, Kitamura H, Basker M, Gojo S, Alwayn IP, et al. Porcine hematopoietic cell xenotransplantation in nonhuman primates is complicated by thrombotic microangiopathy. Bone Marrow Transplant, 2001;27:1227-36.
41. Alwayn IP, Buhler L, Basker M, Goepfert C, Kawai T, Kozlowski T, et al. Coagulation/ thrombotic disorders associated with organ and cell xenotransplantation. Transplant Proc, 2000;32:1099.
42. Nishitai R, Plummer TB, Platt JL. Detection of albumin synthesis in transplanted porcine hepatocytes in mice. Liver Transplantation, 2002;8:972-4.
43. Smolenski RT, Raisky O, Kalsi KK, Abunasra H, Jayakumar J, Suzuki K, et al. Enhanced endogenous adenosine production and protection of the heart after transplantation. Adv Exp Med Biol, 2000;486:167-70.
44. Cozzi E, Bhatti F, Schmoeckel M, Chavez G, Smith KG, Zaidi A, et al. Long-term survival of nonhuman primates receiving life-supporting transgenic porcine kidney xenografts. Transplantation, 2000;70:15-21.
45. Wen D, Boissel J, Tracy TE, Gruninger RH, Mulcahy LS, Czelusniak J, et al. Erythropoietin structure-function relationships: high degree of sequence homology among mammals. Blood, 1993;82:1507-16.
46. Takeuchi Y, Weiss RA. Xenotransplantation: reappraising the risk of retroviral zoonosis. Curr Opin Immunol, 2000;12:504-7.
47. Asano M, Gundry SR, Izutani H, Cannarella SN, Fagoaga O, Bailey LL. Baboons undergoing orthotopic concordant cardiac xenotransplantation surviving more than 300 days: effect of immunosuppressive regimen. J Thorac Cardiovasc Surg, 2003; 125:60-9.
48. Kostopanagiotou G, Smyrniotis V, Arkadopoulos N, Theodoraki K, Papadimitriou L, Papadimitriou J. Anesthetic and perioperative management of adult transplant recipients in nontransplant surgery. Anesth Analg, 1999;89:613-22.
49. Johnston TD, Katz SM. Special considerations in the transplant patient requiring other surgery. Surg Clin North Am, 1994;74: 1211-21.
50. Black AE. Anesthesia for pediatric patients who have had a transplant. Int Anesthesiol Clin, 1995;33:107-23.
51. Cascalho M, Platt JL. Xenotransplantation and other means of organ replacement. Nat Rev Immunol, 2001;1:154-60.
52. Liu J, Weintraub A, Holgersson J. "Multivalent Galα1,3Gal-substitution makes recombinant mucinimmunoglobulins efficient absorbers of anti-pig antibodies". Xenotransplantation, 2003; 10:149-63.
53. Cooper DK, Keogh AM, Brink J, Corris PA, Klepetko W, Pierson RN, et al. Report of the Xenotransplantation Advisory Committee of the International Society for Heart and Lung Transplantation: the present status of xenotransplantation and its potential role in the treatment of end-stage cardiac and pulmonary diseases. J Heart Lung Transplant, 2000;19:1125-65.
54. Platt J, DiSesa V, Gail D, Massicot-Fisher J. Recommendations of the National Heart, Lung, and Blood Institute Heart and Lung Xenotransplantation Working Group. Circulation, 2002;106: 1043-7.
55. Ekblom P. Formation of basement membranes in the embryonic kidney: an immunohistological study. J Cell Biol, 1981;91:1-10.
56. Grobstein C. Inductive epithelio-mesenchymal interaction in cultured organ rudiments of the mouse. Science, 1953;118:52-5.

18 CHAPTER Anesthesia for Intestinal Transplantation

Jayashree Sood

INTRODUCTION

The first intestinal transplant was performed in late 1980s and is now recognized as the primary therapeutic indication for patients with irreversible intestinal failure (IF). Intestinal transplant has been performed in more than 3,000 patients worldwide. This surgery is usually done in patients with short bowel syndrome (SBS) and those who develop cholestatic liver disease from total parenteral nutrition (TPN). Intestinal transplant restores the digestive and absorptive properties of the intestines and so the patient is relieved of the TPN. It is usually considered in those patients who develop serious complications related to TPN, e.g. most of the sites used for TPN (jugular, subclavian vein) become inaccessible due to thrombosis and catheter related sepsis.

The incidence of intestinal transplant is increasing. The 2001 Center for Medicare and Medicaid Services (CMS) has recognized intestinal transplant as the standard of care for patients with IF.[1]

Advances in immunosuppressive therapy, surgical and anesthesia techniques have improved short and long term survival rates after intestinal transplant. The 2003 report of the Intestinal Transplant Registry (ITR) highlighted a new era of IT with improved surgical outcome.[2] The patient and graft survival at 1 year has been reported to be 81% and 74% respectively. A successful intestinal transplant beyond 3 years, is a cost effective alternative to parenteral nutrition.[3]

INDICATIONS

Short bowel syndrome in pediatric population is seen in necrotizing enterocolitis, intestinal atresia, gastroschisis, midgut volvulus and congenital anomalies.

In adults, the indications are several. Short gut syndrome is seen in Crohn's disease and in those who have undergone multiple surgeries; defective motility as in Hirschsprung's disease, impaired absorptive capacity as in massive intestinal polyposis and inflammatory bowel disease.[4]

Indications are depletion of central venous access sites, multiple episodes of catheter related sepsis, dehydration and electrolyte disturbances.

Intestinal transplantation may be done along with liver transplant or as a part of multivisceral transplant of liver, spleen, kidney, stomach, duodenum and colon.

CONTRAINDICATIONS

History of malignancy, infection, major neurological and psychiatric disorders, immune disorders and any co-morbidity restricting life expectancy to <5 years.

DONOR SPECIFICATIONS

The donor should be <45 years, <75 kg and matched to provide a graft 25–50% smaller than would be predicted by recipient height alone.

While elective living related donors are also increasing, the donors are usually the heart beating decreased donors with no intestinal pathology. The procedure involves harvesting of a segment of terminal ileum, 20 cms proximal to the donor's ileocaecal valve (200 cms for adult recipients and 150–180 cm for pediatric recipients). Atleast 60% of the small intestine should be left intact.

Living related donation will help increase the pool of donor organs, thus reducing waiting list mortality.[5]

PREOPERATIVE EVALUATION

A thorough preoperative assessment is mandatory, like other organ transplant recipients. The multidisciplinary team should include the transplant surgeon and anesthesiologist, the gastroenterologist, cardiologist, dental surgeon, psychologist, dietician and psychiatrist.

A battery of laboratory tests including Hb, hematocrit, serum electrolytes, blood grouping, HLA tissue typing and estimation of Vitamin A, B6, D and E levels; urinalysis including culture should be done. Serology including CMV

IgG, EBV IgG, HSV IgG, HIV, HbsAg, HbsAb, HCV, syphilis IgG and VZV IgG are mandatory.[6]

Screening swabs for MRSA should be done.

Radiology investigations include chest X-ray, liver and abdominal ultrasonography, central vein mapping, MRI venography or Doppler ultrasonography, CT scan abdomen and pelvis, barium studies and MR of small bowel and bone density. Cardiopulmonary assessment includes ECG, PFT, coronary angiography; and GI investigations including esophago-gastro-duodenoscopy, colonoscopy and liver biopsy should be done.

SURGICAL STEPS

Isolated small bowel transplantation involves 3 stages.[7]

1. The dissection stage

   Dissection may result in extensive blood loss due to numerous adhesions and contracted abdominal cavity. Abdominal infection may release endotoxins which may produce cardiovascular instability. This stage involves isolation of recipient's infrarenal aorta and part of portomesentric venous system or infrarenal IVC.

2. The anastomotic stage

   After partial clamping of the aorta, the donor's superior mesenteric artery (SMA) is connected to the recipient's infrarenal aorta, and the superior mesenteric vein (SMV) to the recipient's portal venous system or the IVC. After the anastomosis, the clamps are released and reperfusion is done (Fig. 18.1).

3. The intestinal reconstructive stage

   The donor's proximal jejunum is anastomosed to the recipient's jejunum, duodenum or stomach and the donor's ileum to the recipient's ileum, transverse or descending colon or rectum. The distal end of the graft is brought out as a standard end ileostomy or loop ileostomy. Then a feeding jejunostomy or gastrostomy is made.

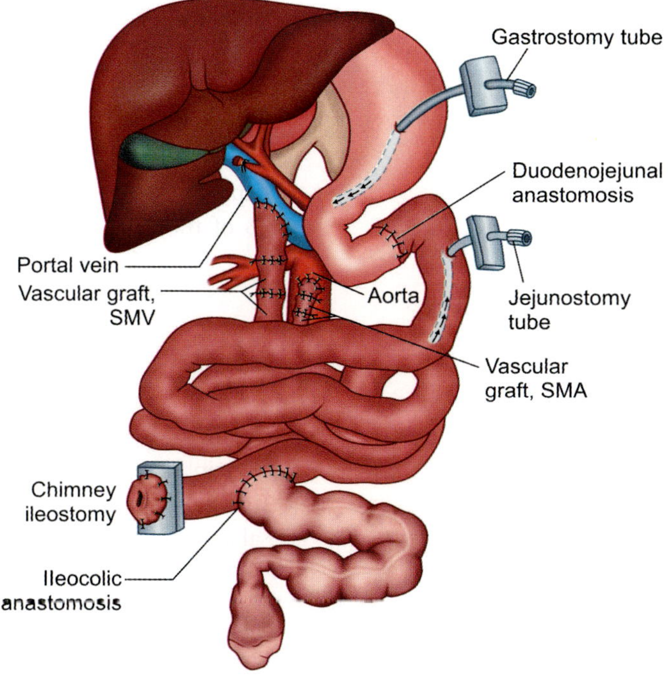

Fig. 18.1: Intestinal transplant

Closure of the abdominal wall may be difficult due to multiple surgeries, infections, scar formation and contracted abdominal cavity. An increase in intra-abdominal pressure may produce intra-abdominal hypertension.

ANESTHETIC IMPLICATIONS[8]

Preoperative Preparation

Adequate blood should be cross matched and kept ready.

Premedication

Prokinetics, e.g. metoclopramide and H_2 receptor antagonist, ranitidine are given due to delayed gastric emptying and reduced intestinal motility.

Anesthetic Technique

A rapid sequence induction is recommended due to delayed gastric emptying and risk of gastric aspiration. Tracheal intubation and controlled ventilation is initiated. A protective lung ventilation strategy targeting volume 6–8 mL/kg with minimal PEEP is provided. Maintenance of anesthesia with a volatile agent along with fentanyl/remifentanil boluses or continuous infusion is done. The risk benefit ratio of insertion of a lumbar epidural for intra and postoperative analgesia should be discussed and done accordingly.

A nasogastric tube is inserted and fixed carefully so that it does not get displaced or else it will require placement under direct vision because of the risk of anastomotic disruption.

The main challenge in intraoperative management is the maintenance of fluid and electrolyte balance and prevention of abdominal viscera edema. Extravasation of fluid takes place due to third space losses and as a consequence, bowel edema may result. Ischemic reperfusion injury also worsens the bowel edema. Therefore a "conservative fluid strategy" with judicious use of inotropes with the help of hemodynamic monitoring is recommended. Balanced crystalloids are infused at the rate of 10 mL/kg/hr.[9]

Reperfusion is a very crucial stage. Methylprednisolone 500 mg should be given atleast 30 minutes before the reperfusion. Reperfusion may result in hyperkalemia and arrhythmias. Intravenous $CaCl_2$ is routinely administered at this stage.

A 'post-reperfusion syndrome' manifested as extreme hypotension and cardiovascular instability is observed several times.

POSTOPERATIVE CARE

At the end of surgery the patient is shifted to the transplant ICU for elective ventilation and postoperative care. The metabolic and coagulation abnormalities are corrected before extubation. Maintenance of adequate perfusion and oxygenation of the graft, prevention of infection and start of nutrition should be ascertained.

Parenteral nutrition is gradually weaned over weeks and jejunal feed started gradually.

POSTOPERATIVE COMPLICATIONS

There are usually surgical—bleeding, thrombosis, anastomotic leaks, infections and rejection of the graft. Infections are the main cause of mortality.

CLINICAL PEARLS

- Intestinal transplant is now accepted as a therapeutic line of management in patients with irreversible intestinal failure
- Indications are patients with irreversible intestinal failure due to short bowel syndrome
- A multidisciplinary team of transplant surgeons, anesthesiologist, gastroenterologist and others involved in management is mandatory

REFERENCES

1. Abu-Elmagd KM, Bond G, Reyes J, Fung J. Intestinal transplantation (a coming of age). Adv Surg, 2002;36:65-101.
2. Grant D, Abu-Elmagd K, Reyes J, Tzakis A, Langnas A, Fishbein T, et al. 2003 Report of the intestine transplant registry (a new are has dewned). Ann Surg, 2005;241:607-613.
3. Abu-Elmagd KM, Starzl TE. Intestinal transplantation for short bowel syndrome and gastrointestinal failure: Current consensus, rewarding outcomes, and practical guidelines. Gastroenterology, 2006;130(2):S132-137.
4. Beebe DS, Belani KG. Anesthesia for kidney, pancreas or other organ transplantation. In: Longnecker De, Brown Dl, Newman MF, Zapol WM, eds. Anaesthesiology New York, NY: McGraw-Hill, Chapter 58,2008;pg1396-418.
5. Pascher A, Kohler S, Neuhaus P, Pratschke J. Present status and future perspectives of intestinal transplantation. Transplant Int, 2008;21:401-14.
6. Raymond M. Planinsic. Anesthetic management for small bowel transplantation. Anesthesiol Clin N Am, 2004;22(4):675-85.
7. Lomax S, Klucniks A, Griffiths J. Anaesthesia for intestinal transplantation. Cont Edu Anaesth Crit Care & Pain, 2011;11(1):1-4.
8. Khan FA, Brown RS Jr., Travis Ac, Selvaggi G. Overview of intestinal and multivisceral transplantation. www.uptodate.com 2013.
9. Jacque JJ. Anesthetic considerations for multivisceral transplantation. Anesthesiol Clin North America, 2004;22:741-751.

19 CHAPTER

Anesthesia for Pancreas Transplantation

Jayashree Sood

INTRODUCTION

Advances in surgical and anesthesia techniques and immunosuppressive therapy have made possible transplantation of pancreas. The first pancreas transplant was done in the USA on 16th December, 1966.[1] It is a well established procedure for patients with Type 1 and Type 2 diabetes. Till last year (2012) more than 26,000 pancreatic transplants have been performed.[2] There are 3 main types of pancreas transplantation (i) Simultaneous pancreas and kidney transplantation (SPK), (ii) Pancreas after kidney (PAK) and (iii) Pancreas alone transplant (PAT).[3] Pancreatic transplants are often done along with a kidney transplant. The International Pancreas Transplant Registry (IPTR) has shown pancreas graft survival rates of 85% for SPK, 77% for PAK and 73% for PAT.[3] Patient survival now reaches over 95% at one year post-transplant and over 83% after 5 years.[4]

INDICATIONS

- SPK and PAK–diabetic who qualifies for a renal transplant
  The outcome of SPK in Type 2 diabetics are comparable to the outcomes in Type 1 diabetics.[5]
- PAT–Type 1–diabetic with labile diabetes mellitus; and inability to tolerate exogenous insulin
  Type 2–diabetic with labile diabetes mellitus; and psychological impairment
- Retransplantation–Chronic rejection and chronic allograft pancreatitis due to non-function of the grafted organ

CONTRAINDICATIONS

The contraindications are similar to those of other transplants, e.g. non-correctable CAD, EF <40%.

PREOPERATIVE EVALUATION

A thorough preoperative evaluation as for any other transplant surgery is essential. Pre-existing co-morbidities and end organ damage as a result of diabetes should be assessed and optimized preoperatively. Longstanding, poorly controlled diabetics often have autonomic dysfunction. This dysfunction is tested by heart rate variability and orthostatic hypotension. Since silent ischemia is known in chronic diabetics, a thorough cardiac risk stratification should be done.[6]

Diabetic nephropathy results in reduced GFR and proteinuria. Microvascular and macrovascular complications should be assessed. Hb_1Ac levels indicate degree of glucose control.

Stiffness at the atlanto-occipital joint leads to a difficult airway. A detailed airway examination is essential in the preoperative examination.

ANESTHETIC TECHNIQUE

General anesthesia with intubation and controlled ventilation is the technique of choice. Rapid sequence intubation is indicated in long standing diabetics, because of chances of gastroparesis and delayed gastric emptying. Suxamethonium or rocuronium are the drugs recommended for intubation. Maintenance of anesthesia with volatile anesthetics including isoflurane or desflurane along with narcotics (intermittent or continuous infusion) is the choice.

MONITORING

Standard monitoring includes, SpO_2, NIBP and ECG. CVP monitoring and radial artery cannulation should be done to assess intravascular volume, administration of IV fluids and drugs and ABG analysis respectively.

After the pancreatic anastomosis and release of clamps, reperfusion results. After graft recirculation, the pancreatic beta cells begin secreting insulin within 5 minutes and therefore meticulous and frequent blood glucose monitoring is emperative.[7]

Blood glucose levels are assessed every 15 minutes for the 1st hour, then every 30 minutes till the completion of surgery.

An insulin infusion should be started to maintain blood sugar in the range of 120–150 mg%.

After skin closure, neuromuscular block is reversed and extubation done on table.

POSTOPERATIVE CARE AND PAIN RELIEF

The patients are shifted to the ICU for further management.

Analgesia can be provided with patient controlled analgesia (PCA). Transversus abdominis plane (TAP) block has been found to be effective.[8]

CLINICAL PEARLS

- Pancreas transplant is performed to achieve euglycemia in patients suffering from Type 1 and Type 2 diabetics. A thorough knowledge of the perioperative management is essential for favorable outcome.

REFERENCES

1. Kelly WD, Lillehei RC, Merkel FK, et al. Allotransplantation of the pancreas and duodenum with the kidney in diabetic nephropathy. Surgery, 1967;61:827-837.
2. Organ Procurement and Transplant.
3. Pancreas transplant outcomes for United States (US) and non-US cases as reported to the International Pancreas Transplant Registry as of October 2002. www.iptr.umn.edu.
4. Transplant Review Guidelines. Solid Organ and Stem Cell Transplantation. United Health Group 2012.
5. Light JA, Barhyte DY. Simultaneous pancreas-kidney transplants in type I and type II diabetic patients with end-stage renal disease: similar 10-year outcomes. Transplant Proc, 2005;37:1283-1284.
6. Van Buren PN, Toto RD. The pathogenesis and management of hypertension in diabetic kidney disease. Med Clin North Am, 2013;97:31-51.
7. Larson-Wadd K, Belani KG. Pancreas and islet cell transplantation. Anesthesiol Clin North America, 2004;22:663-674.
8. Aniskevich S, Clendenen SR, Torp KD. Bilateral transversus abdominis plane block for managing pain after a pancreas transplant. Exp Clin Transplant, 2011;9:277-278.

Index

Page numbers followed by '*f*' and '*t*' indicate figures and tables respectively.

D